Molecular Aspects of Innate and Adaptive Immunity

Molecular Aspects of Innate and Adaptive Immunity

Editor: Riona Moran

hayle medical
New York

Hayle Medical,
750 Third Avenue, 9th Floor,
New York, NY 10017, USA

Visit us on the World Wide Web at:
www.haylemedical.com

ISBN 978-1-64647-572-8 (Hardback)

Cataloging-in-Publication Data

Molecular aspects of innate and adaptive immunity / edited by Riona Moran.
p. cm.
Includes bibliographical references and index.
ISBN 978-1-64647-572-8
1. Natural immunity. 2. Immune response. 3. Molecular immunology. 4. Immunology.
5. Immune system. I. Moran, Riona.
QR185.2 .M65 2023
616.079--dc23

Contents

Preface

Immunity refers to the ability of a body to defend itself against disease causing organisms. The immune system can be categorized into innate immune system and adaptive immune system. The innate immune system is an evolutionary defense system, which is a principal immune system response identified in insects, plants, primitive multicellular organisms and fungi. Its primary functions include activating the adaptive immune system with the help of antigen presentation, and recruiting immune cells to infection sites by generating chemical factors and chemical mediators such as cytokines. The adaptive immune system refers to a subsystem of the immune system, consisting of systematic processes and cells, which eliminate and inhibit pathogen growth. It has both cell-mediated and humoral immunity components, which help in destroying the invading pathogens. This book is a vital tool for all researching and studying the molecular aspects of innate and adaptive immunity. It presents researches and studies performed by experts across the globe. This book provides significant information to help develop a good understanding of innate and adaptive immunity.

The information contained in this book is the result of intensive hard work done by researchers in this field. All due efforts have been made to make this book serve as a complete guiding source for students and researchers. The topics in this book have been comprehensively explained to help readers understand the growing trends in the field.

I would like to thank the entire group of writers who made sincere efforts in this book and my family who supported me in my efforts of working on this book. I take this opportunity to thank all those who have been a guiding force throughout my life.

Editor

1

Interferon Regulatory Factor 9 Structure and Regulation

Alvin Paul, Thean Hock Tang and Siew Kit Ng*

Advanced Medical and Dental Institute, Universiti Sains Malaysia, Penang, Malaysia

***Correspondence:**
Siew Kit Ng
skng@usm.my

Interferon regulatory factor 9 (IRF9) is an integral transcription factor in mediating the type I interferon antiviral response, as part of the interferon-stimulated gene factor 3. However, the role of IRF9 in many important non-communicable diseases has just begun to emerge. The duality of IRF9's role in conferring protection but at the same time exacerbates diseases is certainly puzzling. The regulation of IRF9 during these conditions is not well understood. The high homology of IRF9 DNA-binding domain to other IRFs, as well as the recently resolved IRF9 IRF-associated domain structure can provide the necessary insights for progressive inroads on understanding the regulatory mechanism of IRF9. This review sought to outline the structural basis of IRF9 that guides its regulation and interaction in antiviral immunity and other diseases.

Keywords: Interferon regulatory factor 9, JAK-STAT, type I interferons, innate immunity, interferon-stimulated genes, antiviral defense

INTRODUCTION

Interferon regulatory factor 9 (IRF9) was first discovered as part of a protein subunit purified from the interferon-stimulated gene factor 3 (ISGF3) complex (1). Early studies have referred IRF9 as ISGF3γ and p48—due to its molecular weight of 48 kDa (1–4). IRF9 is best characterized as a transcription factor that mediates (as part of ISGF3) the type I interferon (IFN) response by regulating the downstream expression of interferon-stimulated genes (ISGs) (5, 6). IRF9 is also involved in regulating cell proliferation (4), tumor formation (7), cardiovascular disease (8), inflammation (9), autoimmune disease (10), and immune cell regulation (11), some of which is not related to ISGF3 complex.

There are nine known members of IRF family in humans; numerically designated IRF1 to IRF9 [reviewed in Ref. (12–15)]. Major functions of IRFs involve transcriptional regulation of the immune system and cell growth. All IRFs share three common domains; an N-terminal helix-turn-helix DNA-binding domain (DBD) containing five conserved tryptophan repeats; a C-terminal IRF-associated domain (IAD) responsible for protein–protein interactions [(5), reviewed in Ref. (14, 16)]; and a linker region. It has been suggested that the ancestral gene of IRFs was already present in the last common ancestor of Metazoa, thus tying the evolution of IRF family with that of multicellular animals (17). The IRF family then further diverge evolutionarily along with the adaptive immune system that emerged in early vertebrates, as reflected in their role at the innate-adaptive immunity interface (18).

IRF1 and IRF2 were the first IRFs to be identified where early studies indicated a "*yin-yang*" relationship of the two, functioning as activator and repressor of IFNα/β genes, respectively (19). IRF3 and IRF7 are important regulators in the type I IFN signaling. IRF3 functions to induce IFN-β genes during the first phase of type I IFN activation and binds with IRF7 in the second phase to induce IFN-α (20). A seminal study by Honda et al. (21) showed that homozygous deletion of *irf7* in mice exhibited no expression of type I IFN genes following viral infection, which indicates a definitive role of IRF7 in IFN signaling. Similarly, IRF5 is also involved in the induction of IFN response. IRF5 is activated downstream through the toll-like receptor (TLR)-MyD88 signaling and TRIF pathway to activate proinflammatory cytokine genes (22, 23). IRF4—expressed primarily in lymphoid cells—is known to interact with the PU.1 transcription factor to regulate the development of hematopoietic cells (24). Similarly, IRF8 is primarily expressed in hematopoietic cells and interacts with PU.1 to regulate IL-18 gene expression (25). Meanwhile IRF6 is required in the regulation of keratinocyte development (26) but its function in innate immunity is not known. Although the role of IRF6 in immune response is undefined, *IRF6* gene mutation in humans could lead to genetic disorders such as Van der Woude syndrome (27) and popliteal pterygium syndrome (28).

Interferon regulatory factor 9 was once dubbed "The forgotten IRF" by Paun and Pitha due to relative lack of studies compared to other IRFs (13). Though, recent advances point toward its apparent conflicting roles in health and diseases [reviewed in Ref. (29)]. A focused review by Suprunenko and Hofer (30) provided an excellent view on the overarching role of IRF9 in biological processes. Here, we attempt to explain on how the structural basis of IRF9 influence its regulation and function. We also briefly discuss the latest relevant research toward understanding of IRF9 beyond its role in ISGF3. This is imperative as IRF9 is increasingly implicated in other conditions beyond Janus kinase–signal transducer and activator of transcription (JAK–STAT) signaling (31).

IRF9 SIGNALING IN JAK–STAT PATHWAY

Activation of the type I IFNs response is mediated *via* JAK–STAT pathway, in a biphasic manner, as described in a compelling perspective review [reviewed in Ref. (32)]. The innate immune recognition of cells can occur in an intrinsic or extrinsic manner *via* pattern recognition receptors (PRRs) [reviewed in Ref. (33)]. Intrinsic recognition occurs in infected cells through PRRs such as NOD-like receptors and RIG-I-like receptors [reviewed in Ref. (34)]. Meanwhile, extrinsic recognition occurs in non-infected immune cells (e.g., macrophages and plasmacytoid dendritic cells) *via* PRRs such as the Toll-like receptors and C-type lectins [reviewed in Ref. (34)]. Both can lead to the induction of many cytokines, including type I IFNs (i.e., IFN-α and IFN-β). In the initial activation phase of innate antiviral immune response, activated TLR induces the production of early phase NF-κB-dependent proinflammatory cytokines, the mitogen-activated protein kinases, and the IRF-dependent antiviral cytokines (i.e., type I IFNs) [reviewed in Ref. (35)]. In the following phase, the secreted type I IFN induces an increased expression of ISGs in surrounding cells *via* JAK–STAT pathway.

In the canonical JAK–STAT pathway (**Figure 1**), binding of type I IFNs to its receptors (IFNAR1 and IFNAR2) leads to the dimerization of both IFNARs [reviewed in Ref. (36)]. This in turn phosphorylates IFNAR1-bound tyrosine kinase 2 (TYK2) which then phosphorylates IFNAR2-bound Janus kinase 1 (JAK1). Then, the receptor-bound kinases phosphorylate STAT1 and STAT2 at amino acid position 701 and 690, respectively. The phosphorylated STAT1 and STAT2 subsequently dimerizes *via* reciprocal SH2-phosphotyrosine interactions [reviewed in Ref. (36)]. Phosphorylated STAT1–STAT2 heterodimer then dissociates from the receptors and recruit IRF9 to form the ISGF3 complex in cytoplasm. ISGF3 will translocate into the nucleus and binds to the promoter region of interferon-stimulated response element (ISRE) to activate the transcription of ISGs (37).

Equally as intriguing, a study has shown that unphosphorylated-ISGF3 (U-ISGF3)—where STAT1 and STAT2 proteins are not phosphorylated—can also induce antiviral effect (38). Nonetheless, a different subset of ISGs was induced by U-ISGF3 compared to those of ISGF3. The U-ISGF3 is suggested to prolong the antiviral response for days beyond the resolution of viral infection (38). The prolonged expression of this subset of ISGs induced by U-ISGF3 ameliorates the response toward IFN-α in HCV-infected liver (39).

IRF9 STRUCTURE

As with the other IRFs, IRF9 consists of distinctive DBD and IAD that are joined through a linker (**Figure 2A**). Instead of forming homodimers, IRF9 forms the ISGF3 complex with STAT1 and STAT2, following induction by type I IFNs. Within the ISGF3 complex, the ISRE consensus sequence 5′-A/GNGA AANNGAAACT-3′ at the promoter region of ISGs is jointly recognized by DBDs of IRF9 and STAT1, while STAT2 DBD interacts with non-consensus sequences (40). The crystal structure of IRF1 bound to DNA revealed a helix-turn-helix DBD attaching to the major groove of the DNA GAAA core sequence, with a slight DNA distortion angled toward IRF1 (41). Likewise, the structure of IRF2 bound to DNA revealed the recognition sequence of AANNGAAA, which similarly show DNA distortion toward IRF2 (42). Subsequent studies on crystal structures of IRF3 (43), IRF4 (44), and IRF7 (45) bound to DNA revealed a similar recognition sequence. As the IRF DBDs are well conserved, there is a significant overlap between the ISGF3 and IRF3/5/7-binding motifs and regulation of various ISGs expression (46, 47). Clearly, DNA-based allostery influences the binding efficiency of these IRFs to specific sequences (46). For example, the -NN- dinucleotide sequence between the GAAA repeats is enriched with -CT- for genes induced by ISGF3, but -TG- for IRF3 homodimers (47).

IRF-associated domain mediates the interaction of IRFs to other factors. Unlike DBD, IAD of all IRFs are not well conserved which subsequently confers specificity to different IRFs. The IRF9 IAD is responsible for binding to the coiled-coil domain of STAT2. The structure of mouse IRF9 IAD generally retains the crescent shape of Mad-homology 2 domain fold, resembling IAD of IRF3 (48). Structure-function analysis shows that IRF3, IRF4, IRF5, and IRF7 have an autoinhibitory domain at their respective C-terminal end, which inherently suppresses the transcriptional activity of the proteins (16, 49–51). For IRF3, IRF5, and IRF7, phosphorylation is necessary to mitigate the autoinhibition. For example, the phosphorylation of IRF5 causes protein conformational changes to unveil previously blocked IAD, allowing IRF5 homodimerization and further binding of CREB-binding protein to IRF5 dimer (16). A similar phosphoactivation mechanism is also predicted for IRF3 (16). On the other hand, IRF4 has a flexible autoinhibitory domain that may abrogate the necessity

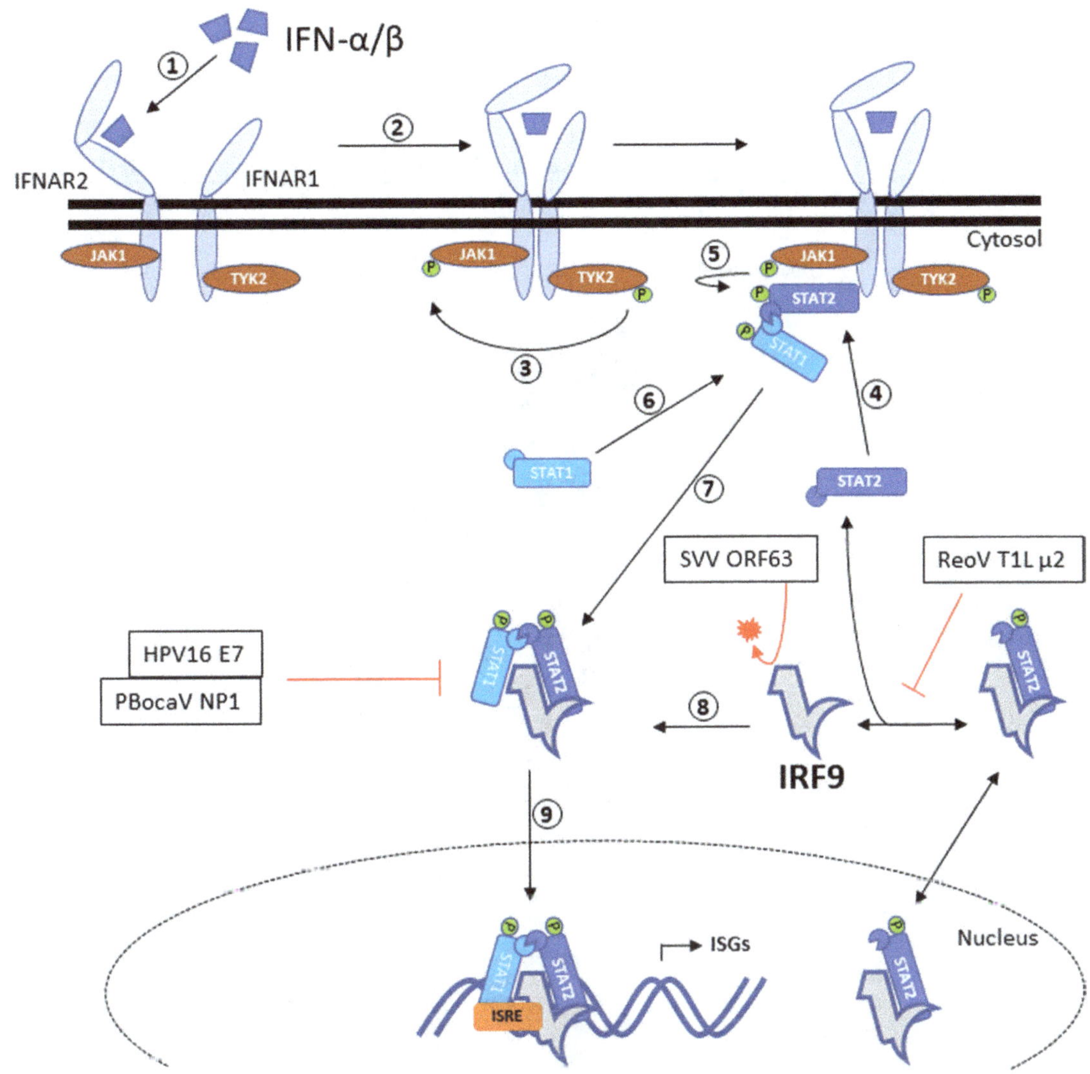

FIGURE 1 | IRF9 signaling *via* the JAK–STAT pathway and antagonism by viral proteins. Recognition of IFN-α/β by IFNAR2 will trigger heterodimerization to IFNAR1, resulting in autophosphorylation of TYK2. Activated TYK2 then phosphorylates the adjacent JAK1. STAT2 recruited by activated IFNAR2 will be phosphorylated by JAK1, thus allowing docking of STAT1 that in turn gets phosphorylated. The phosphorylated STAT1–STAT2 heterodimer then dissociates from the IFNARs and forms the ISGF3 complex with IRF9. ISGF3 complex is then translocated into the nucleus and bind to the ISRE promoter sequence to initiate the transcription of ISGs. IRF9 has been shown to associate with STAT2 and shuttles between the cytoplasm and nucleus. Also annotated are the viral antagonisms directed toward IRF9. HPV16 E7, ReoV T1L μ2, and PBocaV NP1 binds to IRF9 and therefore prevents the formation of ISGF3 complex. Meanwhile, SVV ORF63 directs the proteasomal degradation of IRF9. Abbreviations: HPV16 E7, human papillomavirus 16 E7; SVV ORF63, simian varicella virus ORF63; ReoV T1L μ2, reovirus T1L μ2; PBocaV NP1, porcine bocavirus NP1; IRF9, interferon regulatory factor 9; IFNAR, IFN alpha receptor; TYK2, tyrosine kinase 2; JAK-STAT, Janus kinase–signal transducer and activator of transcription; ISGF3, interferon-stimulated gene factor 3; ISGs, interferon-stimulated genes; ISRE, interferon-stimulated response element.

of phosphorylation in IRF4 activation (51). The linker domain of IRF4 is predicted to be in a compact domain-like conformation, and is involved in the regulation of IRF4 (51). That said, while superposition of the IRF9 IAD to IAD of IRF3, IRF4 and IRF5 reveals general structural homology, the autoinhibitory domain was not identified within the IRF9 IAD (**Figure 2B**) (48). Therefore, it is plausible that IRF9 is constitutively active, whereas post-translational modifications may induce inactivation instead. For example, the phosphorylation of S123, S173, and T180 at the linker domain of IRF3 disrupts its transactivation activity (52).

IRF9 REGULATION

Regulation by Post-Translational Modification

Major post-translational modifications that regulate innate immune proteins include phosphorylation, polyubiquitination, SUMOylation, acetylation, methylation, and succinylation [reviewed in Ref. (53)]. All three components of ISGF3 are acetylated by the cytoplasmic CREB-binding protein (54). Acetylation of IRF9 at residue Lys81 is required for DNA binding

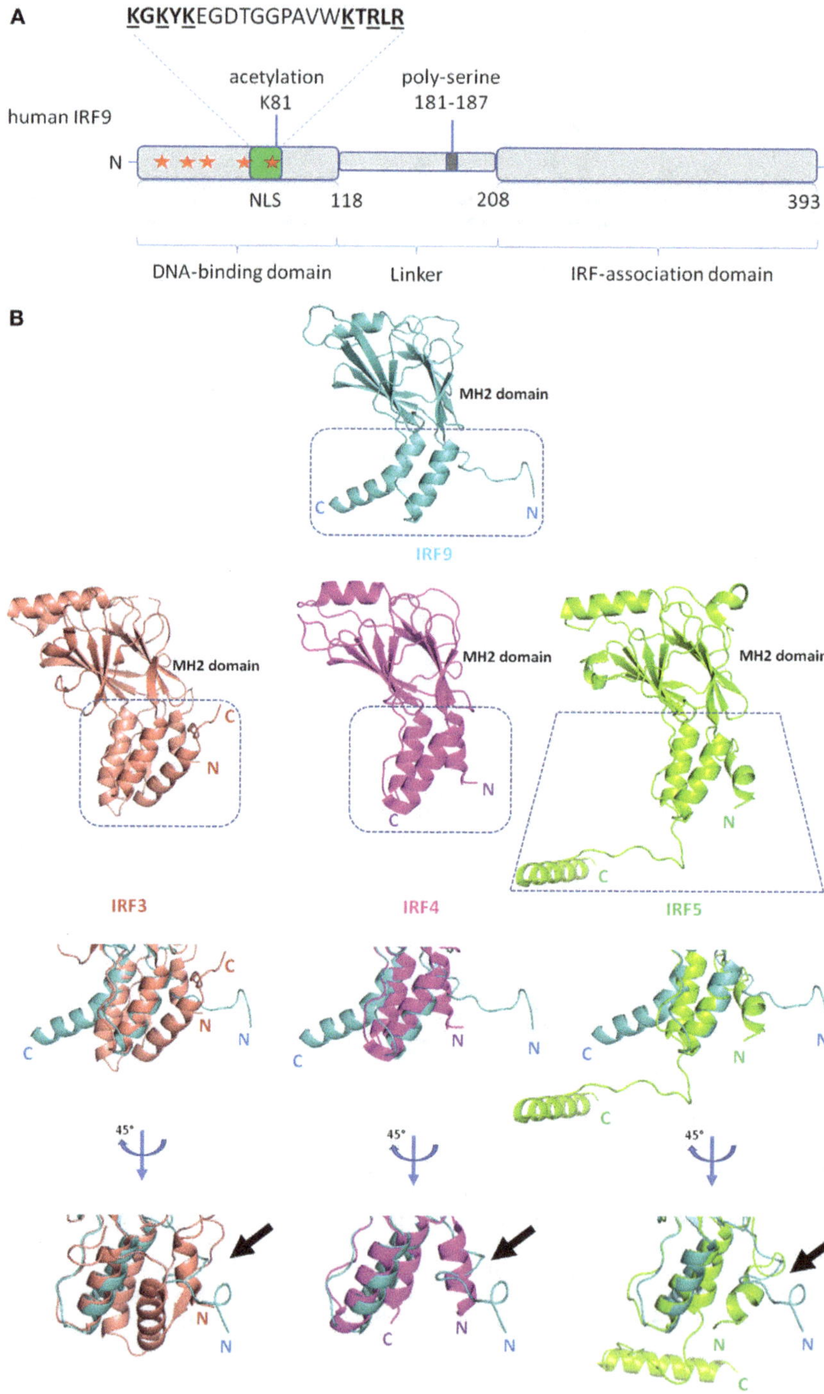

FIGURE 2 | Schematic diagram of interferon regulatory factor 9 (IRF9) and structure of IRF9 IRF-associated domain (IAD). **(A)** Domain organization of the full length human IRF9 shown in a schematic representation. The conserved tryptophan pentad (labeled red stars) of IRF9 are located at amino acid positions 15, 30, 42, 62, and 80 within the DNA-binding domain. Green box indicates the position (a.a. 66–85) of nuclear localization signal (NLS) of IRF9. The largely basic bipartite NLS is characterized as KGKYK separated by a spacer sequence of 10 amino acids followed by KTRLR (basic amino acids are shown underlined). **(B)** Crystal structures of the IAD of IRF9 [Protein Data Bank (PDB) ID code 5OEM], IRF3 (PDB ID code 3A77), IRF4 (PDB ID code 5BVI), IRF5 (PDB ID code 3DSH) show similarity in tertiary structure between all four proteins. The Mad-homology 2 fold (β-sheets, center core) is visibly conserved in the IAD of all four IRFs. Close-up structural superposition between IRF9 against IRF3, IRF4, and IRF5 disclose the absence of N-terminal autoinhibitory helical structure (α1 helix) in the IAD of IRF9 (see black arrow). Therefore, IRF9 could be constitutively active.

and is critical in the ISGF3 complex formation during antiviral response signaling (54). However, there has been no follow-up reports ever since. All IRF family members involved in antiviral immunity are known to be regulated by phosphorylation, except for IRF9 (13). The absence of autoinhibitory region from the IRF9 IAD crystal structure reaffirmed previous notions that activation by phosphorylation may not be necessary for IRF9's association with STAT2 (48). That said, an early paper suggested that IRF9 can be phosphorylated constitutively within the DBD in the absence of IFN stimuli (55). Dephosphorylation of IRF9 *in vitro* by calf intestinal phosphatase abolishes ISRE binding, which suggests a function of IRF9 phosphorylation in DNA association (55). This could represent a yet-to-be characterized mechanism regulating the ISGs expression. To the best of our knowledge, there has been no other report pursuing this interesting find. Therefore, the modulation of IRF9 by post-translational modifications ought to be thoroughly investigated for better understanding of this protein.

Regulation by MicroRNA

Interferon regulatory factor 9 is also subject to regulation by miRNAs such as miR-93 and miR-302d. The inhibition of *IRF9* mRNA by miR-93 results in the decrease of IRG1-itaconic acid, which in turn enhances angiogenesis, arteriogenesis, and perfusion recovery in ischemic muscles (56). On the other hand, monocytes of systemic lupus erythematosus patients have reduced level of miR-302d expression, resulting in increased IRF9 expression (10). Increased expression of type I IFNs and ISGs are among the hallmarks of lupus disease progression (57), consequently leading to high production of IRF9-mediated IgG autoantibodies (58). Nevertheless, *in vivo* transfection of miR-302d mimic was sufficient to reduce ISGs expression *via* inhibition of IRF9-mediated signaling (10).

IRF9 PROTEIN INTERACTION DICTATES ITS OTHER FUNCTIONS

IRF9–STAT2

In addition to JAK–STAT pathway, IRF9 was also shown to constitutively bind to STAT2 in the cytoplasm under non-stimulated condition (59) and that it is necessary for regular nuclear-cytoplasm shuttling [reviewed in Ref. (60, 61)]. The interacting domains were initially predicted (62) and mapped to the STAT2 coiled-coil domain (133–315 a.a.) and IRF9 IAD (182–385 a.a.) (48). IRF9 lacks the nuclear export signal while possessing the classical bipartite nuclear localization signal (NLS) between amino acid residues 66 and 85 within its DBD (59). Conversely, STAT2 lacks the NLS but maintains functionality of its nuclear export signal. As a result, in the absence of STAT2, IRF9 localizes in the nucleus (59). The IRF9–STAT2 dimer localizes to the nucleus by interaction of IRF9 NLS to importin-α/importin-β1 complex (60). However, nuclear localization of ISGF3 is mediated by the interaction of STAT1 NLS to importin-α5/importin β1 complex (60, 63). This switch in importin binding is likely due to change in protein conformation. Indeed, a rendered model of ISGF3 bound to DNA (48) indicates the NLS of IRF9 becoming inaccessible due to its protein conformation, whereas the STAT1 NLS is exposed hence allowing for nuclear transporter binding. Interestingly, IRF9 fused with STAT2 transactivation domain alone can induce antiviral state (64). Other studies have also revealed important regulatory functions of IRF9–STAT2, which includes gene expression of retinoic acid-induced gene G (65), prolonging the ISGF3-like transcriptional activity (66) and drives the IL-6 expression (67)—a proinflammatory cytokine whose elevated serum level is associated with various cancers (68). On a different note, one study reported fewer ISGs being expressed in STAT1- or STAT2-deficient murine glial cells compared to IRF9-deficient cells upon IFN-α stimulation, reflecting the dominant role of STATs in non-canonical IFN signaling (69).

IRF9–Cyclophilin A (CypA)

Proinflammatory cytokines are a subset of ISGs being regulated by IRF9 (70). CypA is a peptidyl-prolyl isomerase involved in the proper folding of proteins and immune cell activation [reviewed in Ref. (71)]. Interestingly, HCV non-structural 5A protein (NS5A) was found to compete with IRF9 for CypA binding *in vitro*, resulting in increased transcriptional activity of IFN-induced ISRE in HepG2 cell lines (72). HCV infection could lead to inflammation and fibrosis in the liver (73). Therefore, the acute liver inflammation associated with early stage of HCV infection may be an inadvertent effect of NS5A sequestration of CypA that is a repressor of IRF9-regulated inflammation. In addition, IRF9-deficient mice were protected from DSS-induced intestinal inflammation, suggesting yet again that IRF9 is pro-inflammation (9).

IRF9 and Peroxisome Proliferator-Activated Receptor α (PPARα)–Sirtuin1 (SIRT1) Axis

Recently, researchers have linked IRF9 to the poor outcome of ischemic reperfusion (IR) injuries (70, 74, 75). Compared to wild-type mice, mice overexpressing IRF9 developed a more severe myocardial damage and exhibited inflammation when challenged with IR, while a reduced response was noticed in IRF9-knockout mice (70). Whereas, liver cells overexpressing IRF9 underwent apoptosis more readily compared to IRF9-deficient cells when subjected to IR challenge (75). In the study, the authors found that IRF9 suppresses gene expression of *SIRT1* responsible for the inhibition of pro-apoptotic protein, p53. In addition, the suppression of *SIRT1* by IRF9 contributes to neointima formation (76).

Meanwhile, the linker region of IRF9 was shown to interact with PPARα to activate PPARα target genes (77). This interaction was found to reduce steatosis, hepatic IR injury, and inflammation (77). Interestingly, the PPARα–SIRT1 axis has been known to mediate cardiac hypertrophy, metabolic dysregulation, inflammation, and anti-aging pathways (74). Together, these studies uncovered a novel role of IRF9 in IR injury progression, steatosis, and inflammation through interaction with the PPARα–SIRT1 axis (**Figure 3**). The seemingly conflicting action of IRF9 on PPARα and SIRT1 necessitate further investigation.

IRF9-Viral Proteins

Massive upregulation of ISGs following activation of the JAK–STAT pathway will establish antiviral state in the infected and neighboring cells. The potency of ISGs against viral infections is highlighted by the many ways viruses have evolved to interfere with IRF9, alone or as part of ISGF3 (**Figure 1**). IRF9 was specifically antagonized by viruses through nuclear sequestration, inhibiting DNA binding of IRF9 and promoting IRF9 degradation.

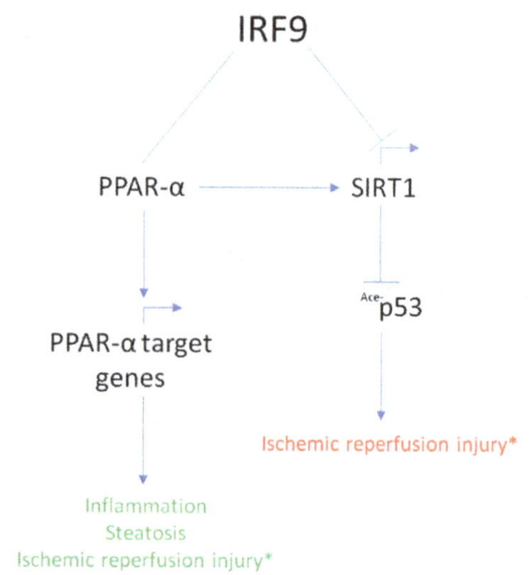

FIGURE 3 | Summary of interferon regulatory factor 9 (IRF9) interaction with the peroxisome proliferator-activated receptor α (PPARα)–Sirtuin1 (SIRT1) axis. IRF9 exerts different effect in its interaction with the PPARα–SIRT1 axis. IRF9 interacts with PPARα and activates PPARα target genes to attenuate inflammation, liver steatosis, and ischemic reperfusion (IR) injury. Whereas, IRF9 inhibits the expression of SIRT1 resulting in augmented acetylation of p53 protein. This results in a poor outcome in IR injury. PPARα is also known to regulate SIRT1 gene expression. **Conflicting roles of IRF9 in the PPARα–SIRT1 axis result in different outcome in IR injury (green font indicates better outcome; red font indicates worst outcome).*

Human papillomavirus 16 produce E7 oncogenes [reviewed in Ref. (78)] that interacts with IRF9 to prevent ISGF3 complex formation and nuclear translocation (79). This interaction occurs between amino acids 25 and 36 of E7 PEST domain and between 327 and 354 of IRF9 IAD domain (80).

Conversely, reovirus type 1 (strain Lang) (T1L) μ2 protein was found to cause IRF9 nuclear accumulation in the absence of IFN stimulation (81). The authors also hypothesized that the T1L μ2 protein prevents IRF9 binding to STAT2. It is of note that a single change of amino acid 208 of T1L μ2 can repress IFN-β signaling (82). However, detailed mechanism on T1L μ2–IRF9 interaction is yet to be defined.

Varicella zoster virus (VZV) is the causative agent of chickenpox in children and establishes latency in the nervous system to cause herpes zoster (shingles) later in adulthood [reviewed in Ref. (83)]. The ORF63 protein of VZV is present during viral lytic phase and is one of immediate early protein expressed in latently infected human ganglia (84). The simian varicella virus (SVV) infection in rhesus macaques has been used as an animal model of VZV infection (83). A recent study shows the SVV ORF63 protein induces specific degradation of IRF9 in a proteasome-dependent manner (85). In rhesus fibroblast cells expressing ORF63, supplementation with proteasome inhibitor MG132 led to increased cellular level of IRF9 compared to non-treated cells (85).

Porcine bocavirus NP1 protein has been reported to bind to the DBD of IRF9, effectively blocking the binding of ISGF3 complex to ISRE promoter, thus reducing ISGs expression (86).

CONCLUSION AND FUTURE DIRECTIONS

Interferon regulatory factor 9 was initially discovered as a component of the potent transcription factor ISGF3 responsible in initiating transcription of hundreds of ISGs to mount antiviral response. IRF9 is further implicated in expansive roles across the pathogenesis and improvement of diseases. Surprisingly, there is limited information on the mechanistic detail of IRF9's various functions, beyond its association with STAT1 and STAT2. Extensive studies are required to elucidate the regulatory mechanisms that govern the IRF9 transcriptional and translational activities, sequestration by protein binding, and compartmentalization. In particular, the dual function of IRF9 in promoting and reducing inflammation requires further investigation. Although not explicitly discussed here, IRF9 is upregulated by c-Myc protooncogene (4) and cell crowding (87), suggesting involvement of IRF9 in oncogenesis. In addition, general screening of candidate genes revealed that increased expression of IRF9 and XRCC1 as genetic biomarkers are predicative of glioblastoma multiform progression (88).

Similarly, further elucidation of virus–host interactions suppressing IRF9-mediated transcription is also an area of intrigue. The genomic sequence of IRF9, though well conserved among mammals, fish, reptiles, and amphibians, is not found in avians (89). The interplay between other immune-regulatory pathways to compensate for absence of IRF9 in birds may shed additional information about the extensive role of IRF9 in other species. Of note, there is a growing interest in IRF9 studies on its broad impact on the antiviral immunity of fishes (90–95).

The knowledge of IRF9 beyond ISGF3 is still at its nascent stage, thus further studies are necessary to explore the molecular function and implication of this key protein in antiviral immunity and beyond. The recent advances in IRF9's structural information will provide better insights in future studies focusing on its wide-ranging function and regulatory role.

AUTHOR CONTRIBUTIONS

AP and SKN prepared the draft manuscript. AP, THT, and SKN revised and edited the final manuscript.

ACKNOWLEDGMENTS

We are very grateful to Yi Jin Liew for critical reading of the draft manuscript and Lee Hung Tey for compiling the literatures. We also thank the members of RNA-Bio Research Group, Advanced Medical and Dental Institute, Universiti Sains Malaysia, for their support and assistance.

FUNDING

AP and SKN received funding from Fundamental Research Grant Scheme (203/CIPPT/6711566) from the Ministry of Higher Education Malaysia, and the Short-Term Research Grant (304/CIPPT/6313229) and Research University Grant for Individual (1001/CIPPT/8012264) from Universiti Sains Malaysia. THT is supported by the Research University Grant for Individual (1001/CIPPT/811319), Fundamental Research Grant Scheme (203/CIPPT/6711510), and eScience Fund (305/CIPPT/613237).

REFERENCES

1. Fu XY, Kessler DS, Veals SA, Levy DE, Darnell JE. ISGF3, the transcriptional activator induced by interferon alpha, consists of multiple interacting polypeptide chains. *Proc Natl Acad Sci U S A* (1990) 87(21):8555–9. doi:10.1073/pnas.87.21.8555
2. Schindler C, Fu XY, Improta T, Aebersold R, Darnell JE. Proteins of transcription factor ISGF-3: one gene encodes the 91-and 84-kDa ISGF-3 proteins that are activated by interferon alpha. *Proc Natl Acad Sci U S A* (1992) 89(16):7836–9. doi:10.1073/pnas.89.16.7836
3. Fu XY, Schindler C, Improta T, Aebersold R, Darnell JE. The proteins of ISGF-3, the interferon alpha-induced transcriptional activator, define a gene family involved in signal transduction. *Proc Natl Acad Sci U S A* (1992) 89(16):7840–3. doi:10.1073/pnas.89.16.7840
4. Weihua X, Lindner DJ, Kalvakolanu DV. The interferon-inducible murine p48 (ISGF3γ) gene is regulated by protooncogene c-myc. *Proc Natl Acad Sci U S A* (1997) 94(14):7227–32. doi:10.1073/pnas.94.14.7227
5. Veals SA, Schindler C, Leonard D, Fu XY, Aebersold R, Darnell JE Jr, et al. Subunit of an alpha-interferon-responsive transcription factor is related to interferon regulatory factor and Myb families of DNA-binding proteins. *Mol Cell Biol* (1992) 12(8):3315–24. doi:10.1128/MCB.12.8.3315
6. Improta T, Schindler C, Horvath CM, Kerr IM, Stark GR, Darnell JE. Transcription factor ISGF-3 formation requires phosphorylated Stat91 protein, but Stat113 protein is phosphorylated independently of Stat91 protein. *Proc Natl Acad Sci U S A* (1994) 91(11):4776–80. doi:10.1073/pnas.91.11.4776
7. Luker KE, Pica CM, Schreiber RD, Piwnica-Worms D. Overexpression of IRF9 confers resistance to antimicrotubule agents in breast cancer cells. *Cancer Res* (2001) 61(17):6540–7.
8. Jiang DS, Luo YX, Zhang R, Zhang XD, Chen HZ, Zhang Y, et al. Interferon regulatory factor 9 protects against cardiac hypertrophy by targeting myocardin. *Hypertension* (2014) 63(1):119–27. doi:10.1161/HYPERTENSIONAHA.113.02083
9. Rauch I, Rosebrock F, Hainzl E, Heider S, Majoros A, Wienerroither S, et al. Noncanonical effects of IRF9 in intestinal inflammation: more than type I and type III interferons. *Mol Cell Biol* (2015) 35(13):2332–43. doi:10.1128/MCB.01498-14
10. Smith S, Fernando T, Wu PW, Seo J, Ní Gabhann J, Piskareva O, et al. MicroRNA-302d targets IRF9 to regulate the IFN-induced gene expression in SLE. *J Autoimmun* (2017) 79:105–11. doi:10.1016/j.jaut.2017.03.003
11. Huber M, Suprunenko T, Ashhurst T, Marbach F, Raifer H, Wolff S, et al. IRF9 prevents CD8+ T cell exhaustion in an extrinsic manner during acute LCMV infection. *J Virol* (2017) 91:e01219–17. doi:10.1128/JVI.01219-17
12. Taniguchi T, Ogasawara K, Takaoka A, Tanaka N. IRF family of transcription factors as regulators of host defense. *Annu Rev Immunol* (2001) 19:623–55. doi:10.1146/annurev.immunol.19.1.623
13. Paun A, Pitha PM. The IRF family, revisited. *Biochimie* (2007) 89(6–7):744–53. doi:10.1016/j.biochi.2007.01.014
14. Tamura T, Yanai H, Savitsky D, Taniguchi T. The IRF family transcription factors in immunity and oncogenesis. *Annu Rev Immunol* (2008) 26:535–84. doi:10.1146/annurev.immunol.26.021607.090400
15. Yanai H, Negishi H, Taniguchi T. The IRF family of transcription factors: inception, impact and implications in oncogenesis. *Oncoimmunology* (2012) 1(8):1376–86. doi:10.4161/onci.22475
16. Chen W, Lam SS, Srinath H, Jiang Z, Correia JJ, Schiffer CA, et al. Insights into interferon regulatory factor activation from the crystal structure of dimeric IRF5. *Nat Struct Mol Biol* (2008) 15:1213. doi:10.1038/nsmb.1496
17. Nehyba J, Hrdličková R, Bose HR. Dynamic evolution of immune system regulators: the history of the interferon regulatory factor family. *Mol Biol Evol* (2009) 26(11):2539–50. doi:10.1093/molbev/msp167
18. Du K, Zhong Z, Fang C, Dai W, Shen Y, Gan X, et al. Ancient duplications and functional divergence in the interferon regulatory factors of vertebrates provide insights into the evolution of vertebrate immune systems. *Dev Comp Immunol* (2018) 81:324–33. doi:10.1016/j.dci.2017.12.016
19. Harada H, Willison K, Sakakibara J, Miyamoto M, Fujita T, Taniguchi T. Absence of the type I IFN system in EC cells: transcriptional activator (IRF-1) and repressor (IRF-2) genes are developmentally regulated. *Cell* (1990) 63(2):303–12. doi:10.1016/0092-8674(90)90163-9
20. Sato M, Suemori H, Hata N, Asagiri M, Ogasawara K, Nakao K, et al. Distinct and essential roles of transcription factors IRF-3 and IRF-7 in response to viruses for IFN-α/β gene induction. *Immunity* (2000) 13(4):539–48. doi:10.1016/S1074-7613(00)00053-4
21. Honda K, Yanai H, Negishi H, Asagiri M, Sato M, Mizutani T, et al. IRF-7 is the master regulator of type-I interferon-dependent immune responses. *Nature* (2005) 434:772. doi:10.1038/nature03464
22. Takaoka A, Yanai H, Kondo S, Duncan G, Negishi H, Mizutani T, et al. Integral role of IRF-5 in the gene induction programme activated by toll-like receptors. *Nature* (2005) 434:243. doi:10.1038/nature03308
23. Ouyang X, Negishi H, Takeda R, Fujita Y, Taniguchi T, Honda K. Cooperation between MyD88 and TRIF pathways in TLR synergy via IRF5 activation. *Biochem Biophys Res Commun* (2007) 354(4):1045–51. doi:10.1016/j.bbrc.2007.01.090
24. Eisenbeis CF, Singh H, Storb U. Pip, a novel IRF family member, is a lymphoid-specific, PU.1-dependent transcriptional activator. *Genes Dev* (1995) 9(11):1377–87. doi:10.1101/gad.9.11.1377
25. Kim Y-M, Kang H-S, Paik S-G, Pyun K-H, Anderson KL, Torbett BE, et al. Roles of IFN consensus sequence binding protein and PU.1 in regulating IL-18 gene expression. *J Immunol* (1999) 163(4):2000–7.
26. Richardson RJ, Dixon J, Malhotra S, Hardman MJ, Knowles L, Boot-Handford RP, et al. Irf6 is a key determinant of the keratinocyte proliferation-differentiation switch. *Nat Genet* (2006) 38:1329. doi:10.1038/ng1894
27. Murray JC, Nishimura DY, Buetow KH, Ardinger HH, Spence MA, Sparkes RS, et al. Linkage of an autosomal dominant clefting syndrome (Van der Woude) to loci on chromosome Iq. *Am J Hum Genet* (1990) 46(3):486–91.
28. Kondo S, Schutte BC, Richardson RJ, Bjork BC, Knight AS, Watanabe Y, et al. Mutations in IRF6 cause Van der Woude and popliteal pterygium syndromes. *Nat Genet* (2002) 32:285. doi:10.1038/ng985
29. Yu WL, Sun Y. Interferon regulatory factor 9 plays a dual function in health and disease. *J Hepatol* (2015) 62(6):1446. doi:10.1016/j.jhep.2015.01.038
30. Suprunenko T, Hofer MJ. The emerging role of interferon regulatory factor 9 in the antiviral host response and beyond. *Cytokine Growth Factor Rev* (2016) 29:35–43. doi:10.1016/j.cytogfr.2016.03.002
31. Majoros A, Platanitis E, Kernbauer-Hölzl E, Rosebrock F, Müller M, Decker T. Canonical and non-canonical aspects of JAK–STAT signaling: lessons from interferons for cytokine responses. *Front Immunol* (2017) 8:29. doi:10.3389/fimmu.2017.00029
32. Stark GR, Darnell JE Jr. The JAK-STAT pathway at twenty. *Immunity* (2012) 36(4):503–14. doi:10.1016/j.immuni.2012.03.013
33. Stetson DB. Connections between antiviral defense and autoimmunity. *Curr Opin Immunol* (2009) 21(3):244–50. doi:10.1016/j.coi.2009.05.005
34. Iwasaki A, Medzhitov R. Regulation of adaptive immunity by the innate immune system. *Science* (2010) 327(5963):291–5. doi:10.1126/science.1183021
35. Kawai T, Akira S. The role of pattern-recognition receptors in innate immunity: update on toll-like receptors. *Nat Immunol* (2010) 11:373. doi:10.1038/ni.1863
36. Stark GR, Kerr IM, Williams BRG, Silverman RH, Schreiber RD. How cells respond to interferons. *Annu Rev Biochem* (1998) 67(1):227–64. doi:10.1146/annurev.biochem.67.1.227
37. Darnell J, Kerr I, Stark G. Jak-STAT pathways and transcriptional activation in response to IFNs and other extracellular signaling proteins. *Science* (1994) 264(5164):1415–21. doi:10.1126/science.8197455
38. Cheon H, Holvey-Bates EG, Schoggins JW, Forster S, Hertzog P, Imanaka N, et al. IFNbeta-dependent increases in STAT1, STAT2, and IRF9 mediate resistance to viruses and DNA damage. *EMBO J* (2013) 32(20):2751–63. doi:10.1038/emboj.2013.203
39. Sung PS, Cheon H, Cho CH, Hong S-H, Park DY, Seo H-I, et al. Roles of unphosphorylated ISGF3 in HCV infection and interferon responsiveness. *Proc Natl Acad Sci U S A* (2015) 112(33):10443–8. doi:10.1073/pnas.1513341112
40. Qureshi SA, Salditt-Georgieff M, Darnell JE. Tyrosine-phosphorylated Stat1 and Stat2 plus a 48-kDa protein all contact DNA in forming interferon-stimulated-gene factor 3. *Proc Natl Acad Sci U S A* (1995) 92(9):3829–33. doi:10.1073/pnas.92.9.3829
41. Escalante CR, Yie J, Thanos D, Aggarwal AK. Structure of IRF-1 with bound DNA reveals determinants of interferon regulation. *Nature* (1998) 391:103. doi:10.1038/34224

42. Fujii Y, Shimizu T, Kusumoto M, Kyogoku Y, Taniguchi T, Hakoshima T. Crystal structure of an IRF-DNA complex reveals novel DNA recognition and cooperative binding to a tandem repeat of core sequences. *EMBO J* (1999) 18(18):5028–41. doi:10.1093/emboj/18.18.5028
43. Panne D, Maniatis T, Harrison SC. Crystal structure of ATF-2/c-Jun and IRF-3 bound to the interferon-β enhancer. *EMBO J* (2004) 23(22):4384–93. doi:10.1038/sj.emboj.7600453
44. Escalante CR, Brass AL, Pongubala JMR, Shatova E, Shen L, Singh H, et al. Crystal structure of PU.1/IRF-4/DNA ternary complex. *Mol Cell* (2002) 10(5):1097–105. doi:10.1016/S1097-2765(02)00703-7
45. Panne D, Maniatis T, Harrison SC. An atomic model of the interferon-β enhanceosome. *Cell* (2007) 129(6):1111–23. doi:10.1016/j.cell.2007.05.019
46. Andrilenas KK, Ramlall V, Kurland J, Leung B, Harbaugh AG, Siggers T. DNA-binding landscape of IRF3, IRF5 and IRF7 dimers: implications for dimer-specific gene regulation. *Nucleic Acids Res* (2018) 46(5):2509–20. doi:10.1093/nar/gky002
47. Ourthiague DR, Birnbaum H, Ortenlof N, Vargas JD, Wollman R, Hoffmann A. Limited specificity of IRF3 and ISGF3 in the transcriptional innate-immune response to double-stranded RNA. *J Leukoc Biol* (2015) 98(1):119–28. doi:10.1189/jlb.4A1014-483RR
48. Rengachari S, Groiss S, Devos JM, Caron E, Grandvaux N, Panne D. Structural basis of STAT2 recognition by IRF9 reveals molecular insights into ISGF3 function. *Proc Natl Acad Sci U S A* (2018) 115:E601–9. doi:10.1073/pnas.1718426115
49. Qin BY, Liu C, Lam SS, Srinath H, Delston R, Correia JJ, et al. Crystal structure of IRF-3 reveals mechanism of autoinhibition and virus-induced phosphoactivation. *Nat Struct Mol Biol* (2003) 10(11):913–21. doi:10.1038/nsb1002
50. Marié I, Smith E, Prakash A, Levy DE. Phosphorylation-induced dimerization of interferon regulatory factor 7 unmasks DNA binding and a bipartite transactivation domain. *Mol Cell Biol* (2000) 20(23):8803–14. doi:10.1128/MCB.20.23.8803-8814.2000
51. Remesh SG, Santosh V, Escalante CR. Structural studies of IRF4 reveal a flexible autoinhibitory region and a compact linker domain. *J Biol Chem* (2015) 290:27779–90. doi:10.1074/jbc.M115.678789
52. Wang J-T, Chang L-S, Chen C-J, Doong S-L, Chang C-W, Chen M-R. Glycogen synthase kinase 3 negatively regulates IFN regulatory factor 3 transactivation through phosphorylation at its linker region. *Innate Immun* (2014) 20(1):78–87. doi:10.1177/1753425913485307
53. Liu J, Qian C, Cao X. Post-translational modification control of innate immunity. *Immunity* (2016) 45(1):15–30. doi:10.1016/j.immuni.2016.06.020
54. Tang X, Gao JS, Guan YJ, McLane KE, Yuan ZL, Ramratnam B, et al. Acetylation-dependent signal transduction for type I interferon receptor. *Cell* (2007) 131(1):93–105. doi:10.1016/j.cell.2007.07.034
55. Veals SA, Santa Maria T, Levy DE. Two domains of ISGF3 gamma that mediate protein-DNA and protein-protein interactions during transcription factor assembly contribute to DNA-binding specificity. *Mol Cell Biol* (1993) 13(1):196–206. doi:10.1128/MCB.13.1.196
56. Ganta VC, Choi MH, Kutateladze A, Fox TE, Farber CR, Annex BH. A microRNA93-IRF9-IRG1-itaconic acid pathway modulates M2-like-macrophage polarization to revascularize ischemic muscle. *Circulation* (2017) 135:2403–25. doi:10.1161/CIRCULATIONAHA.116.025490
57. Baechler EC, Batliwalla FM, Karypis G, Gaffney PM, Ortmann WA, Espe KJ, et al. Interferon-inducible gene expression signature in peripheral blood cells of patients with severe lupus. *Proc Natl Acad Sci U S A* (2003) 100(5):2610–5. doi:10.1073/pnas.0337679100
58. Thibault DL, Chu AD, Graham KL, Balboni I, Lee LY, Kohlmoos C, et al. IRF9 and STAT1 are required for IgG autoantibody production and B cell expression of TLR7 in mice. *J Clin Invest* (2008) 118(4):1417–26. doi:10.1172/JCI30065
59. Lau JF, Parisien JP, Horvath CM. Interferon regulatory factor subcellular localization is determined by a bipartite nuclear localization signal in the DNA-binding domain and interaction with cytoplasmic retention factors. *Proc Natl Acad Sci U S A* (2000) 97(13):7278–83. doi:10.1073/pnas.97.13.7278
60. Banninger G, Reich NC. STAT2 nuclear trafficking. *J Biol Chem* (2004) 279(38):39199–206. doi:10.1074/jbc.M400815200
61. Fink K, Grandvaux N. STAT2 and IRF9: beyond ISGF3. *JAKSTAT* (2013) 2(4):e27521. doi:10.4161/jkst.27521
62. Martinez-Moczygemba M, Gutch MJ, French DL, Reich NC. Distinct STAT structure promotes interaction of STAT2 with the p48 subunit of the interferon-α-stimulated transcription factor ISGF3. *J Biol Chem* (1997) 272(32):20070–6. doi:10.1074/jbc.272.32.20070
63. Melén K, Fagerlund R, Franke J, Köhler M, Kinnunen L, Julkunen I. Importin α nuclear localization signal binding sites for STAT1, STAT2, and influenza A virus nucleoprotein. *J Biol Chem* (2003) 278(30):28193–200. doi:10.1074/jbc.M303571200
64. Kraus TA, Lau JF, Parisien J-P, Horvath CM. A hybrid IRF9-STAT2 protein recapitulates interferon-stimulated gene expression and antiviral response. *J Biol Chem* (2003) 278(15):13033–8. doi:10.1074/jbc.M212972200
65. Lou Y-J, Pan X-R, Jia P-M, Li D, Xiao S, Zhang Z-L, et al. IFR-9/STAT2 functional interaction drives retinoic acid-induced gene G expression independently of STAT1. *Cancer Res* (2009) 69(8):3673–80. doi:10.1158/0008-5472.CAN-08-4922
66. Blaszczyk K, Olejnik A, Nowicka H, Ozgyin L, Chen YL, Chmielewski S, et al. STAT2/IRF9 directs a prolonged ISGF3-like transcriptional response and antiviral activity in the absence of STAT1. *Biochem J* (2015) 466(3):511–24. doi:10.1042/BJ20140644
67. Nan J, Wang Y, Yang J, Stark GR. IRF9 and unphosphorylated STAT2 cooperate with NF-κB to drive IL6 expression. *Proc Natl Acad Sci U S A* (2018) 115(15):3906–11. doi:10.1073/pnas.1714102115
68. Roberto S, Sara J, Ina B, Peter VD, Peter V, Eric VM, et al. Circulating interleukin-6 predicts survival in patients with metastatic breast cancer. *Int J Cancer* (2003) 103(5):642–6. doi:10.1002/ijc.10833
69. Li W, Hofer MJ, Songkhunawej P, Jung SR, Hancock D, Denyer G, et al. Type I interferon-regulated gene expression and signaling in murine mixed glial cells lacking signal transducers and activators of transcription 1 or 2 or interferon regulatory factor 9. *J Biol Chem* (2017) 292(14):5845–59. doi:10.1074/jbc.M116.756510
70. Zhang Y, Liu X, She ZG, Jiang DS, Wan N, Xia H, et al. Interferon regulatory factor 9 is an essential mediator of heart dysfunction and cell death following myocardial ischemia/reperfusion injury. *Basic Res Cardiol* (2014) 109(5):434. doi:10.1007/s00395-014-0434-9
71. Satoh K, Shimokawa H, Berk BC. Cyclophilin A: promising new target in cardiovascular therapy. *Circ J* (2010) 74(11):2249–56. doi:10.1253/circj.CJ-10-0904
72. Bobardt M, Hopkins S, Baugh J, Chatterji U, Hernandez F, Hiscott J, et al. HCV NS5A and IRF9 compete for CypA binding. *J Hepatol* (2013) 58(1):16–23. doi:10.1016/j.jhep.2012.08.007
73. Yin C, Goonawardane N, Stewart H, Harris M. A role for domain I of the hepatitis C virus NS5A protein in virus assembly. *PLoS Pathog* (2018) 14(1):e1006834. doi:10.1371/journal.ppat.1006834
74. Chen H-Z, Guo S, Li Z-Z, Lu Y, Jiang D-S, Zhang R, et al. A critical role for interferon regulatory factor 9 in cerebral ischemic stroke. *J Neurosci* (2014) 34(36):11897–912. doi:10.1523/JNEUROSCI.1545-14.2014
75. Wang PX, Zhang R, Huang L, Zhu LH, Jiang DS, Chen HZ, et al. Interferon regulatory factor 9 is a key mediator of hepatic ischemia/reperfusion injury. *J Hepatol* (2015) 62(1):111–20. doi:10.1016/j.jhep.2014.08.022
76. Zhang SM, Zhu LH, Chen HZ, Zhang R, Zhang P, Jiang DS, et al. Interferon regulatory factor 9 is critical for neointima formation following vascular injury. *Nat Commun* (2014) 5:5160. doi:10.1038/ncomms6160
77. Wang X-A, Zhang R, Jiang D, Deng W, Zhang S, Deng S, et al. Interferon regulatory factor 9 protects against hepatic insulin resistance and steatosis in male mice. *Hepatology* (2013) 58(2):603–16. doi:10.1002/hep.26368
78. Hausen Hz, Villiers E-MD. Human papilloma viruses. *Annu Rev Microbiol* (1994) 48(1):427–47. doi:10.1146/annurev.mi.48.100194.002235
79. Barnard P, McMillan NAJ. The human papillomavirus E7 oncoprotein abrogates signaling mediated by interferon-α. *Virology* (1999) 259(2):305–13. doi:10.1006/viro.1999.9771
80. Antonsson A, Payne E, Hengst K, McMillan DNAJ. The human papillomavirus type 16 E7 protein binds human interferon regulatory factor-9 via a novel PEST domain required for transformation. *J Interferon Cytokine Res* (2006) 26(7):455–61. doi:10.1089/jir.2006.26.455
81. Zurney J, Kobayashi T, Holm GH, Dermody TS, Sherry B. Reovirus μ2 protein inhibits interferon signaling through a novel mechanism involving nuclear accumulation of interferon regulatory factor 9. *J Virol* (2009) 83(5):2178–87. doi:10.1128/JVI.01787-08

82. Irvin SC, Zurney J, Ooms LS, Chappell JD, Dermody TS, Sherry B. A single-amino-acid polymorphism in reovirus protein μ2 determines repression of interferon signaling and modulates myocarditis. *J Virol* (2012) 86(4):2302–11. doi:10.1128/JVI.06236-11
83. White TM, Gilden DH, Mahalingam R. An animal model of varicella virus infection. *Brain Pathol* (2001) 11(4):475–9. doi:10.1111/j.1750-3639.2001.tb00416.x
84. Mahalingam R, Wellish M, Cohrs R, Debrus S, Piette J, Rentier B, et al. Expression of protein encoded by varicella-zoster virus open reading frame 63 in latently infected human ganglionic neurons. *Proc Natl Acad Sci U S A* (1996) 93(5):2122–4. doi:10.1073/pnas.93.5.2122
85. Verweij MC, Wellish M, Whitmer T, Malouli D, Lapel M, Jonjic S, et al. Varicella viruses inhibit interferon-stimulated JAK-STAT signaling through multiple mechanisms. *PLoS Pathog* (2015) 11(5):e1004901. doi:10.1371/journal.ppat.1004901
86. Zhang R, Fang L, Wang D, Cai K, Zhang H, Xie L, et al. Porcine bocavirus NP1 negatively regulates interferon signaling pathway by targeting the DNA-binding domain of IRF9. *Virology* (2015) 485:414–21. doi:10.1016/j.virol.2015.08.005
87. Kolosenko I, Fryknäs M, Forsberg S, Johnsson P, Cheon H, Holvey-Bates EG, et al. Cell crowding induces interferon regulatory factor 9, which confers resistance to chemotherapeutic drugs. *Int J Cancer* (2015) 136(4):E51–61. doi:10.1002/ijc.29161
88. Qian X, Tan H, Zhang J, Liu K, Yang T, Wang M, et al. Identification of biomarkers for pseudo and true progression of GBM based on radiogenomics study. *Oncotarget* (2016) 7(34):55377–94. doi:10.18632/oncotarget.10553
89. Huang B, Qi ZT, Xu Z, Nie P. Global characterization of interferon regulatory factor (IRF) genes in vertebrates: glimpse of the diversification in evolution. *BMC Immunol* (2010) 11(1):22. doi:10.1186/1471-2172-11-22
90. Shi J, Zhang Y-B, Liu T-K, Sun F, Gui J-F. Subcellular localization and functional characterization of a fish IRF9 from crucian carp *Carassius auratus*. *Fish Shellfish Immunol* (2012) 33(2):258–66. doi:10.1016/j.fsi.2012.05.014
91. Shi J, Zhang Y-B, Zhang J-S, Gui J-F. Expression regulation of zebrafish interferon regulatory factor 9 by promoter analysis. *Dev Comp Immunol* (2013) 41(4):534–43. doi:10.1016/j.dci.2013.07.017
92. Hu G-B, Zhao M-Y, Lin J-Y, Liu Q-M, Zhang S-C. Molecular cloning and characterization of interferon regulatory factor 9 (IRF9) in Japanese flounder, *Paralichthys olivaceus*. *Fish Shellfish Immunol* (2014) 39(2):138–44. doi:10.1016/j.fsi.2014.05.002
93. Sobhkhez M, Skjesol A, Thomassen E, Tollersrud LG, Iliev DB, Sun B, et al. Structural and functional characterization of salmon STAT1, STAT2 and IRF9 homologs sheds light on interferon signaling in teleosts. *FEBS Open Bio* (2014) 4:858–71. doi:10.1016/j.fob.2014.09.007
94. Yang Q, Cui J, Song W, Zhao X, Xu T. The evolution and functional characterization of miiuy croaker interferon regulatory factor 9 involved in immune response. *Fish Shellfish Immunol* (2017) 66:524–30. doi:10.1016/j.fsi.2017.05.053
95. Zhan F-B, Liu H, Lai R-F, Jakovlić I, Wang W-M. Expression and functional characterization of interferon regulatory factors (irf2, irf7 and irf9) in the blunt snout bream (*Megalobrama amblycephala*). *Dev Comp Immunol* (2017) 67:239–48. doi:10.1016/j.dci.2016.09.014

2

Direct Inhibition of IRF-Dependent Transcriptional Regulatory Mechanisms Associated with Disease

Aleksandra Antonczyk [1†], ***Bart Krist*** [1†], ***Malgorzata Sajek*** [1], ***Agata Michalska*** [1], ***Anna Piaszyk-Borychowska*** [1], ***Martyna Plens-Galaska*** [1], ***Joanna Wesoly*** [2] ***and Hans A. R. Bluyssen*** [1*]

[1] Department of Human Molecular Genetics, Faculty of Biology, Institute of Molecular Biology and Biotechnology, Adam Mickiewicz University, Poznań, Poland, [2] Laboratory of High Throughput Technologies, Faculty of Biology, Institute of Molecular Biology and Biotechnology, Adam Mickiewicz University, Poznań, Poland

***Correspondence:**
Hans A. R. Bluyssen
h.bluyss@amu.edu.pl

[†] These authors have contributed equally to this work

Interferon regulatory factors (IRFs) are a family of homologous proteins that regulate the transcription of interferons (IFNs) and IFN-induced gene expression. As such they are important modulating proteins in the Toll-like receptor (TLR) and IFN signaling pathways, which are vital elements of the innate immune system. IRFs have a multi-domain structure, with the N-terminal part acting as a DNA binding domain (DBD) that recognizes a DNA-binding motif similar to the IFN-stimulated response element (ISRE). The C-terminal part contains the IRF-association domain (IAD), with which they can self-associate, bind to IRF family members or interact with other transcription factors. This complex formation is crucial for DNA binding and the commencing of target-gene expression. IRFs bind DNA and exert their activating potential as homo or heterodimers with other IRFs. Moreover, they can form complexes (e.g., with Signal transducers and activators of transcription, STATs) and collaborate with other co-acting transcription factors such as Nuclear factor-κB (NF-κB) and PU.1. In time, more of these IRF co-activating mechanisms have been discovered, which may play a key role in the pathogenesis of many diseases, such as acute and chronic inflammation, autoimmune diseases, and cancer. Detailed knowledge of IRFs structure and activating mechanisms predisposes IRFs as potential targets for inhibition in therapeutic strategies connected to numerous immune system-originated diseases. Until now only indirect IRF modulation has been studied in terms of antiviral response regulation and cancer treatment, using mainly antisense oligonucleotides and siRNA knockdown strategies. However, none of these approaches so far entered clinical trials. Moreover, no direct IRF-inhibitory strategies have been reported. In this review, we summarize current knowledge of the different IRF-mediated transcriptional regulatory mechanisms and how they reflect the diverse functions of IRFs in homeostasis and in TLR and IFN signaling. Moreover, we present IRFs as promising inhibitory targets and propose a novel direct IRF-modulating strategy employing a pipeline approach that combines comparative *in silico* docking to the IRF-DBD with *in vitro* validation of IRF inhibition. We hypothesize that our methodology will enable the efficient identification of IRF-specific and pan-IRF inhibitors that can be used for the treatment of IRF-dependent disorders and malignancies.

Keywords: IRF, interferon, TLR, transcriptional regulation, inflammation, inhibition

INTRODUCTION

In 1988 the first interferon regulatory factor (IRF) was identified and named IRF1 (1, 2). Since then, a total of nine IRFs (IRF1-9) have been characterized in mammals. Recently, the presence of IRF10 has been documented in fish and birds, however they were found neither in human nor in mouse (3). Surprisingly, an additional member, IRF11 was identified only in teleost fish (3). Three decades of research has allowed the determination of basic physiological function for each family member. In *Homo sapiens* IRFs are key mediators of signal transduction associated with host immune response, immunomodulation and hematopoietic differentiation. Accordingly, five functional subgroups can be distinguished: IRF1&2, IRF3&7, IRF4&8, IRF5&6, and IRF9 as a part of the Interferon stimulated gene factor 3 (ISGF3) complex. IRF1 and IRF2 promote the response of Th1 immune cells, whereas IRF3 and IRF7 are engaged in antibacterial and antiviral innate immunity. Expression of IRF4 and IRF8 is restricted to the lymphoid and myeloid lineages of the immune system (4), whereas they are crucial for B lymphocyte development and Th cell differentiation. In addition to a pro-inflammatory role, IRF5 is also involved in the regulation of apoptosis. Structurally similar IRF6 regulates proliferation and differentiation of keratinocytes (4). IRF9 together with members of the Signal transducers and activators of transcription (STAT) family, STAT1 and STAT2, forms the ISGF3 complex and transmits IFN type I and III induced signals (5). Based on a comparison of the C-terminal region of the IRF proteins, five members (IRF1, IRF3, IRF5, IRF7, and IRF9) were described as activators, whilst IRF2 and IRF8 as repressors. Furthermore, IRF2, IRF4, IRF5, IRF7, and IRF8 have been recognized as multifunctional agents, which both activate and repress gene transcription (6). In order to clarify the evolutionary relationship between IRFs we conducted phylogenetic analysis of IRF DNA binding domains (DBD). IRF-like proteins have been characterized in non-vertebrate deuterostomes, including the hemichordate—acorn worm, the echinoderm—sea urchin, the cephalochordate—lancelet and the urochordate—sea squirt (7). Based on our analysis vertebral IRFs can be divided into four subfamilies: IRF1 subfamily (including IRF1 and IRF2), IRF3 subfamily (including IRF3 and IRF7) IRF4 subfamily (including IRF4, IRF8, and IRF9) and IRF5 subfamily, which comprises of IRF5 and 6 (**Figure 1A**). This analysis is in agreement with previously published data on evolutionary conservation of the IRF family (7, 8).

All IRF family members are characterized by a multi-domain structure, which consists of: N-terminal DNA binding domain (DBD), a peptide Linker (LK) and IRF-association domain (IAD)1 or IAD2 within the C terminal activation domain (AD) (**Figure 1B**). A linker region connecting the DBD and IAD domains most likely folds into a domain rather than staying in extended form. A subset of IRF proteins (IRF3, 4, 5, and 7) contains an Auto-inhibitory region (AR) in their structure. This AR regulates their activity via different mechanisms involving conformational changes dependent or independent of phosphorylation events (9). Within the highly homologous DBD there are 5 precisely spaced tryptophan repeats forming the "helix-turn-helix" fold, essential for the recognition of similar DNA motifs with conserved GAAA repeats. The IFN regulatory element (IRE, NAANNGAAA) and the IFN-stimulated response element (ISRE, A/GNGAAANNGAAACT) are present in the regulatory regions of IFN-Is and IFN-stimulated genes (ISGs), respectively. IRF1 and IRF2 possess an approximately 177 amino acid long IAD2, while the rest of IRFs contain a conserved IAD1 (10). The more variable IAD is critical in mediating protein-protein interactions and thus defines the functionality of IRF family members.

As mentioned above, IRFs closely control transcriptional activation of IFN-Is and ISGs. As such they are crucial modulators of Toll-like receptor (TLR) and IFN signaling, key pathways of the innate immune system. Upon binding of Pathogen-associated molecular patterns (PAMPs) to the TLRs, or IFNs to the IFN receptors, a signaling cascade causes IRF activation and re-localization to the nucleus where they activate gene expression. IRFs exert the ability to interact with numerous transcriptional partners, including IRF family members, STATs as well as other co-acting transcription factors such as NF-κB (e.g., with IRF1 or IRF3) and PU.1 (with IRF4 and IRF8). These interactions allow IRFs to activate a broad spectrum of genes and control diverse transcriptional programs. Despite the clear similarity between IRF-DBD structures and the fact that they recognize the same consensus DNA-binding site, there are major differences in DNA binding affinities between family members. Moreover, depending on the binding partner, IRFs exhibit various DNA binding modes (**Figure 1C**). The ISRE binding site consists of two spaced GAAA elements, or ISRE half-sites, 2 or 3 bp apart. Activated IRFs might bind the ISRE as homo- and heterodimers. It has been reported that each of the IRFs forming a dimer bind the ISRE half-site on opposite sides of the DNA, in a proximal orientation (11) (**Figure 1C**). Based on the recently described crystal structure and binding models for STAT2 and IRF9 (12), we propose that within the ISGF3 complex, IRF9 interacts with one GAAA ISRE half-site, whereas the STAT1/STAT2 heterodimer via STAT1 binds the adjacent GAAA element spaced by 2bp (**Figure 1C**). An overview of the PU.1-IRF4/DNA complex provided by Escalante et al. revealed that PU.1 E26 transformation specific (ETS) and IRF4-DBD bind to a composite binding site formed on the opposite faces of the DNA in a head-to-tail orientation (**Figure 1C**). NF-κB, consisting of a p50/p65 heterodimer, specifically recognizes the NF-κB DNA element with the consensus sequence of GGGRNYYYCC (13), which is placed in such a way that IRF and NF-κB rest next to each other (or in close vicinity) on the DNA

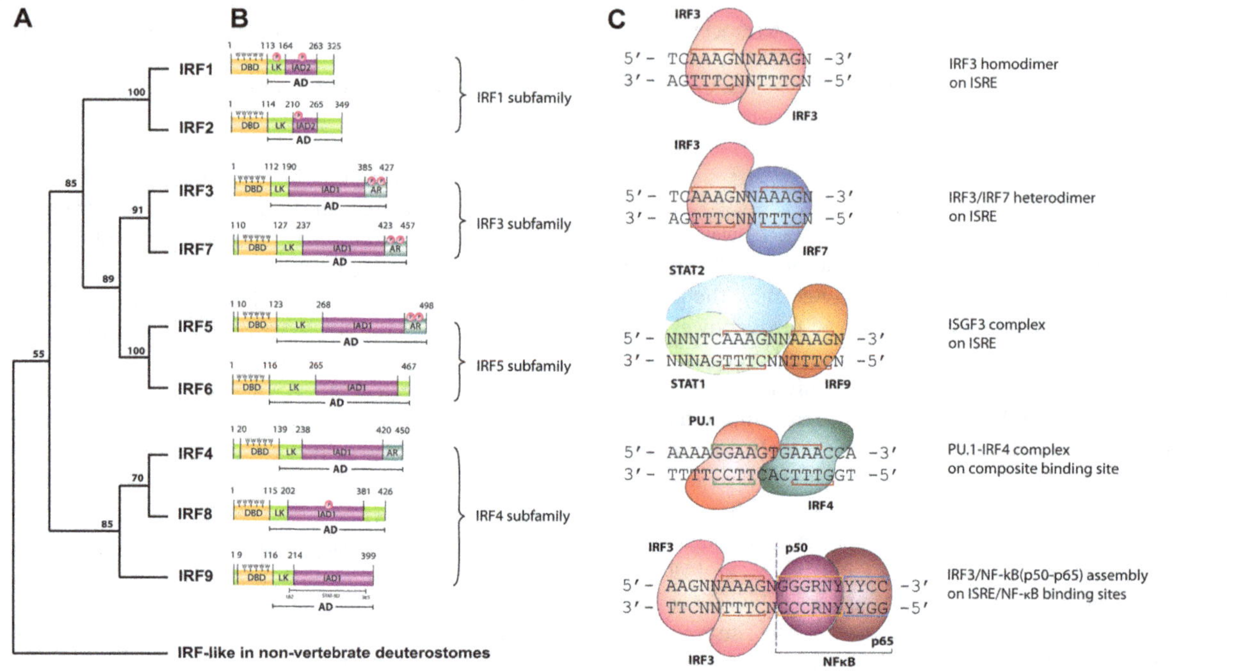

FIGURE 1 | (A) Phylogenetic tree of the DNA-binding domain of IRF family proteins in vertebrates. Homologous protein sequences were searched using the NCBI BLAST server and aligned using ClustalW. Phylogenetic analyses were performed using the Neighbor-Joining method within the Mega 7.0 program. Data were analyzed using Poisson correction, and gaps were removed by pairwise deletion. The bootstrap values of the branches were obtained by testing the tree 10,000 times. Bootstrap values larger than 70% are shown next to the branches based on 10,000 replications. **(B)** Functional domains of human IRF proteins. DBD, DNA-binding domain; AD, activation domain; LK, linker region; IAD, IRF association domain type 1 (IAD1) or type 2 (IAD2); AR, auto-inhibitory region; P, phosphorylation site; 5W, five tryptophan repeats—"tryptophan cluster"; STAT-BD, STAT-binding domain. **(C)** DNA binding modes of IRFs. LINE—nucleotides involved in interaction with IRF—DBD; N, any nucleotide; R, purine; Y, pyrimidine. IRF3 homodimer, IRF3/IRF7 heterodimer and ISGF3 are bound to the consensus ISRE sequence with two ISRE half-sited "GAAA." IRF4/PU.1 complex bind to the composite binding site, while NF-κB binds κB DNA element.

(**Figure 1C**). The DNA-binding specificity and affinity differences of these complexes collectively shape the transcriptional activity of IRFs.

Activation of IRFs is crucial in numerous essential signaling cascades. Thus, abnormalities of IRFs regulatory functions have been confirmed to play a key role in development of disease in all major areas, including acute and chronic inflammatory diseases, autoimmune diseases and multiple types of cancer. Accumulating evidence also suggests that different IRF dependent transcriptional mechanisms may be involved in the pathogenesis of these diseases. Participation of IRFs in divergent and overlapping molecular programs linked to their disease-specific functional role has motivated us to investigate IRFs as interesting therapeutic targets. Surprisingly, until now no direct inhibition strategies targeting IRFs have been reported. Known indirect IRF inhibitory strategies target IRF-dependent signaling at different levels, including inhibition of TLR or IFN receptors, IRF activators, IRF binding partners as well as blocking transcriptional or translational events. Nevertheless, none of these approaches proved to be effective enough to enter clinical trials. Over the years, structural models of IRF-DBDs and IRF-IADs have been systematically appearing in the PDB database. Available structures can be additionally divided into free cytoplasmic apo- and DNA bound nuclear holo-forms. Further investigating the architecture of IRFs, their possible interactions and IRF-mediated transcriptional regulatory mechanisms allowed us to propose a novel direct IRF-modulating strategy. This strategy employs our previously described pipeline approach Comparative Approach for Virtual Screening (CAVS) that combines comparative *in silico* docking to the IRF-DBD with *in vitro* validation of IRF inhibition (10).

With this review, we summarize the current knowledge of the different IRF-mediated transcriptional regulatory mechanisms and their role in health disorders. We postulate that specific target genes activated by the different IRF dependent transcriptional mechanisms have potential as promising novel disease markers. Going a step further, we hypothesize that the presented IRF-specific and pan-IRF inhibition strategies might represent the future for treating numerous immunological diseases. Hence, better understanding of IRF-dependent transcriptional programs and development of direct IRF inhibition approaches, could provide novel insight in the therapeutic, diagnostic and prognostic space occupied by IRFs.

IRFs IN THE IFN AND TLR PATHWAYS

IFN Signaling

IRFs are crucial modulators of production and IFN signaling. IFNs are a group of cytokines which regulate inflammation, cell proliferation, and apoptosis. IFNs are part of the first line of defense of the body against viral infections (14, 15). IFNs are divided into three subfamilies: Type I, Type II, and Type III IFNs. The Type I (IFN-I) subfamily consist of all subtypes of IFNα, and IFNβ, IFNκ, IFNω, IFNε, and signal via a receptor consisting of two subunits, interferon-alpha/beta receptor (IFNAR)−1 and IFNAR-2, which are expressed in nearly all cell types and tissues and are known to be paramount for a robust host response against viral infection (16). The Type II (IFN-II) subfamily consists of a single IFNγ (16) and acts via a receptor which consist of two interferon gamma receptor (IFNγR)-1 and two IFNγR-2 chains. IFN-II is mostly produced as a response to foreign antigens by T lymphocytes and natural killer cells. Finally, the third group of IFNs is the Type III (IFN-III) subfamily which uses the interferon lambda receptor (IFNLR) consisting of IL10R2 and IFNLR1 and is made up of IFNλ1, IFNλ2, IFNλ3 [reviewed in (17)] and the more recently discovered IFNλ4 (18). Like IFN-I, IFN-III possess potent antiviral activity (19).

All types of IFN activate pathways based on Janus kinases (JAKs) and STAT signaling. While the signaling of IFNAR and IFNLR relies on juxta positioning and phosphorylation of JAK1 and tyrosine kinase 2 TYK2 (20), the IFNγR triggers STAT signaling via phosphorylation of JAK1 and JAK2 (21) (**Figure 2**). Subsequent JAK1 and TYK2-dependent phosphorylation of both receptor chains of IFNAR and IFNLR creates docking sites for

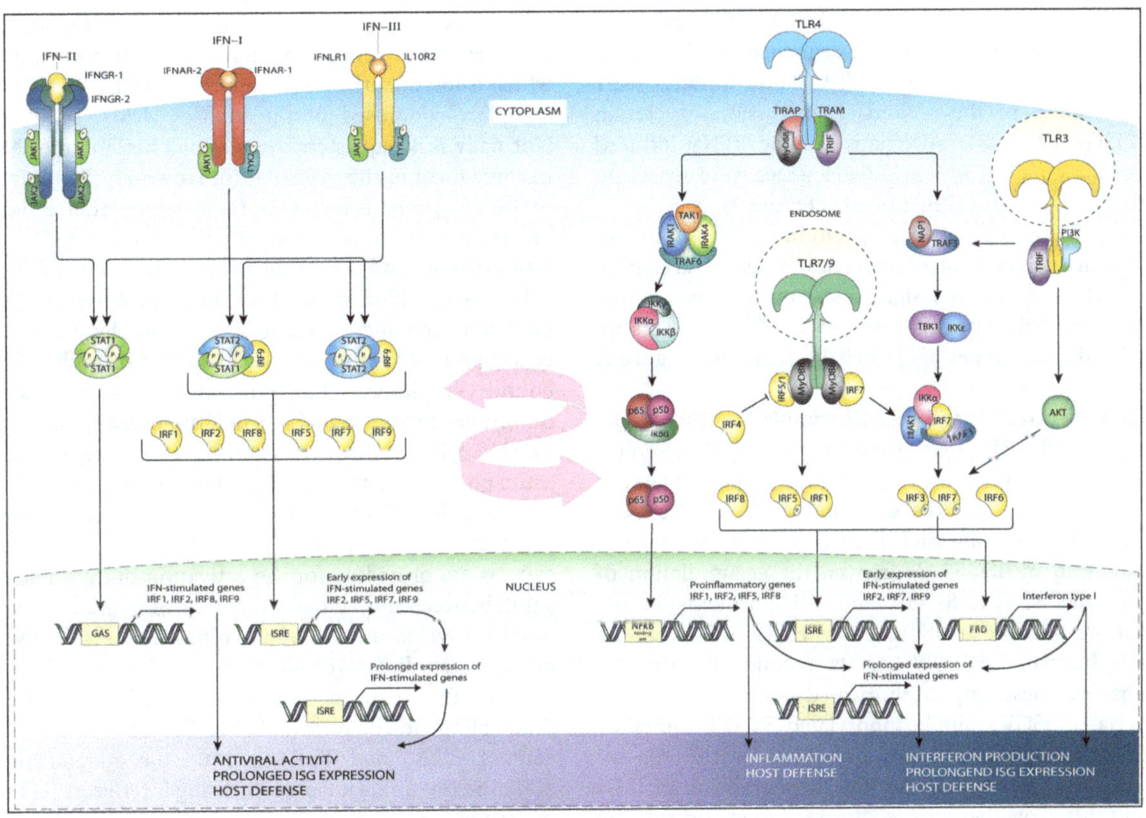

FIGURE 2 | Schematic representation of IRFs in the TLR and IFN pathways**.** The three subfamilies of IFN signal through distinct receptors: IFN-II signals via a receptor which consist of two interferon gamma receptor (IFNγR)-1 and two IFNγR-2 chains (first left). IFN-I signal via the IFNAR receptor expressed in nearly all cell types and tissues (second left). IFN-III subfamily uses the interferon lambda receptor consisting of IL10R2 and IFNLR1 (third from left). While the signaling of IFNAR and IFN-lambda relies on phosphorylation of JAK1 and tyrosine kinase 2 TYK2, the interferon gamma receptor triggers STAT signaling via phosphorylation of JAK1 and JAK2. IFN-II specifically triggers STAT1 homodimer formation (most left), while IFN-I and IFN-III trigger ISGF3, (second from left), or STAT2/IRF9 in absence of ISGF3 (third of left). These complexes translocate to the nucleus to bind DNA on recognition sequences (GAS or ISRE, see bottom-left). The initial IFN stimulation leads to the early expression of ISGs and the transcription of IRF1/5/7/8/9 and STAT1, STAT2. The accumulation of newly synthesized transcription factors leads to a secondary, prolonged wave of ISG expression (bottom-left), contributing to antiviral activity and host defense. TLR4 signaling occurs through a MyD88-dependent (middle-right) and MyD88 independent (right) signaling cascade. In the MyD88 dependent signaling MyD88 recruits IRAK4 and IRAK1 leading to their phosphorylation, which in turn associates IRAK with TRAF6. TRAF6 activates TAK1, which in turn leads to phosphorylation of IKKα/β. The phosphorylation of these proteins results in their degradation and enables the translocation of NF-κB to the nucleus where it binds NF-κB binding sites (middle-right). The MyD88 independent signaling activates TRIF, which in turn via IKKε and TBK1 signaling phosphorylate IRF3 and IRF7 at their C-terminal serine/threonine cluster (right). Upon phosphorylation these IRFs translocate to the nucleus and bind ISRE or PRD sites on the DNA. TLR3 (most-right) also signals through TRAF and IRF3, or via the PI3K-Akt pathway. TLR7 and 9 signaling (right, down) goes via MyD88, TRAF, and IRF7, or via phosphorylation of IRF5. Down below in the figure the subsequent DNA recognition sites are listed, together with the general biological effects of gene activation, such as interferon production, prolonged ISG production and host defense. TLR3 and 4 signaling leads to upregulation of IFN beta, triggering the IFN-I pathway. This, together with the IRFs whose expression is upregulated by pathway activation (listed down below in the figure) provide cross-talk between the TLR and IFN pathways (pink arrow).

STAT1 and STAT2 (22). Receptor bound STATs are activated via phosphorylation of tyrosine residue (Tyr)701 of STAT1 and Tyr690 of STAT2, which leads to heterodimerization and together with IRF9 to the formation of ISGF3. This heterotrimeric complex translocates to the nucleus and binds the ISRE sequence present in more than 300 ISGs, such as *ISG15*, *OAS1-3*, *IFIT1-3*, or *MX1* and *2*, which all are crucial in mediating antiviral activity (20). In a similar manner, but only in response to IFN-I, IRF9 and STAT2 homodimers can form an ISGF3-like complex (STAT2-IRF9) that can reinstate ISG expression in the absence of STAT1 (23–25).

The IFN-II pathway relies on the docking and phosphorylation of STAT1, but not STAT2. Therefore, IFN-II specifically triggers STAT1 homodimer formation known as IFN gamma activating factor (GAF). GAF translocates into the nucleus to activate genes containing the IFN gamma activating site (GAS) DNA element [consensus sequence: TTCN (2–4) GAA; (20, 22, 26)]. GAS binding of STAT1 also initiates IRF1 expression, resulting in the secondary expression of certain groups of ISGs (27, 28). Alternatively, the IFNγ-induced expression of the *CIITA*, *Gbp1*, and *Gp19* genes were shown to depend on both STAT1 and IRF1 (29–31) (**Figure 2**).

IFN-III signal via its distinct heterodimeric receptor to activate antiviral transcriptional responses largely overlapping with those of IFNAR in IFN-I signaling. However, were IFNα receptors are expressed on nearly all cell types, IFNλ receptors are mainly restricted to cell types of epithelial origin (19) (**Figure 2**, left side).

The initial IFN-I, IFN-II and IFN-III stimulation leads to the transcription of IRF1, IRF5, IRF7, IRF8 and even STAT1, STAT2, and IRF9 themselves (4, 6, 26). As IRFs bind a specific GAAA motif (IRF element; IRE), IRFs can bind positive regulatory domains (PRD-I) containing such IREs as well as ISREs. IREs are not recognized by ISGF3. Moreover, the accumulation of newly synthesized STAT1, STAT2 and IRF9 proteins in the cytoplasm can lead to the creation of new transcription factors in an unphosphorylated form. When the amount of phospho-proteins subsides, these unphosphorylated complexes such as unphosphorylated ISGF3, unphosphorylated STAT1 dimer or STAT2/IRF9 complex can support or take over the role of phosphorylated complexes in sustaining the expression of ISGs [reviewed in (26)]. Together, this feedforward loop controls the prolonged expression of many ISGs instrumental in generating a potent antiviral response and host defense.

TLR Signaling

As mentioned above IRFs are also instrumental in the action of TLRs. As part of the innate immune system, TLRs are one of the earliest surveillance systems and line of defense against primary infections by pathogens (32, 33). Currently 10 distinct TLRs have been identified in humans. These TLRs recognize a wide range of PAMPs (e.g., Bacterial lipopolysaccharides) and tissue damage associated molecular patterns (DAMPs; e.g., Heat-shock proteins, uric acid and ATP). In response to these PAMPs or DAMPs, TLRs initiate an inflammatory signaling cascade which in most cells leads to a swift and potent upregulation of inflammatory gene expression. These inflammatory genes include endothelial adhesion molecules, chemokines, and inflammatory cytokines among others (34).

From all TLRs, the most well-known is TLR4, that recognizes lipopolysaccharide (LPS), a component of many bacteria. Besides LPS, other TLR4 ligands include several viral proteins and a variety of endogenous proteins such as low-density lipoprotein, beta-defensins, and heat shock proteins (35). TLR4 is activated upon ligand binding. As such TLR4 downstream signaling pathways either work in a manner dependent on the universal adapter protein called Myeloid differentiation primary response 88 (MyD88), or in a MyD88-independent way (**Figure 2**, right side). In the MyD88-dependent arm of TLR4 signaling, MyD88 recruits IL-1R-associated kinase 4 (IRAK4), and IRAK1 which leads to their phosphorylation and in turn results in the association of IRAK with the ubiquitin ligase Tumor necrosis factor (TNF) receptor-associated factor 6 (TRAF6). TRAF6 then activates transforming growth factor-β activating kinase (TAK1), which subsequently leads to phosphorylation of IκB protein complex, composed of the kinases IKKα, IKKβ, and IKKγ. Normally IκB sequesters the p50-p65 heterodimer NF-κB in an inactive form in the cytosol (36). However, the phosphorylation of the IκB proteins results in their degradation and this enables the translocation of NF-κB to the nucleus (37). NF-κB is a transcription and signaling protein complex of proteins that regulates cytokine production and cell survival (38). All NF-κB family members contain a Rel homology domain in their N terminus, allowing for the formation of multi-protein DNA-bound complexes (39). Upon NF-κB nuclear translocation it can induce expression of pro-inflammatory cytokine genes, such as TNFα, IL-6, and IL-12p40, crucial for the generation of the acute phase response, and the differentiation of neutrophills and natural killer cells (40, 41). Moreover, NF-κB also binds to the promoters of *IRF1*, *IRF2*, *IRF5*, and *IRF8*, upregulating their expression, providing for the activation of ISGs and so forming a link between the TLR and IFN pathways (42).

The MyD88-independent pathway was initially postulated based on studies revealing that both TLR3 and TLR4 ligands are still able to upregulate the expression of IFN-I and IFN inducible genes in mice deficient for MyD88 (43, 44). In this context, TLR3 and TLR4 activate the adapter protein TIR-domain-containing adapter-inducing interferon-β (TRIF), which in turn via IKK kinase signaling activate IRF3 (45). IKK kinases IKK-1 and TANK-binding kinase 1 (TBK1) phosphorylate IRF3 and IRF7 at their C-terminal serine/threonine cluster [(46); see further down below]. IRF3 is constitutively expressed and resides in the cytoplasm, but gets internalized to the nucleus upon phosphorylation. Here, IRF3 will initiate the transcription of *IFNβ*, which in an autocrine fashion through the IFNAR complex further stimulates ISGF3-dependent ISG expression (**Figure 2**; middle part) (26). Endocytosis of the TLR4 complex has been suggested to play a role in determining the order in which the MyD88 dependent and independent pathways are induced, with the first being activated at the plasma membrane, and the latter from early endosomes (47).

Other TLR pathways in which IRFs play a role are TLR3, 7, and 9. TLR3 recognizes double-stranded RNA and therefore is crucial in the host response against viral infection (43). An example of a double-stranded RNA virus is the Reoviridae, a common cause of gastroentritis in children (48). TLR3 mediates TRIF induced phosphorylation of IRF3, similar to the MyD88 independent signaling in TLR4. Moreover, TLR3 can also interact with PI3K and phosphorylate Akt, which leads to further activation of IRF3 and IRF7 [reviewed in (33)]. IRF6 has recently been revealed to play a role in TLR3 signaling in keratinocytes (49). TLR3 stimulation in these epithelial cells enhanced the expression of IFNβ, IL-23p19, IL-8, and CCL5. Silencing of IRF6 resulted in an even higher expression of IFNβ, but a decrease in IL-23p19 (49).

TLR7 and TLR9 are strongly expressed in plasmacytoid dendritic cells (pDCs), where they are responsible for a high level of IFN-I expression in response to viral infection (50, 51). TLR7 recognizes single stranded RNA, and is thus of great importance in host defense against viral infection with HIV or Hepatitis C virus (HCV) (52, 53). TLR9 is a receptor for unmethylated CpG DNA, commonly found in bacteria (54). Both these TLRs rely solely on MyD88 for their downstream signaling. Protein kinases from the IRAK family are important for the MyD88—IRF interactions and subsequent activation. MyD88, TRAF6, and IRAK4 form a complex in the endosomal vesicles of pDCs (55), and there interact with IRF7. IRF7 is constitutively present in the cytoplasm, but upon phosphorylation moves to nucleus and activates the expression of different *IFNα* subspecies (56). In an effort to elucidate the underlying mechanisms of MyD88-mediated TLR signaling, Takaoka et al. discovered a role for IRF5 in this process (57). The IRF5 deficient mice used in this study showed an impaired induction of inflammatory cytokines such as IL-6, IL-12, and TNF after stimulation with several TLR ligands. Other studies found IRF5 to be induced by TLR7 signaling (58). Using *in vivo* reporter assays, Schoenemeyer et al. demonstrated that TLR7 activates IRF5 and IRF7 but not IRF3. They further demonstrated via IRF5 knockdown that TLR7 signaling through IRF7 requires IRF5 to activate IFN-Is (58). Indeed, in 2013 Yasuda et al. confirmed IRF5 importance by demonstrating that this IRF was required for TLR7 and TLR9 induced pro-inflammatory cytokine IL-6 and IFNα/β production in dendritic cells (59). Together, the conclusions of these studies implicate IRF5 and IRF7 as critical mediators of TLR7 and TLR9 signaling.

Signaling through the TLR pathways induces transcription of IFNα, IFNβ, and IRF1,2,5,7,8, and 9 (**Figure 2**). The promoters of *IFNα* and *IFNβ* genes have IRE containing PRD-I, making them susceptible to IRF-induced upregulation (1, 2). Moreover, NF-κB also binds a PRD site in the promoters of *IFNβ* and further enhances transcription of this gene (60). Indeed, in the *IFNβ* promoter, PRD-I or PRD-IV bind IRF3 and 7, PRD-II NF-κB, and PRD-IV binds ATF-2/c-Jun, which all together form the *IFNβ* enhanceosome that has been proven to be an essential component for virus-induced *IFNβ* transcription (60–62). This increased IFNα/β production will trigger the subsequent IFN-I signaling pathway to upregulate ISG expression and so further enhance the host immune response. Indeed, many ISGs exhibit binding sites not only for IRFs and STATs, but also for NF-κB, mediating their cooperation in response to TLR and IFN signaling (28, 63). Moreover, the IRFs produced in the initial wave of TLR signaling further fortify the expression of ISGs and so facilitate prolonged pathway activation and expression during inflammation. The fact that most of the IRFs used in both TLR and IFN pathways overlap, allows for further cross-talk, synergy, and signal integration between these pathways, which is an important aspect of the host defense against pathogens (**Figure 2**).

Although this review focuses on TLR and IFN-mediated IRF activation, Retinoic acid inducible gene I (RIG-I)-like receptors (RLRs) also utilize IRFs to induce the expression of cytokines, or exert gene expression independent effects. These pattern recognition receptors are also of great importance for antiviral responses and are addressed in more detail elsewhere (64–67).

IRF DIMERS IN DNA BINDING AND TRANSCRIPTIONAL ACTIVATION

IRFs activated in the TLR and IFN signaling pathways bind the ISRE as homo- and heterodimers, in which each IRF contact the ISRE half-site on opposite sides of the DNA, in a proximal orientation (11) (**Figure 1C**). A deeper understanding of dimerization of IRFs and DNA binding, comes from the analysis of structural data provided in the literature by means of X-ray crystallography or NMR. Crystal structures of IRF1, 2, 3, and 7 have been used to describe their DNA binding modes. The crystal structure of the *Mus musculus* IRF1-DBD in complex with a 13nt DNA fragment from a PRD1 element containing GAAA core sequence was solved in 1998 (PDB Id 1IF1). Topologically the IRF1 DNA-binding region is similar to a helix-turn-helix DNA-binding domain and includes a four-stranded antiparallel β-sheet and three large loops (L1-L3) connecting the different secondary structure elements, but its mode of DNA interaction is distinct. Thus, four amino acids mediate contact with DNA in the major groove (Arg82, Cys83, Asn86, and Ser87). Additionally, three tryptophan residues (Trp11, Trp38, and Trp58) are involved in hydrogen bonds and van der Waals contacts with the sugar-phosphate backbone (68). The IRF2-DBD-DNA complex reveals a very similar spatial structure, that could be explained by 80% sequence identity with IRF1 within the first 113aa, responsible for DNA binding. This structural similarity results in very similar binding affinities for both proteins (69, 70).

To date, the crystal structures for the majority of the IRF-DBDs were deposited in the PDB, including IRF3- (*Mus musculus*–3QU6), IRF4- (*Homo sapiens*–2DLL), and IRF7-DBDs (*Mus musculus*–3QU3). Despite the significant similarity between DBD structures of different IRFs and the fact that they all recognize the same consensus DNA binding site, there are major differences in DNA binding affinities between family members. Analysis of the DBDs from IRF3 and IRF7 reveals that this phenomenon can be explained by differences in flexibility and conformational changes in the loops, in particular L1. In IRF3 this loop is disordered in the apo-form and becomes ordered, when DNA is contacted. In contrast to IRF3, IRF7 L1 is ordered and stabilized by two hydrophobic residues (Phe45 and Leu50) that fold back into the core of the protein in the apo-form and during

DNA-binding a 2Å rigid body transition is observed (71). Taken together, variable intrinsic loop flexibility of IRFs may determine their binding specificity and differences in binding affinities.

IRF3 is known to form homodimers upon viral infection [reviewed in (72, 73)]. Crystal structures of the IRF3 transactivation domain reveal a unique auto-inhibitory mechanism. As such the auto-inhibitory elements surrounding the IAD, in a closed condensed form, create a hydrophobic core that maintains the protein in an inactive state. Release of the hydrophobic active site upon phosphorylation leads to a conformational change, unveils the DBD and enables DNA binding (74, 75). Moreover, phosphorylation-dependent IRF3 dimerization results in a unique acidic pocket formation, serving as a binding site for other transcription factors such as CREB-binding protein (CBP)/p300 (75, 76). Transcriptional activity of IRF3 is controlled by phosphorylation events on Ser385 or Ser386 induced by viruses and/or dsRNA (46, 76, 77). Additionally, phosphorylation mediated by the IKK related kinases, targets the C-terminal serine/threonine cluster between aa 396-405 (46, 77). This IRF3 homodimer is seen as the master and primary transcription activator of *IFNβ* and *IFNα4* genes, leading to the activation of the IFN-I pathway and subsequent ISG expression [reviewed in (72)]. The proposed model of transcriptional activation of IRF5 and IRF7, similar to IRF3, involves conformational changes induced by C-terminal phosphorylation followed by homo- and heterodimerization and translocation to the nucleus. However, it seems that other IRF family members may work through different activation systems independent of phosphorylation. For example IRF4, which is characterized by low affinity DNA binding, possesses an AR covering the last 30 amino acids of the IAD. In an auto-inhibitory mechanism model proposed by Remesh et al., it was suggested that the AR directly interacts with the DBD and leaves the protein in an auto-inhibited, inactive state. Upon interaction with a binding partner, the protein structure is reorganized, unmasking the DBD and allowing IRF4 to contact DNA. The same group presented a structural characterization of full-length IRF4 based on SAXS (small angle X-ray scattering) studies, which revealed that the flexible linker between DBD and IAD forms rather a domain-like structure that maintains in an extended form. Moreover, it may play a crucial role in regulation of IRF4 function. Due to the high structural similarity, it can be speculated that the regulation of IRF8 activity proceeds in a comparable manner (9, 78) (**Figure 3**).

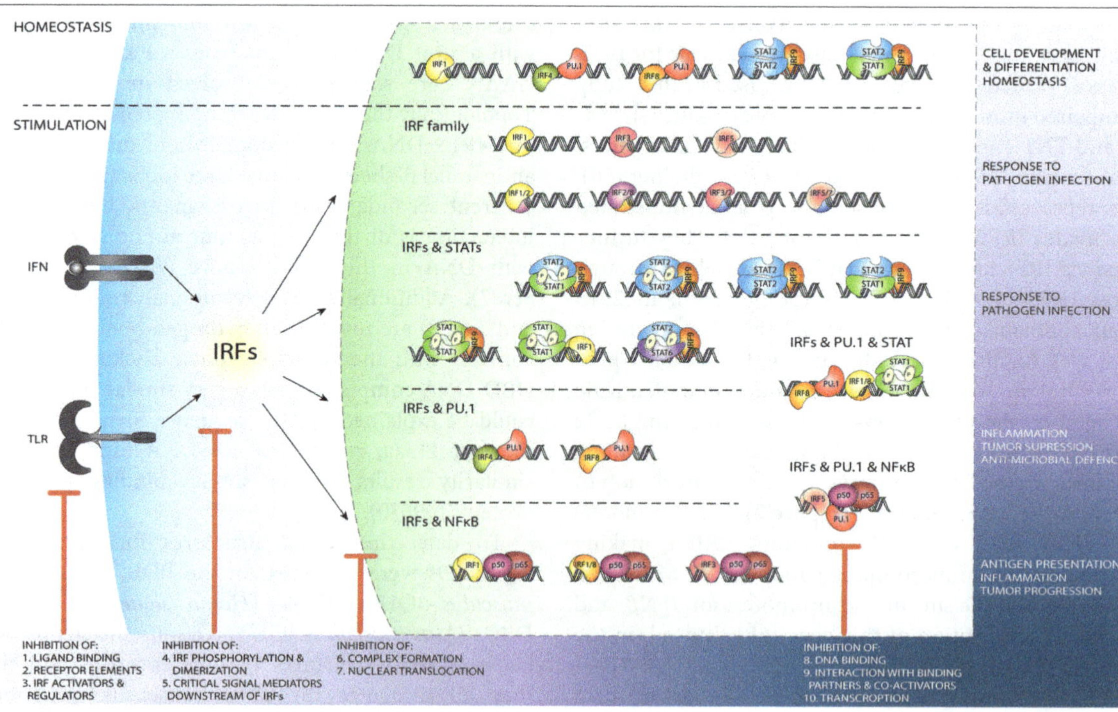

FIGURE 3 | Schematic representation of the wide variety of IRF-mediated transcriptional regulatory mechanisms and their function. Independent of TLR and IFN stimulation, PU.1/IRF binding regulates leukocyte development and differentiation, while IRF1 homodimers, u-ISGF3 and u-STAT2/IRF9 maintain ISG expression in homeostasis (upper panel). After stimulation of the TLR and IFN pathways, DNA binding of IRF homo- and heterodimers (second panel from above), IRF/STAT complexes (middle panel), IRF/PU.1 complexes (second panel from bottom), or NF-κB/IRF (bottom panel) dependent mechanisms initiate or enhance ISG transcription. Potential IRF inhibition strategies. Red sticks indicate several points at which IRFs activity might be blocked by targeting: (1) ligand binding to the receptor e.g., TLR; (2) active components of the receptors, such as Jak2; (3) important IRF regulators and activators, such as NF-κB; (4) events such as phosphorylation, homo- and hetero- dimers formation; (5) critical mediators downstream of IRFs; (6) complex formation with other TF such as STATs; (7) IRFs ability to translocate to the nucleus. IRFs activity might be also modulated by preventing DNA binding, either directly (8) or by blocking interaction with binding partners (9) such as PU.1 or NF-κB. IRFs transcription (10) can be disrupted by RNAi and ncRNA mechanisms.

A genome-wide study in which protein-binding microarrays were used to characterize the DNA binding of IRF3/5/7 homodimers revealed that besides common binding sites, a large number of dimer-specific DNA binding sites are present in the human genome. This suggests that dimer specific binding can result in dimer-specific gene regulation (11). Similar to homodimers, IRF heterodimers form a complex with one IRF on each side of the DNA helix, both contacting the full length ISRE sequence. Both IRF5 and IRF7 are expressed constitutively in monocytes, B lymphocytes, and precursors of dendritic cells (DCs). When IRF7 gets phosphorylated, it can interact with IRF5 and form a heterodimer (**Figure 3**). Through mapping of the interaction domain, Barnes et al. showed with the use of fibrosarcoma and lymphoma cells that IRF5/IRF7 heterodimers are formed through the amino terminus and masks the DNA binding domain, resulting in an alteration in the enhanceosome complex of IFNα activated gene sets (79). In this way, the IRF5 and IRF7 heterodimer can play a critical role in the induction of IFNα genes in infected cells. Genes expressed after IRF5/7 heterodimer initiation were not only encoding inflammatory and antiviral proteins, but also pro-apoptotic proteins and proteins of other functional categories (80, 81). IRF1 and IRF2 are also known to form a heterodimer which has been shown to regulate transcription of the Epstein-Barr virus EBNA1 gene in infected fibroblasts (82). Moreover, IRF1 and IRF2 are both bound to and regulate *Cox-2* an prostaglandin E2 genes upon IFNγ or LPS stimulation (83). Chromatin immunoprecipitation and RNA sequencing studies of genes bound and activated by IRF8, IRF1, PU.1, and STAT1, revealed the existence of an IRF1/IRF8 regulome, which plays critical roles in inflammatory and antimicrobial defense, such as neuroinflammation and tuberculosis (84). Furthermore, the expression of IL-1β in IRF8-expressing reactive microglia in Peripheral nerve injury is dependent on IRF1 further suggesting the existence of an IRF1/8 regulome (85).

The most recognized IRF heterodimer is IRF3/IRF7. At specific stages during inflammation, IRF3 and IRF7 physically interact. In human fibroblast cell lines viral infection activated IRF7 and consequently upregulated MAP3K8, a kinase inhibiting IRF3 dimer formation and promoting the formation of IRF3-IRF7 heterodimers (86). These heterodimers were necessary for limiting viral replication *in vitro* (86).

IRFs IN COMPLEX FORMATION WITH OTHER TRANSCRIPTIONAL REGULATORS

IRFs exert the ability to interact with numerous transcriptional partners, not only within the IRF family but also outside with STATs as well as other co-acting transcriptional regulators such as PU.1. These interactions allow IRFs to activate a broad spectrum of genes and control diverse transcriptional programs.

STATs

The ISGF3 complex (assembly of IRF9, STAT1 and STAT2), recognizing the ISRE element, is an example of a cooperativity between IRF and STAT transcription factors. The direct interaction between the STAT2 coiled-coil domain (STAT2-CCD) and the IRF9-IAD is critical for the function of ISGF3 and the antiviral response. Studies by Rengachari et al. showed that the overall architecture of these domains is similar to that of other STATs and IRFs (12). Crystal structures of the STAT2-CCD/IRF9-IAD complex (*Mus musculus*–5OEN) solved by Panne's group revealed several important adaptations that explain the selective interaction between STAT2 and IRF9. Indeed, the IRF9-IAD is missing the regulatory apparatus that is used for IRF auto-inhibition in the latent form, and in the activated state enables IRF dimerization and interaction with the transcriptional co-activators CBP/p300. Accordingly, IRF9 interacts with the tip of the STAT2-CCD using the convex surface of the β-sandwich core of the IAD domain. While the same surface is available in other IRFs, amino acid substitutions at the key anchoring points account for the preferential IRF9-STAT2 interaction. Taken together, these adaptations explain why IRF9 binds constitutively and selectively to STAT2 and demonstrate that the observed interface is required for ISGF3 function in many cells (**Figures 1C, 3**).

Together with others, our group described the existence of an ISGF3-like complex of IRF9 and STAT2 (STAT2/IRF9), which in absence of STAT1 restores IFN-I responses. STAT2/IRF9, like ISGF3 also recognizes the ISRE sequence (23–25) and upregulates a similar subset of IFN-stimulated genes as compared to ISGF3 in STAT1 deficient cells (87). However, the genes which were activated by both ISGF3 and the STAT2/IRF9 complexes did differ in expression profiles: ISGF3 driven activation appeared to be early and transient, while STAT2/IRF9 gave rise to a delayed but prolonged activation profile (26, 87, 88). A STAT2/STAT6/IRF9 protein complex has also been described. It was found specifically in B-lymphocytes after IFNα stimulation. In these cells, IFN stimulation lead to the activation of STAT6 and the formation of STAT2/STAT6/IRF9 complexes, which may allow for cell-specific modulation of gene expression (87, 89). Furthermore, the existence of another IFN-responsive protein, ISGF2 was hypothesized (90). However, this later was shown to be IRF1 (91). STAT1 homodimers are also known to form transcription complexes together with IRF1. Genome-wide studies to the extent of STAT1 and IRF1 cooperation in HeLa cells showed that co-binding of STAT1 and IRF1 to proximal or distal ISRE and GAS motifs occurs twice as often as STAT1 alone, and even 6 times more in the *MHC I* locus, crucial for antigen presentation. Also, dual binding of IRF1 and STAT1 vs. single binding of IRF1 distinguished IFNγ induced ISGs vs. cell-specific IFNγ resistant ISGs (92).

In an unstimulated state, some ISG expression is present and known to be crucial for controlling cellular susceptibility to viral infection (93). Under these conditions, unphosphorylated (U-)ISGF3, but also U-STAT1 and U-STAT2/IRF9 are proposed to mediate constitutive IFN-independent expression of ISGs to protect against viral infection [reviewed in (26); **Figure 3**, upper panel]. Our group has shown that U-STAT2/IRF9 increases basal expression of several ISGs including IFN-induced apoptosis mediator IFI27, activator of viral RNA degradation OAS2, double-stranded RNA binding protein OASL, and the Hepatitis C associated IFI44 in STAT1-knockout (KO) cells overexpressing

STAT2 and IRF9 (87). Furthermore, basal DNA-binding of U-STAT1 in combination with IRF1 is connected to the constitutive expression of some targets, including the Proteasome subunit LMP2 and cellular membrane transporter TAP2, to maintain their constitutive expression (94).

PU.1

The transcription factor PU.1 (also known as Spi-1) is a protein of the ETS family, and has an ETS domain with which it can bind DNA at a sequence known as the PU box [a core RGAA DNA motif situated within a longer sequence; (95, 96)]. PU.1 is expressed in leukocytes such as macrophages, osteoclasts, neutrophils, and B-lymphocytes (97). Gene activation through IRF & PU.1 happens during homeostasis or is upregulated by transcription factors such as Nrf2 (98) (**Figure 3**). Due to a characteristic low DNA binding affinity and presence of an AR, IRF4 requires interaction with different binding partners, such as PU.1, to effectively bind DNA (99). Escalante et al. reported the structure of a ternary complex formed with the DNA binding domains of PU.1 and IRF4 on a composite DNA element (structure not available in RCSB PDB). The DNA contacted by this complex contorts into an unusual S shape that juxtaposes PU.1 and IRF4 for selective electrostatic and hydrophobic interactions across the central minor groove (99). Considering that PU.1 recruits IRF4 or IRF8 to DNA, and exhibits an anti-cooperative interaction with IRF1 and IRF2, structural characteristics of the IRF4-PU.1 complex with DNA provides insight into the structural basis of cooperativity and anti-cooperativity between ETS and IRF factors. The proposed IRF4 auto-inhibitory strategy suggests that the AR directly interacts with the DBD and leaves the protein in an auto-inhibited, inactive state. Upon interaction with a binding partner, the protein structure is reorganized, unmasking the DBD and allowing IRF4 to contact DNA. Due to the high structural similarity, it can be speculated that the regulation of IRF8 activity proceeds in a comparable manner (9, 78). These complexes can be formed independently of the TLR and IFN activated pathways, as IRF4/PU.1 and IRF8/PU.1 are crucial for leukocyte development (100). However, PU.1 can also be phosphorylated and activated on Ser148 in its PEST region by LPS treatment (101) (**Figure 3**), and by the IFN-pathway signaling protein JAK2 (102), JNK1 (103), as well as IFNα (104). The corresponding IRF4/PU.1 and IRF8/PU.1 co-activating complexes recognize and bind to the PU.1/ISRE binding motif, a variation of the classical ISRE sequence, which has a 5′RRRGAAGT-GAAANY 3′ consensus motif (105–107). Indeed, IRF4 and IRF8 were found to co-operate with PU.1 to activate specific inflammatory genes such as CD20, Ig light chain enhancers, IL-18 and IL-1β (105–107). PU.1 binds the PU.1/ISRE binding motif in gene promoters or enhancer regions, and then recruits IRF4 or IRF8 which interact with PU.1 on a phosphorylated PEST domain, a part of the PU.1 peptide sequence rich in proline, glutamic acid, serine, and threonine (105, 108). The PU.1-IRF4 dimer can potently represses the expression of the immunoglobulin lambda gene (the small polypeptide subunit of any antibody), and thus is of critical importance in the regulation of B cell gene expression (108). On the other hand, PU.1/IRF8 activity is necessary for the regulation of the macrophage expressed cytokine IL-18 (109). Mancino et al. demonstrated a distinct difference in gene regulation by basal IRF8-PU.1 compared to LPS induced complexes. Basal IRF8-PU.1 binding upregulated a broad panel of genes essential for macrophage functions, while after LPS stimulation increased IRF8 expression together with other IRFs or AP-1 family members could activate other genes not premarked by PU.1 (110). Both IRF4-PU.1 and IRF8-PU.1 are able to bind to a PU.1-IRF composite element in the promoter of *IL-1β*. However, when IRF1 or IRF2 were co-expressed with IRF4-PU.1 or IRF8-PU.1, the *IL-1β* promoter activity was increased over 100-fold as compared to that observed in cells with IRF4-PU.1 or IRF8-PU.1 alone (111). These studies provide evidence for an enhancing role of IRF co-activating complexes. A more in-depth study of PU.1-IRF dependent transcriptional mechanisms is presented in the review of Marecki et al. (111) (**Figure 3**).

CREB & BATF

CREB is a transcription factor which recognizes and bind cAMP response elements (CRE, consensus sequenc e 5′-TGACGTCA-3′) on the DNA (112, 113). After CRE binding, CREB needs to be co-activated by CBP before gene activation can commence (114). Both CBP and p300 exert histone acetyltransferase activity, allowing for the stabilization and interaction of additional proteins with the transcription complex (115). CBP and p300 are paralogs and thus highly similar in build-up (116). CREB and CBP/p300 were found to have an important co-activating role in IFNβ regulation. They do so via the recognition element PRD-IV [sequence TGACGTC/A A/G; (117)]. Binding of ATF-2 or CREB-1 proteins to this element was found to be required for virus induced IFNβ expression (117). IRF1 and CREB also form an activating complex upon stimulation with leptin, which can bind the distal promoter of trombosponin-1 and activate the transcription of this gene (118). High level of this gene is associated with vascular injury, diabetes and atherosclerosis (118).

In macrophage and DC differentiation, in which IRF4 and IRF8 are known to play crucial regulatory roles. A chromatin immunoprecipitation study revealed that IRF4 together with The Basic leucine zipper transcription factor (BATF) bound DNA in close proximity of DNA sequences that recognize AP-1 family members (119, 120). BATFs are proteins belonging to the larger AP-1/ATF superfamily of transcription factors, able to dimerize with proteins from the Jun family (121). When B-Jun and BATF form a dimer, they are able to bind DNA on an AICE motif (5′-TGAnTCA/GAAA-3′), and subsequently recruit IRF4 or IRF8 to this site to initiate promoter activation (119, 120). Indeed, knockout studies have shown that BATF binding was diminished in IRF4 deficient T lymphocytes, and IRF4 binding was diminished in BATF deficient T lymphocytes (122). In this manner, BATF-IRF4 and BATF-IRF8 complexes can regulate a narrow set of genes necessary for leukocyte differentiation in a specific manner. BATF2, one of the lesser known BATF family members has been shown to play roles in T-lymphocyte, B-lymphocyte, and DC differentiation (123), and was shown to be highly expressed in IFNγ stimulated M1 type macrophages, contrary to M2 type macrophages (124). Furthermore, BATF2 regulated genes were demonstrated to be enriched with IRF1 binding motifs, while co-immunoprecipitation studies showed an association between BATF2 and IRF1 (124).

IRFs IN CO-BINDING MECHANISMS OF TRANSCRIPTIONAL REGULATION

Another layer of transcriptional regulation in which IRFs play a role can be found in enhancing and co-binding mechanisms. Transcription factors including IRF3/IRF7, ATF-2/c-Jun, NF-κB and architectural protein HMGI(Y) assemble together to form an enhanceosome (62, 77). Cooperative binding of transcription factors to the IFNβ enhancer region stimulates transcription of the *IFNβ* gene. It has been observed that binding-induced changes in DNA conformation and not the surface of protein-protein interactions is crucial for cooperative binding and transcriptional activation. Detailed analysis of this enhanceosome assembly was conducted on crystal structures of the DNA-binding domains of human IRF3, IRF7, and NF-κB bound to the *IFNβ* enhancer (PDB IDs–1T2K, 2O61, 2O6G) (62, 125). Additionally, IRF3 has been shown to interact with CBP, STING, MAVS, and TRIF adaptor proteins. Studies on the structure of the IRF3 phosphomimetic mutant S386/396E bound to CBP (5JEM) suggested that a conserved *pLxIS* motif is responsible for this cooperation.

A wide range of studies have identified a plethora of genes which are upregulated by the co-activating effects of NF-κB and IRFs. The first suggestion of such co-activating effects was of IRF1 and NF-κB, present within the IFN regulatory element (IRE) of the *IFNβ* promoter. NF-κB upregulates IFNβ gene expression by binding two recognition sites in its promoter. These recognition sites flank the PRD-I motif on which IRF1 binds (1, 126, 127). IRF1/NF-κB co-activation therefore relies on both ISRE and κB binding, in which IRFs and NfκB sit next to each other on the DNA (**Figures 1C, 3**). IRF1 by itself is enough to upregulate IFNβ after Newcastle Disease viral infection, while NF-κB alone was shown not to induce upregulation. However, as mentioned before, the upregulation of IFNβ was far more potent when IRF1 and NF-κB bound simultaneously to its promoter region (1).

Cross-regulation between NF-κB and IRF3-activated signaling pathways is also evidenced by the presence of multiple κB and ISRE binding sites in gene regulatory regions (42). The mechanism of IRF3/NF-κB is the same as described for IRF1/NF-κB. Concerted action of NF-κB and IRF3 is mandatory for transcriptional activation of multiple genes, including chemokines *Cxcl10* and *Ccl5*, activator of inflammasome *Gbp5*, Immune-Responsive Gene 1, and *IFNβ1*. Detailed activation kinetics analysis suggested that individual genes within this small cluster use distinct regulatory mechanisms (128, 129). Moreover, virus-induced genome-wide occupancy of IRF3 and p65/RelA binding sites correlated with co-binding of other antiviral transcription factors (130). Mechanistically, NF-κB was found in a genome-wide study of Wienerroither et al. to recruit the mediator kinase module of the transcription complex, while STATs in ISGF3 contact the core mediator module of the transcription complex, both necessary for successful gene transcription (131). Indeed, other genome-wide studies established that also in genes activated by IRF3 and RelA binding, MED1 and Polymerase II binding occurred at overlapping positions in the promoters, suggesting their roles in transcription complex recruitment (130).

More recently, interplay between IRF5 and NF-κB has also been revealed. The induction of the TLR7 pathway by Imiquimod lead to the upregulation of IRF5 via the activation of NF-κB and PU.1, which were found to bind to the first two exons of the IRF5 gene (132). Moreover, NF-κB plays a role in the recruitment of IRF5 to the non-canonical composite PU.1-ISRE binding sites in promoters of inflammatory genes in macrophages after LPS stimulation (133).

Together, these studies suggest that IRFs collaborate globally with NF-κB and other co-activators utilizing diverse regulatory mechanisms to precisely induce distinct transcriptional regulatory networks.

IRFs IN INFLAMMATION, IMMUNOLOGICAL DISORDERS AND CANCER

TLR and IFN signaling cascades are well-ordered processes, regulated by multiple transcription factors, including IRFs. As a consequence, impaired activity of IRFs and the resulting aberrant ISG expression is implicated in a broad range of inflammatory and immunological diseases and cancer.

IRF1 & 2

IRF1 is implicated in many diseases. Extensive studies have been carried out concentrating on the role of this IRF in viral and bacterial infections. For example, polymorphisms in the *Irf1* gene are reliable indicators for susceptibility to the development of chronic hepatitis B and C (134). Moreover, IRF1 has been implicated in the development of gastritis and atrophy in *Helicobacter pylori*-infected wild type (WT) mice (135). IRF1 DNA binding was also enhanced in macrophages *ex vivo* infected with *Mycobacterium tuberculosis*, and IRF1 mRNA expression was elevated in bronchoalveolair lavage samples of tuberculosis patients compared to samples of healthy volunteers (136). Furthermore, mice lacking IRF1 which were infected with *M. tuberculosis* displayed a diminished level of pulmonary inducible NO synthase (iNOS) mRNA expression and significantly increased CD4/CD8 ratio as compared to WT mice (137, 138). Moreover, IRF1 activity has been implicated in the expression of classic and non-classic MHC class I and MHC class II genes and subsequent development of thymic CD8+ T-cells. Thus, implying a role for IRF1 in antigen presentation (139, 140).

IRF1 is also connected to a variety of cancers. IRF1 KO mice studies provided proof for IRF1 antitumor functions (141, 142) (**Figure 3**). IRF1 KO mouse embryonic fibroblasts (MEFs) are more susceptible to oncogene-induced cell transformation (143). Moreover, they do not undergo cell cycle arrest in response to DNA damage (141). *IRF2* originally identified as an IRF1 antagonist acts as an oncogene, promoting cellular transformation. Its role in suppression of IFN-I signals has also been well-documented (144). Moreover, IRF2 was found to repress NF-κB induced *MHC-I* gene expression, involving more IRF family members in the low-MHC-I mediated Neuroblastoma disease progression (145). Another target of IRF1 and IRF2 that is implicated in neuroblastoma is Caspase-8 and its family member Caspase-7. Caspase-7 & 8 are involved in the early stages of apoptosis signaling by death receptors, and silencing this genes have been proposed to play a crucial role in tumor progression (146–148). Indeed, the restoration of Caspase 8 expression sensitized Neuroblastoma cells to death receptor signaling and cytotoxic drugs (149).

Our group and others, have studied to the role of STATs and IRFs in atherosclerosis [reviewed in (10, 63, 150)]. IRF1 is an important regulatory factor in the protection against vessel wall damage. Mice deficient in IRF1 were highly susceptible to neointima formation after vessel injury. IRF1 phosphorylation correlated with cell cycle arrest in coronary artery smooth muscle cells (151). Moreover, IRF1 induced nitric oxide production, which is known to attenuate endothelial dysfunction (152). Finally, increased expression of IRF1 mediates the endogenous IFNγ-promoted intimal thickening in immune-deficient Rag-1 KO mice after vascular injury (152, 153). STAT1 has also been identified as an important regulator of foam-cell formation and atherosclerotic lesion development in mice models (154). Increased STAT1 activity also resulted in VSMCs proliferation and neointimal hyperplasia (155). Interestingly, the *IRF1* promoter contains sequences that are recognized by both STAT1 and NF-κB. Detailed promoter analysis of differentially expressed inflammatory genes in coronary and carotid plaques in our recent data mining studies of atherosclerotic plaque transcriptomes predicted cooperative involvement of NF-κB, STATs, and IRFs (on ISRE, GAS, ISRE/GAS, ISRE/NF-κB, or GAS/NF-κB binding sites) in regulation of their expression in different cell types present in human atherosclerotic plaques (63, 156) (**Figure 3**). As such, the IRF-STAT-NFκB transcriptional mechanisms are a promising therapeutic target for the alleviation of atherosclerosis.

IRF3 & 7

The IRF3/IRF7 heterodimer is widely implicated in viral infection, inflammatory diseases and plays an important role in promoting septic shock (157). Indeed, IRF3 and the closely related IRF7 are key regulators of IFN production induction and for this reason the majority of IRF3 and IRF7 KO mice studies were dedicated to understand their involvement in cell responses to pathogens, most of all viruses (**Figure 3**). Absence of IRF3 and IRF7 disrupts production of IFN-I and significantly increases pathogenesis (77). Mice deficient in both IRF3 and IRF7 exhibited an astonishing 1,000 to 150,000 fold higher level of viral RNA in their tissues after Dengue virus (DENV) infection than their WT counterparts (158). Shilte et al. showed that the lack of both IRF3 and IRF7 resulted in lethal infection in adult mice after exposure to West Nile virus (159). Moreover, a diminished IFN-I induced gene expression and higher viral burden was observed in response to Herpes simplex virus (HSV) or DENV infection in mice deficient in IRF3 and IRF7 (158, 160). HCV mutation studies have also shown that IRF3 and IRF7 are crucial for IFNλ2 and IFNλ3 transcription in HCV infected hepatocytes. Moreover, HCV is able to target and impair the expression of IRF3 via interaction with the basic amino acid region 1 of the HCV core protein. This action resulted in a lower expression of IRF3, and less dimer formation, enabling a persistent infection (161).

Following carotid artery injury, a significant decrease of IRF7 expression was observed in vascular smooth muscle cells (162). Mice overexpressing IRF7 in their smooth muscle cells specifically exhibited reduced neointima formation compared with their non-transgenic controls, while experiments with IRF7 deficient mice revealed an opposite effect (162). These results suggest that IRF7 is a modulator of neointima formation during atherosclerosis.

In addition, IRF7 regulated genes were highly expressed in breast cancer patients with a prolonged metastasis-free survival, suggesting diagnostic potential for this IRF family member (163). A more complete overview of involvement of IRF7 in cancer can be found in the review of Yanai et al. (164).

Systemic lupus erythematosus (SLE) is a common systemic autoimmune disease which affects a variety of organs, including skin, joints, lungs, kidneys, and nervous system (165). Many of the inflammatory cytokines released by leukocytes during SLE disease progression, such as IL-12, IL-6, IL-23, and IL-10 have ISRE sequences and are likely regulated by IRFs (166, 167). Indeed, IRF7 was found to be critical for the TLR9 pathway activation and the high production of IFN-I, observed in experimental SLE (168).

IRF5 & 6

Recent studies in SLE and Rheumatoid Arthritis (RA), concluded that disease-associated atherosclerosis is mediated through IRF5. Likewise, mice deficient in IRF5 presented increased atherosclerosis and also exhibited hyperlipidemia, increased adiposity, and insulin resistance compared to WT controls (169). Moreover, IRF5 polymorphisms are implicated in several autoimmune diseases. In patients with SLE, genome-wide association studies showed that *IRF5* polymorphisms associated with disease risk (170–174). In RA, two polymorphisms of *IRF5* (rs2004640 GG and rs10954213 GG) revealed a protective effect against the risk of atherosclerosis and cardiovascular disease risk (175). Moreover, recently it was demonstrated that IRF5 is a target of the oncogene BCR-ABL kinase and restoration of IRF5 expression reduces Chronic myeloid leukemia (CML) cell proliferation (176).

IRF6 has recently been connected to TLR3 signaling in keratinocytes (49). TLR3 activation in these epithelial cells enhanced the expression of IFNβ, IL-23p19, IL-8, and CCL5. Silencing of IRF6 lead to an even higher expression of IFNβ, but a decrease in IL-23p19 (49). IRF6 has also been implicated in breast cancer, where it interacts with the mammary serine proteinase inhibitor (maspin), which is known to act as a tumor suppressor (177) (**Figure 3**). Moreover, IRF6 also has shown to bind the enhancer sequence of the p63 tumor suppressor gene (178).

IRF4, 8 & 9

As IRF4, IRF8, and PU.1 are implicated in leukocyte development, it comes as no surprise that these co-activating complexes were found to be implicated in leukemia. IRF4 has been recognized to exhibit both oncogenic and tumor suppressor functions (179). Polymorphisms in the *IRF4* gene contribute to elevated IRF4 expression in cells from patients with multiple myeloma (180, 181). IRF4 deficient mice are characterized by normal distribution of B and T cells in earlier development with progressing lymphadenopathy throughout differentiation stages. IRF4 has been described as being essential for proper functioning and maintaining homeostasis of mature B and T cells (182) (**Figure 3**).

Proper activity of IRF8 is crucial for the regulation of apoptosis, mainly through activation of the Bcl-xL, Bax, and Fas genes in CML, although this anti-apoptotic potential of IRF8 is not limited to CML only (183, 184). Indeed, IRF8 deficient mice developed a syndrome resembling human chronic myelogenous leukemia (185). IRF8 has also been recognized as a key mediator of the cross-talk between cancer and immune cells (186). A Chinese study identified three SNPs in the *IRF8* gene (rs925994, rs11117415, and rs10514611) to be associated with susceptibility to tuberculosis (187). Together with the finding of Langlais et al., that in macrophages, IRF1/8 regulome transcripts appeared to be significantly enriched in genes commonly activated in tuberculosis infections (84), and the above mentioned involvement of IRF1 in tuberculosis, a significant role can be postulated e achfor IRF1/8 dimer activated gene expression in this disease too.

Analysis of IRF4,8 DKO mice fail to generate functional B cells due to arrest at the cycling pre-B-cell stage, and revealed that both transcription factors are relevant for DNA sequential rearrangement of immunoglobulins associated with B lymphocyte development (188). Inhibition of IRF4 accelerated c-Myc induced B-cell Leukemia in mice, suggesting its protective role by suppressing c-Myc gene transcription (189).

Studies in IRF9 KO mice models revealed that IRF9 and STAT1 are required for the production of IgG autoantibodies in the pristane-induced mouse model of SLE (190). The expression of NF-κB, along with TNFR1, and MCP-1 was increased locally in SLE associated skin lesions (191). Moreover, higher levels of NF-κB expression in SLE patients is linked to thrombosis formation [reviewed in (192)].

Based on their roles in these inflammatory diseases, IRFs and IRF-mediated transcriptional regulatory mechanisms represent interesting targets for therapeutic inhibition (**Figure 3**).

CURRENT IRF INHIBITORY STRATEGIES

There are several levels at which the activity of IRFs might be interrupted in a therapeutically advantageous manner (**Figure 3**). Indirect modulation might be achieved by targeting known activators and regulators of IRF expression as well as critical pathways downstream of IRFs. Most of the strategies currently known to modify the expression level of IRF proteins are based on the indirect effect of small natural or synthetic compounds. They act on TLRs or IFN receptors, by blocking ligand binding or preventing phosphorylation and downstream signaling (**Figure 3**, left side). Compounds may also inhibit formation of dimers or interaction of IRFs with other transcription factors or with co-activators. Blocking of IRF binding to target DNA sequences or preventing activation of transcription would be possible by direct binding of the inhibitory compounds to the IRF DBD or IAD domains (**Figure 3**, right side).

The inhibitory effect of several compounds on IRF1, 3 and IRF4 has been presented in relation to chronic inflammation and autoimmune disorders. The mechanisms of action of these compounds are mainly indirect, with the majority of them acting on components upstream of IRF signaling pathways (**Figure 3**). For example, Donepezil (DP) is an acetylcholinesterase inhibitor, approved by the FDA as a drug for alleviation of dementia in Alzheimer's patients. It exhibits inhibitory activity against IRF1 and its target matrix metalloproteinase13 (MMP13) involved in degradation of collagen, a root cause of osteoarthritis (OA). Thus, DP presents itself as a potentially effective therapeutic in OA treatment (193). VB-201, an oxidized phospholipid small molecule has been proposed as an effective atherosclerosis treatment agent *in vitro* and *in vivo*, due to its ability to directly bind to TLR2 and simultaneously inhibit IRF1 mediated signaling (194). A group of inhibitors specific toward either NOS2 (pyrrolidine dithiocarbamate, PDTC) or protein kinases (genistein—tyrosine kinase inhibitor; PD98059 and SB203580—MAP kinase inhibitors) has been described to modulate IRF1 expression (195). Leflunomide, a drug responsible for immunomodulation, also exhibits an inhibitory effect on MEK/MAP and thus on IRF1 (196). Several antipsychotic drugs, such as sertraline, trifluoperazine and fluphenazine were identified as specific inhibitors of the TLR3-IRF3 signal transduction pathway (197). Ruiz et al. characterized the anti-inflammatory role of flavonoids (apigenin, luteolin, genistein, 3′-hydroxy-flavone, and flavone) in relation to chronic intestinal inflammation. It revealed an inhibitory effect of these polyphenolic compounds on TNFα-induced NF-κB transcriptional activity and a subsequent decrease in *CXCL10* expression. Moreover, it was observed that luteolin and 3′-hydroxy-flavone induce IRF1 degradation (198). Anti-inflammatory and neuroprotective properties of luteolin have been confirmed in microglia. Luteolin exerted an inhibitory effect on NF-κB, STAT1 and IRF1, thus attenuating inflammatory responses of brain microglial cells (199). TNFα-dependent activation of IRF1 and transcription of the pro-inflammatory gene *CXCL10* is also repressed by the natural plant derivative Compound A (CpdA), which has been tested as a potent therapeutic agent for asthma (200).

Fungi and plants can also produce IRF3 modulating compounds. Zhankuic acid A (ZAA), a major pharmacologically active compound in fruiting bodies of *Taiwanofungus camphoratus*, acts as a JAK2 inhibitor that inhibits downstream signaling mediated by STATs and IRFs. Anti-inflammatory and hepatoprotective functions of ZAA have been evaluated in mice with acute hepatitis, leaving ZAA as a potential therapeutic agent for the treatment of inflammatory diseases (201). Thymoquinone

(TQ) is a compound derived from black cumin, which indirectly inhibits IRF3 by affecting NF-κB and Activator protein 1 (AP1). Moreover, TQ targets the auto-phosphorylation of TBK1, an upstream key enzyme responsible for IRF3 activation (202). iNOS, an important inflammatory mediator, is linked to several inflammatory diseases and cancers. iNOS inhibitors (pinosylvin and BAY11-7082 – IKK inhibitor) have been shown to simultaneously block expression of IRF3 (203, 204). NSC95397 (2,3-bis-[(2-hydroxyethyl)thio]-1,4-naphthoquinone), as a multi-kinase inhibitor exhibits anti-cancer properties. This compound blocks activation of TNFα, AP1, and IRF3 in LPS-treated RAW264.7 cells and TRIF- and MyD88-overexpressing HEK293 cells (205).

More specialized IRF inhibitory mechanisms by direct disruption of transcription, nuclear translocation or DNA-binding have also been documented (**Figure 3**, right side). For example, the highly virulent bacterium *Francisella tularensis* uses its components to block NF-κB p65 activity, IRF1 translocation and binding of IRF1 and IRF8 to the Ets2 element in the promoter region of the IL-12 gene (206). IRF-dependent expression of IL-12 is also suppressed by adenylate cyclase toxin (CyaA) from *Bordetella pertussis* in DCs (207). Minocycline, a tetracycline antibiotic derived from fungi, experimentally used for treatment of many CNS disorders due to its anti-inflammatory properties have been shown to inhibit nuclear translocation of IRF1 (208). Also, Human Papilloma Virus core proteins have been recognized to mediate suppression of IRFs, in this case IRF1 synthesis at the transcriptional level. Subsequent repression of several ISGs, including Il-12 and Il-15, allows the virus to deceive the host organism and carry out an effective invasion (209).

Viruses have developed numerous strategies of direct interaction with IRFs to avoid and inhibit induction of innate immunity responses (**Figure 3**, left side). The human tumor-inducing herpesvirus, Karposi's sarcoma-associated herpesvirus (KSHV), successfully modulates the host IFN-mediated immune response. A unique evasion mechanism of KSHV reveals that this virus incorporates viral homologs of IRFs (vIRFs) to inhibit IRF7 DNA binding by blocking either the DBD or IAD of IRF7 (210) (**Figure 3**, right side). In a parallel study by Zhu et al., another inhibitory mechanism of KSHV has been reported. Namely, it demonstrated that ORF45 in association with virions interacts with IRF7 and subsequently blocks its phosphorylation and nuclear translocation (211). Further studies by this group revealed that ORF45 interacts with the inhibitory domain (ID) of IRF7 and keeps the protein in a closed, inactive form (212). Cai et al. reported that KSHV encoded Latency-associated nuclear antigen (LANA) evades MHC II presentation and blocks transcription of MHC II trans-activator (CIITA) by direct interaction with IRF4. The mechanism of inhibition is not fully understood, nevertheless it is documented that LANA blocks IRF4 DNA binding ability at promoter regions of CIITA (213). The group of Xing et al. reported that the HSV-1 encoded protein VP16 blocks the production of IFNβ by inhibiting NF-κB activation and preventing IRF3 from recruiting its co-activator CREB binding protein (CBP) (214). The Varicella-zoster virus (VZV) is known to antagonize the IFNβ pathway in the IRF3 branch. It has been demonstrated that VZV immediate-early protein ORF61 mediates degradation of IRF3 via direct interaction. Interestingly, it has been shown that ORF61 only targets the phosphorylated form of IRF3 and not the unphosphorylated IRF3 in uninfected cells (215). Another example is the HCV, which targets IFN signaling pathways through a mechanism based on the inhibition of IRF3 phosphorylation and activity by non-structural viral proteins (216). It was shown that NS3/4A, a serine protease, can successfully block IFNβ production by suppressing RIG-I and IRF3 activation (217). Moreover, the HCV NS5A protein was able to block IRF7-mediated IFNα promoter activation, which might be in part responsible for the successful establishment of chronic HCV infection (218).

Finally, molecular biology tools of gene silencing, including RNAi technology and ncRNA, have been employed in IRF targeting for cancer treatment (**Figure 3**, right side). High expression of *IRF1* and *IRF2* have been observed in human leukemic TF-1 cells. The group of Choo et al. developed a novel screening protocol in order to identify effective siRNAs targeting IRF2 in leukemic cells (219). IRF4 activity has been linked to a number of germinal center (GC) and post-GC B lineage subset malignancies (179). In 2010 microRNAs essential for plasma differentiation mediated by IRF4 were identified. Moreover, microRNA 125b was characterized to inhibit B cell differentiation in GCs (220). Another group reported that expression of *IRF4* inversely correlated with microRNA (miR)-125b in multiple melanoma patients. Positive inhibitory effects of this synthetic microRNA have been confirmed *in vitro* and *in vivo*, leaving IRF4 as an interesting multiple myeloma therapeutic target (221).

A DIRECT IRF-TARGETING STRATEGY TO IDENTIFY SPECIFIC- AND PAN-IRF INHIBITORY COMPOUNDS

Despite the large number of described compounds indirectly modulating IRF activity, there are still no effective strategies based on direct inhibition. None of the strategies studied so far have relied on the use of directly interacting compounds, which would affect the IRF protein structure. Moreover, no potential inhibitory binding sites in IRF-DBD or IAD have been proposed in the existing literature. The direct modulation of IRFs has not been attempted previously due to several reasons. Above all, to overcome possible variations between conformational differences under physiological vs. *in silico* conditions, we considered both apo- and holo- forms of IRF DBD in this approach. There are two types of IRF-DBD structures deposited in PDBe or RCSB PDB; inactive cytoplasmic free forms and active nuclear DNA bound forms. Under physiological conditions IRFs undergo major conformational changes when they transform from inactive to the active state. To efficiently inhibit IRFs, it is essential to identify compounds which would bind to the inactive form and block conformational changes and DNA binding. We propose the IRF DNA binding site as the most promising active site for inhibition. Moreover, we believe that the good quality models presented here supported by our previously described pipeline approach CAVS, which combines comparative *in silico* docking to the IRF-DBD with *in vitro* validation of potential inhibition will prove to be successful in the search for effective inhibitory compounds. Only after thorough *in vitro* validation we will be able to prove effectiveness of *in silico* selected compounds as potential IRF inhibitors, as well as asses their possible cytotoxicity. Taken together, an in-depth understanding of the IRF protein structure and the mechanisms involved in the binding of these transcription factors to DNA will allow the development of potent and effective inhibition strategies.

For this reason, we generated 3D structure models for IRF1, 2 and 8 DBDs (10), presented in two distinct conformations essential to the function of IRFs. Namely, non-DNA-bound cytoplasmic conformations known as apo-forms, and DNA-bound nuclear conformations or holo-forms. In our effort to identify specific inhibitors for different STATs, we developed a five-step comparative virtual screening tool, CAVS (222). Subsequently, we utilized this *in silico* screening method to identified potential specific IRF1-DBD and IRF8-DBD inhibitors (10). The basic assumption of the system is the adaptation of two main selection criteria to evaluate virtual screening results: Comparative Binding Affinity Value (CBAV)—a measurement of the binding quality between different IRFs, and Ligand Binding Pose Variation (LBPV), which reflects compound binding specificity (222). The LBPV ratio (from 0 to 1) represents the conformational conservation of all 20 output conformations obtained from docking. Previously we presented top-scored IRF1-specific and IRF8-specific inhibitors in apoDBD of IRF1, IRF2, and IRF8, where IRF2, as a closest correlate to IRF1, was used as a control for comparison. CBAV-IRF(1-2), CBAV-IRF(1-8), and CBAV-IRF(8-2) were determined to compare the binding affinities between IRF1, IRF2, and IRF8 for both compounds. Consequently, we obtained 60 top hits for IRF1-DBD and 7 top hits for IRF8-DBD (data not shown). The compounds were ordered based on descending CBAV-IRF(1-2) and CBAV-IRF(8-2) values, which allowed to select the most potent IRF1 and IRF8 targeting molecules displaying at the same time low affinity to the IRF2-DBD control. Here we present the top 3 IRF1-specific and IRF8-specific compounds (**Table 1**) and the graphical representation of ZINC20112987 and ZINC95910680 fitted into the binding cavities of IRF1 and IRF8 in a new graphic design mode (**Figures 4A,B**). High CBAV values (>3) of compounds ZINC20112987 (4, 82), ZINC08623925 (4, 42), and ZINC20112989 (4, 25) confirm their high binding affinity toward IRF1 and not IRF8. Analogously, CBAV values of compounds ZINC20112987 (4, 26), ZINC08623925 (3, 36) and ZINC20112989 (3, 01) point to their possible specificity toward IRF8 (**Table 1**). For example, ZINC20112987 has IRF1-LBPV of 0.75 meaning high conformational conservation toward IRF1-DBD and subsequent significantly lower IRF8-LBPV. Likewise, ZINC95910680 (IRF8-LBPV = 0.85) displays high conformational conservation toward IRF8-DBD, but low conservation within IRF1-DBD (**Table 1**).

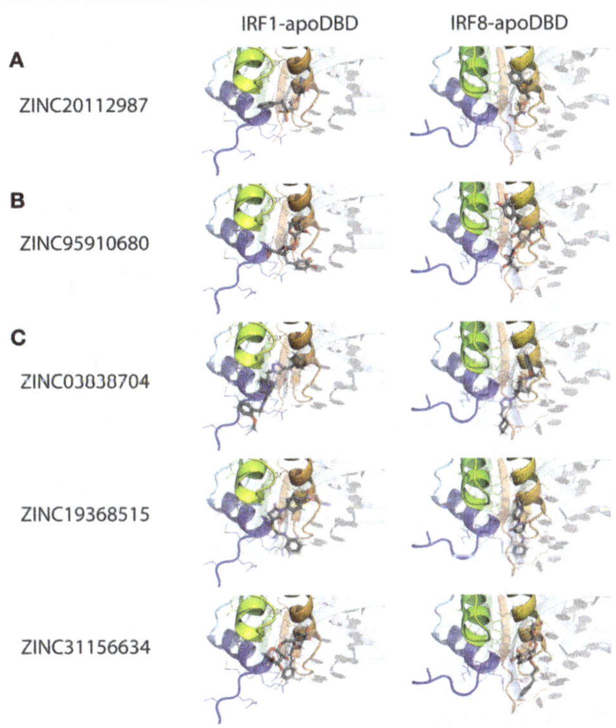

FIGURE 4 | Binding conformations of pre-selected compounds from Natural Products ZINC database subset in different IRF DNA-binding domains. **(A)** Top-scored IRF1-specific binding compounds in apo-DBD of IRF1 and IRF8; **(B)** Top-scored IRF8-specific binding compounds in apo-DBD of IRF1 and IRF8; **(C)** Top-scored pan-IRF1/8 binding compounds in apo-DBD of IRF1 and IRF8. Graphical representation, that has been used, describes in detail binding mode of top-scored conformation of the inhibitor in the active pocket of apoIRF-DBD. dsDNA fragment of the respective holoIRF-DBD/IRE complexes superimposed on the apo-form implicates the position of selected target cavity for inhibitory compound. The best binding conformation of each potential inhibitor is shown in stick representation (carbon—gray; oxygen—red; nitrogen—blue; phosphorus—orange and hydrogen—white). IRF1 and IRF8 apo-DBDs are in the cartoon representation with visible secondary structure, multi-colored with amino acid side chains that interact with compounds shown as lines. dsDNA fragment of the respective IRF-holo-DBD/IRE complexes is shown in 60%-transparent cartoon representation and colored in pale-cyan with nucleobases colored in light-pink. Ligand docking results were obtained using Surflex-Dock 2.6 software.

Moreover, by adapting the comparative docking and selection of STAT inhibitory compounds, CAVS (223), we recently re-evaluated previously considered STAT3-specific inhibitors STATTIC and STX-0119 as pan-STAT1/2/3 inhibitors in vascular inflammation (224). Analysis of the corresponding total binding score values (BS) and CBAVs of STATTIC and STX-0119 calculated for each individual STAT, points to their equal binding affinities for STAT1, STAT2, and STAT3 (222). In the same study, we described a novel pan-STAT1/2/3 inhibitor, C01L_F03, with similar characteristics (225). We proposed that this novel class of inhibitors could be implemented in a multi-STAT inhibitory strategy with great promise for the treatment of Cardiovascular diseases (CVDs) (225). Accordingly, blocking of IRF-DNA binding by IRF-specific or pan-IRF inhibitors presents itself as a promising therapeutic tool to combat a wide range of immunological diseases. In case of disorders where only one specific member of the IRF family is involved in disease development, usage of compounds specific toward this particular IRF would be the most suitable. Such an IRF-specific inhibitor

TABLE 1 | Potential pan-IRF1/8-DBD; IRF1-DBD specific and IRF8-DBD specific inhibitors.

Ligand	IRF1-BS	IRF8-BS	CBAV	IRF1 LBPV	IRF8 LBPV
pan-IRF1/8-DBD[a]					
ZINC03838704	7.736	7.7377	−0.0017	0.4/0.3	0.4/0.35
ZINC19368515	7.4603	7.4238	0.0365	0.2/0.25	0.3/0.35
ZINC31156634	8.514	8.4656	0.0484	0.25/0.15	0.5/0.15
IRF1-DBD SPECIFIC[b]					
ZINC20112987	12.6694	7.8452	4.8242	0.75	0.4
ZINC08623925	11.0354	6.611	4.4244	0.9	0.4
ZINC20112989	12.6045	8.3569	4.2476	1.0	0.8
IRF8-DBD SPECIFIC[c]					
ZINC95910680	7.4184	11.6812	4.2628	0.3	0.85
ZINC35465373	4.7842	8.144	3.3598	0.2	0.75
ZINC85542529	3.6799	6.6869	3.007	0.35	0.7

Comparative docking characteristics: pgeom algorithm, CBAV and LBPV of top selected compounds from Natural Products screen bound to IRF1- and IRF8-DBD domain. In silico calculations were performed by Surflex-Dock 2.6. BS, binding score; CBAV, comparative binding score value; LBPV, ligand binding pose variation.
[a]CBAV(pan-IRF1/8) = BS(IRF1) − BS(IRF8).
[b]CBAV(IRF1spec) = BS(IRF1) − BS(IRF8).
[c]CBAV(IRF8spec) = BS(IRF8) − BS(IRF1).

based approach, could be applied for many previously described infectious diseases and cancers. Nevertheless, many disorders are dependent on aberrant interaction of two or more IRFs at the same time. A representative example of an autoimmune disease where the use of a pan-IRF inhibitor could be advantageous is SLE, in which combined action of IRF5 and IRF7 has been documented (168, 169). A similar strategy could be applied for numerous chronic inflammatory diseases, such as RA or atherosclerosis. Several studies (169, 226, 227) pointed to the role of IRF1 as well as IRF5 in OA or RA, while IRF1, 5, 7, and 8 are recognized as key factors contributing to development and progression of atherosclerotic plaques (156, 169, 175).

STAT family members together with IRF1 and IRF8 were identified as key mediators of inflammation associated with CVDs. Therefore, going a step further, we used described 3D models of IRF1 and IRF8-DBD apo-forms, as the molecular targets for a virtual screening strategy, in order to identify pan-IRF1/8 inhibitors. Herein, we present a list of the top 3 compounds with a high inhibitory potential toward both IRF1 and IRF8 (**Table 1** and **Figure 4C**). The five-step docking procedure, subsequently resulted in a list of 20 optimized conformations for each selected compound, with supporting BS, CBAVs and LBPVs for each IRF. **Table 1** shows the top IRF1-BS and IRF8-BS of ZINC03838704, ZINC19368515 and ZINC31156634, as well as CBAV-IRF(1-8). In an ideal situation, the value of CBAV parameter for pan-inhibitors is equal or close to 0. After analysis of corresponding CBAV (−0.01 - 0.04) values it becomes clear that presented compounds exhibited nearly identical binding affinity to the IRF1 and IRF8 DBD. Compounds are presented according to ascending CBAV values, which allowed to select the most potent pan-IRF1/8-DBD targeting molecules. **Figure 4C** illustrates the top scored conformation of ZINC03838704, ZINC19368515 and ZINC31156634 compounds in IRF1- and IRF8-DBD, as representative pan-IRF1/8-DBD inhibitors. While for IRF-specific inhibitors one dominant pose represented the compounds' conformational tendency, for pan-IRF inhibitors it was common that two dominant binding conformations oriented in opposite directions were observed, which results in two LBPV values calculated. LBPV in the range of 0.8; 1.0 represented low conformer diversity and significant binding specificity of the compound to IRF-DBD, whereas the range of 0.0; 0.2 denotes high conformer diversity and poor binding specificity. Low-throughput *in vitro* cell-based multiple activation and IRF inhibition should be used to validate the effect of pre-selected inhibitory compounds on cytokine-induced IRF action and target gene expression in different cell types.

DIAGNOSTICS, THERAPEUTICS & FUTURE PERSPECTIVES

IRFs in Diagnostics

IRFs have an important role in various diseases. In recent years their clinical relevance was established by genome-wide association studies (GWAS). Applying genome-wide SNP association studies, it was demonstrated that IRF4 is strongly associated with susceptibility to Chronic lymphocytic leukemia (CLL), with risk loci identified at 6p25.3 (rs872071, IRF4) (228). IRF5 and IRF7 alleles rs2004640 and rs1131665 predispose to the development of SLE (173, 174, 224). Acknowledging the implications of IRF4, IRF5, and IRF7 polymorphisms and aberrant expression in autoimmune diseases like SLE, RA and cancer, prognostic screening could provide insights in disease severity (**Figure 5**).

Changes in IRF expression could be a prognostic factor in several human diseases. For instance, IRF1, IRF4, and IRF8 are significantly downregulated in failing human hearts compared with healthy controls (229, 230), whereas IRF3 is profoundly

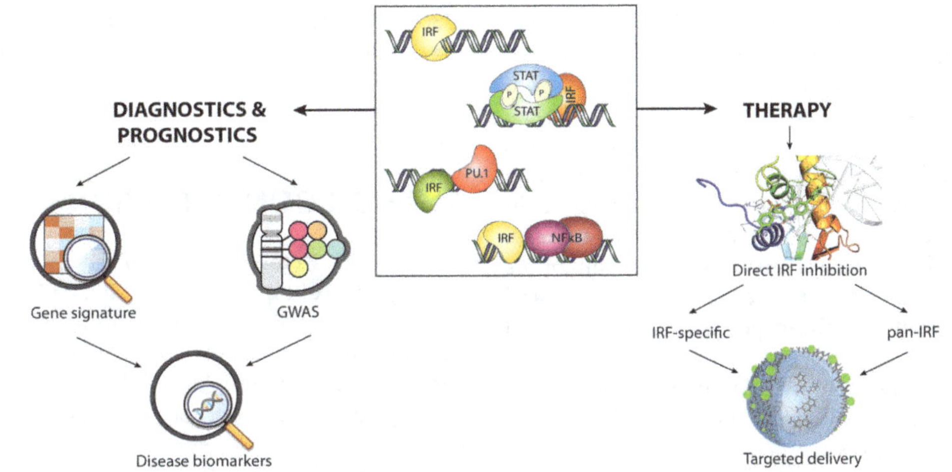

FIGURE 5 | Therapeutic, diagnostic, and prognostic space occupied by IRFs and IRF-mediated transcription regulatory mechanisms. IRF-containing complexes involved in transcriptional regulation, including IRF homodimers, STAT/IRF, PU.1/IRF, and NF-κB/IRF (central), can serve as diagnostic and therapeutic targets in different ways. The analysis of IRFs transcriptional mechanisms together with GWAS and characterization of gene expression signatures might provide disease diagnostic and prognostic markers (left side). Novel IRF-specific and pan-IRF inhibitors combined with an appropriate delivery system have the potential to be effective therapeutic agents for numerous immune related diseases (right side). We propose nanoparticles as promising tool for IRF inhibitory compound administration.

upregulated in the hearts of patients with dilated or hypertrophic cardiomyopathy (231). IRF1 and IRF2 expression is associated with prognosis and tumor invasion in hepatocellular carcinoma (HCC). Supporting this notion, the IRF2/IRF1 ratio positively correlated with tumor metastatic potential in the metastatic model of HCC cell lines—HCCLM3 (232). Hence, IRF expression can be used as viable prognostic markers in SLE and several types of cancer (**Figure 5**).

Not only IRF expression itself, but downstream ISG expression provides interesting markers for diagnostic use. With the demonstrated variety in IRF-mediated transcriptional regulatory mechanisms implicated in diseases, leading to the upregulation of specific subsets of ISGs, several applications can be envisioned (**Figure 5**). Indeed, specific subsets of ISGs are already being proposed for use in assays for the prediction of recurrence risk in patients with colon cancer and assays assessing the risk of transplant rejection (233, 234). In previous work our group identified a 72 gene "plaque signature" that predominantly consisted of STAT1 and IRF8-target genes which could be of use as a novel diagnostic tool to monitor and diagnose plaque phenotype in human atherosclerosis (156).

IRF in Therapeutics

Dysregulation of IRF function is critical in the development of immune system-originated diseases. Therefore, investigating the regulatory mechanisms mediated by IRFs and modulating IRFs expression might be crucial for disease treatment (**Figure 5**).

So far, IRFs have not been pursued as drug targets in terms of direct and selective inhibition. Current IRF inhibitory strategies are mainly limited to indirect modulation of their expression and function. Only direct inhibition strategies, which target IRFs transcription by siRNA or miRNA have been employed. Preventing IRF binding to DNA could serve as another potential therapeutically advantageous way to inhibit IRFs. An in-depth understanding of the IRF protein structure and the mechanisms involved in the binding of these transcription factors to DNA will allow the development of effective inhibition strategies. Moreover, the fact that many IRFs require a binding partner, such as PU.1, to effectively contact DNA can be used to develop a potent inhibitory system for IRFs. In addition, formation of homo- and heterodimers or cooperative DNA binding with co-activators, both promoted by the IAD in the C-terminal region can be directly blocked by inhibitory compounds.

We postulate that successful targeting of IRF-DBDs using small molecule inhibitors provides hope that IRFs can be "attacked" directly and used for the treatment of IRF-dependent disorders and malignancies. Considering the similarities and differences between the individual IRFs, in particular two directly modulating IRF DNA binding strategies can be proposed (**Figure 5**). The first approach would be based on the specific inhibition of IRF responsible for the development of the disease. Selective targeting of the IRF-DBD could lead to overcoming viral or bacterial infections as well as cancers. The second strategy would be designed to trigger a pan-IRF effect and inhibit two or more causative IRFs e.g., in SLE treatment. In addition, existing protein-DNA and protein-protein interfaces of human IRFs can be screened for potential cavities selectively binding inhibitory compounds.

Future Perspectives

In this review, we have summarized the current knowledge of the different IRF-mediated transcriptional regulatory mechanisms and how they reflect the diverse functions of IRFs in homeostasis and in TLR and IFN signaling. IRFs orchestrate expression of distinct subsets of ISGs via dimer formation, their involvement in transcriptional complexes, and co-binding with other transcription factors. ISG subset expression, as well as the expression of IRFs or the SNPs they contain might be exploited in future diagnostic arrays for the assessment of disease progression of a wide variety of (auto)immune diseases and cancer.

Several STAT inhibitors, including synthetic small compounds, natural products and oligonucleotide decoys, in recent (pre)clinical trials prove that strategies targeting transcription factors might find their way to the clinic in the near future. Therefore, we postulate that successful targeting of IRF-DBDs using small-molecule inhibitors provides hope that IRFs can be "attacked" directly and used for the treatment of IRF-dependent disorders and malignancies (**Figure 5**).

In vitro and *in vivo* validation of IRF inhibitory compounds has to prove their hypothesized effectiveness, as well as assess potential cytotoxicity before these products can move to clinical studies. Another challenge for the use of inhibitory strategies in therapeutics is the administration of such compounds. Systemic administration of IRF inhibitors is undesirable, because of possible unforeseen side effects. Therefore, either local injection/release or targeted administration with labeled compounds will be more effective as inhibition therapy. Nanotechnology might offer novel ways of drug administration (**Figure 5**). Antibody-conjugated nanoparticles have previously been used experimentally (235), and already several studies with nanoparticle based administration of inhibitory drugs have been published, such as inhibition of PI3K or the apoptotic regulator protein survivin in several types of cancer (236, 237). The results reported in such studies strengthen the feasibility of a nanomedicine targeted approach to IRF inhibition.

AUTHOR CONTRIBUTIONS

AA and BK were equally involved in concept development, writing and editing the manuscript. MS generated 3D models of IRFs DBD domains and performed *in silico* analysis and described the results. AM took part in figures preparation and concept development. AP-B, MP-G, and JW participated in development of the concept and critically evaluated and edited the manuscript. HB developed the concept and was involved in writing and editing the manuscript and coordinated input from all co-authors.

ACKNOWLEDGMENTS

We would like to thank members of the Department of Human Molecular Genetics for their critical discussion and input. We apologize to colleagues whose work could not be cited due to space constraints.

REFERENCES

1. Fujita T, Sakakibara J, Sudo Y, Miyamoto M, Kimura Y, Taniguchi T. Evidence for a nuclear factor(s), IRF-1, mediating induction and silencing properties to human IFN-beta gene regulatory elements. *EMBO J.* (1988) 7:3397–405. doi: 10.1002/j.1460-2075.1988.tb03213.x
2. Miyamoto M, Fujita T, Kimura Y, Maruyama M, Harada H, Sudo Y, et al. Regulated expression of a gene encoding a nuclear factor, IRF-1, that specifically binds to IFN-β gene regulatory elements. *Cell.* (1988) 54:903–13. doi: 10.1016/S0092-8674(88)91307-4
3. Suzuki Y, Yasuike M, Kondo H, Aoki T, Hirono I. Molecular cloning and expression analysis of interferon regulatory factor 10 (IRF10) in Japanese flounder, *Paralichthys olivaceus. Fish Shellfish Immunol.* (2011) 30:67–76. doi: 10.1016/j.fsi.2010.09.010
4. Taniguchi T, Ogasawara K, Takaoka A, Tanaka N. IRF family of transcription factors as regulators of host defense. *Annu Rev Immunol.* (2001) 19:623–55. doi: 10.1146/annurev.immunol.19.1.623
5. Levy DE, Kessler DS, Pine R, Darnell JE. Cytoplasmic activation of ISGF3, the positive regulator of interferon-alpha-stimulated transcription, reconstituted *in vitro. Genes Dev.* (1989) 3:1362–71. doi: 10.1101/gad.3.9.1362
6. Barnes B, Lubyova B, Pitha PM. On the role of IRF in host defense. *J Interferon Cytokine Res.* (2002) 22:59–71. doi: 10.1089/107999002753452665
7. Huang B, Qi ZT, Xu Z, Nie P. Global characterization of interferon regulatory factor (IRF) genes in vertebrates: glimpse of the diversification in evolution. *BMC Immunol.* (2010) 11:22. doi: 10.1186/1471-2172-11-22
8. Zhu Y, Qi C, Shan S, Zhang F, Li H, An L, et al. Characterization of common carp (*Cyprinus carpio* L.) interferon regulatory factor 5 (IRF5) and its expression in response to viral and bacterial challenges. *BMC Vet Res.* (2016) 12:127. doi: 10.1186/s12917-016-0750-4
9. Remesh SG, Santosh V, Escalante CR. Structural studies of IRF4 reveal a flexible autoinhibitory region and a compact linker domain. *J Biol Chem.* (2015) 290:27779–90. doi: 10.1074/jbc.M115.678789
10. Szelag M, Piaszyk-Borychowska A, Plens-Galaska M, Wesoly J, Bluyssen HAR. Targeted inhibition of STATs and IRFs as a potential treatment strategy in cardiovascular disease. *Oncotarget.* (2016) 7:48788–812. doi: 10.18632/oncotarget.9195
11. Andrilenas KK, Ramlall V, Kurland J, Leung B, Harbaugh AG, Siggers T. DNA-binding landscape of IRF3, IRF5 and IRF7 dimers: implications for dimer-specific gene regulation. *Nucleic Acids Res.* (2018) 46:2509–20. doi: 10.1093/nar/gky002
12. Rengachari S, Groiss S, Devos JM, Caron E, Grandvaux N, Panne D. Structural basis of STAT2 recognition by IRF9 reveals molecular insights into ISGF3 function. *Proc Natl Acad Sci USA.* (2018) 115:E601–9. doi: 10.1073/pnas.1718426115
13. Chen FE, Huang D-B, Chen Y-Q, Ghosh G. Crystal structure of p50/p65 heterodimer of transcription factor NF-κB bound to DNA. *Nature.* (1998) 391:410. doi: 10.1038/34956
14. Gibbert K, Schlaak JF, Yang D, Dittmer U. IFN-α subtypes: distinct biological activities in antiviral therapy. *Br J Pharmacol.* (2013) 168:1048–58. doi: 10.1111/bph.12010
15. Nagarajan U. Induction and function of IFNβ during viral and bacterial infection. *Crit Rev Immunol.* (2011) 31:459–74. doi: 10.1615/CritRevImmunol.v31.i6.20
16. Pestka S, Krause CD, Walter MR. Interferons, interferon-like cytokines, and their receptors. *Immunol Rev.* (2004) 202:8–32. doi: 10.1111/j.0105-2896.2004.00204.x
17. Fensterl V, Sen GC. Interferons and viral infections. *BioFactors.* (2009) 35:14–20. doi: 10.1002/biof.6

18. Prokunina-Olsson L, Muchmore B, Tang W, Pfeiffer RM, Park H, Dickensheets H, et al. A variant upstream of *IFNL3* (*IL28B*) creating a new interferon gene *IFNL4* is associated with impaired clearance of hepatitis C virus. *Nature Genet.* (2013) 45:164–71. doi: 10.1038/ng.2521
19. Donnelly RP, Kotenko SV. Interferon-lambda: a new addition to an old family. *J Interferon Cytokine Res.* (2010) 30:555–64. doi: 10.1089/jir.2010.0078
20. Levy DE, Darnell JE Jr. STATs: transcriptional control and biological impact. *Nat Rev Mol Cell Biol.* (2002) 3:651. doi: 10.1038/nrm909
21. Stark GR, Kerr IM, Williams BR, Silverman RH, Schreiber RD. How cells respond to interferons. *Annu Rev Biochem.* (1998) 67:227–64. doi: 10.1146/annurev.biochem.67.1.227
22. Platanias LC. Mechanisms of type-I- and type-II-interferon-mediated signalling. *Nat Rev Immunol.* (2005) 5:375. doi: 10.1038/nri1604
23. Poat B, Hazari S, Chandra PK, Gunduz F, Alvarez X, Balart LA, et al. Intracellular expression of IRF9 Stat fusion protein overcomes the defective Jak-Stat signaling and inhibits HCV RNA replication. *Virol J.* (2010) 7:265. doi: 10.1186/1743-422X-7-265
24. Kraus TA, Lau JF, Parisien J-P, Horvath CM. A hybrid IRF9-STAT2 protein recapitulates interferon-stimulated gene expression and antiviral response. *J Biol Chem.* (2003) 278:13033–8. doi: 10.1074/jbc.M212972200
25. Bluyssen HA, Levy DE. Stat2 is a transcriptional activator that requires sequence-specific contacts provided by stat1 and p48 for stable interaction with DNA. *J Biol Chem.* (1997) 272:4600–5. doi: 10.1074/jbc.272.7.4600
26. Michalska A, Blaszczyk K, Wesoly J, Bluyssen HAR. A positive feedback amplifier circuit that regulates interferon (IFN)-stimulated gene expression and controls type I and type II IFN responses. *Front Immunol.* (2018) 9:1135. doi: 10.3389/fimmu.2018.01135
27. Schroder K, Hertzog PJ, Ravasi T, Hume DA. Interferon-gamma: an overview of signals, mechanisms, and functions. *J Leukoc Biol.* (2004) 75:163–89. doi: 10.1189/jlb.0603252
28. Sikorski K, Chmielewski S, Olejnik A, Wesoly JZ, Heemann U, Baumann M, et al. STAT1 as a central mediator of IFNγ and TLR4 signal integration in vascular dysfunction. *JAKSTAT.* (2012) 1:241–9. doi: 10.4161/jkst.22469
29. Ramsauer K, Farlik M, Zupkovitz G, Seiser C, Kroger A, Hauser H, et al. Distinct modes of action applied by transcription factors STAT1 and IRF1 to initiate transcription of the IFN- -inducible gbp2 gene. *Proc Natl Acad Sci USA.* (2007) 104:2849–54. doi: 10.1073/pnas.0610944104
30. Morris AC, Beresford GW, Mooney MR, Boss JM. Kinetics of a gamma interferon response: expression and assembly of CIITA promoter IV and inhibition by methylation. *Mol Cell Biol.* (2002) 22:4781. doi: 10.1128/MCB.22.13.4781-4791.2002
31. Kumatori A, Yang D, Suzuki S, Nakamura M. Cooperation of STAT-1 and IRF-1 in interferon-γ-induced transcription of the gp91 *phox* gene. *J Biol Chem.* (2002) 277:9103–11. doi: 10.1074/jbc.M109803200
32. Erridge C. The roles of Toll-like receptors in atherosclerosis. *J Innate Immun.* (2009) 1:340–9. doi: 10.1159/000191413
33. Moynagh PN. TLR signalling and activation of IRFs: revisiting old friends from the NF-kappaB pathway. *Trends Immunol.* (2005) 26:469–76. doi: 10.1016/j.it.2005.06.009
34. Kawai T, Akira S. The role of pattern-recognition receptors in innate immunity: update on Toll-like receptors. *Nat Immunol.* (2010) 11:373–84. doi: 10.1038/ni.1863
35. Brubaker SW, Bonham KS, Zanoni I, Kagan JC. Innate immune pattern recognition: a cell biological perspective. *Annu Rev Immunol.* (2015) 33:257–90. doi: 10.1146/annurev-immunol-032414-112240
36. Yi A-K, Krieg AM. CpG DNA rescue from anti-IgM-induced WEHI-231 B lymphoma apoptosis via modulation of IκBα and IκBβ and sustained activation of nuclear factor-κB/c-Rel. *J Immunol.* (1998) 160:1240.
37. Medzhitov R, Preston-Hurlburt P, Janeway CA Jr. A human homologue of the drosophila toll protein signals activation of adaptive immunity. *Nature.* (1997) 388:394. doi: 10.1038/41131
38. Gilmore TD. Introduction to NF-kappaB: players, pathways, perspectives. *Oncogene.* (2006) 25:6680–4. doi: 10.1038/sj.onc.1209954
39. Wolberger C. Combinatorial transcription factors. *Curr Opin Genet Dev.* (1998) 8:552–9. doi: 10.1016/S0959-437X(98)80010-5
40. Colonna M. TLR pathways and IFN-regulatory factors: to each its own. *Eur J Immunol.* (2007) 37:306–9. doi: 10.1002/eji.200637009
41. Martin MU, Wesche H. Summary and comparison of the signaling mechanisms of the Toll/interleukin-1 receptor family. *Biochim Biophys Acta.* (2002) 1592:265–80. doi: 10.1016/S0167-4889(02)00320-8
42. Iwanaszko M, Kimmel M. NF-κB and IRF pathways: cross-regulation on target genes promoter level. *BMC Genom.* (2015) 16:307. doi: 10.1186/s12864-015-1511-7
43. Alexopoulou L, Holt AC, Medzhitov R, Flavell RA. Recognition of double-stranded RNA and activation of NF-kappaB by Toll-like receptor 3. *Nature.* (2001) 413:732–8. doi: 10.1038/35099560
44. Kawai T, Adachi O, Ogawa T, Takeda K, Akira S. Unresponsiveness of MyD88-deficient mice to endotoxin. *Immunity.* (1999) 11:115–22. doi: 10.1016/S1074-7613(00)80086-2
45. Fitzgerald KA, McWhirter SM, Faia KL, Rowe DC, Latz E, Golenbock DT, et al. IKKε and TBK1 are essential components of the IRF3 signaling pathway. *Nat Immunol.* (2003) 4:491. doi: 10.1038/ni921
46. Sharma S, tenOever BR, Grandvaux N, Zhou G-P, Lin R, Hiscott J. Triggering the interferon antiviral response through an IKK-related pathway. *Science.* (2003) 300:1148–51. doi: 10.1126/science.1081315
47. Kagan JC, Su T, Horng T, Chow A, Akira S, Medzhitov R. TRAM couples endocytosis of Toll-like receptor 4 to the induction of interferon-beta. *Nat Immunol.* (2008) 9:361–8. doi: 10.1038/ni1569
48. Patton JT, Spencer E. Genome replication and packaging of segmented double-stranded RNA viruses. *Virology.* (2000) 277:217–25. doi: 10.1006/viro.2000.0645
49. Ramnath D, Tunny K, Hohenhaus DM, Pitts CM, Bergot A-S, Hogarth PM, et al. TLR3 drives IRF6-dependent IL-23p19 expression and p19/EBI3 heterodimer formation in keratinocytes. *Immunol Cell Biol.* (2015) 93:771–9. doi: 10.1038/icb.2015.77
50. Diebold SS, Kaisho T, Hemmi H, Akira S, Reis e Sousa C. Innate antiviral responses by means of TLR7-mediated recognition of single-stranded RNA. *Science.* (2004) 303:1529–31. doi: 10.1126/science.1093616
51. Bauer S, Kirschning CJ, Häcker H, Redecke V, Hausmann S, Akira S, et al. Human TLR9 confers responsiveness to bacterial DNA via species-specific CpG motif recognition. *Proc Natl Acad Sci USA.* (2001) 98:9237–42. doi: 10.1073/pnas.161293498
52. Zhang Y, El-Far M, Dupuy FP, Abdel-Hakeem MS, He Z, Procopio FA, et al. HCV RNA activates APCs via TLR7/TLR8 while virus selectively stimulates macrophages without inducing antiviral responses. *Sci Rep.* (2016) 6:29447. doi: 10.1038/srep29447
53. Heil F, Hemmi H, Hochrein H, Ampenberger F, Kirschning C, Akira S, et al. Species-specific recognition of single-stranded RNA via toll-like receptor 7 and 8. *Science.* (2004) 303:1526–9. doi: 10.1126/science.1093620
54. Ashkar AA, Rosenthal KL. Toll-like receptor 9, CpG DNA and innate immunity. *Curr Mol Med.* (2002) 2:545–56. doi: 10.2174/1566524023362159
55. Latz E, Schoenemeyer A, Visintin A, Fitzgerald KA, Monks BG, Knetter CF, et al. TLR9 signals after translocating from the ER to CpG DNA in the lysosome. *Nat Immunol.* (2004) 5:190–8. doi: 10.1038/ni1028
56. Kawai T, Sato S, Ishii KJ, Coban C, Hemmi H, Yamamoto M, et al. Interferon-alpha induction through Toll-like receptors involves a direct interaction of IRF7 with MyD88 and TRAF6. *Nat Immunol.* (2004) 5:1061–8. doi: 10.1038/ni1118
57. Takaoka A, Yanai H, Kondo S, Duncan G, Negishi H, Mizutani T, et al. Integral role of IRF-5 in the gene induction programme activated by Toll-like receptors. *Nature.* (2005) 434:243–9. doi: 10.1038/nature03308
58. Schoenemeyer A, Barnes BJ, Mancl ME, Latz E, Goutagny N, Pitha PM, et al. The interferon regulatory factor, IRF5, is a central mediator of toll-like receptor 7 signaling. *J Biol Chem.* (2005) 280:17005–12. doi: 10.1074/jbc.M412584200
59. Yasuda K, Nündel K, Watkins AA, Dhawan T, Bonegio RG, Ubellacker JM, et al. Phenotype and function of B cells and dendritic cells from interferon regulatory factor 5-deficient mice with and without a mutation in DOCK2. *Int Immunol.* (2013) 25:295–306. doi: 10.1093/intimm/dxs114
60. Wang J, Basagoudanavar SH, Wang X, Hopewell E, Albrecht R, García-Sastre A, et al. NF-κB RelA subunit is crucial for early IFN-β expression and resistance to RNA virus replication. *J Immunol.* (2010) 185:1720–9. doi: 10.4049/jimmunol.1000114

61. Thanos D, Maniatis T. Virus induction of human IFN beta gene expression requires the assembly of an enhanceosome. *Cell.* (1995) 83:1091–100. doi: 10.1016/0092-8674(95)90136-1
62. Panne D, Maniatis T, Harrison SC. An atomic model of the interferon-beta enhanceosome. *Cell.* (2007) 129:1111–23. doi: 10.1016/j.cell.2007.05.019
63. Chmielewski S, Piaszyk-Borychowska A, Wesoly J, Bluyssen HAR. STAT1 and IRF8 in vascular inflammation and cardiovascular disease: diagnostic and therapeutic potential. *Int Rev Immunol.* (2016) 35:434–54. doi: 10.3109/08830185.2015.1087519
64. Kawai T, Akira S. Toll-like receptor and RIG-I-like receptor signaling. *Ann N Y Acad Sci.* (2008) 1143:1–20. doi: 10.1196/annals.1443.020
65. Weber F. The catcher in the RIG-I. *Cytokine.* (2015) 76:38–41. doi: 10.1016/j.cyto.2015.07.002
66. Chattopadhyay S and Ganes C. dsRNA-Activation of TLR3 and RLR signaling: gene induction-dependent and independent effects. *J Interferon Cytokine Res.* (2014) 34: 427–36. doi: 10.1089/jir.2014.0034
67. Chattopadhyay S, Sen GC. RIG-I-like receptor-induced IRF3 mediated pathway of apoptosis (RIPA): a new antiviral pathway. *Protein Cell.* (2017) 8:165–8. doi: 10.1007/s13238-016-0334-x
68. Escalante CR, Yie J, Thanos D, Aggarwal AK. Structure of IRF-1 with bound DNA reveals determinants of interferon regulation. *Nature.* (1998) 391:103–6. doi: 10.1038/34224
69. Fujii Y, Shimizu T, Kusumoto M, Kyogoku Y, Taniguchi T, Hakoshima T. Crystal structure of an IRF-DNA complex reveals novel DNA recognition and cooperative binding to a tandem repeat of core sequences. *EMBO J.* (1999) 18:5028–41. doi: 10.1093/emboj/18.18.5028
70. Furui J, Uegaki K, Yamazaki T, Shirakawa M, Swindells MB, Harada H, et al. Solution structure of the IRF-2 DNA-binding domain: a novel subgroup of the winged helix-turn-helix family. *Structure.* (1998) 6:491–500. doi: 10.1016/S0969-2126(98)00050-1
71. De Ioannes P, Escalante CR, Aggarwal AK. Structures of apo IRF-3 and IRF-7 DNA binding domains: effect of loop L1 on DNA binding. *Nucleic Acids Res.* (2011) 39:7300–7. doi: 10.1093/nar/gkr325
72. Wang Z, Ji J, Peng D, Ma F, Cheng G, Qin FX-F. Complex regulation pattern of IRF3 activation revealed by a novel dimerization reporter system. *J Immunol.* (2016) 196:4322–30. doi: 10.4049/jimmunol.1502458
73. Yoneyama M, Suhara W, Fujita T. Control of IRF-3 activation by phosphorylation. *J Interferon Cytokine Res.* (2002) 22:73–6. doi: 10.1089/107999002753452674
74. Qin BY, Liu C, Lam SS, Srinath H, Delston R, Correia JJ, et al. Crystal structure of IRF-3 reveals mechanism of autoinhibition and virus-induced phosphoactivation. *Nat Struct Biol.* (2003) 10:913–21. doi: 10.1038/nsb1002
75. Takahasi K, Suzuki NN, Horiuchi M, Mori M, Suhara W, Okabe Y, et al. X-ray crystal structure of IRF-3 and its functional implications. *Nat Struct Biol.* (2003) 10:922–7. doi: 10.1038/nsb1001
76. Takahasi K, Horiuchi M, Fujii K, Nakamura S, Noda NN, Yoneyama M, et al. Ser386 phosphorylation of transcription factor IRF-3 induces dimerization and association with CBP/p300 without overall conformational change. *Genes Cell.* (2010) 15:901–10. doi: 10.1111/j.1365-2443.2010.01427.x
77. Hiscott J. Triggering the innate antiviral response through IRF-3 activation. *J Biol Chem.* (2007) 282:15325–9. doi: 10.1074/jbc.R700002200
78. Perkel JM, Atchison ML. A two-step mechanism for recruitment of Pip by PU.1. *J Immunol.* (1998) 160:241–52.
79. Barnes BJ, Field AE, Pitha-Rowe PM. Virus-induced heterodimer formation between IRF-5 and IRF-7 modulates assembly of the IFNA enhanceosome in vivo and transcriptional activity of IFNA genes. *J Biol Chem.* (2003) 278:16630–41. doi: 10.1074/jbc.M212609200
80. Barnes BJ, Richards J, Mancl M, Hanash S, Beretta L, Pitha PM. Global and distinct targets of IRF-5 and IRF-7 during innate response to viral infection. *J Biol Chem.* (2004) 279:45194–207. doi: 10.1074/jbc.M400726200
81. Li Q, Tang L, Roberts PC, Kraniak JM, Fridman AL, Kulaeva OI, et al. Interferon regulatory factors IRF5 and IRF7 inhibit growth and induce senescence in immortal Li-Fraumeni fibroblasts. *Mol Cancer Res.* (2008) 6:770–84. doi: 10.1158/1541-7786.MCR-07-0114
82. Schaefer BC, Paulson E, Strominger JL, Speck SH. Constitutive activation of Epstein-Barr virus (EBV) nuclear antigen 1 gene transcription by IRF1 and IRF2 during restricted EBV latency. *Mol Cell Biol.* (1997) 17:873–86. doi: 10.1128/MCB.17.2.873
83. Blanco JC, Contursi C, Salkowski CA, DeWitt DL, Ozato K, Vogel SN. Interferon regulatory factor (IRF)-1 and IRF-2 regulate interferon gamma-dependent cyclooxygenase 2 expression. *J Exp Med.* (2000) 191:2131–44. doi: 10.1084/jem.191.12.2131
84. Langlais D, Barreiro LB, Gros P. The macrophage IRF8/IRF1 regulome is required for protection against infections and is associated with chronic inflammation. *J Exp Med.* (2016) 213:585–603. doi: 10.1084/jem.20151764
85. Masuda T, Iwamoto S, Mikuriya S, Tozaki-Saitoh H, Tamura T, Tsuda M, et al. Transcription factor IRF1 is responsible for IRF8-mediated IL-1β expression in reactive microglia. *J Pharmacol Sci.* (2015) 128:216–20. doi: 10.1016/j.jphs.2015.08.002
86. Schmid S, Sachs D, tenOever BR. Mitogen-activated protein kinase-mediated licensing of interferon regulatory factor 3/7 reinforces the cell response to virus. *J Biol Chem.* (2014) 289:299–311. doi: 10.1074/jbc.M113.519934
87. Blaszczyk K, Nowicka H, Kostyrko K, Antonczyk A, Wesoly J, Bluyssen HAR. The unique role of STAT2 in constitutive and IFN-induced transcription and antiviral responses. *Cytokine Growth Factor Rev.* (2016) 29:71–81. doi: 10.1016/j.cytogfr.2016.02.010
88. Bluyssen H. STAT2-directed pathogen responses. *Oncotarget.* (2015) 6:28525–26. doi: 10.18632/oncotarget.5266
89. Gupta S, Jiang M, Pernis A. IFN-α activates Stat6 and leads to the formation of Stat2: Stat6 complexes in B cells. *J Immunol.* (1999) 163:3834–41.
90. Levy DE, Kessler DS, Pine R, Reich N, Darnell JE. Interferon-induced nuclear factors that bind a shared promoter element correlate with positive and negative transcriptional control. *Genes Dev.* (1988) 2:383–93. doi: 10.1101/gad.2.4.383
91. Pine R, Decker T, Kessler DS, Levy DE, Darnell JE. Purification and cloning of interferon-stimulated gene factor 2 (ISGF2): ISGF2 (IRF-1) can bind to the promoters of both beta interferon- and interferon-stimulated genes but is not a primary transcriptional activator of either. *Mol Cell Biol.* (1990) 10:2448–57. doi: 10.1128/MCB.10.6.2448
92. Abou El Hassan M, Huang K, Eswara MBK, Xu Z, Yu T, Aubry A, et al. Properties of STAT1 and IRF1 enhancers and the influence of SNPs. *BMC Mol Biol.* (2017) 18:6. doi: 10.1186/s12867-017-0084-1
93. Randall RE, Goodbourn S. Interferons and viruses: an interplay between induction, signalling, antiviral responses and virus countermeasures. *J Gen Virol.* (2008) 89:1–47. doi: 10.1099/vir.0.83391-0
94. Chatterjee-Kishore M, Wright KL, Ting JP, Stark GR. How Stat1 mediates constitutive gene expression: a complex of unphosphorylated Stat1 and IRF1 supports transcription of the LMP2 gene. *EMBO J.* (2000) 19:4111–22. doi: 10.1093/emboj/19.15.4111
95. Moreau-Gachelin F. Spi-1/PU.1: an oncogene of the Ets family. *Biochim Biophys Acta.* (1994) 1198:149–63. doi: 10.1016/0304-419X(94)90011-6
96. Wasylyk B, Hahn SL, Giovane A. The Ets family of transcription factors. *Eur J Biochem.* (1993) 211:7–18. doi: 10.1111/j.1432-1033.1993.tb19864.x
97. Fisher RC, Scott EW. Role of PU.1 in hematopoiesis. *Stem Cells.* (1998) 16:25–37. doi: 10.1002/stem.160025
98. Staitieh BS, Fan X, Neveu W, Guidot DM. Nrf2 regulates PU.1 expression and activity in the alveolar macrophage. *Am J Physiol Lung Cell Mol Physiol.* (2015) 308:L1086–93. doi: 10.1152/ajplung.00355.2014
99. Escalante CR, Shen L, Escalante MC, Brass AL, Edwards TA, Singh H, et al. Crystallization and characterization of PU.1/IRF-4/DNA ternary complex. *J Struct Biol.* (2002) 139:55–9. doi: 10.1016/S1047-8477(02)00514-2
100. Marecki S, Fenton MJ. The role of IRF-4 in transcriptional regulation. *J Interferon Cytokine Res.* (2002) 22:121–33. doi: 10.1089/107999002753452737
101. Lodie TA, Savedra R, Golenbock DT, Van Beveren CP, Maki RA, Fenton MJ. Stimulation of macrophages by lipopolysaccharide alters the phosphorylation state, conformation, and function of PU.1 via activation of casein kinase II. *J Immunol.* (1997) 158:1848–56.
102. Irino T, Uemura M, Yamane H, Umemura S, Utsumi T, Kakazu N, et al. JAK2 V617F-dependent upregulation of PU.1 expression in the peripheral blood of myeloproliferative neoplasm patients. *PLoS ONE.* (2011) 6:e22148. doi: 10.1371/journal.pone.0022148
103. Mao C, Ray-Gallet D, Tavitian A, Moreau-Gachelin F. Differential phosphorylations of Spi-B and Spi-1 transcription factors. *Oncogene.* (1996) 12:863–73.

104. Gutiérrez P, Delgado MD, Richard C, Moreau-Gachelin F, León J. Interferon induces up-regulation of Spi-1/PU.1 in human leukemia K562 cells. *Biochem Biophys Res Commun.* (1997) 240:862–8. doi: 10.1006/bbrc.1997.7760
105. Pongubala JM, Nagulapalli S, Klemsz MJ, McKercher SR, Maki RA, Atchison ML. PU.1 recruits a second nuclear factor to a site important for immunoglobulin kappa 3' enhancer activity. *Mol Cell Biol.* (1992) 12:368–78. doi: 10.1128/MCB.12.1.368
106. Eklund EA, Jalava A, Kakar R. PU.1, interferon regulatory factor 1, and interferon consensus sequence-binding protein cooperate to increase gp91(phox) expression. *J Biol Chem.* (1998) 273:13957–65. doi: 10.1074/jbc.273.22.13957
107. Eisenbeis CF, Singh H, Storb U. Pip, a novel IRF family member, is a lymphoid-specific, PU.1-dependent transcriptional activator. *Genes Dev.* (1995) 9:1377–87. doi: 10.1101/gad.9.11.1377
108. Brass AL, Zhu AQ, Singh H. Assembly requirements of PU.1-Pip (IRF-4) activator complexes: inhibiting function in vivo using fused dimers. *EMBO J.* (1999) 18:977–91. doi: 10.1093/emboj/18.4.977
109. Kim YM, Kang HS, Paik SG, Pyun KH, Anderson KL, Torbett BE, et al. Roles of IFN consensus sequence binding protein and PU.1 in regulating IL-18 gene expression. *J Immunol.* (1999) 163:2000–7.
110. Mancino A, Termanini A, Barozzi I, Ghisletti S, Ostuni R, Prosperini E, et al. A dual cis-regulatory code links IRF8 to constitutive and inducible gene expression in macrophages. *Genes Dev.* (2015) 29:394–408. doi: 10.1101/gad.257592.114
111. Marecki S, Fenton MJ. PU.1/Interferon regulatory factor interactions: mechanisms of transcriptional regulation. *Cell Biochem Biophys.* (2000) 33:127–48. doi: 10.1385/CBB:33:2:127
112. Carlezon WA, Duman RS, Nestler EJ. The many faces of CREB. *Trends Neurosci.* (2005) 28:436–45. doi: 10.1016/j.tins.2005.06.005
113. Bourtchuladze R, Frenguelli B, Blendy J, Cioffi D, Schutz G, Silva AJ. Deficient long-term memory in mice with a targeted mutation of the cAMP-responsive element-binding protein. *Cell.* (1994) 79:59–68. doi: 10.1016/0092-8674(94)90400-6
114. Chrivia JC, Kwok RP, Lamb N, Hagiwara M, Montminy MR, Goodman RH. Phosphorylated CREB binds specifically to the nuclear protein CBP. *Nature.* (1993) 365:855–9. doi: 10.1038/365855a0
115. Ogryzko VV, Schiltz RL, Russanova V, Howard BH, Nakatani Y. The transcriptional coactivators p300 and CBP are histone acetyltransferases. *Cell.* (1996) 87:953–9. doi: 10.1016/S0092-8674(00)82001-2
116. Wojciak JM, Martinez-Yamout MA, Dyson HJ, Wright PE. Structural basis for recruitment of CBP/p300 coactivators by STAT1 and STAT2 transactivation domains. *EMBO J.* (2009) 28:948–58. doi: 10.1038/emboj.2009.30
117. Du W, Maniatis T. An ATF/CREB binding site is required for virus induction of the human interferon beta gene [corrected]. *Proc Natl Acad Sci USA.* (1992) 89:2150–4. doi: 10.1073/pnas.89.6.2150
118. Sahu S, Ganguly R, Raman P. Leptin augments recruitment of IRF-1 and CREB to thrombospondin-1 gene promoter in vascular smooth muscle cells in vitro. *Am J Physiol Cell Physiol.* (2016) 311:C212–24. doi: 10.1152/ajpcell.00068.2016
119. Sahoo A, Alekseev A, Tanaka K, Obertas L, Lerman B, Haymaker C, et al. Batf is important for IL-4 expression in T follicular helper cells. *Nat Commun.* (2015) 6:7997. doi: 10.1038/ncomms8997
120. Glasmacher E, Agrawal S, Chang AB, Murphy TL, Zeng W, Vander Lugt B, et al. A genomic regulatory element that directs assembly and function of immune-specific AP-1-IRF complexes. *Science.* (2012) 338:975–80. doi: 10.1126/science.1228309
121. Dorsey MJ, Tae HJ, Sollenberger KG, Mascarenhas NT, Johansen LM, Taparowsky EJ. B-ATF: a novel human bZIP protein that associates with members of the AP-1 transcription factor family. *Oncogene.* (1995) 11:2255–65.
122. Li P, Spolski R, Liao W, Wang L, Murphy TL, Murphy KM, et al. BATF-JUN is critical for IRF4-mediated transcription in T cells. *Nature.* (2012) 490:543–6. doi: 10.1038/nature11530
123. Guler R, Roy S, Suzuki H, Brombacher F. Targeting Batf2 for infectious diseases and cancer. *Oncotarget.* (2015) 6:26575–82. doi: 10.18632/oncotarget.5576
124. Roy S, Guler R, Parihar SP, Schmeier S, Kaczkowski B, Nishimura H, et al. Batf2/Irf1 induces inflammatory responses in classically activated macrophages, lipopolysaccharides, and mycobacterial infection. *J Immunol.* (2015) 194:6035–44. doi: 10.4049/jimmunol.1402521
125. Panne D, Maniatis T, Harrison SC. Crystal structure of ATF-2/c-Jun and IRF-3 bound to the interferon-beta enhancer. *EMBO J.* (2004) 23:4384–93. doi: 10.1038/sj.emboj.7600453
126. Lenardo MJ, Fan CM, Maniatis T, Baltimore D. The involvement of NF-kappa B in beta-interferon gene regulation reveals its role as widely inducible mediator of signal transduction. *Cell.* (1989) 57:287–94. doi: 10.1016/0092-8674(89)90966-5
127. Visvanathan KV, Goodbourn S. Double-stranded RNA activates binding of NF-kappa B to an inducible element in the human beta-interferon promoter. *EMBO J.* (1989) 8:1129–38. doi: 10.1002/j.1460-2075.1989.tb03483.x
128. Tong A-J, Liu X, Thomas BJ, Lissner MM, Baker MR, Senagolage MD, et al. A stringent systems approach uncovers gene-specific mechanisms regulating inflammation. *Cell.* (2016) 165:165–79. doi: 10.1016/j.cell.2016.01.020
129. Leung TH, Hoffmann A, Baltimore D. One nucleotide in a kappaB site can determine cofactor specificity for NF-kappaB dimers. *Cell.* (2004) 118:453–64. doi: 10.1016/j.cell.2004.08.007
130. Freaney JE, Kim R, Mandhana R, Horvath CM. Extensive cooperation of immune master regulators IRF3 and NFκB in RNA Pol II recruitment and pause release in human innate antiviral transcription. *Cell Rep.* (2013) 4:959–73. doi: 10.1016/j.celrep.2013.07.043
131. Wienerroither S, Shukla P, Farlik M, Majoros A, Stych B, Vogl C, et al. Cooperative transcriptional activation of antimicrobial genes by STAT and NF-κB pathways by concerted recruitment of the mediator complex. *Cell Rep.* (2015) 12:300–12. doi: 10.1016/j.celrep.2015.06.021
132. Clark DN, Read RD, Mayhew V, Petersen SC, Argueta LB, Stutz LA, et al. Four promoters of IRF5 respond distinctly to stimuli and are affected by autoimmune-risk polymorphisms. *Front Immunol.* (2013) 4:360. doi: 10.3389/fimmu.2013.00360
133. Saliba DG, Heger A, Eames HL, Oikonomopoulos S, Teixeira A, Blazek K, et al. IRF5:RelA interaction targets inflammatory genes in macrophages. *Cell Rep.* (2014) 8:1308–17. doi: 10.1016/j.celrep.2014.07.034
134. Korachi M, Ceran N, Adaleti R, Nigdelioglu A, Sökmen M. An association study of functional polymorphic genes IRF-1, IFNGR-1, and IFN-γ with disease progression, aspartate aminotransferase, alanine aminotransferase, and viral load in chronic hepatitis B and C. *Int J Infect Dis.* (2013) 17:e44–9. doi: 10.1016/j.ijid.2012.08.004
135. Sommer F, Faller G, Röllinghoff M, Kirchner T, Mak TW, Lohoff M. Lack of gastritis and of an adaptive immune response in interferon regulatory factor-1-deficient mice infected with *Helicobacter pylori*. *Eur J Immunol.* (2001) 31:396–402. doi: 10.1002/1521-4141(200102)31:2<396::AID-IMMU396>3.0.CO;2-Y
136. Pine R. IRF and tuberculosis. *J Interferon Cytokine Res.* (2002) 22:15–25. doi: 10.1089/107999002753452629
137. Yamada H, Mizuno S, Sugawara I. Interferon regulatory factor 1 in mycobacterial infection. *Microbiol Immunol.* (2002) 46:751–60. doi: 10.1111/j.1348-0421.2002.tb02760.x
138. Reis LF, Ruffner H, Stark G, Aguet M, Weissmann C. Mice devoid of interferon regulatory factor 1 (IRF-1) show normal expression of type I interferon genes. *EMBO J.* (1994) 13:4798–806. doi: 10.1002/j.1460-2075.1994.tb06805.x
139. Lefebvre S, Berrih-Aknin S, Adrian F, Moreau P, Poea S, Gourand L, et al. A specific interferon (IFN)-stimulated response element of the distal HLA-G promoter binds IFN-regulatory factor 1 and mediates enhancement of this nonclassical class I gene by IFN-beta. *J Biol Chem.* (2001) 276:6133–9. doi: 10.1074/jbc.M008496200
140. Hobart M, Ramassar V, Goes N, Urmson J, Halloran PF. IFN regulatory factor-1 plays a central role in the regulation of the expression of class I and II MHC genes *in vivo*. *J Immunol.* (1997) 158:4260–9.
141. AbuSara N, Razavi S, Derwish L, Komatsu Y, Licursi M, Hirasawa K. Restoration of IRF1-dependent anticancer effects by MEK inhibition in human cancer cells. *Cancer Lett.* (2015) 357:575–81. doi: 10.1016/j.canlet.2014.12.017

142. Mamane Y, Heylbroeck C, Génin P, Algarté M, Servant MJ, LePage C, et al. Interferon regulatory factors: the next generation. *Gene.* (1999) 237:1–14. doi: 10.1016/S0378-1119(99)00262-0
143. Tanaka N, Ishihara M, Taniguchi T. Suppression of c-myc or fosB-induced cell transformation by the transcription factor IRF-1. *Cancer Lett.* (1994) 83:191–6. doi: 10.1016/0304-3835(94)90318-2
144. Minamino K, Takahara K, Adachi T, Nagaoka K, Iyoda T, Taki S, et al. IRF-2 regulates B-cell proliferation and antibody production through distinct mechanisms. *Int Immunol.* (2012) 24:573–81. doi: 10.1093/intimm/dxs060
145. Drew PD, Franzoso G, Becker KG, Bours V, Carlson LM, Siebenlist U, et al. NF kappa B and interferon regulatory factor 1 physically interact and synergistically induce major histocompatibility class I gene expression. *J Interferon Cytokine Res.* (1995) 15:1037–45. doi: 10.1089/jir.1995.15.1037
146. Kim PKM, Armstrong M, Liu Y, Yan P, Bucher B, Zuckerbraun BS, et al. IRF-1 expression induces apoptosis and inhibits tumor growth in mouse mammary cancer cells in vitro and in vivo. *Oncogene.* (2004) 23:1125–35. doi: 10.1038/sj.onc.1207023
147. Teitz T, Wei T, Valentine MB, Vanin EF, Grenet J, Valentine VA, et al. Caspase 8 is deleted or silenced preferentially in childhood neuroblastomas with amplification of MYCN. *Nat Med.* (2000) 6:529–35. doi: 10.1038/75007
148. Doherty GM, Boucher L, Sorenson K, Lowney J. Interferon regulatory factor expression in human breast cancer. *Ann Surg.* (2001) 233:623–9. doi: 10.1097/00000658-200105000-00005
149. Fulda S, Küfer MU, Meyer E, van Valen F, Dockhorn-Dworniczak B, Debatin KM. Sensitization for death receptor- or drug-induced apoptosis by re-expression of caspase-8 through demethylation or gene transfer. *Oncogene.* (2001) 20:5865–77. doi: 10.1038/sj.onc.1204750
150. Chmielewski S, Olejnik A, Sikorski K, Pelisek J, Błaszczyk K, Aoqui C, et al. STAT1-dependent signal integration between IFNγ and TLR4 in vascular cells reflect pro-atherogenic responses in human atherosclerosis. *PLoS ONE.* (2014) 9:e113318. doi: 10.1371/journal.pone.0113318
151. Wessely R, Hengst L, Jaschke B, Wegener F, Richter T, Lupetti R, et al. A central role of interferon regulatory factor-1 for the limitation of neointimal hyperplasia. *Hum Mol Genet.* (2003) 12:177–87. doi: 10.1093/hmg/ddg018
152. Kusaba K, Kai H, Koga M, Takayama N, Ikeda A, Yasukawa H, et al. Inhibition of intrinsic interferon-gamma function prevents neointima formation after balloon injury. *Hypertension.* (2007) 49:909–15. doi: 10.1161/01.HYP.0000259668.37901.8c
153. Dimayuga PC, Li H, Chyu K-Y, Fredrikson GN, Nilsson J, Fishbein MC, et al. T cell modulation of intimal thickening after vascular injury: the bimodal role of IFN-gamma in immune deficiency. *Arterioscler Thromb Vasc Biol.* (2005) 25:2528–34. doi: 10.1161/01.ATV.0000190606.41121.00
154. Agrawal S, Febbraio M, Podrez E, Cathcart MK, Stark GR, Chisolm GM. Signal transducer and activator of transcription 1 is required for optimal foam cell formation and atherosclerotic lesion development. *Circulation.* (2007) 115:2939–47. doi: 10.1161/CIRCULATIONAHA.107.696922
155. Torella D, Curcio A, Gasparri C, Galuppo V, De Serio D, Surace FC, et al. Fludarabine prevents smooth muscle proliferation *in vitro* and neointimal hyperplasia *in vivo* through specific inhibition of STAT-1 activation. *Am J Physiol Heart Circ Physiol.* (2007) 292:H2935–43. doi: 10.1152/ajpheart.00887.2006
156. Sikorski K, Wesoly J, Bluyssen HAR. Data mining of atherosclerotic plaque transcriptomes predicts STAT1-dependent inflammatory signal integration in vascular disease. *Int J Mol Sci.* (2014) 15:14313–31. doi: 10.3390/ijms150814313
157. Chattopadhyay S, Veleeparambil M, Poddar D, Abdulkhalek S, Bandyopadhyay SK, Fensterl V, et al. EGFR kinase activity is required for TLR4 signaling and the septic shock response. *EMBO Rep.* (2015) 16:1535–47. doi: 10.15252/embr.201540337
158. Chen H-W, King K, Tu J, Sanchez M, Luster AD, Shresta S. The roles of IRF-3 and IRF-7 in innate antiviral immunity against dengue virus. *J Immunol.* (2013) 191:4194–201. doi: 10.4049/jimmunol.1300799
159. Schilte C, Buckwalter MR, Laird ME, Diamond MS, Schwartz O, Albert ML. Cutting edge: independent roles for IRF-3 and IRF-7 in hematopoietic and nonhematopoietic cells during host response to Chikungunya infection. *J Immunol.* (2012) 188:2967–71. doi: 10.4049/jimmunol.1103185
160. Murphy AA, Rosato PC, Parker ZM, Khalenkov A, Leib DA. Synergistic control of herpes simplex virus pathogenesis by IRF-3, and IRF-7 revealed through noninvasive bioluminescence imaging. *Virology.* (2013) 444:71–9. doi: 10.1016/j.virol.2013.05.034
161. Inoue K, Tsukiyama-Kohara K, Matsuda C, Yoneyama M, Fujita T, Kuge S, et al. Impairment of interferon regulatory factor-3 activation by hepatitis C virus core protein basic amino acid region 1. *Biochem Biophys Res Commun.* (2012) 428:494–9. doi: 10.1016/j.bbrc.2012.10.079
162. Huang L, Zhang S-M, Zhang P, Zhang X-J, Zhu L-H, Chen K, et al. Interferon regulatory factor 7 protects against vascular smooth muscle cell proliferation and neointima formation. *J Am Heart Assoc.* (2014) 3:e001309. doi: 10.1161/JAHA.114.001309
163. Bidwell BN, Slaney CY, Withana NP, Forster S, Cao Y, Loi S, et al. Silencing of Irf7 pathways in breast cancer cells promotes bone metastasis through immune escape. *Nat Med.* (2012) 18:1224–31. doi: 10.1038/nm.2830
164. Yanai H, Negishi H, Taniguchi T. The IRF family of transcription factors: Inception, impact and implications in oncogenesis. *Oncoimmunology.* (2012) 1:1376–86. doi: 10.4161/onci.22475
165. Rothfield N. Clinical aspects and treatment of systemic lupus erythematosus. *Curr Opinion Rheumatol.* (1989) 1:327. doi: 10.1097/00002281-198901030-00014
166. Dennehy KM, Willment JA, Williams DL, Brown GD. Reciprocal regulation of IL-23 and IL-12 following co-activation of Dectin-1 and TLR signaling pathways. *Eur J Immunol.* (2009) 39:1379–86. doi: 10.1002/eji.200838543
167. Napolitani G, Rinaldi A, Bertoni F, Sallusto F, Lanzavecchia A. Selected Toll-like receptor agonist combinations synergistically trigger a T helper type 1-polarizing program in dendritic cells. *Nat Immunol.* (2005) 6:769–76. doi: 10.1038/ni1223
168. Honda K, Yanai H, Negishi H, Asagiri M, Sato M, Mizutani T, et al. IRF-7 is the master regulator of type-I interferon-dependent immune responses. *Nature.* (2005) 434:772–7. doi: 10.1038/nature03464
169. Watkins AA, Yasuda K, Wilson GE, Aprahamian T, Xie Y, Maganto-Garcia E, et al. IRF5 deficiency ameliorates lupus but promotes atherosclerosis and metabolic dysfunction in a mouse model of lupus-associated atherosclerosis. *J Immunol.* (2015) 194:1467–79. doi: 10.4049/jimmunol.1402807
170. Li Y, Chen S, Li P, Wu Z, Li J, Liu B, et al. Association of the IRF5 rs2070197 polymorphism with systemic lupus erythematosus: a meta-analysis. *Clin Rheumatol.* (2015) 34:1495–501. doi: 10.1007/s10067-015-3036-5
171. Tang L, Chen B, Ma B, Nie S. Association between IRF5 polymorphisms and autoimmune diseases: a meta-analysis. *Genet Mol Res.* (2014) 13:4473–85. doi: 10.4238/2014.June.16.6
172. Hellquist A, Järvinen TM, Koskenmies S, Zucchelli M, Orsmark-Pietras C, Berglind L, et al. Evidence for genetic association and interaction between the TYK2 and IRF5 genes in systemic lupus erythematosus. *J Rheumatol.* (2009) 36:1631–8. doi: 10.3899/jrheum.081160
173. Graham RR, Kyogoku C, Sigurdsson S, Vlasova IA, Davies LRL, Baechler EC, et al. Three functional variants of IFN regulatory factor 5 (IRF5) define risk and protective haplotypes for human lupus. *Proc Natl Acad Sci USA.* (2007) 104:6758–63. doi: 10.1073/pnas.0701266104
174. Sigurdsson S, Nordmark G, Göring HHH, Lindroos K, Wiman A-C, Sturfelt G, et al. Polymorphisms in the tyrosine kinase 2 and interferon regulatory factor 5 genes are associated with systemic lupus erythematosus. *Am J Hum Genet.* (2005) 76:528–37. doi: 10.1086/428480
175. García-Bermúdez M, López-Mejías R, Genre F, Castañeda S, Llorca J, González-Juanatey C, et al. Interferon regulatory factor 5 genetic variants are associated with cardiovascular disease in patients with rheumatoid arthritis. *Arthritis Res Ther.* (2014) 16:R146. doi: 10.1186/ar4608
176. Manzella L, Tirrò E, Pennisi MS, Massimino M, Stella S, Romano C, et al. Roles of interferon regulatory factors in chronic myeloid leukemia. *Curr Cancer Drug Targets.* (2016) 16:594–605. doi: 10.2174/1568009616666160105105857
177. Bailey CM, Abbott DE, Margaryan NV, Khalkhali-Ellis Z, Hendrix MJC. Interferon regulatory factor 6 promotes cell cycle arrest and is regulated by the proteasome in a cell cycle-dependent manner. *Mol Cell Biol.* (2008) 28:2235–43. doi: 10.1128/MCB.01866-07
178. Moretti F, Marinari B, Lo Iacono N, Botti E, Giunta A, Spallone G, et al. A regulatory feedback loop involving p63 and IRF6 links the pathogenesis of 2 genetically different human ectodermal dysplasias. *J Clin Invest.* (2010) 120:1570–7. doi: 10.1172/JCI40267

179. Simonetti G, Carette A, Silva K, Wang H, De Silva NS, Heise N, et al. IRF4 controls the positioning of mature B cells in the lymphoid microenvironments by regulating NOTCH2 expression and activity. *J Exp Med.* (2013) 210:2887–902. doi: 10.1084/jem.20131026
180. Shaffer AL, Emre NCT, Romesser PB, Staudt LM. IRF4: immunity. malignancy! therapy? *Clin Cancer Res.* (2009) 15:2954–61. doi: 10.1158/1078-0432.CCR-08-1845
181. Wang S, Yan Q, Chen P, Zhao P, Gu A. Association of interferon regulatory factor 4 gene polymorphisms rs12203592 and rs872071 with skin cancer and haematological malignancies susceptibility: a meta-analysis of 19 case-control studies. *BMC Cancer.* (2014) 14:410. doi: 10.1186/1471-2407-14-410
182. Ochiai K, Maienschein-Cline M, Simonetti G, Chen J, Rosenthal R, Brink R, et al. Transcriptional regulation of germinal center B and plasma cell fates by dynamical control of IRF4. *Immunity.* (2013) 38:918–29. doi: 10.1016/j.immuni.2013.04.009
183. Hu X, Bardhan K, Paschall AV, Yang D, Waller JL, Park MA, et al. Deregulation of apoptotic factors Bcl-xL and Bax confers apoptotic resistance to myeloid-derived suppressor cells and contributes to their persistence in cancer. *J Biol Chem.* (2013) 288:19103–15. doi: 10.1074/jbc.M112.434530
184. Yang J, Hu X, Zimmerman M, Torres CM, Yang D, Smith SB, et al. Cutting edge: IRF8 regulates Bax transcription *in vivo* in primary myeloid cells. *J Immunol.* (2011) 187:4426–30. doi: 10.4049/jimmunol.1101034
185. Holtschke T, Löhler J, Kanno Y, Fehr T, Giese N, Rosenbauer F, et al. Immunodeficiency and chronic myelogenous leukemia-like syndrome in mice with a targeted mutation of the ICSBP gene. *Cell.* (1996) 87:307–17. doi: 10.1016/S0092-8674(00)81348-3
186. Mattei F, Schiavoni G, Sestili P, Spadaro F, Fragale A, Sistigu A, et al. IRF-8 controls melanoma progression by regulating the cross talk between cancer and immune cells within the tumor microenvironment. *Neoplasia.* (2012) 14:1223–35. doi: 10.1593/neo.121444
187. Ding S, Jiang T, He J, Qin B, Lin S, Li L. Tagging single nucleotide polymorphisms in the IRF1 and IRF8 genes and tuberculosis susceptibility. *PLoS ONE.* (2012) 7:e42104. doi: 10.1371/journal.pone.0042104
188. Ma S, Turetsky A, Trinh L, Lu R. IFN regulatory factor 4 and 8 promote Ig light chain kappa locus activation in pre-B cell development. *J Immunol.* (2006) 177:7898–904. doi: 10.4049/jimmunol.177.11.7898
189. Pathak S, Ma S, Trinh L, Eudy J, Wagner K-U, Joshi SS, et al. IRF4 is a suppressor of c-Myc induced B cell leukemia. *PLoS ONE.* (2011) 6:e22628. doi: 10.1371/journal.pone.0022628
190. Thibault DL, Chu AD, Graham KL, Balboni I, Lee LY, Kohlmoos C, et al. IRF9 and STAT1 are required for IgG autoantibody production and B cell expression of TLR7 in mice. *J Clin Invest.* (2008) 118:1417–26. doi: 10.1172/JCI30065
191. Liu L, Xu G, Dou H, Deng G-M. The features of skin inflammation induced by lupus serum. *Clin Immunol.* (2016) 165:4–11. doi: 10.1016/j.clim.2016.02.007
192. Metoni A, Mambet C, Necula LG, Aldea IM, Neagu AI, Matei L, et al. Mechanisms of thrombosis in systemic lupus erythematosus. *Roum Arch Microbiol Immunol.* (2014) 73:92–8. doi: 10.1016/j.berh.2017.09.008
193. Zhang D, Zhou Y. The protective effects of donepezil (DP) against cartilage matrix destruction induced by TNF-α. *Biochem Biophys Res Commun.* (2014) 454:115–18. doi: 10.1016/j.bbrc.2014.10.046
194. Mendel I, Feige E, Yacov N, Salem Y, Levi I, Propheta-Meiran O, et al. VB-201, an oxidized phospholipid small molecule, inhibits CD14- and Toll-like receptor-2-dependent innate cell activation and constrains atherosclerosis. *Clin Exp Immunol.* (2014) 175:126–37. doi: 10.1111/cei.12212
195. Faure V, Hecquet C, Courtois Y, Goureau O. Role of interferon regulatory factor-1 and mitogen-activated protein kinase pathways in the induction of nitric oxide synthase-2 in retinal pigmented epithelial cells. *J Biol Chem.* (1999) 274:4794–800. doi: 10.1074/jbc.274.8.4794
196. Jankovic V, Samardzic T, Stosic-Grujicic S, Popadic D, Trajkovic V. Cell-specific inhibition of inducible nitric oxide synthase activation by leflunomide. *Cell Immunol.* (2000) 199:73–80. doi: 10.1006/cimm.1999.1600
197. Zhu J, Smith K, Hsieh PN, Mburu YK, Chattopadhyay S, Sen GC, et al. High-throughput screening for TLR3–IFN regulatory factor 3 signaling pathway modulators identifies several antipsychotic drugs as TLR inhibitors. *J Immunol.* (2010). 184:5768–76. doi: 10.4049/jimmunol.0903559
198. Ruiz PA, Haller D. Functional diversity of flavonoids in the inhibition of the proinflammatory NF-kappaB, IRF, and Akt signaling pathways in murine intestinal epithelial cells. *J Nutr.* (2006) 136:664–71. doi: 10.1093/jn/136.3.664
199. Kao T-K, Ou Y-C, Lin S-Y, Pan H-C, Song P-J, Raung S-L, et al. Luteolin inhibits cytokine expression in endotoxin/cytokine-stimulated microglia. *J Nutr Biochem.* (2011) 22:612–24. doi: 10.1016/j.jnutbio.2010.01.011
200. Gavrila A, Chachi L, Tliba O, Brightling C, Amrani Y. Effect of the plant derivative Compound A on the production of corticosteroid-resistant chemokines in airway smooth muscle cells. *Am J Respir Cell Mol Biol.* (2015) 53:728–37. doi: 10.1165/rcmb.2014-0477OC
201. Chen Y-F, Wang S-H, Chang S-J, Shiau A-L, Her L-S, Shieh G-S, et al. Zhankuic acid A as a novel JAK2 inhibitor for the treatment of concanavalin A-induced hepatitis. *Biochem Pharmacol.* (2014) 91:217–30. doi: 10.1016/j.bcp.2014.06.026
202. Aziz N, Son Y-J, Cho JY. Thymoquinone suppresses IRF-3-mediated expression of type I interferons via suppression of TBK1. *Int J Mol Sci.* (2018) 19:1355. doi: 10.3390/ijms19051355
203. Lee J, Rhee MH, Kim E, Cho JY. BAY 11-7082 is a broad-spectrum inhibitor with anti-inflammatory activity against multiple targets. *Mediators Inflamm.* (2012) 2012:416036. doi: 10.1155/2012/416036
204. Park E-J, Min H-Y, Chung H-J, Ahn Y-H, Pyee J-H, Lee SK. Pinosylvin suppresses LPS-stimulated inducible nitric oxide synthase expression via the MyD88-independent, but TRIF-dependent downregulation of IRF-3 signaling pathway in mouse macrophage cells. *Cell Physiol Biochem.* (2011) 27:353–62. doi: 10.1159/000327961
205. Yang Y, Yang WS, Yu T, Yi Y-S, Park JG, Jeong D, et al. Novel anti-inflammatory function of NSC95397 by the suppression of multiple kinases. *Biochem Pharmacol.* (2014) 88:201–15. doi: 10.1016/j.bcp.2014.01.022
206. Ireland R, Wang R, Alinger JB, Small P, Bosio CM. *Francisella tularensis* SchuS4 and SchuS4 lipids inhibit IL-12p40 in primary human dendritic cells by inhibition of IRF1 and IRF8. *J Immunol.* (2013) 191:1276–86. doi: 10.4049/jimmunol.1300867
207. Hickey FB, Brereton CF, Mills KHG. Adenylate cycalse toxin of Bordetella pertussis inhibits TLR-induced IRF-1 and IRF-8 activation and IL-12 production and enhances IL-10 through MAPK activation in dendritic cells. *J Leukoc Biol.* (2008) 84:234–43. doi: 10.1189/jlb.0208113
208. Nikodemova M, Watters JJ, Jackson SJ, Yang SK, Duncan ID. Minocycline down-regulates MHC II expression in microglia and macrophages through inhibition of IRF-1 and protein kinase C (PKC)alpha/betaII. *J Biol Chem.* (2007) 282:15208–16. doi: 10.1074/jbc.M611907200
209. Ciccaglione AR, Stellacci E, Marcantonio C, Muto V, Equestre M, Marsili G, et al. Repression of interferon regulatory factor 1 by hepatitis C virus core protein results in inhibition of antiviral and immunomodulatory genes. *J Virol.* (2007) 81:202–14. doi: 10.1128/JVI.01011-06
210. Joo CH, Shin YC, Gack M, Wu L, Levy D, Jung JU. Inhibition of interferon regulatory factor 7 (IRF7)-mediated interferon signal transduction by the Kaposi's sarcoma-associated herpesvirus viral IRF homolog vIRF3. *J Virol.* (2007) 81:8282–92. doi: 10.1128/JVI.00235-07
211. Zhu FX, Yuan Y. The ORF45 protein of Kaposi's sarcoma-associated herpesvirus is associated with purified virions. *J Virol.* (2003) 77:4221–30. doi: 10.1128/JVI.77.7.4221-4230.2003
212. Sathish N, Yuan Y. Evasion and subversion of interferon-mediated antiviral immunity by Kaposi's sarcoma-associated herpesvirus: an overview. *J Virol.* (2011) 85:10934–44. doi: 10.1128/JVI.00687-11
213. Cai Q, Banerjee S, Cervini A, Lu J, Hislop AD, Dzeng R, et al. IRF-4-mediated CIITA transcription is blocked by KSHV encoded LANA to inhibit MHC II presentation. *PLoS Pathog.* (2013) 9:e1003751. doi: 10.1371/journal.ppat.1003751
214. Xing J, Ni L, Wang S, Wang K, Lin R, Zheng C. Herpes simplex virus 1-encoded tegument protein VP16 abrogates the production of beta interferon (IFN) by inhibiting NF-κB activation and blocking IFN regulatory factor 3 to recruit its coactivator CBP. *J Virol.* (2013) 87:9788–801. doi: 10.1128/JVI.01440-13
215. Zhu H, Zheng C, Xing J, Wang S, Li S, Lin R, Mossman KL. Varicella-zoster virus immediate-early protein ORF61 abrogates the IRF3-mediated innate

immune response through degradation of activated IRF3. *J Virol.* (2011) 85:11079–89. doi: 10.1128/JVI.05098-11.
216. Foy E, Li K, Wang C, Sumpter R, Ikeda M, Lemon SM, et al. Regulation of interferon regulatory factor-3 by the hepatitis C virus serine protease. *Science.* (2003) 300:1145–8. doi: 10.1126/science.1082604
217. Kaukinen P, Sillanpää M, Kotenko S, Lin R, Hiscott J, Melén K, et al. Hepatitis C virus NS2 and NS3/4A proteins are potent inhibitors of host cell cytokine/chemokine gene expression. *Virol J.* (2006) 3:66. doi: 10.1186/1743-422X-3-66
218. Chowdhury JB, Kim H, Ray R, Ray RB. Hepatitis C virus NS5A protein modulates IRF-7-mediated interferon-α signaling. *J Interferon Cytokine Res.* (2014) 34:16–21. doi: 10.1089/jir.2013.0038
219. Choo A, Palladinetti P, Holmes T, Basu S, Shen S, Lock RB, et al. siRNA targeting the IRF2 transcription factor inhibits leukaemic cell growth. *Int J Oncol.* (2008) 33:175–83. doi: 10.3892/ijo.33.1.175
220. Gururajan M, Haga CL, Das S, Leu C-M, Hodson D, Josson S, et al. MicroRNA 125b inhibition of B cell differentiation in germinal centers. *Int Immunol.* (2010) 22:583–92. doi: 10.1093/intimm/dxq042
221. Morelli E, Leone E, Cantafio MEG, Di Martino MT, Amodio N, Biamonte L, et al. Selective targeting of IRF4 by synthetic microRNA-125b-5p mimics induces anti-multiple myeloma activity *in vitro* and *in vivo*. *Leukemia.* (2015) 29:2173–83. doi: 10.1038/leu.2015.124
222. Czerwoniec A, Szelag M, Juszczak K, Wesoly J, Bluyssen HAR. CAVS—Novel *in silico* selection strategy of specific STAT inhibitory compounds. *J Comput Sci.* (2015) 10:186–94. doi: 10.1016/j.jocs.2015.03.001
223. Szelag M, Czerwoniec A, Wesoly J, Bluyssen HAR. Identification of STAT1 and STAT3 specific inhibitors using comparative virtual screening and docking validation. *PLoS ONE.* (2015) 10:e0116688. doi: 10.1371/journal.pone.0116688
224. Cunninghame Graham DS, Manku H, Wagner S, Reid J, Timms K, Gutin A, et al. Association of IRF5 in UK SLE families identifies a variant involved in polyadenylation. *Hum Mol Genet.* (2007) 16:579–91. doi: 10.1093/hmg/ddl469
225. Plens-Galaska M, Szelag M, Collado A, Marques P, Vallejo S, Ramos-González M, et al. Genome-wide inhibition of pro-atherogenic gene expression by multi-STAT targeting compounds as a novel treatment strategy of CVDs. *Front Immunol.* (2018) 9:2141. doi: 10.3389/fimmu.2018.02141
226. Marotte H, Tsou P-S, Rabquer BJ, Pinney AJ, Fedorova T, Lalwani N, et al. Blocking of interferon regulatory factor 1 reduces tumor necrosis factor α-induced interleukin-18 bioactivity in rheumatoid arthritis synovial fibroblasts by induction of interleukin-18 binding protein a: role of the nuclear interferon regulatory factor 1-NF-κB-c-jun complex. *Arthritis Rheum.* (2011) 63:3253–62. doi: 10.1002/art.30583
227. Sweeney SE, Mo L, Firestein GS. Antiviral gene expression in rheumatoid arthritis: role of IKKepsilon and interferon regulatory factor 3. *Arthritis Rheum.* (2007) 56:743–52. doi: 10.1002/art.22421
228. Di Bernardo MC, Crowther-Swanepoel D, Broderick P, Webb E, Sellick G, Wild R, et al. A genome-wide association study identifies six susceptibility loci for chronic lymphocytic leukemia. *Nat Genet.* (2008) 40:1204–10. doi: 10.1038/ng.219
229. Jiang D-S, Bian Z-Y, Zhang Y, Zhang S-M, Liu Y, Zhang R, et al. Role of interferon regulatory factor 4 in the regulation of pathological cardiac hypertrophy. *Hypertension.* (2013) 61:1193–202. doi: 10.1161/HYPERTENSIONAHA.111.00614
230. Jiang D-S, Li L, Huang L, Gong J, Xia H, Liu X, et al. Interferon regulatory factor 1 is required for cardiac remodeling in response to pressure overload. *Hypertension.* (2014) 64:77–86. doi: 10.1161/HYPERTENSIONAHA.114.03229
231. Lu J, Bian Z-Y, Zhang R, Zhang Y, Liu C, Yan L, et al. Interferon regulatory factor 3 is a negative regulator of pathological cardiac hypertrophy. *Basic Res Cardiol.* (2013) 108:326. doi: 10.1007/s00395-012-0326-9
232. Yi Y, Wu H, Gao Q, He H-W, Li Y-W, Cai X-Y, et al. Interferon regulatory factor (IRF)-1 and IRF-2 are associated with prognosis and tumor invasion in HCC. *Ann Surg Oncol.* (2013) 20:267–76. doi: 10.1245/s10434-012-2487-z
233. You YN, Rustin RB, Sullivan JD. Oncotype DX(®) colon cancer assay for prediction of recurrence risk in patients with stage II and III colon cancer: A review of the evidence. *Surg Oncol.* (2015) 24:61–6. doi: 10.1016/j.suronc.2015.02.001
234. Khatri P, Roedder S, Kimura N, De Vusser K, Morgan AA, Gong Y, et al. A common rejection module (CRM) for acute rejection across multiple organs identifies novel therapeutics for organ transplantation. *J Exp Med.* (2013) 210:2205–21. doi: 10.1084/jem.20122709
235. Cardoso MM, Peça IN, Roque ACA. Antibody-conjugated nanoparticles for therapeutic applications. *Curr Med Chem.* (2012) 19:3103–27. doi: 10.2174/092986712800784667
236. Pandey A, Kulkarni A, Roy B, Goldman A, Sarangi S, Sengupta P, et al. Sequential application of a cytotoxic nanoparticle and a PI3K inhibitor enhances antitumor efficacy. *Cancer Res.* (2014) 74:675–85. doi: 10.1158/0008-5472.CAN-12-3783
237. Wang S, Xu Y, Chan HF, Kim H-W, Wang Y, Leong KW, et al. Nanoparticle-mediated inhibition of survivin to overcome drug resistance in cancer therapy. *J Contr Rel.* (2016) 240:454–64. doi: 10.1016/j.jconrel.2016.04.018

3

Immunotolerant p50/NFκB Signaling and Attenuated Hepatic IFNβ Expression Increases Neonatal Sensitivity to Endotoxemia

*Sarah McKenna, Taylor Burey, Jeryl Sandoval, Leanna Nguyen, Odalis Castro, Suma Gudipati, Jazmin Gonzalez, Karim C. El Kasmi and Clyde J. Wright**

Section of Neonatology, Department of Pediatrics, University of Colorado School of Medicine, Aurora, CO, United States

Correspondence:
Clyde J. Wright
clyde.wright@ucdenver.edu

Sepsis is a major cause of neonatal morbidity and mortality. The current paradigm suggests that neonatal susceptibility to infection is explained by an innate immune response that is functionally immature. Recent studies in adults have questioned a therapeutic role for IFNβ in sepsis; however, the role of IFNβ in mediating neonatal sensitivity to sepsis is unknown. We evaluated the transcriptional regulation and expression of IFNβ in early neonatal (P0) and adult murine models of endotoxemia (IP LPS, 5 mg/kg). We found that hepatic, pulmonary, and serum IFNβ expression was significantly attenuated in endotoxemic neonates when compared to similarly exposed adults. Furthermore, endotoxemia induced hepatic p65/NFκB and IRF3 activation exclusively in adults. In contrast, endotoxemia induced immunotolerant p50/NFκB signaling in neonatal mice without evidence of IRF3 activation. Consistent with impaired IFNβ expression and attenuated circulating serum levels, neonatal pulmonary STAT1 signaling and target gene expression was significantly lower than adult levels. Using multiple *in vivo* approaches, the source of hepatic IFNβ expression in endotoxemic adult mice was determined to be the hepatic macrophage, and experiments in RAW 264.7 cells confirmed that LPS-induced IFNβ expression was NFκB dependent. Finally, treating neonatal mice with IFNβ 2 h after endotoxemia stimulated pulmonary STAT1 signaling and STAT1 dependent gene expression. Furthermore, IFNβ treatment of endotoxemic neonatal animals resulted in significantly improved survival following exposure to lethal endotoxemia. In conclusion, endotoxemia induced IFNβ expression is attenuated in the early neonatal period, secondary to impaired NFκB-p65/IRF3 signaling. Pre-treatment with IFNβ decreases neonatal sensitivity to endotoxemia. These results support further study of the role of impaired IFNβ expression and neonatal sensitivity to sepsis.

Keywords: neonate, endotoxemia, interferon beta, IRF3, STAT-1, NF-kappa B

INTRODUCTION

Worldwide, sepsis is a leading killer of neonates (1). The current paradigm suggests that neonatal susceptibility to infection is explained by an innate immune response that is functionally immature, limited in its ability to mount efficient response, and "biased against the production of pro-inflammatory cytokines" (2–9). Thus, understanding the mechanisms that contribute to impaired production of the mediators of the innate immune response may reveal therapeutic targets meant to improve the outcomes of septic neonates.

The role of IFNβ in the pathogenesis of sepsis in adults is controversial. Produced by most nucleated cells, IFNβ ultimately activates immune cells, cytokine/chemokine production, and links the early innate and later adaptive immune response (10). It is well established that in adult murine models of endotoxemic shock, the transcription factors NFκB and IRF3 work together to induce IFNβ expression (11). IRF3 null, IFNβ null, IFN-α/β receptor (IFNAR) null, STAT1 null, and pharmacologic inhibition of the IFNAR improve protect adult mice from mortality with endotoxemic shock (12–15). Importantly, attenuating IFNβ activity has been proposed as a potential therapeutic target to treat in endotoxemia in experimental animals and in sepsis in humans (11).

In contrast to these findings, some experimental data support a protective role played by IFNβ in endotoxemia and sepsis. Type 1 IFN expression is required to limit viral infections, and its activation results in multiple anti-bacterial effects (16). Absent Type 1 interferon signaling increases mortality in adult murine polymicrobial sepsis (13). Importantly, downregulation of IFNβ has been implicated the period of immunosupression following the acute pro-inflammatory period of sepsis (17). Specifically, monocytes from immunosuppressed septic patients demonstrate attenuated IFNβ expression (18). These findings have led some to propose treating septic patients with IFNβ to restore the deactivated immune response (19).

It has been hypothesized that there may be common mechanisms underlying innate immune tolerance and the "developmentally immature immune response" that contributes to increased mortality in pediatric sepsis. If that were true, linking the mechanisms underlying impaired innate immune response and tolerance may reveal therapeutic targets to treat neonatal and pediatric sepsis. Altered signaling dynamics of the transcription factor NFκB have been implicated in mediating macrophage tolerance. Specifically, following TLR4 stimulation, tolerant macrophages demonstrate nuclear translocation of inhibitory p50 homodimers (20). Importantly, downregulation of LPS-induced IFN expression is mediated by transition from activating p65/p50 NFκB dimers to inhibitory p50 homodimers at the IFNβ promoter (18). Of note, LPS-induced IFNβ expression is impaired in neonatal blood (21). However, whether tolerant p50 dominant NFκB signaling results in impaired IFNβ expression and contributes to worse neonatal and pediatric outcomes in endotoxemia and sepsis is unknown.

Therefore, we hypothesized that the increased mortality seen in endotoxemic neonatal mice is due in part to impaired IFNβ expression. Furthermore, we hypothesized that similar to tolerant macrophages, that predominant inhibitory p50 NFκB signaling would underlie impaired IFNβ expression. In this study, we found significantly attenuated expression of hepatic IFNβ in endotoxemia neonatal mice when compared to similarly exposed adults. In the neonatal liver, this was associated with exclusive p50-NFκB activation, whereas the adult liver demonstrated nuclear translocation of both p50, p65, and p-IRF3. As evidence of impaired IFNβ expression in neonatal mice, we found impaired pulmonary STAT1 signaling and gene expression. Finally, treating endotoxemic neonatal mice with IFNβ restored pulmonary STAT1 signaling, gene expression and significantly decreased mortality. These results justify further investigation into the role of IFNβ in treating neonatal and pediatric sepsis.

MATERIALS AND METHODS

Murine Model of Endotoxemia

Neonatal (P0) and adult (8–10 weeks, male) ICR mice were exposed to LPS (Sigma L2630, 5 mg/kg, IP) for 0–24 h. Additional neonatal mice were treated with IFNβ (R and D Systems 8234-MB/CF, 0–100 U/g, IP) 2 h after a lethal dose of LPS (10 mg/kg, IP). Intrahepatic leukocytes were isolated, and hepatic macrophages were ablated with clodronate as previously described to assess their role in IFNβ production (22). All procedures were approved by the IACUC at the University of Colorado (Aurora, CO) and care and handling of the animals was in accord with the National Institutes of Health guidelines for ethical animal treatment.

Cell Culture, Exposures, and Pharmacologic NFκB Inhibition

RAW 264.7 murine macrophages (ATCC) were cultured according to the manufacturer's instructions. Cells were exposed to LPS (1 μg/ml, Sigma L6529) or Interferon-β (100–1,000 U/ml, R and D systems). To pharmacologically inhibit NFκB activation, cells were exposed to BAY 11-7085 (1–20 μM, Sigma) for 1 h prior to LPS exposure.

IκBα Overexpression

RAW 264.7 cells were transfected with wild-type IκBα vectors (Clontech) as previously described (22).

Pulmonary Lysate, Cytosolic, and Nuclear Protein Extraction

Pulmonary tissue was homogenized using the Bullet Blender (NextAdvance) and pulmonary whole cell lysates were collected in T-PER (Thermo Fisher Scientific). Cytosolic and nuclear extracts were prepared using the NE-PER kit (ThermoFisher Scientific).

Immunoblot Analysis

Lysates, cytosolic, and nuclear extracts were electrophoresed on a 4–12% polyacrylamide gel (Invitrogen) and proteins were transferred to an Immobilon membrane (Millipore) and blotted with antibodies (**Supplementary Table 1**). Blots were imaged using the LiCor Odyssey imaging system and densitometric analysis was performed using ImageStudio (LiCor). Full blot images are found in **Supplementary Figures 1–5**.

Analysis of Relative mRNA Levels by RT-qPCR

Pulmonary mRNA was collected using the RNeasy Mini Kit (Qiagen) according to the manufacturer's instructions. RNA was assessed for purity and concentration using the NanoDrop (ThermoFisher Scientific), and cDNA synthesized using the Verso cDNA synthesis Kit (ThermoFisher Scientific). Relative mRNA levels were evaluated by quantitative real-time PCR using exon spanning primers (**Supplementary Table 2**) and the TaqMan gene expression and StepOnePlus Real-Time PCR System (Applied Biosystems). Relative quantitation was performed via normalization to the endogenous control 18S using the cycle threshold ($\Delta\Delta$Ct) method.

ELISA

Neonatal and adult serum levels of IFNβ were measured by ELISA (PBL Assay Science).

Statistical Analysis

For comparison between treatment groups, the null hypothesis that no difference existed between treatment means was tested by Student's *t*-test for two groups and two-way ANOVA for multiple groups with potentially interacting variables (organ, age, duration of exposure), with statistical significance between and within groups determined by means of Bonferroni method of multiple comparisons (InStat, GraphPad Software, Inc.,). Statistical significance was defined as $p < 0.05$.

RESULTS

Endotoxemia Induces Hepatic IFNβ Expression in Adult but Not Neonatal Mice

First, we sought to determine whether endotoxemia induced IFNβ expression in neonatal mice. Consistent with previous reports, levels of circulating IFNβ were significantly higher in endotoxemic adult mice when compared to controls (**Figure 1A**). Following IP injection, LPS enters the portal circulation and stimulates hepatic macrophages (23). Thus, we assessed whether hepatic IFNβ expression increased with endotoxemia. Hepatic IFNβ mRNA expression significantly increased in both neonatal and adult liver after 1 h of endotoxemia (**Figure 1B**). However, at this time point, adult hepatic IFNβ mRNA induction was significantly higher compared to neonatal mice (**Figure 1B**). Consistent with impaired induction of IFNβ in endotoxemic neonatal mice, hepatic IFNβ protein expression (**Figures 1C,D**) and circulating serum levels (**Figure 1A**) were not significantly increased at this early time point in neonatal mice. In contrast, both hepatic protein (**Figures 1C–E**) and circulating serum levels (**Figure 1A**) were significantly increased in endotoxemic adult mice (**Figures 1C–E**). These results demonstrate that in contrast to observations made in adult mice, circulating IFNβ levels and hepatic IFNβ protein do not increase in endotoxemic neonatal mice.

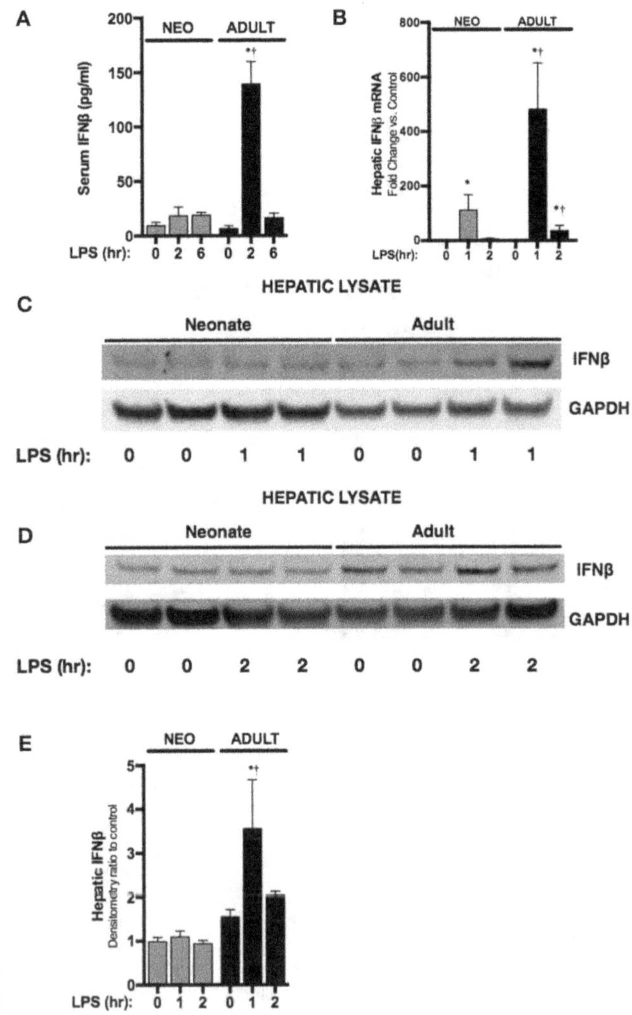

FIGURE 1 | Neonates demonstrate attenuated LPS-induced hepatic IFNβ expression. **(A)** Serum levels of IFNβ in neonatal or adult mice following LPS exposure (0–6 h, 5 mg/kg). *$p < 0.05$ vs. control; $^{\dagger}p < 0.05$ vs. LPS-exposed neonate. Values shown as means ± SEM; $n = 3$–4/timepoint. **(B)** Fold-increase in gene expression of IFNβ in neonatal and adult liver following LPS exposure (0–2 h, 5 mg/kg). *$p < 0.05$ vs. control; $^{\dagger}p < 0.05$ vs. LPS-exposed neonate. Values shown as means ± SEM; $n = 5$–6/timepoint. **(C,D)** Representative Western blots showing IFNβ protein in neonatal and adult hepatic lysate following 1 h **(C)** or 2 h **(D)** of LPS exposure (5 mg/kg) with GAPDH shown as loading control. **(E)** Densitometry ratio to control of neonatal and adult hepatic IFNβ. *$p < 0.05$ vs. control; $^{\dagger}p < 0.05$ vs. LPS-exposed neonate. Values shown as means ± SEM; $n = 2$–3/timepoint.

Endotoxemia Induces Hepatic IRF3 Activity in Adult but Not Neonatal Mice

Having observed attenuated IFNβ expression in endotoxemic neonatal mice, we next investigated its transcriptional regulation. The transcription factor IRF3 is a known inducer of IFNβ expression. Importantly, IRF3 is expressed at easily detectable levels in both the neonatal and adult liver (**Figure 2K**). In the nuclear extracts isolated from endotoxemic adult mice, we observed significant increases in p-IRF3 (**Figures 2A,B**). This was associated with increased expression of IRF3 dependent genes IFIT1 (**Figure 2C**) and IRG1 (**Figure 2D**). Furthermore, hepatic expression of IKKε, the kinase responsible for phosphorylating and activating IRF3, was significantly increased in endotoxemic adult mice (**Figure 2E**). In contrast, we found evidence of absent or attenuated hepatic IRF3

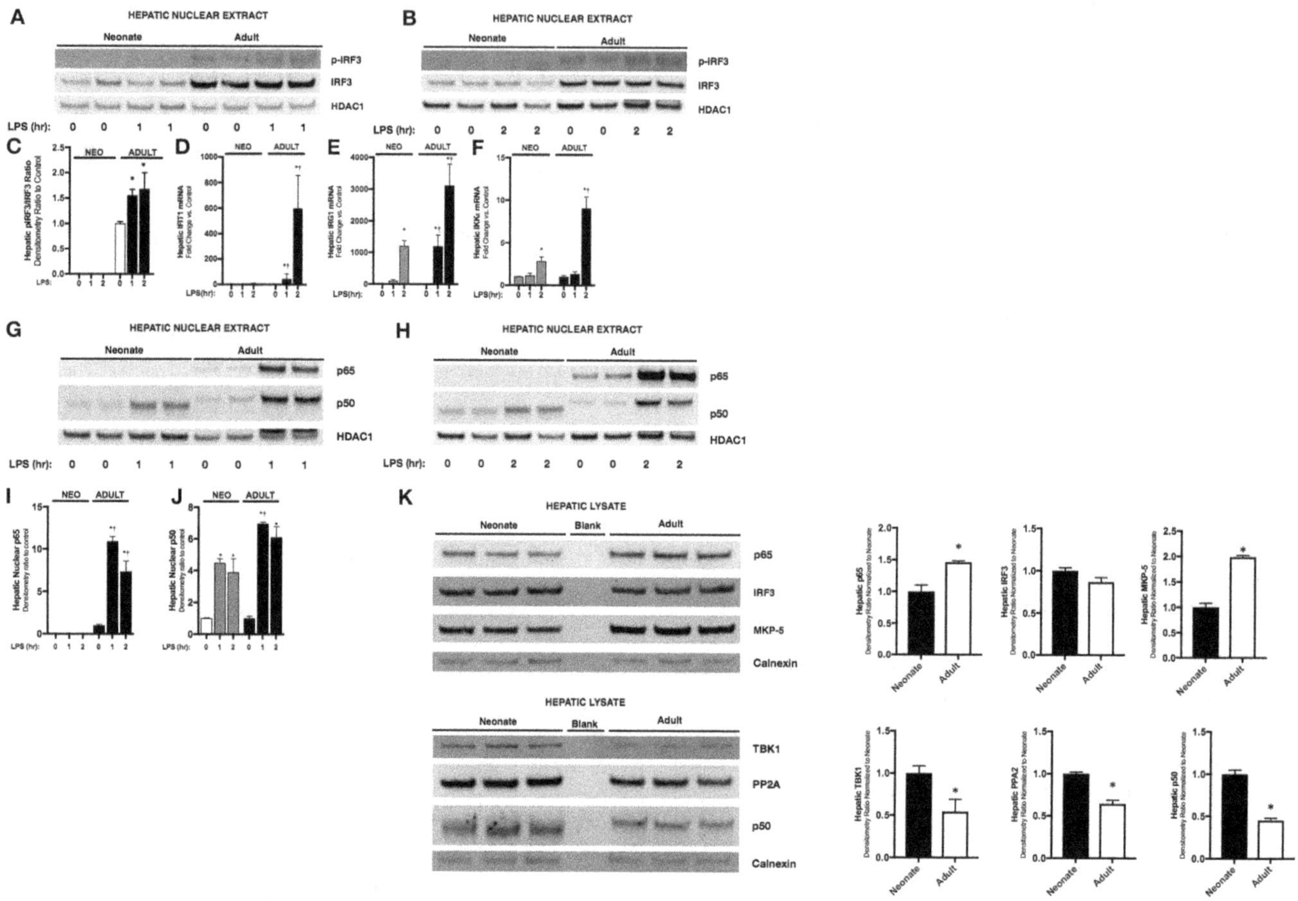

FIGURE 2 | Neonates demonstrate attenuated LPS-induced hepatic IRF3 and p50/NFκB activation. **(A,B)** Representative Western Blot showing neonatal and adult hepatic nuclear extracts following 1 h **(A)** or 2 h **(B)** of LPS exposure (5 mg/kg) for phosphorylated and total IRF3 with HDAC1 shown as loading control. **(C)** Densitometry ratio to control of adult hepatic pIRF3. *$p < 0.05$ vs. control. Values shown as means ± SEM; $n = 3$/timepoint **(D–F)** Fold-increase in gene expression in neonatal and adult hepatic IFIT1, IRG1, and IKKε following LPS exposure (0–2 h, 5 mg/kg) *$p < 0.05$ vs. control; $^{\dagger}p < 0.05$ vs. LPS-exposed neonate. Values shown as means ± SEM; $n = 3$–6/timepoint. **(G, H)** Representative Western Blots showing neonatal and adult hepatic nuclear extract following 1 h **(G)** or 2 h **(H)** LPS exposure (5 mg/kg) for NFκB subunits p65 and p50 with HDAC1 shown as loading control. **(I,J)** Densitometry ratio to control of p65 or p50 in neonatal and adult hepatic nuclear extract following LPS exposure (0–2 h). *$p < 0.05$ vs. control; $^{\dagger}p < 0.05$ vs. LPS-exposed neonate. Values shown as means ± SEM; $n =$ 5–6/timepoint. **(K)** Representative Western Blots showing neonatal and adult hepatic whole cell lysate for total IRF3 and the NFκB subunits p65 and p50, the kinase TBK1, and the IRF3 phosphatases PP2A catalytic subunit and MKP-5, with calnexin shown as loading control. Densitometry ratio normalized to neonatal control is provided. *$p < 0.05$ vs. neonatal control.

activation in endotoxemic neonatal mice. Hepatic nuclear extracts isolated from endotoxemic neonatal mice did not demonstrate presence of p-IRF3 (**Figures 2A,B**), and expression of IRF3 dependent genes was variably absent (IFIT1, **Figure 2D**) or attenuated compared to adult mice (IRG1, **Figure 2E**). Of note, hepatic expression of the activating kinase IKKε was also attenuated in endotoxemic neonatal mice (**Figure 2F**). Furthermore, we could not detect decreased levels of the IRF3 kinase TBK1, or increased levels of the IRF3 phosphatases PP2A (24) and MKP-5 (25), findings that if present may help explain the mechanisms underlying lack of p-IRF3 in the LPS-exposed neonatal hepatic nuclear extracts (**Figure 2K**). These results demonstrate that activation of the transcription factor responsible for IFNβ expression is attenuated in endotoxemic neonatal mice.

Endotoxemia Induces Hepatic p65 and p50 Nuclear Translocation in Adults, and Exclusively p50 in Neonatal Mice

Previous studies have shown that downstream of TLR4 stimulation, IFNβ upregulation is dependent upon both IRF3 and the NFκB dimers containing the subunit p65 (26). Thus, we sought to determine whether there were differences between NFκB subunits in hepatic nuclear extracts isolated from endotoxemic neonatal and adult mice. Importantly, p65 is expressed in both the neonatal and adult liver, although levels in the adult liver are significantly higher (**Figure 2K**). Furthermore, p50 is expressed in both the neonatal and adult liver, however levels in the neonatal liver are significantly higher (**Figure 2K**). Interestingly, we found that hepatic NFκB signaling was distinct in

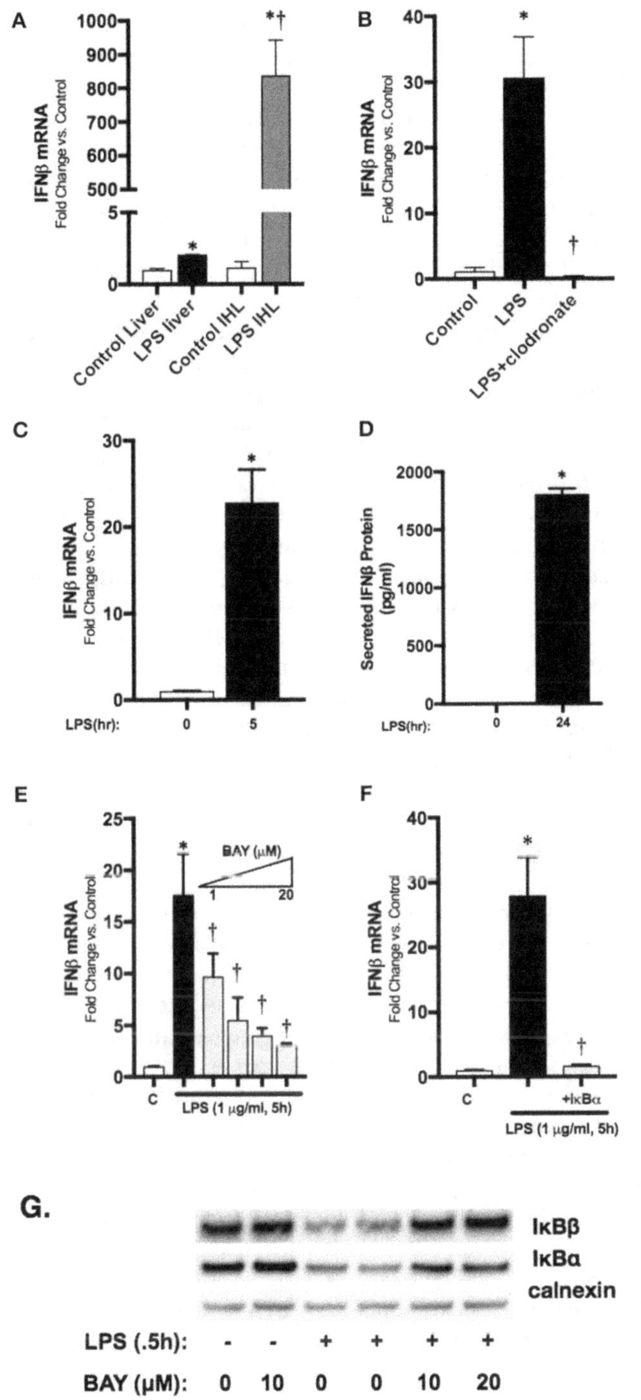

FIGURE 3 | Macrophage-derived, LPS-induced IFNβ stimulates STAT1 activation *in vitro*. **(A)** Fold-increase in gene expression of IFNβ in adult whole liver or isolated intrahepatic leukocytes following LPS exposure (2 h, 50 mg/kg). $^{*}p < 0.05$ vs. control; $^{\dagger}p < 0.05$ vs. LPS-exposed whole liver. Values shown as means ± SEM; n = 4–6/timepoint. **(B)** Fold-increase in gene expression of IFNβ in adult liver following LPS exposure or clodronate pretreatment (24 h) with LPS exposure (4 h, 3 mg/kg). $^{*}p < 0.05$ vs. control; $^{\dagger}p < 0.05$ vs. LPS-exposed. Values shown as means ± SEM; n = 4–6/timepoint **(C)** Fold-increase in gene expression of IFNβ in RAW 264.7 macrophages following LPS exposure (0–5 h, 1 μg/ml).

(Continued)

FIGURE 3 | $^{*}p < 0.05$ vs. control. Values shown as means ± SEM; n = 4/timepoint **(D)** Secreted IFNβ protein measurement in RAW 264.7 culture supernatant following LPS exposure (0–24 h, 1 μg/ml). $^{*}p < 0.05$ vs. control. Values shown as means ± SEM; n = 4/timepoint **(E)** Fold-increase in gene expression of IFNβ in RAW 264.7 macrophages following LPS exposure (0–5 h, 1 μg/ml) or BAY 11-7085 pretreatment (1 h, 1–20 μM) and LPS exposure. $^{*}p < 0.05$ vs. control; $^{\dagger}p < 0.05$ vs. LPS-exposed. Values shown as means ± SEM; n = 4/timepoint. **(F)** Fold-increase in gene expression of IFNβ following LPS exposure (1 μg/ml, 5 h) or IκBα overexpression and LPS exposure. $^{*}p < 0.05$ vs. control; $^{\dagger}p < 0.05$ vs. LPS-exposed Values shown as means ± SEM; n = 4/timepoint. **(G)** Representative Western blot showing IκBα and IκBβ in cytosolic fractions following exposure to LPS (0.5 h), or LPS after pretreatment (1 h) with BAY 11-7085 (1–20 μM) with calnexin as loading control.

endotoxemic neonatal and adult mice. In endotoxemic adult mice, there was nuclear translocation of p65 and p50 at 1 and 2 h of exposure (**Figures 2G–J**). In contrast, no p65 nuclear translocation was observed in endotoxemic neonatal mice (**Figures 2G–I**). However, we did observe significant nuclear translocation of p50 in endotoxemic neonatal mice (**Figures 2G,H,J**). These results suggest that the impaired IFNβ expression observed in endotoxemic neonatal mice is due to absence of both nuclear p-IRF3 (**Figures 2A,B**) and p65 (**Figures 2F–H**).

LPS-Induced IFNβ Expression in Macrophages Is NFκB Regulated

To localize hepatic IFNβ expression, we determined IFNβ mRNA expression in purified intrahepatic mononuclear cells (ihMNCs) isolated from livers of endotoxemic adult mice. This population of ihMNCs is inclusive of macrophage populations (27). Compared to the significant ~2-fold increased IFNβ expression in whole liver from LPS-exposed mice, expression of IFNβ in ihMNCs was increased ~800-fold compared to ihMNCs from untreated mice (**Figure 3A**). In addition, clodronate-mediated ablation of hepatic macrophages completely abrogated LPS-induced hepatic IFNβ expression (**Figure 3B**). These results identify hepatic macrophages as a potential source of circulating IFNβ observed in endotoxemic adult mice.

Having identified the hepatic macrophage as a potential source of circulating IFNβ, we next sought to link LPS-induced NFκB signaling to IFNβ expression in macrophages. For these *in vitro* experiments we used immortalized murine macrophages (RAW 264.7). In cultured RAW 264.7 cells, LPS induced significant expression of IFNβ mRNA by 5 h of expression (**Figure 3C**), and levels could be measured in the cell media at 24 h (**Figure 3D**). Our previous work has shown that LPS-induced p65 nuclear translocation occurs in RAW 264.7 cells by 2 h of exposure (22). To confirm that LPS-induced NFκB activation regulates IFNβ in RAW 264.7 macrophages, cells were pretreated with the pharmacologic NFκB inhibitor BAY 11-7085 for 1 h prior to LPS (1 μg/ml, 1 h) exposure. Pre-treatment with BAY 11-7085 inhibited LPS-induced degradation of the NFκB inhibitory proteins IκBα and IκBβ (**Figure 3G**), and inhibited expression the IFNβ in a dose-dependent manner

(**Figure 3E**). To rule out off-target effects of BAY 11-7085 on IFNβ expression independent of NFκB signaling, we transfected RAW 264.7 cells with plasmids overexpressing wild-type (WT) IκBα. Following exposure to LPS, IFNβ expression was significantly attenuated in cells overexpressing the inhibitory protein WT IκBα (**Figure 3F**). These results implicate LPS-induced NFκB activation in the transcriptional regulation of IFNβ in macrophages.

LPS-Induced JAK/STAT Signaling Is Impaired in the Neonatal Lung With Endotoxemia

Next, we sought to understand the systemic implications of impaired hepatic IFNβ expression observed in neonatal mice. IFNβ is a known inducer of STAT1 activation (10), and pulmonary STAT1 activation is known to occur with endotoxemia (28). Consistent with previous reports, we found STAT1 phosphorylation in the pulmonary lysates of endotoxemic adult mice (**Figures 4A,B**). In contrast, STAT1 phosphorylation, while present, was attenuated in degree and duration in the lungs of endotoxemic neonatal mice (**Figures 4A,B**). It is likely that the hepatic derived IFNβ results in pulmonary STAT1 signaling, as LPS-induced hepatic IFNβ expression is significantly higher than pulmonary induction (**Figure 4C**). Additionally, we could not detect any IFNβ in pulmonary lysates from endotoxemic neonatal or adult mice (**Figure 4D**). These results demonstrate that in endotoxemic adult mice, hepatic IFNβ expression is temporally associated with pulmonary STAT1 signaling. This signaling is attenuated in duration and degree in endotoxemic neonatal mice.

Stat Dependent Gene Expression Is Attenuated in the Neonatal Lung With Endotoxemia

Having observed attenuated STAT1 signaling in the neonatal lung, we next checked the expression of interferon stimulated genes previously shown to be dependent upon JAK/STAT signaling (29–31). Consistent with attenuated IFNβ-stimulated pulmonary STAT signaling, we found significantly attenuated expression of multiple STAT-dependent genes in the neonatal lung. These included IP10 (**Figure 4E**), MCP1 (**Figure 4F**), IRF7 (**Figure 4G**), MDA5 (**Figure 4H**), and OAS2 (**Figure 4I**). Furthermore, IFNβ/STAT1 activation are responsible for LPS-induced iNOS gene expression (32). Consistent with impaired LPS-induced STAT-1 signaling in the neonatal lung, we found significantly lower iNOS expression when compared to similarly exposed adults (**Figure 4J**).

IFNβ Treatment Restores Pulmonary STAT1 Signaling and Improves Survival of Endotoxemic Neonatal Mice

Previous studies have demonstrated that absence of STAT1 activity exacerbates lung injury associated with endotoxemia (33, 34). We next sought to determine whether we could augment neonatal pulmonary STAT signaling by bypassing impaired LPS-induced hepatic IFNβ expression through direct administration of IFNβ after the induction of endotoxemia. First, we sought to determine if this was possible in cell culture. In RAW 264.7 cells, LPS induces STAT1 phosphorylation (**Figure 5A**). Importantly, LPS-induced STAT1 activation is completely inhibited by the NFκB inhibitor BAY 11-7085 (**Figure 5B**), likely due to impaired NFκB-regulated IFNβ expression (**Figure 3E**). We then demonstrated that exposing RAW 264.7 cells to IFNβ in the absence of LPS resulted in dose-dependent increase in STAT1 activation (**Figure 5C**). These results demonstrate macrophages respond directly to IFNβ with STAT1 signaling in the absence of LPS-TLR4 mediated NFκB activation.

Next, we sought to determine the effect of administering IFNβ to endotoxemic neonatal mice. Neonatal (P0) mice were exposed to endotoxemia (10 mg/kg) and experienced ~75% mortality (**Figure 5D**). When administered 2 h after LPS, IFNβ at a dose of 50 U/g had no effect on survival. In contrast, a dose of 100 U/g significantly improved survival to >50%. Importantly, administration of IFNβ after 2 h of endotoxemia induced pulmonary STAT1 signaling (**Figure 5E**). The IFNβ dependent induction of pulmonary STAT1 signaling significantly increased pulmonary expression of STAT1-dependent genes including IP10, MCP1, IRF7, OAS2, MDA5, and iNOS when compared to LPS alone (**Figures 5F–K**). These results demonstrate that in neonatal endotoxemia, IFNβ treatment improves survival and that this is associated with increased pulmonary STAT1 signaling and gene expression.

DISCUSSION

Our study revealed attenuated IFNβ expression in endotoxemic neonatal mice when compared to similarly exposed adults. In endotoxemic adult mice, activation of the NFκB-p65 and IRF3 transcription factors is associated with hepatic IFNβ expression, and occurs in the hepatic macrophage. In the setting of hepatic IFNβ expression in adult mice, pulmonary STAT1 signaling and increased expression of STAT1-dependent genes occurs. In contrast to these findings in adults, endotoxemic neonatal mice demonstrate attenuated hepatic IFNβ expression. We could find no evidence of hepatic IRF3 or p65-NFκB activation in endotoxemic neonatal mice. In contrast, hepatic p50-NFκB signaling was observed. In the absence of hepatic IFNβ expression, we observed attenuated pulmonary STAT1 signaling and target gene expression in neonatal mice. By treating endotoxemic neonatal mice with IFNβ, pulmonary STAT1 signaling was restored and this was associated with a significant decrease in mortality.

The type 1 response to endotoxemia and sepsis in adults has been an area of intense study and has been offered as a therapeutic target (11). Early reports showed that IRF3 null, IFNβ null, IFN-α/β receptor (IFNAR) null, STAT1 null, and pharmacologic inhibition of the IFNAR improve outcomes in endotoxemic adult mice (12–15). However, IFNβ affects the immune system via multiple mechanisms, such that it has been concluded that "IFN-1 are neither "good" nor "bad" regulators of inflammation, but that their protective or adverse character

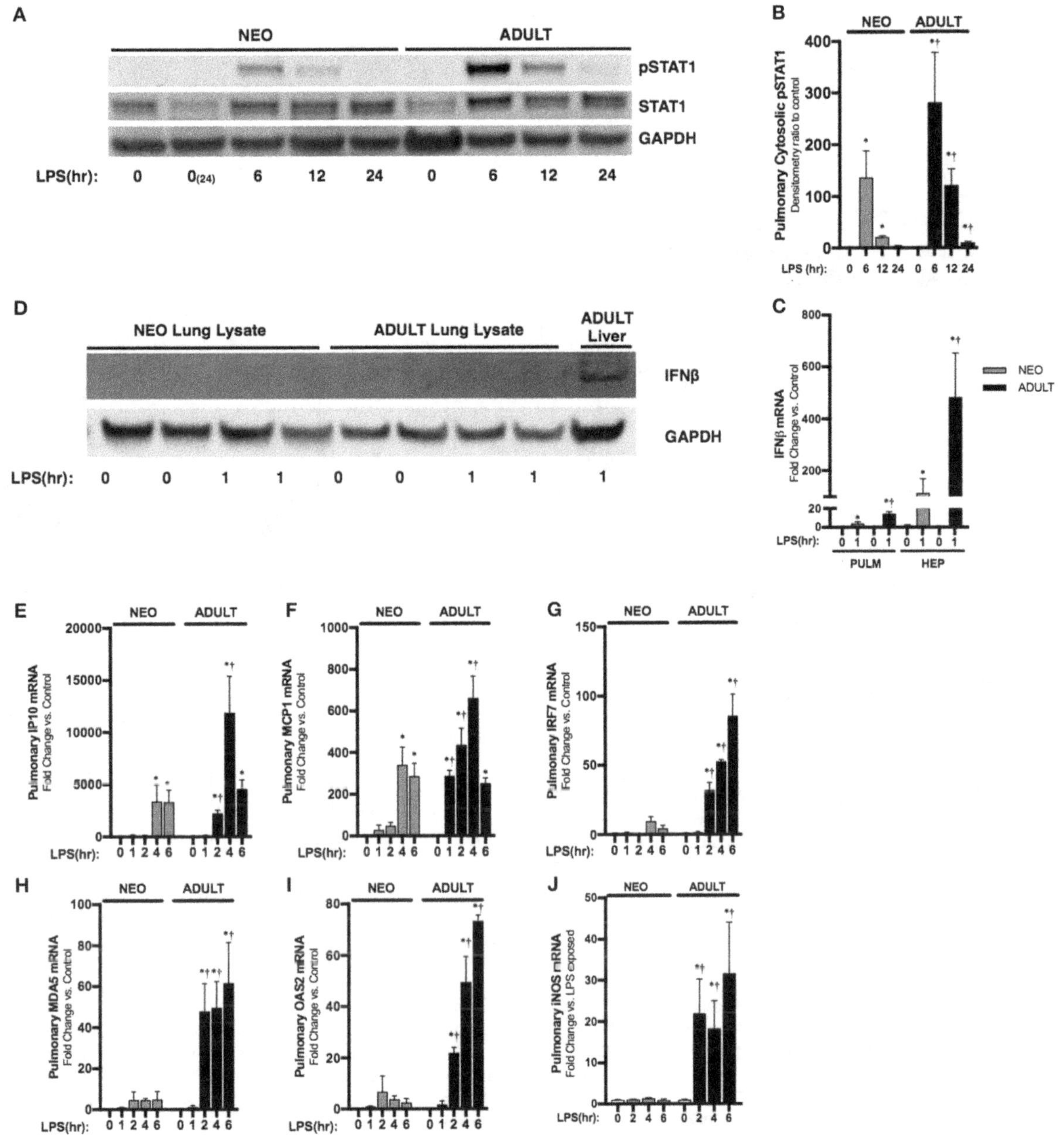

FIGURE 4 | Neonates demonstrate attenuated LPS-induced pulmonary STAT1 activation downstream of hepatic IRF3 activation and IFNβ secretion. **(A)** Representative Western Blot of neonatal and adult pulmonary cytosolic extracts following LPS exposure (0–24 h, 5 mg/kg) for phosphorylated and total STAT1 with GAPDH shown as loading control; two neonatal controls shown to reflect baseline conditions on PN0 and after 24 h of life, at the completion of the exposure period. **(B)** Densitometry ratio to control of phosphorylated STAT1 in neonatal and adult pulmonary cytosolic extracts following LPS exposure. $^{*}p < 0.05$ vs. control; $^{\dagger}p < 0.05$ vs. LPS-exposed neonate. Values shown as means ± SEM; $n = 3$–4/timepoint. **(C)** Fold-increase in gene expression of neonatal and adult pulmonary and hepatic IFNβ following LPS exposure (0–1 h, 5 mg/kg). $^{*}p < 0.05$ vs. control; $^{\dagger}p < 0.05$ vs. LPS-exposed neonate. Values shown as means ± SEM; $n =$ 5–6/timepoint. **(D)** Representative Western Blot of neonatal and adult pulmonary lysate following LPS exposure (0–1 h, 5 mg/kg) for IFNβ with adult LPS-exposed liver lysate provided as positive control and GAPDH shown as loading control. **(E–J)** Fold-increase in gene expression of STAT1 target genes **(E)** IP10, **(F)** MCP1, **(G)** IRF7, **(H)** MDA5, **(I)** OAS2, and **(J)** iNOS in neonatal and adult pulmonary tissue following LPS exposure (0–6 h, 5 mg/kg). $^{*}p < 0.05$ vs. control; $^{\dagger}P < 0.05$ vs. LPS-exposed neonate. Values shown as means ± SEM; $n =$ 5–6 per timepoint.

varies with more or less pronounce inflammatory environments." (35) This may explain somewhat conflicting data in the literature regarding the role of interferons in mediating the response to endotoxemia and/or sepsis. For example, IFNAR1 mice have shown both increased resistance and sensitivity to polymicrobial sepsis (13, 15). Furthermore, recent reports have demonstrated that IFNβ may protect adult mice against lethal endotoxemia (36). These nuanced findings may have particular relevance

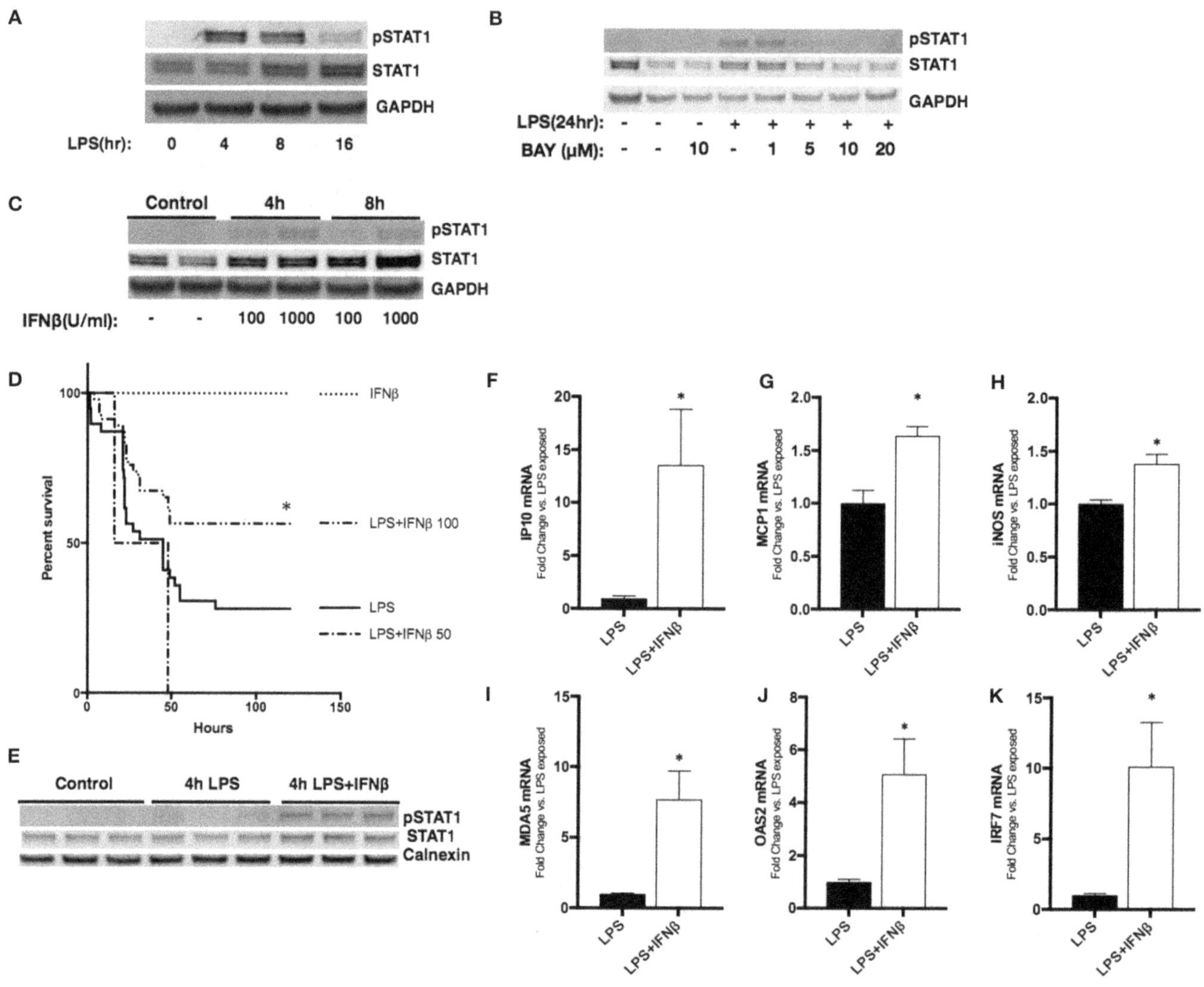

FIGURE 5 | Treatment with IFNβ following LPS exposure reduces mortality and activates pulmonary STAT1 signaling in neonatal mice. **(A)** Representative Western Blot of phosphorylated and total STAT1 in RAW 264.7 macrophage lysate following LPS exposure (1 μg/ml, 0–16 h) with GAPDH shown as loading control. **(B)** Representative Western Blot of phosphorylated and total STAT1 in RAW 264.7 lysates following LPS exposure (1 μg/ml, 0–24 h) or BAY 11-7085 pretreatment (1–20 μM, 1 h) and LPS exposure with GAPDH shown as loading control. **(C)** Representative Western Blot of phosphorylated and total STAT1 in RAW 264.7 lysates following IFNβ exposure (100–1,000 μ/ml, 0–8 h) with GAPDH shown as loading control. **(D)** Kaplan-Meier curve analysis of neonatal mice exposed to IFNβ (100 μ/g; $n = 7$), LPS (10 mg/kg; $n = 39$), or LPS and IFNβ (50 ($n = 7$) or 100 μ/g ($n = 46$), administered 2 h post-LPS. *$p < 0.05$ vs. LPS-exposed; $n = 7$–40 per group. **(E)** Representative Western Blot of phosphorylated and total STAT1 in neonatal pulmonary lysates following LPS exposure (5 mg/kg, 4 h) or LPS exposure and IFNβ exposure (100 μ/g, administered 2 h post-LPS). $n = 3$/timepoint **(F–K)** Fold-increase in gene expression of STAT1 target genes IP10, MCP1, iNOS, OAS2, MDA5, and IRF7 in neonatal lung following LPS (5 mg/kg, 4 h) or LPS exposure and IFNβ exposure (100 μ/g, 2 h post-LPS). Values shown as means of fold induction normalized to mean LPS-induced fold induction ± SEM. *$p < 0.05$ vs. LPS-exposed; $n = 3$–5/timepoint.

in understanding the role of IFNβ in mediating the neonatal response to endotoxemia and sepsis.

Neonates and adults display markedly different susceptibilities to endotoxemia and sepsis. Neonatal animals (mice, rats, guinea pigs) demonstrate increased mortality when compared to adults following exposure to bacterial endotoxin shock (37–44). Multiple recent reviews of early life immunity conclude that this is in part due to an impaired ability to mount a pro-inflammatory innate immune response in the perinatal period (2, 4–6, 8, 9). Of note, previous studies have demonstrated that adult ICR mice demonstrate less sensitivity to endotoxemia when exposed to the exposure doses used in the current study (45, 46). Our work adds to a growing body of literature demonstrating that impaired IFNβ expression in the perinatal period contributes to these findings. *In vitro* work has showed that LPS-induced IFNβ expression is blunted in neonatal cord blood cells (21), and this observation is true following exposure to other TLR ligands (47). Of note, completely absent IFNβ signaling (IFNβ null and IFNα/β receptor null) in neonatal mice leads to 100% mortality following GBS infection (48) Furthermore, studies in adult mice demonstrate that IFNβ plays a protective role against infections common in the perinatal period, including Group B streptococcus and *E. coli* (49). Our report provides evidence that impaired LPS-induced IFNβ expression in the early neonatal period may contribute to increased susceptibility to certain infections.

Our results demonstrate that there are fundamental differences between neonatal and adult LPS-induced hepatic NFκB signaling and target gene expression. Previous studies have demonstrated that LPS/TLR4 mediated IRF3/ISRE activation is p65 dependent (26), and that IFNβ is an NFκB target gene (50). Our results clearly demonstrate a lack of p65/NFκB signaling in the neonatal liver following exposure to LPS (**Figure 3**). In contrast, the adult liver demonstrates robust p65/NFκB signaling and associated IRF3 activation (**Figure 2**) and IFNβ expression (**Figure 1**). Interestingly, the p50/NFκB signaling observed in the neonatal liver has been implicated in macrophage tolerance and M2 polarization (18, 20). Importantly, p50/NFκB signaling attenuates IFNβ expression and drives a macrophage tolerance and an M2 phenotype. Additionally, it should be noted that the p50 in neonatal hepatic nuclear extracts consistently migrates further when subjected to electrophoresis through a 4-12% polyacrylamide gel (**Figures 2G,H**). We hypothesize that this difference is due to post-translational modification of the p50 subunit in the adult liver. Of note, other groups have identified sites subject to post-translational modification on the p50 subunit (51). The implications of these potential modifications remain to be discovered. Further work is needed to understand whether these post-translational modifications explain our findings, and whether what we have observed in the neonatal endotoxemia model is a true "recapitulation of immune tolerance" (9).

This study has a number of limitations. Specifically, only one LPS dose (5 mg/kg, IP) was used for neonatal and adult endotoxin exposure; importantly, our lab has identified this as a dose that results in ~25% mortality in neonatal mice (52); thus, it is possible that alterations in IFNβ expression and STAT1 signaling might be observed at increasingly lethal LPS doses. Additionally, samples were collected at relatively early timepoints following LPS exposure, and there may be differences in neonatal and adult IFNβ expression at later time points. However, IFNβ is a primary response gene and previous publications have shown early and robust upregulation in endotoxemia (53). Our study did not specifically interrogate other tissues beyond the lung and liver as potential sources of IFNβ. However, LPS exposure results in widespread systemic effects, and significant IFNβ release may occur in other organs. However, we did assess circulating IFNβ levels in endotoxemic adult and neonatal mice, and regardless of expression in other organs, our observations in the liver and lung are valid. Finally, while treating endotoxemic neonatal mice with IFNβ resulted in pulmonary STAT1 activation and increased target gene expression, the direct mechanisms contributing to improved survival are unknown. Finally, *in vitro* experiments linking LPS-induced NFκB activity and IFNβ expression in macrophages were not performed in primary cell lines, but rather in immortalized murine macrophages (RAW 264.7, **Figures 3C–H**). We chose to use this cell line given the difficulty in transfecting primary cell lines and their susceptibility to pharmacologic agents.

CONCLUSIONS

We conclude that LPS-induced hepatic IFNβ expression is attenuated in neonatal animals when compared to similarly exposed adults. Our data suggest that this is associated with LPS-induced p50-NFκB signaling and impaired IRF3 activation. These results are interesting known mechanistic role played by p50 in mediating macrophage phenotype and tolerance. Our findings support the hypothesis that in the neonatal period, there are shared mechanisms between an impaired innate immune response and immune tolerance. Treating endotoxemic neonatal mice with IFNβ restores pulmonary STAT1 signaling, STAT1 dependent gene expression and improves survival. These results justify further investigation into the role of both IFNβ and STAT1 signaling in treating neonatal and pediatric sepsis.

AUTHOR CONTRIBUTIONS

CW and SM conception and design of research. SM, TB, JS, LN, OC, SG, JG, KE, and CW performed the experiments. SM, TB, JS, LN, OC, SG, JG, KE, and CW analyzed data; SM, TB, JS, OC, SG, JG, KE, and CW interpreted results of the experiments. SM and CW edited and revised the manuscript. SM, TB, JS, LN, OC, SG, JG, KE, and CW approved the final version of the manuscript. SM and CW prepared the figures. CW drafted the manuscript.

REFERENCES

1. GBD 2015 Child Mortality Collaborators. Global, regional, national, and selected subnational levels of stillbirths, neonatal, infant, and under-5 mortality, 1980-2015: a systematic analysis for the Global Burden of Disease Study 2015. *Lancet* (2016) 388:1725–74. doi: 10.1016/S0140-6736(16) 31575-6
2. Strunk T, Currie A, Richmond P, Simmer K, Burgner D. Innate immunity in human newborn infants: prematurity means more than immaturity. *J Matern Fetal Neonatal Med.* (2011) 24:25–31. doi: 10.3109/14767058.2010.482605
3. Levy O. Innate immunity of the newborn: basic mechanisms and clinical correlates. *Nat Rev Immunol.* (2007) 7:379–90. doi: 10.1038/nri2075
4. Kollmann TR, Levy O, Montgomery RR, Goriely S. Innate immune function by Toll-like receptors: distinct responses in newborns and

the elderly. *Immunity* (2012) 37:771–83. doi: 10.1016/j.immuni.2012.10.014

5. Adkins B. Neonatal immunology: responses to pathogenic microorganisms and epigenetics reveal an "immunodiverse" developmental state. *Immunol Res.* (2013) 57:246–57. doi: 10.1007/s12026-013-8439-2
6. Cuenca AG, Wynn JL, Moldawer LL, Levy O. Role of innate immunity in neonatal infection. *Am J Perinatol.* (2013) 30:105–12. doi: 10.1055/s-0032-1333412
7. Levy O, Wynn JL. A prime time for trained immunity: innate immune memory in newborns and infants. *Neonatology* (2014) 105:136–41. doi: 10.1159/000356035
8. Dowling DJ, Levy O. Ontogeny of early life immunity. *Trends Immunol.* (2014) 35:299–310. doi: 10.1016/j.it.2014.04.007
9. Maddux AB, Douglas IS. Is the developmentally immature immune response in paediatric sepsis a recapitulation of immune tolerance? *Immunology* (2015) 145:1–10. doi: 10.1111/imm.12454
10. Ivashkiv LB, Donlin LT. Regulation of type I interferon responses. *Nat Rev Immunol.* (2014) 14:36–49. doi: 10.1038/nri3581
11. Mahieu T, Libert C. Should we inhibit type I interferons in sepsis? *Infect Immun.* (2007) 75:22–9. doi: 10.1128/IAI.00829-06
12. Karaghiosoff M, Steinborn R, Kovarik P, Kriegshauser G, Baccarini M, Donabauer B, et al. Central role for type I interferons and Tyk2 in lipopolysaccharide-induced endotoxin shock. Nature immunology. (2003) 4:471–7. doi: 10.1038/ni910
13. Kelly-Scumpia KM, Scumpia PO, Delano MJ, Weinstein JS, Cuenca AG, Wynn JL, et al. Type I interferon signaling in hematopoietic cells is required for survival in mouse polymicrobial sepsis by regulating CXCL10. *J Exp Med.* (2010) 207:319–26. doi: 10.1084/jem.20091959
14. Sakaguchi S, Negishi H, Asagiri M, Nakajima C, Mizutani T, Takaoka A, et al. Essential role of IRF-3 in lipopolysaccharide-induced interferon-beta gene expression and endotoxin shock. *Biochem Biophys Res Commun.* (2003) 306:860–6. doi: 10.1016/S0006-291X(03)01049-0
15. Dejager L, Vandevyver S, Ballegeer M, Van Wonterghem E, An LL, Riggs J, et al. Pharmacological inhibition of type I interferon signaling protects mice against lethal sepsis. *J Infect Dis.* (2014) 209:960–70. doi: 10.1093/infdis/jit600
16. Trinchieri G. Type I interferon: friend or foe? *J Exp Med.* (2010) 207:2053–63. doi: 10.1084/jem.20101664
17. Delano MJ, Ward PA. Sepsis-induced immune dysfunction: can immune therapies reduce mortality? *J Clinical Invest.* (2016) 126:23–31. doi: 10.1172/JCI82224
18. Rackov G, Hernandez-Jimenez E, Shokri R, Carmona-Rodriguez L, Manes S, Alvarez-Mon M, et al. p21 mediates macrophage reprogramming through regulation of p50-p50 NF-kappaB and IFN-beta. *J Clin Invest.* (2016) 126:3089–103. doi: 10.1172/JCI83404
19. Rackov G, Shokri R, De Mon MA, Martinez AC, Balomenos D. The role of IFN-beta during the course of sepsis progression and its therapeutic potential. *Front. Immunol.* (2017) 8:493. doi: 10.3389/fimmu.2017.00493
20. Porta C, Rimoldi M, Raes G, Brys L, Ghezzi P, Di Liberto D, et al. Tolerance and M2 (alternative) macrophage polarization are related processes orchestrated by p50 nuclear factor kappaB. *Proc Natl Acad Sci USA.* (2009) 106:14978–83. doi: 10.1073/pnas.0809784106
21. Aksoy E, Albarani V, Nguyen M, Laes JF, Ruelle JL, De Wit D, et al. Interferon regulatory factor 3-dependent responses to lipopolysaccharide are selectively blunted in cord blood cells. *Blood* (2007) 109:2887–93. doi: 10.1182/blood-2006-06-027862
22. McKenna S, Gossling M, Bugarini A, Hill E, Anderson AL, Rancourt RC, et al. Endotoxemia induces IkappaBbeta/NF-kappaB-dependent endothelin-1 expression in hepatic macrophages. *J Immunol.* (2015) 195:3866–79. doi: 10.4049/jimmunol.1501017
23. Lukas G, Brindle SD, Greengard P. The route of absorption of intraperitoneally administered compounds. *J Pharmacol Exp Ther.* (1971) 178:562–4.
24. Long L, Deng Y, Yao F, Guan D, Feng Y, Jiang H, et al. Recruitment of phosphatase PP2A by RACK1 adaptor protein deactivates transcription factor IRF3 and limits type I interferon signaling. Immunity (2014) 40:515–29. doi: 10.1016/j.immuni.2014.01.015
25. James SJ, Jiao H, Teh HY, Takahashi H, Png CW, Phoon MC, et al. MAPK phosphatase 5 expression induced by influenza and other RNA virus infection negatively regulates IRF3 activation and type I interferon response. *Cell Rep.* (2015) 10:1722–34. doi: 10.1016/j.celrep.2015.02.030
26. Wietek C, Miggin SM, Jefferies CA, O'Neill LA. Interferon regulatory factor-3-mediated activation of the interferon-sensitive response element by Toll-like receptor (TLR) 4 but not TLR3 requires the p65 subunit of NF-kappa. *J Biol Chem.* (2003) 278:50923–31. doi: 10.1074/jbc.M308135200
27. Petrasek J, Bala S, Csak T, Lippai D, Kodys K, Menashy V, et al. IL-1 receptor antagonist ameliorates inflammasome-dependent alcoholic steatohepatitis in mice. *J Clin Invest.* (2012) 122:3476–89. doi: 10.1172/JCI60777
28. Severgnini M, Takahashi S, Rozo LM, Homer RJ, Kuhn C, Jhung JW, et al. Activation of the STAT pathway in acute lung injury. *Am J Physiol Lung Cell Mol Physiol.* (2004) 286:L1282–92. doi: 10.1152/ajplung.00349.2003
29. Rani MR, Shrock J, Appachi S, Rudick RA, Williams BR, Ransohoff RM. Novel interferon-beta-induced gene expression in peripheral blood cells. *J Leukoc Biol.* (2007) 82:1353–60. doi: 10.1189/jlb.0507273
30. Satoh J, Tabunoki H. A comprehensive profile of ChIP-Seq-based STAT1 target genes suggests the complexity of STAT1-mediated gene regulatory mechanisms. *Gene Regul Syst Biol.* (2013) 7:41–56. doi: 10.4137/GRSB.S11433
31. Schoggins JW, Wilson SJ, Panis M, Murphy MY, Jones CT, Bieniasz P, et al. A diverse range of gene products are effectors of the type I interferon antiviral response. *Nature* (2011) 472:481–5. doi: 10.1038/nature09907
32. Gao JJ, Filla MB, Fultz MJ, Vogel SN, Russell SW, Murphy WJ. Autocrine/paracrine IFN-alphabeta mediates the lipopolysaccharide-induced activation of transcription factor Stat1alpha in mouse macrophages: pivotal role of Stat1alpha in induction of the inducible nitric oxide synthase gene. *J Immunol.* (1998) 161:4803–10.
33. Jones MR, Quinton LJ, Simms BT, Lupa MM, Kogan MS, Mizgerd JP. Roles of interleukin-6 in activation of STAT proteins and recruitment of neutrophils during *Escherichia coli* pneumonia. *J Infect Dis.* (2006) 193:360–9. doi: 10.1086/499312
34. Lee YJ, Han JY, Byun J, Park HJ, Park EM, Chong YH, et al. Inhibiting Mer receptor tyrosine kinase suppresses STAT1, SOCS1/3, and NF-kappaB activation and enhances inflammatory responses in lipopolysaccharide-induced acute lung injury. *J Leukoc Biol.* (2012) 91:921–32. doi: 10.1189/jlb.0611289
35. Rauch I, Muller M, Decker T. The regulation of inflammation by interferons and their STATs. *Jak Stat.* (2013) 2:e23820. doi: 10.4161/jkst.23820
36. Yoo CH, Yeom JH, Heo JJ, Song EK, Lee SI, Han MK. Interferon beta protects against lethal endotoxic and septic shock through SIRT1 upregulation. Scientific reports. (2014) 4:4220. doi: 10.1038/srep04220
37. Zhao J, Kim KD, Yang X, Auh S, Fu YX, Tang H. Hyper innate responses in neonates lead to increased morbidity and mortality after infection. *Proc Natl Acad Sci USA.* (2008) 105:7528–33. doi: 10.1073/pnas.0800152105
38. Cusumano V, Mancuso G, Genovese F, Cuzzola M, Carbone M, Cook JA, et al. Neonatal hypersusceptibility to endotoxin correlates with increased tumor necrosis factor production in mice. *J Infect Dis.* (1997) 176:168–76. doi: 10.1086/514019
39. Cochran JB, Chen H, La Via M, Cusumano V, Teti G, Cook JA. Age-related mortality and adherent splenic cell mediator production to endotoxin in the rat. *Shock* (1995) 4:450–4.
40. Fitzgerald M, Zeller WP, Goto M, Anderson CL, Hurley RM. Concurrent clinical and metabolic derangements in the newborn rat: a late phase sepsis model. *Ann Clin Lab Sci.* (1988) 18:229–34.
41. Porter PJ, Spievack AR, Kass EH. The effect of neonatal thymectomy on susceptibility to bacterial endotoxin. *J Lab Clin Med.* (1966) 68:455–62.
42. Zeller WP, Goto M, Witek-Janusek L, Hurley RM. Mortality, temporal substrate and insulin responses to endotoxic shock in zero, ten and twenty-eight day old rats. *Surg Gynecol Obstet.* (1991) 173:375–83.
43. Mancuso G, Tomasello F, von Hunolstein C, Orefici G, Teti G. Induction of tumor necrosis factor alpha by the group- and type-specific polysaccharides from type III group B streptococci. *Infect Immun.* (1994) 62:2748–53.
44. Uhr JW. The effect of bacterial endotoxin on the newborn guinea pig. *J Exp Med.* (1962) 115:685–94. doi: 10.1084/jem.115.4.685

45. Kang YJ, Seo SJ, Yun-Choi HS, Lee DH, Kim YM, Chang KC. A synthetic isoquinoline alkaloid, 1-(beta-naphthylmethyl)-6,7-dihydroxy-1,2,3,4-tetrahydroisoquinoline (YS 51), reduces inducible nitric oxide synthase expression and improves survival in a rodent model of endotoxic shock. *J Pharmacol Exp Ther.* (2002) 301:561–7. doi: 10.1124/jpet.301.2.561
46. Tateda K, Matsumoto T, Miyazaki S, Yamaguchi K. Lipopolysaccharide-induced lethality and cytokine production in aged mice. *Infect Immun.* (1996) 64:769–74.
47. Danis B, George TC, Goriely S, Dutta B, Renneson J, Gatto L, et al. Interferon regulatory factor 7-mediated responses are defective in cord blood plasmacytoid dendritic cells. *Eur J Immunol.* (2008) 38:507–17. doi: 10.1002/eji.200737760
48. Mancuso G, Midiri A, Biondo C, Beninati C, Zummo S, Galbo R, et al. Type I IFN signaling is crucial for host resistance against different species of pathogenic bacteria. *J Immunol.* (2007) 178:3126–33. doi: 10.4049/jimmunol.178.5.3126
49. McNab F, Mayer-Barber K, Sher A, Wack A, O'Garra A. Type I interferons in infectious disease. *Nat Rev Immunol.* (2015) 15:87–103. doi: 10.1038/nri3787
50. Lenardo MJ, Fan CM, Maniatis T, Baltimore D. The involvement of NF-kappa B in beta-interferon gene regulation reveals its role as widely inducible mediator of signal transduction. *Cell* (1989) 57:287–94. doi: 10.1016/0092-8674(89)90966-5
51. Christian F, Smith EL, Carmody RJ. The regulation of NF-kappaB subunits by phosphorylation. *Cells* (2016) 5:E12. doi: 10.3390/cells5010012
52. McKenna S, Butler B, Jatana L, Ghosh S, Wright CJ. Inhibition of IkappaBbeta/NFkappaB signaling prevents LPS-induced IL1beta expression without increasing apoptosis in the developing mouse lung. *Pediatr Res.* (2017) 82:1064–72. doi: 10.1038/pr.2017.182
53. Samarajiwa SA, Mangan NE, Hardy MP, Najdovska M, Dubach D, Braniff SJ, et al. Soluble IFN receptor potentiates *in vivo* type I IFN signaling and exacerbates TLR4-mediated septic shock. *J Immunol.* (2014) 192:4425–35. doi: 10.4049/jimmunol.1302388

4

Therapeutic Targeting of IRFs: Pathway-Dependence or Structure-Based?

*Cherrie D. Thompson, Bharati Matta and Betsy J. Barnes**

Center for Autoimmune Musculoskeletal and Hematopoietic Diseases, Feinstein Institute for Medical Research, Manhasset, NY, United States

Correspondence:
Betsy J. Barnes
bbarnes1@northwell.edu

The interferon regulatory factors (IRFs) are a family of master transcription factors that regulate pathogen-induced innate and acquired immune responses. Aberration(s) in IRF signaling pathways due to infection, genetic predisposition and/or mutation, which can lead to increased expression of type I interferon (IFN) genes, IFN-stimulated genes (ISGs), and other pro-inflammatory cytokines/chemokines, has been linked to the development of numerous diseases, including (but not limited to) autoimmune and cancer. What is currently lacking in the field is an understanding of how best to therapeutically target these transcription factors. Many IRFs are regulated by post-translational modifications downstream of pattern recognition receptors (PRRs) and some of these modifications lead to activation or inhibition. We and others have been able to utilize structural features of the IRFs in order to generate dominant negative mutants that inhibit function. Here, we will review potential therapeutic strategies for targeting all IRFs by using IRF5 as a candidate targeting molecule.

Keywords: IRF5, inhibition, negative regulation, positive regulation, autoimmunity

INTRODUCTION

Interferon Regulatory Factors (IRFs) are a family of transcription factors that signal downstream of multiple pathways, including Toll-like receptor (TLR), retinoic acid-inducible gene I (RIG-I), melanoma differentiation associated gene 5 (MDA5), and B cell receptor (BCR) signaling pathways to regulate gene expression involved in both innate and adaptive immunity (1–3). IRFs are also known to play central roles in cell differentiation and development, cell proliferation, apoptosis, DNA damage response and tumor suppression (2–9). There are currently 9 mammalian IRFs-IRF1, IRF2, IRF3, IRF4/PIP/ICSAT, IRF5, IRF6, IRF7, IRF8/ICSBP, and IRF9/p48/ISGF3γ (3). This family of transcription factors is generally localized to the cytoplasm of an unstimulated cell, in which they exist in their inactive monomeric form. Induction of the different signaling cascades leads to the recruitment of adaptor molecules that in turn regulate a cascade of signals to promote IRF activation and nuclear translocation. This process ultimately leads to the downstream production of cytokines, chemokines and other transcription factors that regulate innate and adaptive immune responses (10, 11).

A key event prior to IRF activation and nuclear translocation is post-translational modification that leads to conformational changes allowing for protein-protein interactions. In the case of IRFs that contain a carboxyl (C)-terminal autoinhibitory domain (AID) (**Figure 1**), post-translational modification leads to disruption of intramolecular association of the AID with the amino (N)-terminal DNA binding domain (DBD) and IRF association domain (IAD) (12–14). Ultimately, these conformational changes enable the IRFs to homo- or hetero-dimerize with each other or another molecule, thus allowing them to translocate to the nucleus and bind to DNA (with other co-factors), resulting in the regulation of gene transcription (15, 16). As in most critical signaling pathways that elicit an immune response, once the response has been elicited and immune cells respond, an intrinsic negative regulatory pathway is expected to be initiated to shut down the originating signal. If activation persists, inflammatory molecules will begin to damage tissues, and/or trigger the development of autoimmunity.

Indeed, hyper-activation of IRFs (most notably IRF1, IRF3, IRF5, IRF7, and IRF9) has been implicated in disease pathogenesis as it leads to unrestricted production of IFNs, which is linked to the development of numerous inflammatory and autoimmune diseases (17, 18). Further, polymorphisms in *IRF* genes show either protection from or increased susceptibility to the development of such diseases (19–23). Thus, the development of small molecules that directly bind to and inhibit IRF function(s) would be extremely valuable to patients with a variety of inflammatory and autoimmune diseases. To date, there are no therapeutic inhibitors of the IRFs. In general, transcription factors are thought to be notoriously difficult to target (24). This certainly holds true for IRFs as we still do not fully understand the physiologic mechanisms that control IRF activation and inhibition in a cell. For many IRF family members, the mechanism of activation depends on the cell type and initiating signaling pathway. Last, crystal structures of full-length IRFs have been difficult to resolve, which when done, will lend valuable insight into the rational targeting of specific structural features inherent to each family member (13, 14). Thus, indirect strategies for inhibiting IRF function(s) have been focused on by targeting molecules that regulate their activities, such as kinases that phosphorylate the IRFs, rather than directly targeting their structure.

Hence, in this review, we will discuss the critical events involved in IRF activation, including mechanisms of post-translational modification, classical IRF signaling pathways, and negative regulatory pathways as methods to indirectly target IRF activation and function. In addition, we will discuss new insights into the direct targeting of IRFs through focused studies on the IRF5 family member. Ultimately, understanding the mechanisms of IRF-mediated inflammatory responses will aid in the identification of new strategies to therapeutically target these critical players.

IMPLICATIONS FOR IRFs IN DISEASE PATHOGENESIS–WHY TARGET THE IRFs?

The role of IRFs and their importance in regulating immunity have been increasingly conspicuous in the last decade. Dysregulation of IRFs can lead to either suppression or hyper-activation, both of which may contribute to disease development. Hence, identifying methods to target the modulation of these transcription factors will provide new avenues of treatment for patients suffering from IRF-mediated diseases. In this section, we will briefly discuss IRF family members and their role(s) in disease pathogenesis.

IRF1 was the first family member to be identified and found to regulate type I IFN gene expression. Recent data from genome wide association studies (GWAS) identified IRF1 as a risk factor for inflammatory bowel disease (25, 26). In mice, IRF1 was shown to promote the severity and incidence of autoimmune diseases like collagen-induced arthritis (CIA) and experimental allergic encephalomyelitis. The incidence and severity of CIA and EAE were significantly reduced mice lacking *Irf1* (27).

Conversely, IRF2 is a negative regulator of IFN-mediated gene expression. IRF2 suppresses the activity of IRF1 by competing for binding sites (28). An increase in the IRF1/IRF2 ratio has been considered an important event needed for the transcriptional activation of IFNα genes required for the development of cellular responses to viruses (29). Limited and not very well-replicated studies have reported an association of *IRF2* polymorphism with susceptibility to the autoimmune disease systemic lupus erythematosus (SLE). The SLE risk haplotype was suggested to be associated with activation of IRF2 (17, 30, 31).

Similarly, *IRF3* polymorphisms were found to be associated with SLE but controversy still exists regarding their role in susceptibility and pathogenesis (17, 23, 32). Studies in a Mexican mestizo cohort found that the rs2304206 gene variant associated with increased IRF3 expression in plasmacytoid dendritic cells (pDCs), with elevated type I IFN expression and dsDNA autoantibodies (32). In a murine model of EAE, $Irf3^{-/-}$ mice showed reduced disease severity due to attenuated Th1 and Th17 type responses (33). Further, IRF3 over-activation was found to contribute to autoinflammatory conditions, such as Aicardi-Goutières syndrome (34–36) and STING-associated vasculopathy of infancy (SAVI) (34, 36). Last, over-active IRF3 in macrophages and enhanced production of type I IFN resulted in fatal inflammatory response to myocardial infarction while $Irf3^{-/-}$ mice were protected from myocardial infarction (36).

In contrast, dysregulated IRF4 has been implicate in multiple myeloma where its expression was found to correlate with malignancy-specific gene expression (37). *IRF4* polymorphisms were also found to contribute to elevated IRF4 expression in cells from multiple myeloma patients (38, 39). Polymorphisms in the *IRF4* gene have also been detected in adult T cell leukemia (40). Under the condition of chronic infection, IRF4 induces the exhaustion of $CD8^+$ T cells and hinders the development of memory T cells (41). More recent findings suggest that *IRF4* polymorphisms are associated with high risk of rheumatoid arthritis (RA) (17, 42, 43) and systemic sclerosis (17, 43).

Mutations in *IRF6* have been shown to contribute to the development of Van der Woude syndrome (VWS) and popliteal pterygium syndrome (PPS). VWS is an autosomal dominant form of cleft lip and PPS is a disorder with a similar orofacial phenotype that includes skin and genital anomalies. Further, increased IRF6 mRNA was found along the medial edge of the fusing palate, tooth buds, hair follicles, genitalia and skin in samples with *IRF6* mutations (44, 45).

IRF7 polymorphisms, like IRF5, are associated with increased risk of SLE (46–49). IRF7 has also been implicated in the

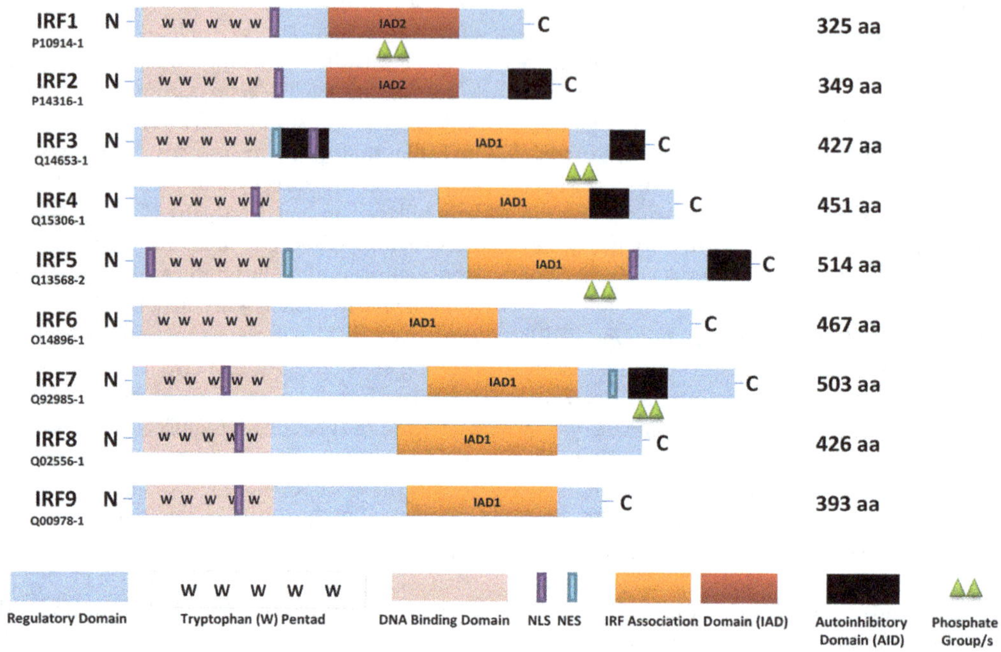

FIGURE 1 | A schematic representation of full-length human IRFs showing different functional domains. All IRFs harbor a DNA binding domain that contains a conserved tryptophan pentad (pink) in the N-terminus. They also contain an IRF activation domain termed either IAD1 (orange) or IAD2 (red). Other domains present are a nuclear localization signal (NLS, purple), nuclear export signal (NES, blue-green), an autoinhibitory domain (black), and a regulatory domain (blue). In this scheme, IRF activation (green triangles) is denoted as phosphorylation. The length of each IRF is indicated by the number of amino acids (aa), as found in Uniprot, with each identifier listed. IRF, interferon regulatory factor; C, carboxy terminus; N, amino terminus.

pathogenesis of type 1 diabetes through the upregulation of inflammatory gene networks (50). Most relevant to the current review is the finding that reduction/inhibition of mucosal IRF7 expression with liposomal *Irf7* siRNA resulted in protection of mice from bacterial infection and renal tissue damage (51). Last, IRF7 expression was recently found to be elevated in PBMC from patients with systemic sclerosis, as compared to healthy donors, due to promoter hypomethylation (52).

IRF8 was recently found to play an important role in the differentiation of IL9-producing T helper cells (Th9). Th9 cells are a subset of CD4^{+} T cells with pro-inflammatory function (53). In the NZB/W F1 model of spontaneous murine lupus, mice lacking *Irf8* failed to produce anti-nuclear, -chromatin and -erythrocyte autoantibodies and had reduced kidney disease (54). Dual and opposing functions for IRF8 were found in Autoimmune Uveitis. Deletion of IRF8 in T cells exacerbated the disease, while loss of IRF8 in retinal cells had a protective effect (55). Additionally, a meta- analysis detected association of *IRF8* genetic variants with susceptibility of Multiple Sclerosis (MS) (56). Last, IRF8-expressing antigen presenting cells in EAE led to disease development by facilitating the onset and expansion of T effector cells and promoting microglial-based neuro-inflammation. Thus, mice lacking *Irf8* are protected from EAE (57).

Although limited reports implicate a direct role for IRF9 in disease pathogenesis that support its therapeutic targeting, IRF9 is well-known to regulate IFN signaling through formation of the ISGF3 complex (58). A recent report by Nan and colleagues, however, found that IRF9 contributes to STAT3 activation by upregulating IL6 expression in cancer cells. IL6 is necessary for some cancer cells to grow and thus inhibition of this pathway could be therapeutic (59).

We have saved IRF5 to discuss last as it has become the most widely implicated IRF in disease pathogenesis. In the last 10 years, numerous studies have reported the association of *IRF5* polymorphisms with autoimmune disease susceptibility. Diseases include, but are not limited to–RA, systemic sclerosis, MS, inflammatory bowel disease and SLE (17, 60–62). In the case of SLE, GWAS across multiple ancestral backgrounds have confirmed that *IRF5* polymorphisms associate with SLE risk [(60, 63–66)]. In SLE patient blood, IRF5 expression and activation were found to be significantly elevated (67–71). Prior to these findings, IRF5 was identified as a critical mediator of MyD88-dependent TLR signaling, leading to the expression/production of multiple pro-inflammatory cytokines including type I IFNs, IL6, TNFα, IL12, IL23, and others implicated in autoimmune disease pathogenesis (62, 72–76).

IRF5 has also been shown to play critical roles during viral infection. IRF5 was recently found to promote the death of protective CD4^{+} T cells during chronic visceral leishmaniasis resulting in the establishment of chronic infection (77). Expression levels of IRF5 and its related downstream inflammatory cytokines were also found to be associated with severity, prognosis, and the causative pathogen of community acquired pneumonia in patients (10). Last, genetic variants of *IRF5* have been associated with chronic hepatitis B infection (78).

In addition to its role(s) in autoimmune and viral disease pathogenesis, the past 5–10 years has brought about a plethora of new data implicating IRF5 in multiple other diseases, including cancer, obesity, neuropathic pain, cardiovascular, and metabolic dysfunction (79–82). For the purpose of this review, we will not be discussing the role of IRF5 in cancer as it tends to act as a tumor suppressor and thus its expression/activation are downregulated (83–87). We instead focus on diseases where IRF5 expression/activation are upregulated. For example, in two distinct models of murine atherosclerosis, murine *Irf5* was recently found to contribute to the formation of atherosclerotic lesions by impairing efferocytosis (88). This effect was due to IRF5's role in promoting the maintenance of pro-inflammatory $CD11c^+$ macrophages within lesions leading to the expansion of the necrotic core. IRF5 also plays a role in liver fibrosis caused by hepatitis C virus or in non-alcoholic fatty liver disease (89). IRF5 expression was significantly higher in liver macrophages from human subjects with liver fibrosis than healthy controls and its expression positively correlated with clinical markers of liver damage. Of note, mice lacking *Irf5* in their myeloid compartment were protected from hepatic fibrosis (89). In a coronary ligation model, high levels of IRF5 expression were detected during the early inflammatory stage (day 4) of wound healing. This phase was then followed by a decrease in IRF5 expression in infarct macrophages skewing them toward an M2 phenotype that is involved in the resolution of inflammation (day 8). Accelerated cutaneous and infarct healing, and attenuated development of post-myocardial infarct heart failure were observed during the second phase of decreased IRF5 expression (81, 90).

IRF5 dysfunction was also recently implicated in neuropathic pain, which plays an important role in the pathogenesis of tactile allodynia induced by nerve injury. IRF5 expression on M1 microglia is upregulated by spinal nerve injury, which in turn induces the expression of ATP receptors to activate microglia and signal neuropathic pain in the spinal cord (91). In spinal cord injury (SCI) there is an acute, long-lasting inflammatory response and macrophages play an important role in persistent inflammation contributing to the pathogenesis of SCI. The first phase after SCI is acute and is characterized by M2 macrophage infiltration that is then followed by a long-lasting phase of M1 macrophages, which slows healing and compromises organ function. IRF5 was shown to play a critical role in this process by up-regulating genes associated with the M1 macrophage phenotype (92).

In the antigen-induced model of arthritis, a population of *Irf5*-positive pro-inflammatory macrophages was found to significantly increase in inflamed knees, suggesting that IRF5 can be used as a marker of inflammatory macrophages in a disease setting (93). Another report from the same group studied the role of IRF5 in a model of acute inflammation and lung injury. Neutrophil influx is known to play a major role in both diseases. Mice lacking *Irf5* had a significant reduction in the number of neutrophils accumulating at the site of infection, and acute lung injury was markedly reduced in *Irf5*-deficient mice (93).

Another important role for IRF5 was identified in patients carrying *IRF5* polymorphism rs3757385 that associates with acute rejection and is considered a risk factor for transplant rejection (94). *IRF5* polymorphisms were also recently identified that associate with asthma and its severity. Interestingly, *IRF5* risk alleles that associate with asthma were found to be almost completely opposite to those for autoimmune disorders, supporting potentially distinct roles for IRF5 in the pathogenesis of asthma and autoimmune disorders (95). Additional work in both human and mouse models of asthma and allergic airway inflammation suggests an important role for Irf5 in driving disease severity (96, 97).

A final example of IRF5 dysregulation in disease comes from the field of hematologic malignancies. Distinct from the multitude of solid cancers and hematologic malignancies that have been shown to have lost IRF5 expression (79, 83, 98), a tumor-promoting role for IRF5 was identified in classical Hodgkin Lymphoma (HL) where IRF5 expression was found to be elevated and over-activated in HL B cells (84, 99).

Given the multitude of studies implicating IRF5 dysregulation in a vast number of diseases, we use this IRF family member as a candidate therapeutic target for drug discovery. Below, we focus on the details of IRF5 structure-function, signaling, post-translational modification and negative regulation that may be used as molecular targets for therapeutic inhibition. Since there is significant homology between IRF family members (**Figure 1**), combined with distinct and overlapping functional roles in the immune system, we anticipate that strategies developed to inhibit IRF5 may be utilized to modulate the function/activity of other IRF family members.

UNDERSTANDING THE MOLECULAR STRUCTURE OF IRF5

IRF family members regulate IFNs and IFN-inducible genes supporting their critical role(s) in the innate immune response against pathogens. All IRFs have a homology of over 115 amino acids in their N-terminal region that harbors the DBD (**Figure 1**). The DBD contains a highly conserved tryptophan (W) repeat forming a helix-turn-helix motif that recognizes DNA sequences referred to as IFN-stimulated response elements (ISRE) (A/GNGAAANNGAAACT) or IRF elements (IRF-E) (5, 9, 17). The C-terminal region, on the other hand, exhibits diversity in all IRFs, which supports their distinct function(s), and could be potentially used for therapeutic inhibition that would provide specificity to each family member. As summarized in **Figure 1**, the IRFs contain a regulatory domain, nuclear localization signal (NLS), nuclear export signal (NES), IRF-association domains (IAD), and some family members (IRF3, IRF5, IRF7) contain an autoinhibitory domain (AID) (48, 100). Each of these regions defines or elicits cell type-specific functions, activation via distinct signaling pathways, and interaction with other proteins.

IRF5 isoform-1 -SGELSWSADSIRLQIS-
IRF5 isoform-2 -SGELSWSADSIRLQIS-
IRF5 isoform-3 -SGELSWSADSIRLQIS-
IRF5 isoform-4 -SGELSWSADSIRLQIS-
IRF5 isoform-5 -SGELSWSADSIRLQIS-
IRF5 isoform-6 -SGELSWSADSIRLQIS-

FIGURE 2 | The Serine Rich Region (SRR) is conserved in all IRF5 isoforms. The C-terminus contains conserved serine (**S**) residues that are targeted for phosphorylation by kinases, such as IKKβ (blue-bolded serine). Red-bolded serines are those originally identified as critical for IRF5 activation (13, 101). Phosphorylation leads to structural changes, including removal of the AID, liberation of the IAD and exposure of the C-terminus for further modification(s) and/or protein interaction. Although IRF5 isoforms range in size, most contain the SRR independent of its numerical amino acid location.

The AID suppresses IRF transcriptional activity. There are two identified AIDs in IRF3 located in the N- and C-terminal regions compared to one AID found in IRF5 and IRF7 (14, 101, 102). The IRF3 crystal structure in its latent (unstimulated or autoinhibited monomer) form revealed the hydrophobic surface and a region essential for CBP/p300 binding that is masked by the AID (14). The presence of two AIDs provides a unique activation conformation upon phosphorylation with the IAD and AID forming a hydrophobic core and realignment of the DBD. The pseudo-phosphorylated IRF5 crystal structure, on the other hand, revealed the AID and key phosphorylation sites (**Figure 2**) as being highly extended allowing for dimerization and/or interaction with CBP/p300 in the hydrophobic region (13).

Insights from the crystal structures, along with data from functional mutagenesis, provides key structural information that can be used to directly target each IRF family member. These models also allow for the further testing of different mechanisms that may lead to IRF activation and conformational changes that liberate the AID and expose critical residues essential for homo- or hetero-dimerization and other protein-protein interactions. Specific phosphorylated residues in the C-terminus, referred to as the serine rich region (SRR, **Figure 2**), contribute to the stabilization of IRF dimers and interaction with DNA. Mutational analysis of the SRR originally identified S425, S427, and S430 of the identical isoform encoded by *IRF5* variants 3 and 4 (**Figure 2**, red-bolded residues) as the critical sites of phosphorylation that are necessary for Newcastle disease virus (NDV)-induced IRF5 activation (101, 103). Later studies from multiple groups confirmed the functional importance of these three residues (13). While protein length and numerical amino acid location varies between IRF5 isoforms (104), the SRR is conserved (**Figure 2**). Given that we still do not know all of the pathways and mechanisms leading to IRF5 activation or inhibition of activation, further studies focused on identifying mutations that lead to either of these outcomes will be essential to our understanding of how better to target these molecules. An example of this was the finding years ago by others and us of dominant negative IRF mutants that lead to the inhibition of IRF transactivation function (104–110). These types of studies suggest that the utilization of small peptides that mimic the IRFs may lead to inhibition. Indeed, two examples of this currently exist for IRF5 that will be discussed in the last section [(111); U.S. Patent No US20160009772A1; (112); U.S. Patent No WO2017044855A2], but are depicted in **Figure 3**.

IRF5 SIGNALING PATHWAYS: THE POSITIVE AND NEGATIVE PARADIGM

The combination of protein-protein interaction, signaling co-factors, adaptor proteins, and cell type specificity will all contribute to determining which IRF family member will be "turned on" in response to stimulation. For instance, IRF3 is ubiquitously expressed in all immune cells while IRF7 is more restricted in cells of lymphoid origin (101). IRF5, on the other hand, is expressed in monocytes, macrophages (Mφ), B cells and dendritic cells (DC) (16, 114).

Innate pattern recognition receptors (PRRs), which include TLRs, C-type lectin receptors (CLRs), RIG-I-like receptors (RLRs), and NOD-like receptors (NLRs), all recognize various pathogen-associated molecular patterns (PAMPs) and danger-associated molecular patterns (DAMPs). In response to these PAMPs and DAMPs, intracellular signaling cascades are differentially triggered that induce the expression and/or activation of IRFs (115). In the case of TLR signaling, activation occurs via binding of ligand to receptor, leading to a conformational change that immediately recruits adaptor proteins. MyD88 is a proximal adaptor protein responsible for the propagation of the innate immune signal transduction downstream of TLR7 and upstream of IRF5 (9, 116). In the MyD88-dependent pathway, MyD88 recruits TNFR-associated factor 6 (TRAF6) and IL-1R-associated kinase 4 (IRAK4) followed by recruitment of IRAK1, IRAK2 or IRAK3 to form a complex called the Myddosome (117). IRF5 activation occurs downstream of this TLR7/8 pathway and has recently been shown to be phosphorylated by IKKβ (**Figure 4**), leading to downstream cytokine and chemokine expression (105, 118, 119). Additional reviews are available that cover in more detail the TLR-IRF signaling pathways (3, 11, 120, 121).

In human primary monocytes and macrophages, induction of IFNβ following infection of Staphylococcus aureus (RNA) was found to require two key signaling molecules in the TLR8-MyD88 pathway–TAK1 and IKKβ (122). Use of an IRAK4 inhibitor revealed that IRAK4 regulates TAK1 and IKKβ activity (123). Inhibition of IRAK4 autophosphorylation led to the inhibition of TAK1 activation, which resulted in the inhibition of IKKβ phosphorylation at S177, and inhibition of IRF5 activation and downstream proinflammatory cytokine production (123). IKKβ was previously identified as a kinase for IRF5 (**Figure 2**, blue-bolded serine) (118, 119).

As for negative regulators of IRF5 function, IRF4 was shown to act as an antagonist of IRF5 in Epstein-Barr Virus (EBV)-transformed cells (124). IRF4 knockdown resulted in elevated IRF5 expression. IRF4 was found to bind to similar IRF5 target genes and compete for binding with IRF5 (124). Further, a few studies reported that IRF4 also competes with IRF5 for MyD88

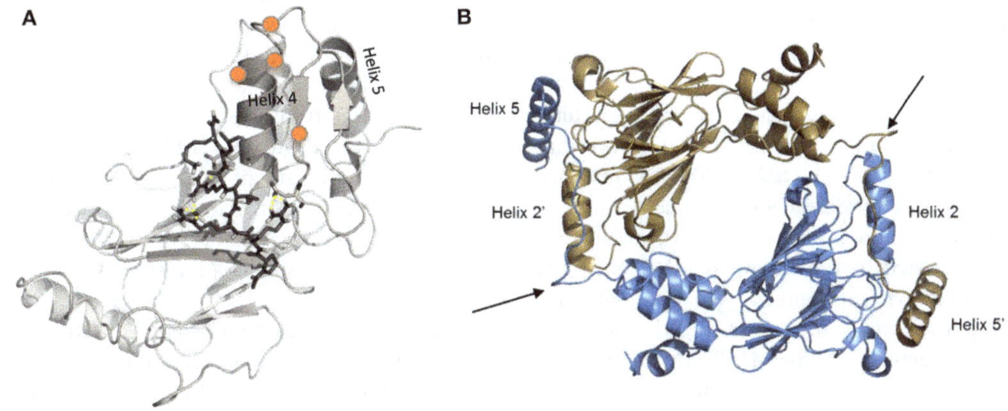

FIGURE 3 | Modified crystal structures of IRF5. **(A)** Homology model of the inactive IRF5 C-terminal domain (variant 5) generated using the monomeric autoinhibited IRF3 C-terminal domain (PDB: 1QWT) as a template (113). Representative image from docking of an inhibitor (112) to the C-terminal SRR of the inactive IRF5 monomer, which results in maintenance of a closed, non-phosphorylated conformation. Orange balls represent phosphorylation sites at the C-terminal SRR. **(B)** Representative image generated from IRF5 crystal structure coordinates (13) showing formation of an IRF5 homodimer. Arrows show critical regions that are being therapeutically targeted to inhibit homodimerization between Helix 2 and Helix 5 (111).

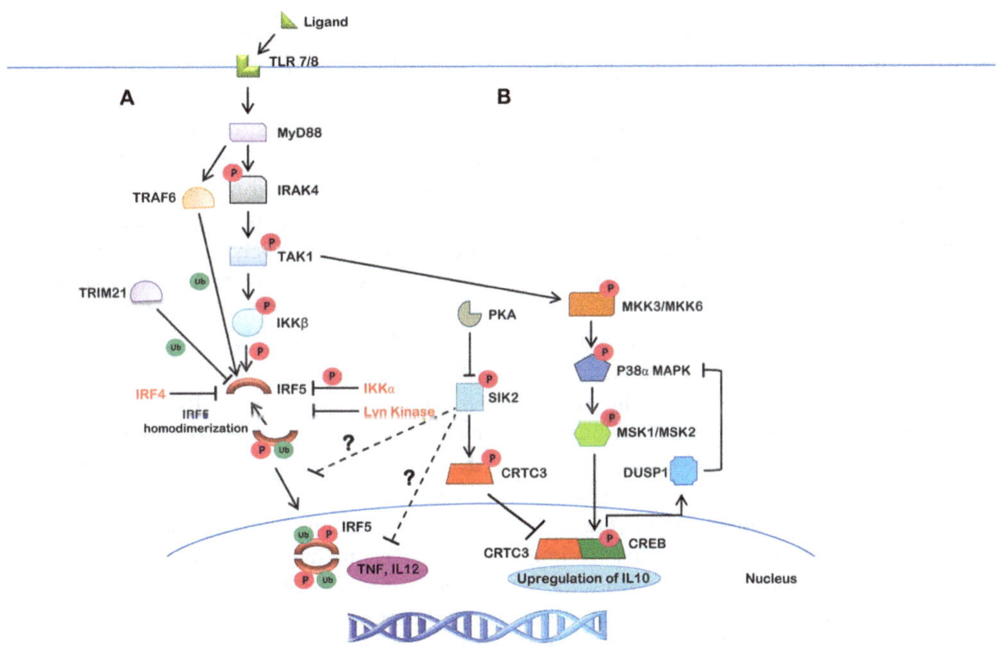

FIGURE 4 | The canonical IRF5 signaling pathway and its negative regulation. **(A)** Upon ligand binding to TLR7/8, MyD88 gets recruited in, along with IRAK1/4 and TRAF6, which leads to the autophosphorylation of IRAK4 and ubiquitination of IRF5 by TRAF6. IRAK4 then activates TAK1, which then phosphorylates IKKβ. The ubiquitinated IRF5 is then phosphorylated by IKKβ (or other kinases). This action results in homodimerization and translocation of the IRF5 homodimer to the nucleus, leading to the production of downstream cytokines. Lyn kinase, IKKα and IRF4, on the other hand, were found to negatively regulate IRF5 activity. TRIM21 is a molecule that targets IRF5 for proteasomal- or lysosomal-mediated degradation. **(B)** A negative feedback loop may also be involved in the suppression of IRF5-mediated inflammatory gene transcription. TAK1 initiates a series of phosphorylation events on different kinases, including MMK3/MKK6, P38α/MAPK, MSK1/MSK2, and CREB, which leads to the upregulation of IL10. SIK2, on the other hand, inhibits CRTC3 activity by phosphorylation leading to its cytosolic localization and inhibition of IL10 expression. SIK2 also inhibits inflammatory molecules, such as TNF and IL12 by unknown mechanisms that may involve inhibition of IRF5 (shown by ?).

interaction, resulting in the negative regulation of downstream IRF5 targets (125, 126). While these are not direct effects on IRF5 itself, subsequent studies identified Lyn kinase as a direct regulator of IRF5 activity. Lyn kinase was found to bind to IRF5 and even phosphorylate it; however, phosphorylation did not alter protein activity (116). Instead, inhibition of IRF5 activity was due to the direct interaction of Lyn with IRF5 resulting in allosteric interaction. Further discussion of Lyn-IRF5 interaction is included below in the section on IRF5 post-translational modification.

Results from independent studies also allow us to speculate on other negative regulatory pathways of inflammatory cytokine expression that may regulate IRF5 (127, 128). For instance, SIK2 was reported to phosphorylate CRTC3, which results in its cytoplasmic localization and inhibition of IL10 expression. SIK2 has also been reported to downregulate TNF and IL12 production via an unknown mechanism. We speculate that components of this pathway may serve as a negative feedback loop that inhibits IRF5 activity (**Figure 4**). TRIM21-mediated dose-dependent degradation of IRF5 was also found to contribute to reduced IRF5 activity and may lead to a mechanism of inhibition (129).

IRF5 POST-TRANSLATIONAL MODIFICATIONS AND KEY MODIFIERS

Post-translational modifications (PTMs) are essential to protein stability and function. A single protein may undergo single or multiple reversible or irreversible PTM(s). Phosphorylation (of serine, threonine or tyrosine) is an important modification required by most IRFs for their activation and/or inhibition. IRFs also undergo either K48- (targeted for proteosomal degradation) or K63-ubiquitination (for intracellular trafficking). Here, we will discuss some of the most important modifiers and PTMs essential for IRF5 activation that could be potential targets for inhibition.

IRF5 can be phosphorylated by IKKβ which leads to homo-dimerization and nuclear translocation to induce IFN activation following viral infection (**Figure 4**) (118, 119). Phosphorylation is required not just for homo- and hetero-dimerization but also for the interaction with histone acetyltransferases (HATs) (70, 71, 130). Two independent studies identified IKKβ as a kinase that phosphorylates a single C-terminal Ser residue in IRF5 (**Figure 2**, blue-bolded serine) (118, 119). Mutation of this residue abrogated IRF5 homodimerization and nuclear translocation. Three additional Ser residues that were previously identified as being important for IRF5 activation (**Figure 2**, red-bolded serines) (101), may also be important for dimerization, based on crystal structure analysis (14, 15, 101, 103). These Ser residues, however, also appear to be essential to the liberation of the AID (13).

Prior to phosphorylation, IRF5 has been shown to undergo ubiquitination which is catalyzed by TRAF6 (98, 131). A few studies mentioned that ubiquitination is not required for IRF5 activation but it appears to be required for phosphorylation (116, 132). In particular, K410 and K411 are essential for IRF5 activation, nuclear translocation and the IFNα promoter-inducing activity (131). TRIM21 has been shown to ubiquitinate IRF5 which reduces or dose-dependently inhibits its activity via proteasomal- or lysosomal-mediated degradation (129).

Lyn kinase phosphorylates IRF5 at Y313 and Y335 but this modification was dispensable as transactivation ability of the double mutant IRF5 (YY313, 335FF) was still inhibited by Lyn (116). Further, a kinase-dead Lyn point mutant (K275D) inhibited IRF5 transcriptional activity. These data show that Lyn negatively regulates IRF5 transcriptional activity via a mechanism independent of its kinase activity and possibly via a direct interaction of Lyn with IRF5. IKKα also inhibits IRF5 function through phosphorylation which can be circumvented by the action of alkaline phosphatase causing it to undergo dephosphorylation (133).

Last, we previously reported that IRF5 activity may also be regulated by acetylation. We found that histone deacetylases (HDACs) and HATs CREB-binding protein (CBP)/p300 interact with IRF5 in response to virus infection, and this was required for IRF5 transactivation (15, 70, 130).

CURRENT THERAPEUTIC STRATEGIES TO INHIBIT IRF5

IRF5 was identified as a key regulatory factor for macrophage polarization. The activation of IRF5 expression in macrophages decides their fate to either be M1 or M2 macrophages. Higher expression of IRF5 leads to M1 polarization whereas reduced or downregulated expression leads to M2 polarization (76). In a SCI mouse model, macrophage activation along with persistent inflammation was found to contribute to severity. After injury, there is an immediate influx of M2-activated macrophages; however, following this, there is a long-lasting phase characterized by an influx of activated M1 macrophages to the site of injury. This long-lasting phase of M1 macrophages causes derailed healing and compromises organ function(s) (92). Since up-regulated IRF5 expression induces the M1 macrophage phenotype, IRF5 siRNA was delivered *in vivo* by lipidoid nanoparticle to silence IRF5 in the macrophages that infiltrated the spinal cord injury wound. Nanoparticle-mediated IRF5 siRNA delivery to the wound resulted in a dramatic change in macrophage phenotype changing from M1 to M2 in the long-lasting phase. Decreased inflammation, attenuation of demyelination and neurofilament loss, and a significant improvement in locomotor function were found (92). A similar study using nanoparticle-mediated IRF5 siRNA delivery *in vivo* into macrophages residing in myocardial infarcts (MI) and in surgically induced skin wounds in mice showed resolution of inflammation and infarct healing. Furthermore, treatment led to the attenuation of post-MI heart failure after coronary ligation (81). Likewise, in the severe acute pancreatitis mouse model there is pancreatitis-induced activation of lung M1 macrophages with high expression of IRF5, TNFα, iNOS and IL10. These macrophages were polarized toward the M2 phenotype after treatment with IRF5 siRNA *in vitro*. Moreover, *in vivo*, treatment with IRF5 siRNA reversed the pancreatitis-induced activation of lung macrophages from M1 phenotype to M2 phenotype (134). Last, selective suppression of IRF5 in microglia cells using gene therapy with homing peptide-siRNA-IRF5 complexes in a mouse model of neuropathic pain resulted in a significant reduction in neuropathic pain (91).

An alternative method of targeting IRF5 was demonstrated using an AAG-rich microsatellite DNA mimicking oligodeoxynucleotide designated as MS19 to inhibit IRF5 activation. LPS stimulated RAW264.7 cells, when cultured along with MS19, resulted in reduced expression of iNOS, IL6, and TNFα along with inhibiting the nuclear translocation of IRF5 *in vitro* detected by western blot of nuclear and cytoplasmic extracts. Bioinformatics analysis revealed the mechanism of action of MS19 to be competition with IRF5 at regulatory consensus sequences in the promoter of target genes. MS19 was further studied in a murine model of septic peritonitis revealing that MS19 prolonged the survival of the mice and down-regulated the expression of iNOS, IRF5, IL6, and TNFα (135). Another interesting study using the natural polyphenol Mangiferin that is a component of Mangifera indica Linn. leaves found a marked reduction in IRF5 expression in macrophages stimulated with LPS/IFNγ. This translated into a significant reduction in pro-inflammatory cytokine expression (136). How Mangiferin down-regulates IRF5 expression is not currently known.

NEW THERAPEUTIC STRATEGIES FOR TARGETING IRF5

Given its role in both innate and adaptive immune signaling, constitutive activation of IRF5, like other IRF family members, can create havoc on immune homeostasis leading to detrimental effects on cellular phenotypic plasticity and the development of autoimmune and inflammatory diseases. In this section, we discuss recent new methods that have been developed by our lab and others that directly target IRF5 activation and speculate on other possible avenues that may lead to IRF5 inhibition.

Some IRF family members regulate the expression and activity of other IRFs. Examples of this are seen with IRF1-IRF2 and IRF4-IRF5 (5, 104, 124, 137–139). These positive and negative feedback mechanisms show vulnerability in the signaling system that could be used for targeting. However, because of these mechanisms of co-regulation, altering the expression of individual IRF family members may lead to non-specific effects on other IRF family members. This may be cell type-dependent since not all IRFs are expressed in every cell type. An example of this methodology was used in cancer cells where inhibition of IRF2 expression/function was induced by upregulation of its antagonist, IRF1 (140). Similarly, IRF4 was identified as a negative regulator of IRF5 transactivation ability (106, 124, 126). Upregulation of these negative regulators would lead to a respective switch from pro-tumorigenic to anti-tumorigenic and pro-inflammatory to anti-inflammatory. Unfortunately, upregulation of these negative regulators may also impact other signaling pathways that could promote the development of other diseases depending on cell type. Another challenge to targeting the IRFs is targeting them in a cell type-specific manner.

Additional negative regulatory pathways of IRF5 are being discovered (127). SIK2 has been implicated as a negative regulator of TNF and IL12 production and CRTC3. Inhibition of CRTC3 prevents it from undergoing nuclear translocation and reduces IL10 expression. These data suggest that SIK2 plays a role in the regulation of pro- and anti-inflammatory signaling and may be a candidate to target therapeutically for the inhibition of autoimmune and inflammatory diseases. We are currently examining whether SIK2 may be a negative regulator of IRF5 (**Figure 4**).

IKKβ, IRAK1/4, and TRAF6 are activators of latent IRF5 that can also be targeted to inhibit its activity. Certainly, these have been the more common strategies in the Pharma industry since enzymes have catalytically active sites that are more readily accessible by small molecular weight compounds. Another possibility is the targeting of phosphatases that lead to the deactivation or inhibition of IRF5. These include A20 (132) and alkaline phosphatase (133). Again, similar to targeting kinases, phosphatases and ligases are not specific for one protein and therefore targeting them would be expected to lead to global changes in gene expression and protein activation. The same is true for other co-activators identified to interact with IRF5, such as CBP/p300 and GCN/PCAF; they are not specific to IRF5.

A number of viruses have now been shown to encode viral IRF (vIRF) homologs, including Kaposi's sarcoma-associated herpesvirus and rhesus monkey rhadinovirus, which function as dominant negative mutants by antagonizing IRF activity (110, 124, 141). Some of these dominant negative mutants lack the IRF DBD that do not allow them to bind to the host DNA, instead they form homo- and hetero-dimers with the IRFs leading to inhibition. Alternatively, C-terminal deletion mutants have been shown to inhibit IRF function by binding directly to host DNA, thus competing out wild-type IRFs (106–108). Although the mechanisms of dominant negative function have not been entirely worked out, given that most IRFs require homo- or hetero-dimerization for function, and/or interaction with other proteins, targeting these types of interactions would be expected to provide enhanced specificity. Additionally, other viral proteins have been found to inhibit IRF function through targeted degradation (142). These viral proteins, and/or sequences within them, may be further developed to inhibit IRF function.

In this regard, we and others have developed novel peptide inhibitors that utilize specific sequences within the IRF5 gene to inhibit activation. In collaboration with colleagues at Roche, a series of peptide inhibitors were developed based on crystal structure data predicting regions in the IRF5 protein that are critical for homo- and hetero-dimerization [(111); U.S. Patent No US20160009772A1]. We found that these inhibitors directly bind to the IRF5 protein, inhibit TLR-induced IRF5 homo-dimerization, nuclear translocation and downstream cytokine production. Independently, we developed another series of peptide inhibitors that are cell permeable, directly bind to full-length endogenous IRF5, and inhibit the development of murine lupus *in vivo* [(112); U.S. Patent No WO2017044855A2]. Results from these two studies support the specific targeting of IRF5 with inhibitors that directly bind to the protein. The value of targeting IRF5 directly rather than mediators of its activation is that specificity will be enhanced and inhibition will be independent of cell type and pathway of activation.

CONCLUSIONS

Given the similarities in IRF crystal structures, mechanisms of activation and necessity of protein-protein interactions for activity, we expect that similar methodologies as those identified to inhibit IRF5 activation can be used to target other IRF family members.

AUTHOR CONTRIBUTIONS

All authors listed have made a substantial, direct and intellectual contribution to the work, and approved it for publication.

ACKNOWLEDGMENTS

We thank members of the Barnes Lab for critical discussion and input. This work was supported in part by grants from the National Institutes of Health NIAMS AR065959, FAMRI 123059, Lupus Research Alliance and the DoD Lupus Research Program LR170107.

REFERENCES

1. De S, Zhang B, Shih T, Singh S, Winkler A, Donnelly R, et al. Cell-intrinsic role for IRF5 in TLR9/BCR-induced human B cell activation, proliferation, and plasmablast differentiation. *Front Immunol.* (2018) 8:1938. doi: 10.3389/fimmu.2017.01938
2. Taniguchi T, Ogasawara K, Takaoka A, Tanaka N. IRF family of transcription factors as regulators of host defense. *Annu Rev Immunol.* (2001) 19:623–55. doi: 10.1146/annurev.immunol.19.1.623
3. Zhao GN, Jiang DS, Li H. Interferon regulatory factors: at the crossroads of immunity, metabolism, and disease. *Biochim Biophys Acta* 1852:365–78. doi: 10.1016/j.bbadis.2014.04.030
4. Kroger A. IRFs as competing pioneers in T-cell differentiation. *Cell Mol Immunol.* (2017) 4:649–51. doi: 10.1038/cmi.2017.37
5. Chen F, Jiang G, Xu K, Zheng J. Function and mechanism by which interferon regulatory factor-1 inhibits oncogenesis (Review). *Oncol Lett.* (2013) 5:417–23. doi: 10.3892/ol.2012.1051
6. Yanai H, Negishi H, Taniguchi T. The IRF family of transcription factors: Inception, impact and implications in oncogenesis. *Oncoimmunology* (2012) 1:1376–86. doi: 10.4161/onci.22475
7. Nam S, Lim JS. Essential role of interferon regulatory factor 4 (IRF4) in immune cell development. *Arch Pharm Res.* (2016) 39:1548–55. doi: 10.1007/s12272-016-0854-1
8. Tamura T, Ozato K. ICSBP/IRF-8: its regulatory roles in the development of myeloid cells. *J Interferon Cytokine Res.* (2002) 22:145–52. doi: 10.1089/107999002753452755
9. Tamura T, Yanai H, Savitsky D, Taniguchi T. The IRF family, transcription factors in immunity and oncogenesis. *Annu Rev Immunol.* (2008) 26:535–84. doi: 10.1146/annurev.immunol.26.021607.090400
10. Wang X, Guo J, Wang Y, Xiao Y, Wang L, Hua S. Expression levels of Interferon Regulatory Factor 5 (IRF5) and related inflammatory cytokines associated with severity, prognosis, and causative pathogen in patients with community-acquired pneumonia. *Med Sci Monit.* (2018) 24:3620–30. doi: 10.12659/MSM.910756
11. Colonna M. TLR pathways and IFN-regulatory factors: to each its own. *Eur J Immunol.* (2007) 37:306–9. doi: 10.1002/eji.200637009
12. Lin R, Mamane Y, Hiscott J. Multiple regulatory domains control IRF-7 activity in response to virus infection. *J Bio Chem.* (2000) 275:34320–7. doi: 10.1074/jbc.M002814200
13. Chen W, Lam SS, Srinath H, Jiang Z, Correia JJ, Schiffer CA, et al. Insights into interferon regulatory factor activation from the crystal structure of dimeric IRF5. *Nat Struct Mol Biol.* (2008) 15:1213–20. doi: 10.1038/nsmb.1496
14. Chen W, Royer WE. Structural insights into interferon regulatory factor activation. *Cell Signal.* (2010) 22:883–7. doi: 10.1016/j.cellsig.2009.12.005
15. Cheng TF, Brzostek S, Ando O, Van Scoy S, Kumar KP, Reich NC. Differential activation of IFN regulatory factor (IRF)-3 and IRF-5 transcription factors during viral infection. *J Immunol.* (2006) 176:7462–70. doi: 10.4049/jimmunol.176.12.7462
16. Barnes BJ, Richards J, Mancl M, Hanash S, Beretta L, Pitha PM. Global and distinct targets of IRF-5 and IRF-7 during innate response to viral infection. *J Biol Chem.* (2004) 279:45194–207. doi: 10.1074/jbc.M400726200
17. Matta B, Song S, Li D, Barnes BJ. Interferon regulatory factor signaling in autoimmune disease. *Cytokine* (2017) 98:15–26. doi: 10.1016/j.cyto.2017.02.006
18. Crow MK. Type I interferon in the pathogenesis of lupus. *J Immunol.* (2014) 192:5459–68. doi: 10.4049/jimmunol.1002795
19. Zervou MI, Dorschner JM, Ghodke-Puranik Y, Boumpas DT, Niewold TB, Goulielmos GN. Association of IRF5 polymorphisms with increased risk for systemic lupus erythematosus in population of Crete, a southern-eastern European Greek island. *Gene* (2017) 610:9–14. doi: 10.1016/j.gene.2017.02.003
20. Hammad A, Mossad YM, Nasef N, Eid R. Interferon regulatory factor 5 gene polymorphism in Egyptian children with systemic lupus erythematosus. *Lupus* (2017) 26:871–80. doi: 10.1177/0961203316686845
21. Eames HL, Corbin AL, Udalova IA. Interferon regulatory factor 5 in human autoimmunity and murine models of autoimmune disease. *Trans Res.* (2016) 167:167–82. doi: 10.1016/j.trsl.2015.06.018
22. Vernerova L, Spoutil F, Vlcek M, Krskova K, Penesova A, Meskova M, et al. A Combination of CD28 (rs1980422) and IRF5 (rs10488631) polymorphisms is associated with seropositivity in rheumatoid arthritis: a case control study. *PLoS ONE* (2016) 11:e0153316. doi: 10.1371/journal.pone.0153316
23. Akahoshi M, Nakashima H, Sadanaga A, Miyake K, Obara K, Tamari M, et al. Promoter polymorphisms in the IRF3 gene confer protection against systemic lupus erythematosus. *Lupus* (2008) 17:568–74. doi: 10.1177/0961203308089340
24. Fontaine F, Overman J, François M. Pharmacological manipulation of transcription factor protein-protein interactions: opportunities and obstacles. *Cell Regeneration.* (2015) 4:2. doi: 10.1186/s13619-015-0015-x
25. Budarf ML, Labbé C, David G, Rioux JD. GWA studies: rewriting the story of IBD. *Trends Genet.* (2009) 25:137–46. doi: 10.1016/j.tig.2009.01.001
26. Jostins L, Ripke S, Weersma RK, Duerr RH, McGovern DP, Hui KY, et al. Host-microbe interactions have shaped the genetic architecture of inflammatory bowel disease. *Nature* (2012) 491:119–24. doi: 10.1038/nature11582
27. Tada Y, Ho A, Matsuyama T, Mak TW. Reduced incidence and severity of antigen-induced autoimmune diseases in mice lacking interferon regulatory factor-1. *J Exp Med.* (1997) 185:231–8. doi: 10.1084/jem.185.2.231
28. Harada H, Fujita T, Miyamoto M, Kimura Y, Maruyama M, Furia A, et al. Structurally similar but functionally distinct factors, IRF-1 and IRF-2, bind to the same regulatory elements of IFN and IFN-inducible genes. *Cell* (1989) 58:729–39. doi: 10.1016/0092-8674(89)90107-4
29. Mukherjee RM, Bansode B, Gangwal P, Jakkampudi A, Reddy PB, Rao PN, et al. Human interferon regulatory factor 2 gene expression is induced in chronic hepatitis C virus infection-A possible mode of viral persistence. *J Clin Exp Hepatol.* (2012) 2:27–34. doi: 10.1016/S0973-6883(12)60080-2
30. Ramos PS, Kelly JA, Gray-McGuire C, Bruner GR, Leiran AN, Meyer CM, et al. Familial aggregation and linkage analysis of autoantibody traits in

pedigrees multiplex for systemic lupus erythematosus. *Genes Immun.* (2006) 7:417–32. doi: 10.1038/sj.gene.6364316

31. Kawasaki A, Furukawa H, Nishida N, Warabi E, Kondo Y, Ito S, et al. Association of functional polymorphisms in interferon regulatory factor 2 (IRF2) with susceptibility to systemic lupus erythematosus: a case-control association study. *PLoS ONE* (2014) 9:e109764. doi: 10.1371/journal.pone.0109764
32. Santana-de Anda K, Gómez-Martín D, Monsivais-Urenda AE, Salgado-Bustamante M, González-Amaro R, Alcocer-Varela J. Interferon regulatory factor 3 as key element of the interferon signature in plasmacytoid dendritic cells from systemic lupus erythematosus patients: novel genetic associations in the Mexican mestizo population. *Clin Exp Immunol.* (2014) 178:428–37. doi: 10.1111/cei.12429
33. Fitzgerald DC, O'Brien K, Young A, Fonseca-Kelly Z, Rostami A, Gran B. Interferon regulatory factor (IRF) 3 is critical for the development of experimental autoimmune encephalomyelitis. *J Neuroinflammation* (2014) 11:130. doi: 10.1186/1742-2094-11-130
34. Liu Y, Jesus AA, Marrero B, Yang D, Ramsey SE, Sanchez GAM, et al. Activated STING in a vascular and pulmonary syndrome. *N Engl J Med.* (2014) 371:507–18. doi: 10.1056/NEJMoa1312625
35. Gall A, Treuting P, Elkon KB, Loo YM, Gale M, Barber GN, et al. Autoimmunity initiates in nonhematopoietic cells and progresses via lymphocytes in an interferon-dependent autoimmune disease. *Immunity* (2012) 36:120–31. doi: 10.1016/j.immuni.2011.11.018
36. King KR, Aguirre AD, Ye YX, Sun Y, Roh JD, Ng RP, et al. IRF3 and type I interferons fuel a fatal response to myocardial infarction. *Nat Med.* (2017) 23:12. doi: 10.1038/nm.4428
37. Wang L, Yao ZQ, Moorman JP, Xu Y, Ning S. Gene expression profiling identifies IRF4-associated molecular signatures in hematological malignancies. *PLoS ONE* (2014) 9:e106788. doi: 10.1371/journal.pone.0106788
38. Shaffer AL, Emre NC, Lamy L, Ngo VN, Wright G, Xiao W, et al. IRF4 addiction in multiple myeloma. *Nature* (2008) 454:226–31. doi: 10.1038/nature07064
39. Agnarelli A, Chevassut T, Mancini EJ. IRF4 in multiple myeloma-Biology, disease and therapeutic target. *LeukRes.* (2018) 72:52–8. doi: 10.1016/j.leukres.2018.07.025
40. Cherian MA, Olson S, Sundaramoorthi H, Cates K, Cheng X, Harding J, et al. An activating mutation of interferon regulatory factor 4 (IRF4) in adult T-cell leukemia. *J Biol Chem.* (2018) 293:6844–58. doi: 10.1074/jbc.RA117.000164
41. Man K, Gabriel SS, Liao Y, Gloury R, Preston S, Henstridge DC, et al. Transcription factor IRF4 promotes $CD8^+$ T cell exhaustion and limits the development of memory-like T cells during chronic infection. *Immunity* 47: 1129–41.e5. doi: 10.1016/j.immuni.2017.11.021
42. Okada Y, Wu D, Trynka G, Raj T, Terao C, Ikari K, et al. Genetics of rheumatoid arthritis contributes to biology and drug discovery. *Nature* (2014) 506:376–81. doi: 10.1038/nature12873
43. López-Isac E, Martín JE, Assassi S, Simeón CP, Carreira P, Ortego-Centeno N, et al. Brief report: IRF4 newly identified as a common susceptibility locus for systemic sclerosis and rheumatoid arthritis in a cross-disease meta-analysis of genome-wide association studies. *Arthritis Rheum.* (2016) 68:2338–44. doi: 10.1002/art.39730
44. Zucchero TM, Cooper ME, Maher BS, Daack-Hirsch S, Nepomuceno B, Ribeiro L, et al. Interferon regulatory factor 6 (IRF6) gene variants and the risk of isolated cleft lip or palate. *N Engl J Med.* (2004) 351:769–80. doi: 10.1056/NEJMoa032909
45. Kondo S, Schutte BC, Richardson RJ, Bjork BC, Knight AS, Watanabe Y, et al. Mutations in IRF6 cause Van der Woude and popliteal pterygium syndromes. *Nat Genet.* (2002) 32:285–9. doi: 10.1038/ng985
46. Fu Q, Zhao J, Qian X, Wong JL, Kaufman KM, Yu CY, et al. Association of a functional IRF7 variant with systemic lupus erythematosus. *Arthritis Rheum.* (2011) 63:749–54. doi: 10.1002/art.30193
47. Xu WD, Zhang YJ, Xu K, Zhai Y, Li BZ, Pan HF, et al. IRF7, a functional factor associates with systemic lupus erythematosus. *Cytokine* (2012) 58:317–20. doi: 10.1016/j.cyto.2012.03.003
48. Ning S, Pagano JS, Barber GN. IRF7: activation, regulation, modification and function. *Genes Immun.* (2011) 12:399–414. doi: 10.1038/gene.2011.21
49. Salloum R, Franek BS, Kariuki SN, Rhee L, Mikolaitis RA, Jolly M, et al. Genetic variation at the IRF7/PHRF1 locus is associated with autoantibody profile and serum interferon-alpha activity in lupus patients. *Arthritis Rheum.* (2010) 62:553–61. doi: 10.1002/art.27182
50. Heinig M, Petretto E, Wallace C, Bottolo L, Rotival M, Lu H, et al. A trans-acting locus regulates an anti-viral expression network and type 1 diabetes risk. *Nature* (2010) 467:460–4. doi: 10.1038/nature09386
51. Puthia M, Ambite I, Cafaro C, Butler D, Huang Y, Lutay N, et al. IRF7 inhibition prevents destructive innate immunity-a target for nonantibiotic therapy of bacterial infections. *Sci Transl Med.* (2016) 8:336ra59. doi: 10.1126/scitranslmed.aaf1156
52. Rezaei R, Mahmoudi M, Gharibdoost F, Kavosi H, Dashti N, Imeni V, et al. IRF7 gene expression profile and methylation of its promoter region in patients with systemic sclerosis. *Int J Rheum Dis.* (2017) 20:1551–61. doi: 10.1111/1756-185X.13175
53. Humblin E, Thibaudin M, Chalmin F, Derangère V, Limagne E, Richard C, et al. IRF8-dependent molecular complexes control the Th9 transcriptional program. *Nat Commun.* (2017) 8:2085. doi: 10.1038/s41467-017-01070-w
54. Baccala R, Gonzalez-Quintial R, Blasius AL, Rimann I, Ozato K, Kono DH, et al. Essential requirement for IRF8 and SLC15A4 implicates plasmacytoid dendritic cells in the pathogenesis of lupus. *Proc Natl Acad Sci USA.* (2013) 110:2940–5. doi: 10.1073/pnas.1222798110
55. Kim SH, Burton J, Yu CR, Sun L, He C, Wang H, et al. Dual function of the IRF8 transcription factor in autoimmune uveitis: loss of IRF8 in T cells exacerbates uveitis, whereas Irf8 deletion in the retina confers protection. *J Immunol.* (2015) 195:1480–8. doi: 10.4049/jimmunol.1500653
56. De Jager PL, Jia X, Wang J, de Bakker PI, Ottoboni L, Aggarwal NT, et al. et al., (2009). Meta-analysis of genome scans and replication identify *CD6, IRF8* and *TNFRSF1A* as new multiple sclerosis susceptibility loci. *Nat. Genet. 41:776–82.* doi: 10.1038/ng.401
57. Yoshida Y, Yoshimi R, Yoshii H, Kim D, Dey A, Xiong H, et al. The transcription factor IRF8 activates integrin-mediated TGF-β signaling and promotes neuroinflammation. *Immunity* (2014) 40:187–98. doi: 10.1016/j.immuni.2013.11.022
58. Ivashkiv LB, Donlin LT. Regulation of type I interferon responses. *Nat. Rev. Immunol.* (2014) 14:36–49. doi: 10.1038/nri3581
59. Nan J, Wang Y, Yang J, Stark GR. IRF9 and unphosphorylated STAT2 cooperate with NF-κB to drive IL6 expression. *Proc Natl Acad Sci USA.* (2018) 115:201714102. doi: 10.1073/pnas.1714102115
60. Tang L, Chen B, Ma B, Nie S. Association between IRF5 polymorphisms and autoimmune diseases: a meta-analysis. *Genet Mol Res.* (2014) 13:4473–85. doi: 10.4238/2014.June.16.6
61. Nordang GB, Viken MK, Amundsen SS, Sanchez ES, Flatø B, Førre OT, et al. Interferon regulatory factor 5 gene polymorphism confers risk to several rheumatic diseases and correlates with expression of alternative thymic transcripts. *Rheumatology* (2012) 51:619–26. doi: 10.1093/rheumatology/ker364
62. Cham CM, Ko K, Niewold TB. Interferon regulatory factor 5 in the pathogenesis of systemic lupus erythematosus. *Clin Dev Immunol.* (2012) 2012:780436. doi: 10.1155/2012/780436
63. Sigurdsson S, Nordmark G, Göring HH, Lindroos K, Wiman AC, Sturfelt G, et al. Polymorphisms in the tyrosine kinase 2 and interferon regulatory factor 5 genes are associated with systemic lupus erythematosus. *Am J Hum Genet.* (2005) 76:528–37. doi: 10.1086/428480
64. Li Y, Chen S, Li P, Wu Z, Li J, Liu B, et al. Association of the IRF5 rs2070197 polymorphism with systemic lupus erythematosus: a meta-analysis.*Clin Rheumatol.* (2015) 34:1495–501. doi: 10.1007/s10067-015-3036-5
65. Graham RR, Kyogoku C, Sigurdsson S, Vlasova IA, Davies LR, Baechler EC, et al. Three functional variants of IFN regulatory factor 5 (IRF5) define risk and protective haplotypes for human lupus. *Proc Natl Acad Sci USA.* (2007) 104:6758–63. doi: 10.1073/pnas.0701266104
66. Hellquist A, Järvinen TM, Koskenmies S, Zucchelli M, Orsmark-Pietras C, Berglind L, et al. Evidence for genetic association and interaction between the TYK2 and IRF5 genes in systemic lupus erythematosus. *J Rheumatol.* (2009) 36:1631–8. doi: 10.3899/jrheum.081160
67. Shu J, Li L, Zhou LB, Qian J, Fan ZD, Zhuang LL, et al. IRF5 is elevated in childhood-onset SLE and regulated by histone acetyltransferase

and histone deacetylase inhibitors. *Oncotarget* (2017) 8:47184–94. doi: 10.18632/oncotarget.17586

68. Stone RC, Feng D, Deng J, Singh S, Yang L, Fitzgerald-Bocarsly P, et al. Interferon regulatory factor 5 activation in monocytes of systemic lupus erythematosus patients is triggered by circulating autoantigens independent of type I interferons. *Arthritis Rheum.* (2012) 64:788–98. doi: 10.1002/art.33395
69. Stone RC, Du P, Feng D, Dhawan K, Rönnblom L, Eloranta ML, et al. RNA-Seq for enrichment and analysis of IRF5 transcript expression in SLE. *PLoS ONE* 8:e54487. doi: 10.1371/journal.pone.0054487
70. Feng D, Sangster-Guity N, Stone R, Korczeniewska J, Mancl ME, Fitzgerald-Bocarsly P, et al. Differential requirement of histone acetylase and deacetylase activities for IRF5-medicated proinflammatory cytokine expression. *J Immunol.* (2010) 185:6003–12. doi: 10.4049/jimmunol.1000482
71. Feng D, Stone RC, Eloranta ML, Sangster-Guity N, Nordmark G, Sigurdsson S, et al. Genetic variants and disease-associated factors contribute to enhanced interferon regulatory factor 5 expression in blood cells of patients with systemic lupus erythematosus. *Arthritis Rheum.* (2010) 62: 562–73. doi: 10.1002/art.27223
72. Feng D, Yang L, Bi X, Stone RC, Patel P, Barnes BJ. Protection of *Irf5*-deficient mice from pristane-induced lupus involves altered cytokine production and class switching. *Eur J Immunol.* (2012) 42:1477–87. doi: 10.1002/eji.201141642
73. Yasuda K, Richez C, Maciaszek JW, Agrawal N, Akira S, Marshak-Rothstein A, et al. Murine dendritic cell type I IFN production induced by human IgG-RNA immune complexes is IFN regulatory factor (IRF)5 and IRF7 dependent and is required for IL-6 production. *J Immunol.* (2007) 178:6876–85. doi: 10.4049/jimmunol.178.11.6876
74. Steinhagen F, McFarland AP, Rodriguez LG, Tewary P, Jarret A, Savan R, et al. IRF-5 and NF-κB p50 co-regulate IFN-β and IL-6 expression in TLR9-stimulated human plasmacytoid dendritic cells. *Eur J Immunol.* (2013) 43:1896–906. doi: 10.1002/eji.201242792
75. Ouyang X, Negishi H, Takeda R, Fujita Y, Taniguchi T, Honda K. Cooperation between MyD88 and TRIF pathways in TLR synergy via IRF5 activation. *Biochem Biophys Res Commun.* (2007) 354:1045–51. doi: 10.1016/j.bbrc.2007.01.090
76. Krausgruber T, Blazek K, Smallie T, Alzabin S, Lockstone H, Sahgal N, et al. IRF5 promotes inflammatory macrophage polarization and TH1-TH17 responses. *Nat Immunol.* (2011) 12:231–8. doi: 10.1038/ni.1990
77. Fabié A, Mai LT, Dagenais-Lussier X, Hammami A, van Grevenynghe J, Stäger S. IRF-5 promotes cell death in CD4 T cells during chronic infection. *Cell Rep.* (2018) 24:1163–75. doi: 10.1016/j.celrep.2018.06.107
78. Sy BT, Hoan NX, Tong HV, Meyer CG, Toan NL, Song LH, et al. Genetic variants of interferon regulatory factor 5 associated with chronic hepatitis B infection. *World J Gastroenterol.* (2018) 24:248–56. doi: 10.3748/wjg.v24.i2.248
79. Barnes BJ, Kellum MJ, Pinder KE, Frisancho JA, Pitha PM. Interferon regulatory factor 5, a novel mediator of cell cycle arrest and cell death. *Cancer Res.* (2003) 63:6424–31.
80. Masuda T, Iwamoto S, Yoshinaga R, Tozaki-Saitoh H, Nishiyama A, Mak TW, et al. Transcription factor IRF5 drives $P2X4R^{+}$-reactive microglia gating neuropathic pain. *Nat Commun.* (2014) 5:3771. doi: 10.1038/ncomms4771
81. Courties G, Heidt T, Sebas M, Iwamoto Y, Jeon D, Truelove J, et al. *In vivo* silencing of the transcription factor IRF5 reprograms the macrophage phenotype and improves infarct healing. *J Am Coll Cardiol.* (2014) 63:1556–66. doi: 10.1016/j.jacc.2013.11.023
82. Watkins AA, Yasuda K, Wilson GE, Aprahamian T, Xie Y, Maganto-Garcia E, et al. IRF5 deficiency ameliorates lupus but promotes atherosclerosis and metabolic dysfunction in a mouse model of lupus-associated atherosclerosis. *J Immunol.* (2015) 194:1467–79. doi: 10.4049/jimmunol.1402807
83. Bi X, Hameed M, Mirani N, Pimenta EM, Anari J, Barnes BJ. Loss of interferon regulatory factor 5 (IRF5) expression in human ductal carcinoma correlates with disease stage and contributes to metastasis. *Breast Cancer Res.* (2011) 13:R111. doi: 10.1186/bcr3053
84. Kreher S, Bouhlel MA, Cauchy P, Lamprecht B, Li S, Grau M, et al. Mapping of transcription factor motifs in active chromatin identifies IRF5 as key regulator in classical Hodgkin lymphoma. *Proc Natl Acad Sci USA.* (2014) 111:E4513–22. doi: 10.1073/pnas.1406985111
85. Pimenta EM, De S, Weiss R, Feng D, Hall K, Kilic S, et al. IRF5 is a novel regulator of CXCL13 expression in breast cancer that regulates CXCR5(+) B- and T-cell trafficking to tumor-conditioned media. *Immunol Cell Biol.* (2015) 93:486–99. doi: 10.1038/icb.2014.110
86. Garaud S, Willard-Gallo K IRF5: a rheostat for tumor-infiltrating lymphocyte trafficking in breast cancer? *Immunol. Cell Biol.* (2015) 93:425–6. doi: 10.1038/icb.2015.39
87. Cevik O, Li D, Baljinnyam E, Manvar D, Pimenta EM, Waris G, et al. Interferon regulatory factor 5 (IRF5) suppresses hepatitis C virus (HCV) replication and HCV-associated hepatocellular carcinoma. *J Biol Chem.* (2017) 292:21676–89. doi: 10.1074/jbc.M117.792721
88. Seneviratne AN, Edsfeldt A, Cole JE, Kassiteridi C, Swart M, Park I, et al. Interferon regulatory factor 5 controls necrotic core formation in atherosclerotic lesions by impairing efferocytosis. *Circulation* (2017) 136:1140–54. doi: 10.1161/CIRCULATIONAHA.117.027844
89. Alzaid F, Lagadec F, Albuquerque M, Ballaire R, Orliaguet L, Hainault I, et al. IRF5 governs liver macrophage activation that promotes hepatic fibrosis in mice and humans. *JCI Insight.* (2016) 1:e88689. doi: 10.1172/jci.insight.88689
90. Hall JL, Wei LN. Could silencing IRF5 improve healing of a myocardial infarct through the reprogramming of the macrophage population? *J Am Coll Cardiol.* (2014) 63:1567–8. doi: 10.1016/j.jacc.2013.11.024
91. Terashima T, Ogawa N, Nakae Y, Sato T, Katagi M, Okano J, et al. Gene therapy for neuropathic pain through siRNA-IRF5 gene delivery with homing peptides to microglia. *Mol Ther Nucleic Acids* (2018) 11:203–15. doi: 10.1016/j.omtn.2018.02.007
92. Li J, Liu Y, Xu H, Fu Q. Nanoparticle-delivered IRF5 siRNA facilitates M1 to M2 transition, reduces demyelination and neurofilament loss, and promotes functional recovery after spinal cord injury in mice. *Inflammation* (2016) 39:1704–17. doi: 10.1007/s10753-016-0405-4
93. Weiss M, Byrne AJ, Blazek K, Saliba DG, Pease JE, Perocheau D, et al. IRF5 controls both acute and chronic inflammation. *Proc Natl Acad Sci USA.* (2015) 112:11001–6. doi: 10.1073/pnas.1506254112
94. Yu X, Wei B, Dai Y, Zhang M, Wu J, Xu X, et al. Genetic polymorphism of interferon regulatory factor 5 (IRF5) correlates with allograft acute rejection of liver transplantation. *PLoS ONE* (2014) 9:e94426. doi: 10.1371/journal.pone.0094426
95. Wang C, Rose-Zerilli MJ, Koppelman GH, Sandling JK, Holloway JW, Postma DS, et al. Evidence of association between interferon regulatory factor 5 gene polymorphisms and asthma. *Gene* (2012) 504:220–5. doi: 10.1016/j.gene.2012.05.021
96. Oriss TB, Raundhal M, Morse C, Huff RE, Das S, Hannum R, et al. IRF5 distinguishes severe asthma in humans and drives Th1 phenotype and airway hyperreactivity in mice. *JCI Insight* (2017) 2:e91019. doi: 10.1172/jci.insight.91019
97. Byrne AJ, Weiss M, Mathie SA, Walker SA, Eames HL, Saliba D, et al. A critical role for IRF5 in regulating allergic airway inflammation. *Mucosal Immunol.* (2017) 10:716–26. doi: 10.1038/mi.2016.92
98. Hu G, Mancl M, Barnes BJ. Signaling through IFN regulatory factor-5 sensitizes p53-deficient tumors to DNA damage-induced apoptosis and cell death. *Canc Res.* (2005) 65:7403–12. doi: 10.1158/0008-5472.CAN-05-0583
99. Babaian A, Romanish MT, Gagnier L, Kuo LY, Karimi MM, Steidl C, et al. Onco-exaptation of an endogenous retroviral LTR drives IRF5 expression in Hodgkin lymphoma. *Oncogene* (2015) 35:2542–6. doi: 10.1038/onc.2015.308
100. Qin BY, Liu C, Lam SS, Srinath H, Delston R, Correia JJ, et al. Crystal structure of IRF-3 reveals mechanism of autoinhibition and virus-induced phosphoactivation. *Nat Struct Bio.* (2003) 10:913–21. doi: 10.1038/nsb1002
101. Barnes BJ, Kellum MJ, Field AE, Pitha PM. Multiple regulatory domains of IRF-5 control activation, cellular localization, and induction of chemokines that mediate recruitment of T lymphocytes. *Mol Cell Biol.* (2002) 22:5721–40. doi: 10.1128/MCB.22.16.5721-5740.2002
102. Lin R, Mamane Y, Hiscott J. A role for casein kinase II phosphorylation in the regulation of IRF-1 transcriptional activity. *Mol Cell Biochem.* (1999) 191:169–80. doi: 10.1023/A:1006850009017
103. Barnes BJ, Moore PA, Pitha PM. Virus-specific activation of novel interferon regulatoy factor-5, results in the induction of distinct interferon alpha genes. *J Biol Chem.* (2001) 276:23382–90. doi: 10.1074/jbc.M101216200

104. Mancl ME, Hu G, Sangster-Guity N, Olshalsky SL, Hoops K, Fitzgerald-Bocarsly P, et al. Two discrete promoters regulate the alternatively spliced human interferon regulatory factor-5 isoforms. Multiple isoforms with distinct cell type-specific expression, localization, regulation, and function. *J Biol Chem.* (2005) 280:21078–90. doi: 10.1074/jbc.M500543200

105. Schoenemeyer A, Barnes BJ, Mancl ME, Latz E, Goutagny N, Pitha PM, et al. The interferon regulatory factor, IRF5, is a central mediator of toll-like receptor 7 signaling. *J Bio Chem.* (2005) 280:17005–12. doi: 10.1074/jbc.M412584200

106. Martin HJ, Lee JM, Walls D, Hayward SD. Manipulation of the toll-like receptor 7 signaling pathway by Epstein-Barr virus. *J Virol.* (2007) 81:9748–58. doi: 10.1128/JVI.01122-07

107. Yang L, Zhao T, Shi X, Nakhaei P, Wang Y, Sun Q, et al. Functional analysis of a dominant negative mutation of interferon regulatory factor 5. *PLoS ONE* (2009) 4:e5500. doi: 10.1371/journal.pone.0005500

108. Ren Z, Wang Y, Tao D, Liebenson D, Liggett T, Goswami R, et al. Overexpression of the dominant-negative form of interferon regulatory factor 1 in oligodendrocytes protects against experimental autoimmune encephalomyelitis. *J Neurosci.* (2011) 31:8329–41. doi: 10.1523/JNEUROSCI.1028-11.2011

109. Kim TY, Lee KH, Chang S, Chung C, Lee HW, Yim J, et al. Oncogenic potential of a dominant negative mutant of interferon regulatory factor 3. *J Biol Chem.* (2003) 278:15272–8. doi: 10.1074/jbc.M205792200

110. Ning S, Huye LE, Pagano JS. Interferon regulatory factor 5 represses expression of the Epstein-Barr Virus oncoprotein LMP1: braking of the IRF7/LMP1 regulatory circuit. *J Virol.* (2005) 79:11671–6. doi: 10.1128/JVI.79.18.11671-11676.2005

111. Demartino J, Fotouhi N, Hoffman A, Huang K-S, Milletti F, Panicker S, et al. *Cell Penetrating Peptides Which Bind to IRF5.* US Patent No WO20145056813A1. Nutley, NJ: U.S. Patent and Trademark Office (2016).

112. Barnes BJ. *Cell Penetrating Peptides that Inhibit IRF5 Nuclear Localization.* U.S. Patent No WO2017/044855A2. New Brunswick, NJ: U.S. Patent and Trademark Office (2017).

113. Takahasi K, Suzuki NN, Horiuchi M, Mori M, Suhara W, Okabe Y, et al. X-ray crystal structure of IRF-3 and its functional implications. *Nat Struct Biol.* (2003) 10:922–7. doi: 10.1038/nsb1001

114. Izaguirre A, Barnes BJ, Amrute S, Yeow WS, Megjugorac N, Dai J, et al. Comparative analysis of IRF and IFN-alpha expression in human plasmacytoid and monocyte-derived dendritic cells. *J Leukoc Biol.* (2003) 74:1125–38. doi: 10.1189/jlb.0603255

115. Ikushima H, Negishi H, Taniguchi T. The IRF family transcription factors at the interface of innate and adaptive immune responses. *Cold Spring Harb Symp Quant Biol.* (2013) 78:105–16. doi: 10.1101/sqb.2013.78.020321

116. Ban T, Sato GR, Nishiyama A, Akiyama A, Takasuna M, Umehara M, et al. Lyn kinase suppresses the transcriptional activity of IRF5 in the TLR-MyD88 pathway to restrain the development of autoimmunity. *Immunity* (2016) 45:319–32. doi: 10.1016/j.immuni.2016.07.015

117. Gillen JG, Nita-Lazar A. Composition of the myddosome during the innate immune response. *J Immunol.* (2017) 198.

118. Ren J, Chen X, Chen ZJ. IKKβ is an IRF5 kinase that instigates inflammation. *PNAS* (2014) 111:17438–43. doi: 10.1073/pnas.1418516111

119. Lopez-Pelaez M, Lamont DJ, Peggie M, Shpiro N, Gray NS, Cohen P. Protein kinase IKKβ-catalyzed phosphorylation of IRF5 at Ser462 induces its dimerization and nuclear translocation in myeloid cells. *PNAS* (2014) 111:17432–7. doi: 10.1073/pnas.1418399111

120. Kawasaki T, Kawai T. Toll-like receptor signaling pathways. *Front Immunol.* (2014) 5:461. doi: 10.3389/fimmu.2014.00461

121. Moynagh PN. TLR signalling and activation of IRFs: revisiting old friends from the NF-κB pathway. *Trends Immunol.* (2005) 26:469–76. doi: 10.1016/j.it.2005.06.009

122. Bergstrøm B, Aune MH, Awuh JA, Kojen JF, Blix KJ, Ryan L, et al. TLR8 senses *Staphylococcus aureus* RNA in human primary monocytes and macrophages and induces IFN-β production via a TAK1-IKKβ-IRF5 signaling pathway. *J Immunol.* (2015) 195:1100–11. doi: 10.4049/jimmunol.1403176

123. Cushing L, Winkler A, Jelinsky SA, Lee K, Korver W, Hawtin R, et al. IRAK4 kinase activity controls toll-like receptor–induced inflammation through the transcription factor IRF5 in primary human monocytes. *J Biol Chem.* (2017) 292:18689–98. doi: 10.1074/jbc.M117.796912

124. Xu D, Meyer F, Ehlers E, Blasnitz L, Zhang L. Interferon regulatory factor 4 (IRF-4) targets IRF-5 to regulate Epstein-Barr virus transformation. *J Biol Chem.* (2011) 286:18261–7. doi: 10.1074/jbc.M110.210542

125. Lech M, Weidenbusch M, Kulkarni OP, Ryu M, Darisipudi MN, Susanti HE, et al. IRF4 deficiency abrogates lupus nephritis despite enhancing systemic cytokine production. *J Am Soc Nephrol.* (2011) 22:1443–52. doi: 10.1681/ASN.2010121260

126. Negishi H, Ohba Y, Yanai H, Takaoka A, Honma K, Yui K, et al. Negative regulation of Toll-like-receptor signaling by IRF-4. *PNAS* (2005) 102:15989–94. doi: 10.1073/pnas.0508327102

127. Cohen P. The TLR and IL-1 signalling network at a glance. *J Cell Sci.* (2014) 127(Pt 11):2383–90. doi: 10.1242/jcs.149831

128. Clark K, Takeuchi O, Akira S, Cohen P. The TRAF-associated protein TANK facilitates cross-talk within the IκB kinase family during Toll-like receptor signaling. *Proc Natl Acad Sci USA.* (2011) 108:17093–8. doi: 10.1073/pnas.1114194108

129. Lazzari E, Korczeniewska J, Ní Gabhann J, Smith S, Barnes BJ, Jefferies CA. TRIpartite motif 21 (TRIM21) differentially regulates the stability of interferon regulatory factor 5 (IRF5) isoforms. *PLoS ONE* (2014) 9:e103609. doi: 10.1371/journal.pone.0103609

130. Masumi A. Histone acetyltransferases as regulators of nonhistone proteins: the role of interferon regulatory factor acetylation on gene transcription. *J Biomed Biotechnol.* (2011) 2011:640610. doi: 10.1155/2011/640610

131. Balkhi MY, Fitzgerald KA, Pitha PM. Functional regulation of MyD88-activated interferon regulatory factor 5 by K63-linked polyubiquitination. *Mol Cell Biol.* (2008) 28:7296–308. doi: 10.1128/MCB.00662-08

132. Chang Foreman HC, Van Scoy S, Cheng TF, Reich NC. Activation of interferon regulatory factor 5 by site specific phosphorylation. *PLoS ONE* (2012) 7:e33098. doi: 10.1371/journal.pone.0033098

133. Balkhi MY, Fitzgerald KA, Pitha PM. IKKalpha negatively regulates IRF-5 function in a MyD88-TRAF6 pathway. *Cell Signal.* (2010) 22:117–27. doi: 10.1016/j.cellsig.2009.09.021

134. Sun K, He SB, Qu JG, Dang SC, Chen JX, Gong AH, et al. IRF5 regulates lung macrophages M2 polarization during severe acute pancreatitis *in vitro*. *World J Gastroenterol.* (2016) 22:9368–77. doi: 10.3748/wjg.v22.i42.9368

135. Gao S, Li X, Nie S, Yang L, Tu L, Dong B, et al. An AAAG-rich oligodeoxynucleotide rescues mice from bacterial septic peritonitis by interfering interferon regulatory factor 5. *Int J Mol Sci.* (2017) 18:1034. doi: 10.3390/ijms18051034

136. Wei Z, Yan L, Chen Y, Bao C, Deng J, Deng J. Mangiferin inhibits macrophage classical activation via downregulating interferon regulatory factor 5 expression. *Mol Med Rep.* (2016) 14:1091–8. doi: 10.3892/mmr.2016.5352

137. Tanaka N, Ishihara M, Kitagawa M, Harada H, Kimura T, Matsuyama T, et al. Cellular commitment to oncogene-induced transformation or apoptosis is dependent on the transcription factor IRF-1. *Cell* (1994) 77:829–39. doi: 10.1016/0092-8674(94)90132-5

138. Ren G, Cui K, Zhang Z, Zhao K. Division of labor between IRF1 and IRF2 in regulating different stages of transcriptional activation in cellular antiviral activities. *Cell Biosci.* (2015) 5:17. doi: 10.1186/s13578-015-0007-0

139. Harada H, Willison K, Sakakibara J, Miyamoto M, Fujita T, Taniguchi T. Absence of the type I IFN system in EC cells: transcriptional activator (IRF-1) and repressor (IRF-2) genes are developmentally regulated. *Cell* (1990) 63:303–12. doi: 10.1016/0092-8674(90)90163-9

140. Sakai T, Mashima H, Yamada Y, Goto T, Sato W. The roles of interferon regulatory factors 1 and 2 in the progression of human pancreatic cancer. *Pancreas* (2014) 43:909–16. doi: 10.1097/MPA.0000000000000116

141. Alexander L, Denekamp L, Knapp A, Auerbach MR, Damania B, Desrosiers RC. The primary sequence of rhesus monkey rhadinovirus isolate 26–95: sequence similarities to Kaposi's sarcoma-associated herpesvirus and rhesus monkey rhadinovirus isolate. *J Virol.* (2000) 74:3388–98. doi: 10.1128/JVI.74.7.3388-3398.2000
142. Melroe GT, Silva L, Schaffer PA, Knipe DM. Recruitment of activated IRF-3 and CBP/p300 to herpes simplex virus ICP0 nuclear foci: potential role in blocking IFN-β induction. *Virology* (2007) 360:305–21. doi: 10.1016/j.virol.2006.10.028

5

IRF4 and IRGs Delineate Clinically Relevant Gene Expression Signatures in Systemic Lupus Erythematosus and Rheumatoid Arthritis

Javier Rodríguez-Carrio [1,2,3], Patricia López [1,2], Mercedes Alperi-López [2,4], Luis Caminal-Montero [2,5], Francisco J. Ballina-García [2,4] and Ana Suárez [1,2]*

[1] Area of Immunology, Department of Functional Biology, Faculty of Medicine, University of Oviedo, Oviedo, Spain, [2] Instituto de Investigación Sanitaria del Principado de Asturias (ISPA), Oviedo, Spain, [3] Bone and Mineral Research Unit, REDinREN del ISCIII, Hospital Universitario Central de Asturias, Oviedo, Spain, [4] Department of Rheumatology, Hospital Universitario Central de Asturias, Oviedo, Spain, [5] Department of Internal Medicine, Hospital Universitario Central de Asturias, Oviedo, Spain

Correspondence:
Javier Rodríguez-Carrio
rodriguezcjavier@uniovi.es

Introduction: Overactivation of the type I interferon (IFN) signature has been observed in several systemic autoimmune conditions, such as Systemic Lupus Erythematosus (SLE) or Rheumatoid Arthritis (RA). Impaired control of Interferon-Responding Genes (IRGs) expression by their regulatory mechanisms, including Interferon Regulatory Factors (IRFs), may underlie these findings and it may explain the heterogeneity observed among these conditions. In the present study we aimed to evaluate the associations between IRF4 gene expression and those of IRGs in SLE and RA patients to gain insight about its links with the IFN signature as well as to explore the potential clinical relevance of these associations.

Methods: The gene expression of IRF4 and IRGs (IFI44, IFI44L, IFI6, and MX1) in peripheral blood was analyzed in 75 SLE patients, 98 RA patients, and 28 healthy controls. A group of 13 biological-naïve RA patients was prospectively followed upon TNFα-blockade. The associations among IRF4 and IRGs were evaluated by principal component analyses (PCA), correlations and network analyses. Publicly available datasets were used for replication.

Results: A broad activation of IRGs was observed in autoimmune patients, although certain heterogeneity can be distinguished, whereas IRF4 was only upregulated in RA. The differential expression of IRF4 in RA was then confirmed in publicly available gene expression datasets. PCA revealed different associations among IRF4 and IRGs in each condition, which was later confirmed by correlation and network analyses. Cluster analysis identified 3 gene expression signatures on the basis of IRF4 and IRGs expression which were differentially used by SLE and RA patients. Cluster III was associated with markers of disease severity in SLE patients. Cluster II, hallmarked by IRF4 upregulation, was linked to clinical stage and mild disease course in RA. TNFα-blockade led to changes in the association between IRF4 and IRGs, whereas increasing IRF4 expression was associated with a good clinical outcome in RA.

Conclusions: The differential expression of IRF4 and IRGs observed in SLE and RA can delineate gene expression signatures associated with clinical features and treatment outcomes. These results support a clinically-relevant phenomenon of shaping of the IFN signature by IRF4 in autoimmune patients.

Keywords: interferon, IFN signature, autoimmunity, systemic lupus erythematosus, arthritis, biomarker

INTRODUCTION

The type I interferons (IFNs) are pleiotropic mediators that play a critical role as regulators of innate and adaptive immune responses (1, 2). Signaling through the type I IFN pathway leads to an increased expression of several IFN-responding genes (IRGs). This global expression profile has been termed as the "IFN signature" (3). There is a compelling body of evidence linking the type I IFNs and the presence of the IFN signature to systemic autoimmune conditions in peripheral blood and target tissues (4–6). Either as biomarkers or as disease targets, several studies have been focused on the role of IRGs and the IFN signature in these rheumatic conditions (7). The identification of biomarkers to assist in patient stratification and therapy response is of upmost relevance in these complex conditions, in order to resolve the clinical heterogeneity that hallmarks these diseases (8, 9). This is especially important for decision-making regarding biological treatments, due to their high costs and moderate clinical response in unselected patient populations (10–13).

Type I IFN production is tightly controlled at the gene expression level in a highly ordered process regulated by multiple transcription factors (14). Then, the aberrant IRG expression in autoimmunity may be caused, at least in part, by an impaired activity of their regulatory factors. However, the mechanisms underlying the abnormal triggering and perpetuation of the type I IFN signature in these conditions are poorly characterized. In recent years, the role of Interferon Regulatory Factors (IRFs) has emerged. IRFs are a family of transcription factors that modulate immune responses through various molecular events related to the IFN signaling pathway (15, 16). Among IRFs, IRF1, IRF3, IRF5, and IRF7 have been previously demonstrated to act as regulators of type I IFNs and IRGs transcription (14). IRF1 was the first family member discovered to activate type I IFN gene promoters (17), although further studies found that type I IFN signaling can be observed in $Irf1^{-/-}$ mouse models (18). Later, IRF5 was linked to the expression of type I IFNs. Indeed, gene variants at the IRF5 loci, which are related to autoimmune disease susceptibility, were found to correlate with type I IFN signature (19). Nevertheless, further studies suggest that IRF5 is dispensable for IRGs induction (20). In recent years, IRF3 and IRF7 have been also related to IRGs responses (21–23), acting as negative regulators, this effect being related to the NFkB pathway (24). However, a recent study has challenged this observation (24). Importantly, by targeting IRF3 and IRF7 signaling, only a partial effect on type I IFNs was observed, hence suggesting that additional mediators could be involved (24). Overall, although there is some evidence that IRFs can modulate the IFN signature, the current evidence is scarce. Nevertheless, despite less attention has been paid in early studies, the potential involvement of other family member, the IRF4, has emerged. More importantly, whether these molecular events play any role in the context of autoimmunity remains unknown.

IRF4 is required for proper maturation and differentiation of immune cells (25, 26). IRF4 is expressed in dendritic cells, monocytes/macrophages, granulocytes and B-cells (27), all cell subsets relevant for IFN signature in autoimmunity (28). Moreover, IRF4 loci has been found to be associated with genetic susceptibility to systemic autoimmune diseases (29, 30). Of note, IRF4 has been also related to NFkB pathway (31). Additionally, IRF4 has been revealed to interact with MyD88, an adaptor protein crucial for the activation of IRGs (32).

All these lines of evidence point to IRF4 as a relevant player for IRGs activation and thus, IFN signature in autoimmunity. Taken all these ideas into account, we hypothesize that IRF4 activation could be related to IRGs expression in systemic autoimmune conditions and that different gene expression signatures may be identified on the basis of their associations. Thus, in the present study we aimed to assess the IRF4 gene expression in SLE, RA patients and HC in order to evaluate (i) its association with IRGs expression in these conditions, (ii) the clinical relevance of IRF4 and IRGs in each condition, and (iii) the changes in IRF4 expression upon TNFα-blockade.

MATERIALS AND METHODS

Ethical Approval

The study was approved by the Institutional Review Board (Comité de Ética de Investigación Clínica del Principado de Asturias, reference PI16/00113) in compliance with the Declaration of Helsinki. Written informed consent was signed from all study subjects prior to study entry.

Abbreviations: ACR, American College of Rheumatology; ACPA, anti-citrullinated peptide antibodies; ANA, antinuclear antibodies; csDMARDs, conventional synthetic DMARDs; DAS28, disease activity score 28-joints; DMARDs, disease-modifying antirheumatic drugs; ENA, extractable nuclear antigens; EULAR, European league against rheumatism; ESR, erythrocyte sedimentation rate; HAQ, health assessment questionnaire; HC, healthy controls; IFI6, interferon alpha inducible protein 6; IFI44, interferon induced protein 44; IFI44L, interferon induced protein 44 like; IFN, interferon; IRF, interferon regulatory factor; IRG, interferon-responding gene; MX1, MX dynamin like GTPase 1; NSAIDs, non-steroidal anti-inflammatory drugs; RA, rheumatoid arthritis; RF, rheumatoid factor; SLE, systemic lupus erythematosus; RNP, ribonucleoproteins; RibP, ribosomal P protein; SLEDAI, systemic lupus erythematosus disease activity index; TNFα, tumor necrosis factor alpha.

Patients and Controls

Our study involved 75 SLE patients [age median 48.40 (range 27–75) years, 70 women], 98 RA patients [age median 52.93 (range 22–87) years, 79 women] and 28 age- and gender-matched healthy volunteers (HC) [age median 49.38 (range 35–60) years, 20 women] recruited from the same population. Additionally, a group of 13 biologicals-naïve RA patients [12 women, age median age 43 (range 30–65), DAS28 5.08(1.93), 38.5% RF+, 46.1% ACPA+], candidates for TNFα-blockers was recruited and prospectively followed up for 3 months. A blood sample was collected from all study subjects by venipuncture. In the prospective study, a blood sample was obtained before (baseline, BL) and 3-months after the initiation of the TNFα-blockade therapy (post-treatment, PT). SLE patients were recruited from the outpatient clinic of the Autoimmune Disease Unit [Department of Internal Medicine, Hospital Universitario Central de Asturias (HUCA)] and fulfilled the American College of Rheumatology (ACR) revised criteria for the SLE classification (33). RA patients were enrolled from the Department of Rheumatology (HUCA) and fulfilled the 2010 ACR/EULAR classification criteria (34). A complete clinical examination, including disease activity score calculation [SLE Disease Activity Index (SLEDAI) or Disease Activity Score 28-joints (DAS28), respectively] was performed on all patients during the clinical appointment at their respective departments. Information on further clinical features, including disease-related autoantibodies and treatments (received during the previous 3 months before sampling) were registered from medical records. RA patients recruited at onset and not being previously exposed to treatments were classified as very early RA (VERA). The clinical response of RA patients upon TNFα-blockade was evaluated by EULAR criteria (35). Patients exhibiting a good response (R) were compared to those with moderate or no response (NR).

RNA Isolation and RT-PCR

Blood samples were immediately processed after collection as previously described (36). Whole blood was mixed with RNA Stabilization Reagent for Blood/Bone Marrow (Roche, Germany) for stabilization and stored at −20°C, in compliance with the instructions provided by the manufacturer. Next, samples were thawed at room temperature and mRNA was isolated using the mRNA Isolation Kit for Blood/Bone Marrow (Roche), according to the protocol provided by the manufacturer. Reverse Transcription (RT) was performed using a High-Capacity cDNA Reverse Transcription Kit (Applied Biosystems).

Gene Expression Assays

A number of IRG was selected from previous studies in the field using peripheral blood (37–41) and later validated in a factor analysis as those that best reflect the global IFN signature (42, 43). Gene expression was evaluated by Real-Time PCR with pre-designed TaqMan Gene Expression Assays (Applied Biosystems, Germany) for the following genes: IRF4 (interferon regulatory factor 4, reference Hs00180031_m1), IFI44 (interferon induced protein 44, reference Hs00197427_m1), IFI44L (interferon induced protein 44 like, reference Hs00915292_m1), MX1 (MX dynamin like GTPase 1, reference Hs00895608_m1), and IFI6 (interferon alpha inducible protein 6, reference Hs00242571_m1). Reactions were performed in TaqMan Gene Expression Master Mix (Applied Biosystems). Real-Time quantitative PCR was performed in an ABI Prism HT7900 (Applied Biosystems) instrument and Ct values were analyzed with the software SDS 2.3. All samples were assayed by triplicate and the average was used. Expression level was evaluated by the $2^{-\Delta Ct}$ method, using the GAPDH gene expression as housekeeping to normalize Ct values. The expression levels were log-transformed and Z-scores were calculated for each gene from the distribution observed in the whole population.

Statistical Analysis

Continuous variables were summarized as median (interquartile range), whereas *n*(%) was used for categorical ones. Differences among groups were analyzed by Kruskal-Wallis (with Dunn-Bonferroni correction for multiple comparisons if significant differences were observed), Wilcoxon test for paired analises or chi-squared tests, according to the distribution of the variables. Correlations were assessed by Spearman ranks' test. Principal Component Analysis (matrix correlation method) was performed with the individual gene expression data and biplots were generated to evaluate the associations among individual genes. Correlograms and network analyses were built to analyze the correlations among genes as well as to visualize the associations among them in the different conditions. A cluster analysis was performed based on squared euclidean distances and Ward's Minimum Variance Method to identify clusters minimizing the loss of information. The R package *heatmap.2* was used to generate the corresponding heatmap. A Correspondence Analysis was used to explore the simultaneous associations among categorical variables (clusters identified vs. disease groups). Since important differences in sizes were observed, the weighted chi-square distance was selected. For the validation of our results, gene expression datasets were downloaded from the publicly available NCBI Gene Expression Omnibus (GEO) repository (44). First, IRF4 expression was checked to be differentially regulated in the patient groups using the GEO2R tool (using *GEOquery* and *limma* R packages) and the corresponding adjusted *p*-value [multiple testing and false discovery rate corrections by the Benjamini & Hochberg method (45)] was calculated. Next, target data were downloaded and presented in graphs (analysis by conventional tests). A $p < 0.050$ was considered as statistically significant. Statistical analyses were performed in SPSS 22.0 (IBM SPSS, NY, USA), R 3.3.1 (R Project) and GraphPad Prism 5.0 (La Jolla, CA, USA) for Windows.

RESULTS

IRF4 and IRGs Expression in SLE and RA Patients

The expression of IRF4 and four IRGs (IFI44, IFI44L, IFI6, and MX1) was quantified in 75 SLE patients (**Supplementary Table 1**), 98 RA patients (**Supplementary Table 2**) and 28 HC. All IRGs were increased in autoimmune patients, to a higher degree in SLE (**Figure 1**). IRF4 expression was found to be increased in RA patients compared

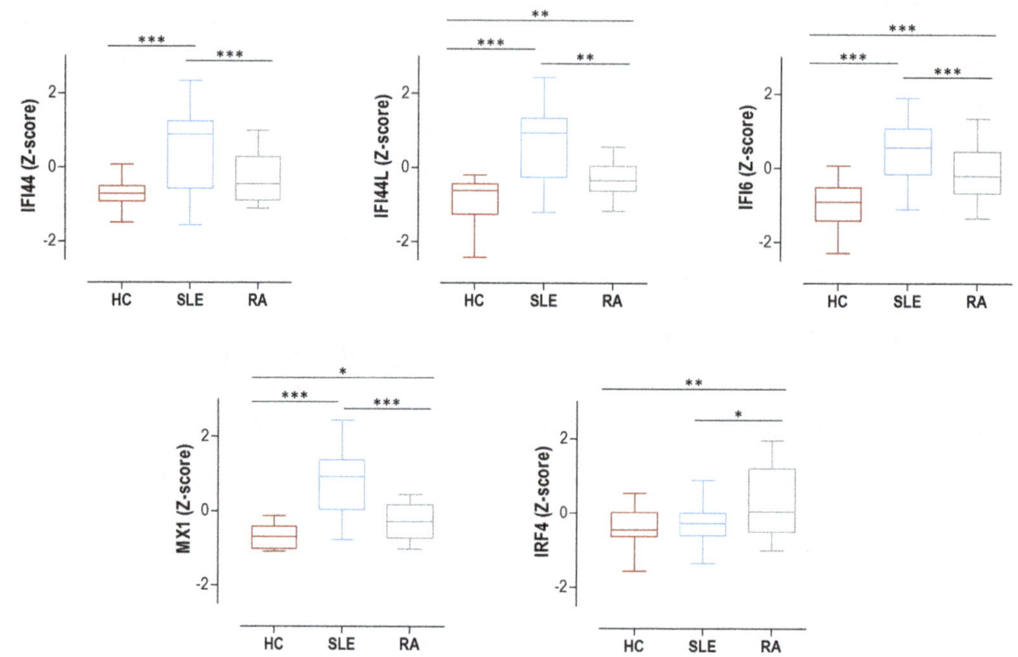

FIGURE 1 | Expression of IRF4 and IRGs in SLE, RA patients and HC. IRF4 and IRGs (IFI44, IFI44L, IFI6, and MX1) gene expression in HC (dark red boxes) ($n = 28$), SLE patients (blue boxes) ($n = 75$), and RA patients (gray boxes) ($n = 98$). Results are shown as box plots, where the boxes represent the 25th and 75th percentiles, the lines within the boxes representing the median, and the lines outside the boxes represent the minimum and maximum values. Differences were assessed by Kruskal-Wallis with Dunn-Bonferroni tests for multiple comparisons. *P*-values correspond to those obtained in the multiple comparisons tests and are indicated as follows: *$p < 0.050$, **$p < 0.010$, and ***$p < 0.001$.

to both SLE patients and HC (**Figure 1**). No differences on IRF4 expression by seropositivity status were found in RA patients (**Supplementary Figure 1**).

To evaluate whether differences in peripheral blood cell composition may account for the differences observed in the expression of IRF4 and IRGs, multiple regression models including the frequency of monocytes, lymphocytes and neutrophils as covariables were carried out for each gene expression. None of the cell populations analyzed were related to gene expression in any condition (all $p > 0.050$, data not shown), hence ruling out the possibility that a differential cell composition underlie these findings.

All these results support a broad activation of IRGs in autoimmune patients, especially in SLE, whereas IRF4 expression was only increased in RA.

IRF4 and IRGs Expression: Global Analysis and Cluster Approach

Based on our previous findings, we aimed to evaluate whether distinct associations between IRF4 and IRGs may underlie the differences observed among RA and SLE patients, leading to the identification of global gene expression signatures.

First, we conducted a PCA with the IRF4 and IRGs expression. PCA revealed a good adequacy of the data (KMO = 0.741, Barlett' spherificity test $p = 8.240{\cdot}10^{-208}$) and identified 2 components that accounted for 90.43% of the total variance. The biplot generated (**Figure 2A**) showed that, although certain degree of overlap existed, different global signatures could be distinguished. Whereas, patients (both SLE and RA) exhibited a different distribution than HC regarding PC1 (horizontal axis), SLE and RA patients diverged from each other in PC2 (vertical axis), hence suggesting that the associations among genes could differ among groups. Then, the associations among IRF4 and IRGs were plotted in correlation graphs (**Figure 2B**). This approach confirmed that gene expression patterns were not homogenous, but different pictures can be distinguished, especially regarding the role of IRF4 and the overall degree of correlation. On the one hand, both SLE and RA exhibited a higher degree of correlation among genes than that of observed in HC. Interestingly, stronger correlations were observed for IRF4 expression in RA, whereas the same was applied to MX1 in SLE. Network graphs plotted to visualize the mutual interactions among independent genes revealed different structures among groups, IRGs following different grouping patterns and IRF4 exhibiting a different relative position depending on disease status (**Figure 2C**). A weaker network was observed in HC, strong correlations being only found among IFI44L, IFI6, and MX1. SLE patients exhibited strong correlations among IFI44, IFI44L, IFI6, and MX1, whereas IRF4 lay apart from this cluster of genes. A different picture was observed in RA, with a concentric network hallmarked by a higher and more uniform degree of correlation among all genes analyzed. These results strengthened our previous observations.

Finally, we performed an unsupervised cluster analysis to assess whether these differences could delineate gene expression signatures related to disease status. Cluster analysis (**Figure 3A**)

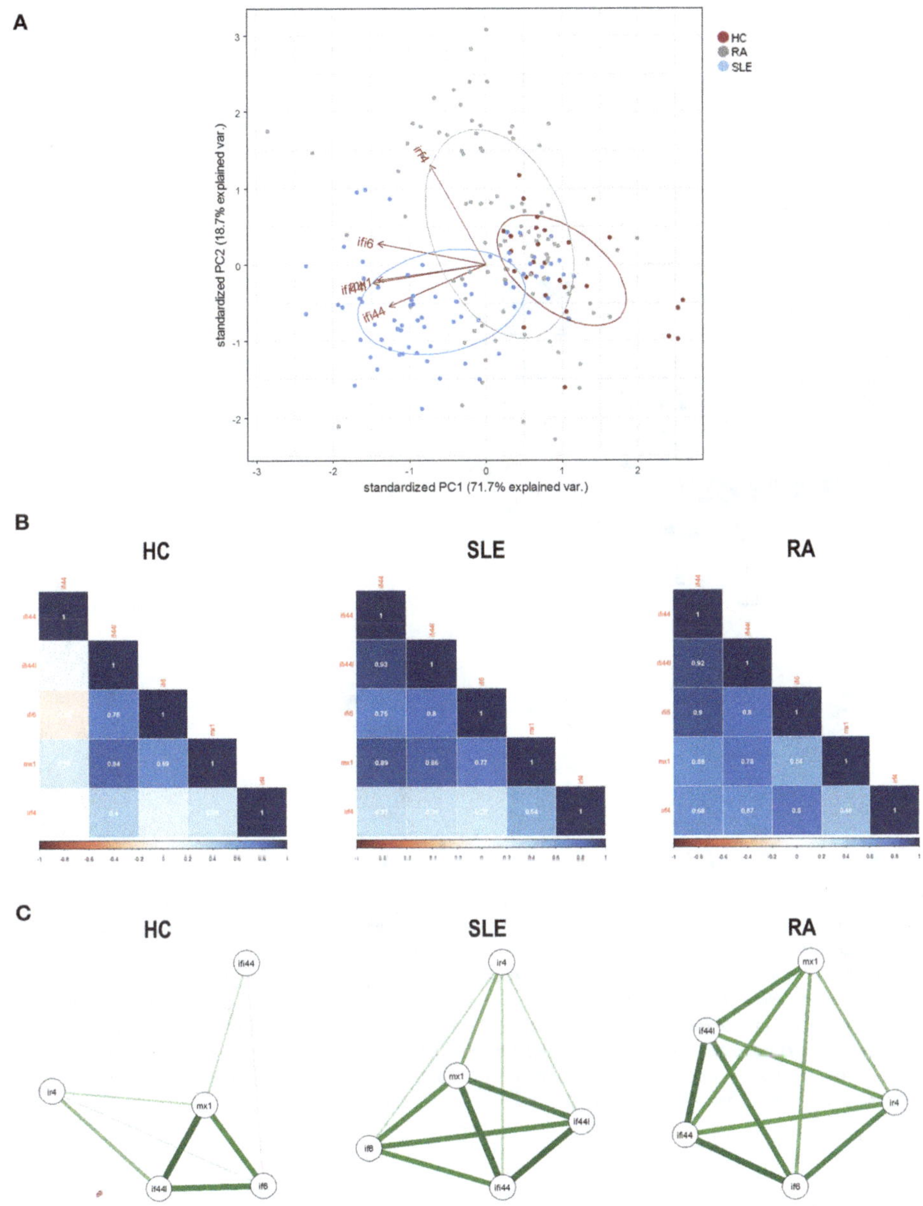

FIGURE 2 | Associations among IRF4 and IRGs in autoimmune patients and HC. **(A)** Biplot originated from the PCA (correlation matrix method) conducted on the study groups recruited [HC (dark), SLE (blue), and RA (gray)]. Arrows delineate the associations among the original variables entered in the analysis (IRF4 and IRGs expression). **(B)** Analysis of the correlations among IRF4 and IRG in the different study groups. Correlation matrices were plotted in correlograms, where the color of the tiles is proportional to the strength of the correlation between each pair of genes. Correlation coefficients were depicted in white. **(C)** Network analyses depicted based on the IRF4 and IRGs expression in the different study groups. Each node corresponds to a single gene and the lines between nodes illustrate the strength (width) and type (green: positive, red: negative) of the correlations between each pair of genes. The relative position of the nodes parallels its degree of correlation that is, nodes more closely correlated locate closer to each other. The architecture defined by IRF4 and IRGs differed among conditions and it went from a weaker structure in HC toward a more concentric and uniform network in RA. The different genes analyzed followed different grouping patterns among disease status.

revealed 3 independent clusters: cluster I, characterized by a low expression of all genes analyzed; cluster II, characterized by a medium expression of IRGs and a high expression of IRF4, and cluster III, characterized by an enhanced expression of IRGs and a low expression of IRF4. Cluster I included all HC and some patients, cluster II only included RA patients and cluster III included mostly SLE and some RA patients. The frequency of each cluster differed by disease status ($p < 0.001$) (**Figure 3B**). Each disease exhibited a predominant cluster, as confirmed by a correspondence analysis (**Figure 3C**), hence demonstrating that SLE patients were closely related to cluster III, whereas RA patients did to cluster II. The individual expression of each gene stratified by clusters and according to disease diagnosis can be observed in **Figure 3D**.

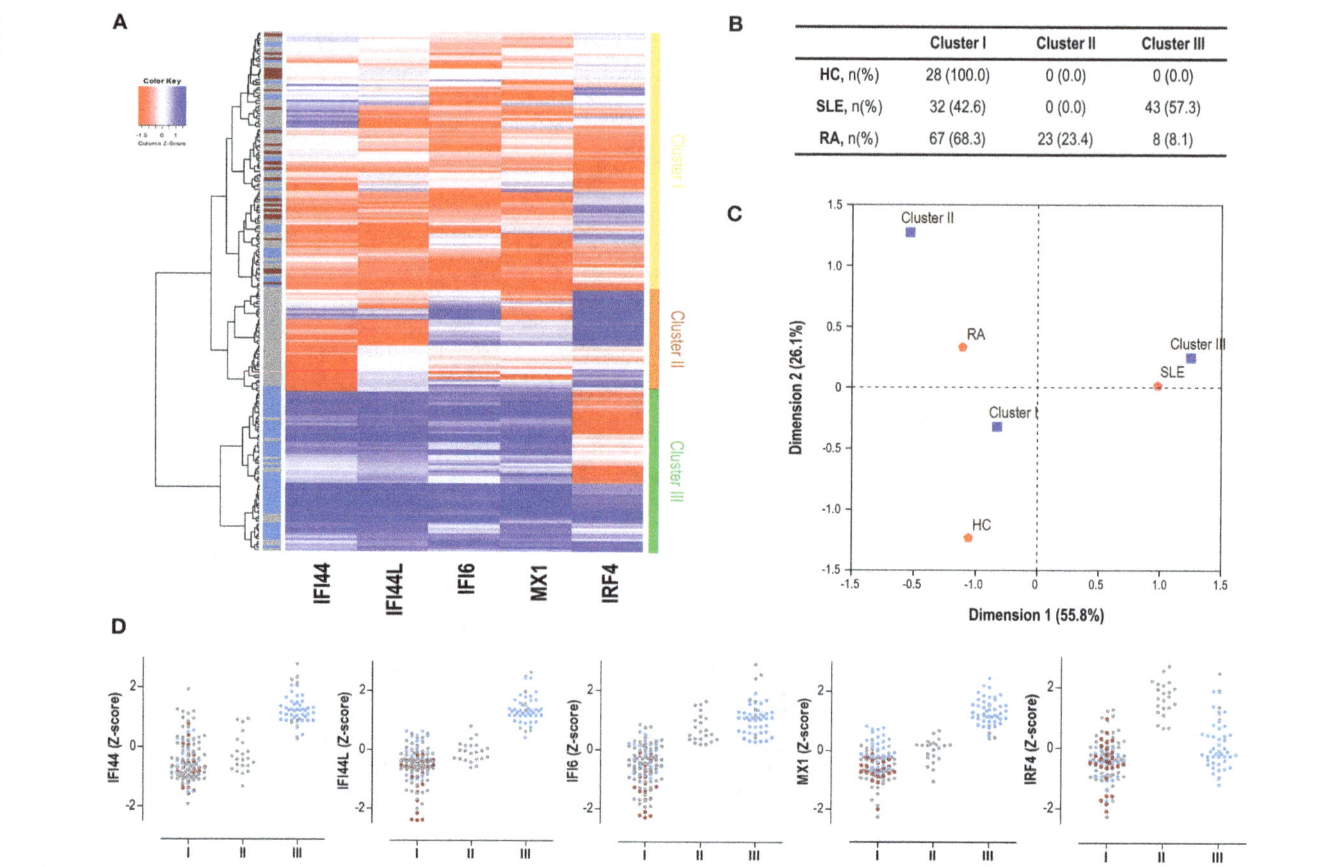

	Cluster I	Cluster II	Cluster III
HC, n(%)	28 (100.0)	0 (0.0)	0 (0.0)
SLE, n(%)	32 (42.6)	0 (0.0)	43 (57.3)
RA, n(%)	67 (68.3)	23 (23.4)	8 (8.1)

FIGURE 3 | Gene signatures defined by IRF4 and IRGs. **(A)** Heatmap and cluster analysis revealing the identification of the three clusters based on the expression of IRF4 and IRGs (columns). Each row represents a study subject. Colors in the vertical left bar denoted HC (dark red), SLE patients (blue), or RA patients (gray). Vertical right bar indicates the clusters identified: cluster I (yellow), cluster II (orange), and cluster III (green). Tiles are colored based on gene expression levels, red and blue indicating low or high levels, respectively, as indicated in the legend (top left). **(B)** Table indicating the number of individuals of each study group (HC, SLE patients, and RA patients) using the different clusters identified. **(C)** Correspondence analysis (weighted chi-square distances) to study the associations between disease status (red signs) and the three clusters identified (blue signs). Axes represent the dimensions derived from the analysis. **(D)** Levels of expression for all the genes analyzed (IRF4 and IRGs) stratified by the clusters identified in the analysis. For each cluster, dots are colored according to disease status as follows: HC (dark red), SLE patients (blue), and RA patients (gray). Each dot represents one individual. These graphs were only included for visualization purposes since they were derived from previously identified expression profiles, based on individual gene expression levels. Then, no statistical analysis was performed.

All these results support that, apart from quantitative differences in gene expression, distinct associations among IRF4 and IRGs can be observed in autoimmune patients. These differences define specific expression signatures which are in turn differentially related to SLE and RA.

IRF4 and IRGs Expression Signatures: Association With Clinical Features

Next, we analyzed whether the different gene signatures identified by cluster analysis were related to clinical features.

SLE patients exhibiting cluster III were younger at the time of diagnosis and were more likely to suffer from lupus nephritis and tended to exhibit elevated ESR than those in cluster I (**Table 1**). Additionally, patients in cluster III exhibited a higher prevalence of anti-SSA/Ro and anti-RNP antibodies than their cluster I counterparts (**Table 1**). As a consequence, the number of ENAs was higher in cluster III than in cluster I SLE patients (1.21 ± 0.91 vs. 0.58 ± 0.71, $p = 0.002$). Importantly, patients between both clusters did not differ in age ($p = 0.114$), gender ($p = 0.582$) or frequency of treatments (**Table 1**).

On the other hand, RA patients were distributed among the 3 clusters identified. A differential distribution of the patients according to disease stages was noted, since the frequency of the VERA group (recruited at onset, untreated) was enriched in cluster I (**Table 2**). Interestingly, lower disease activity score, joint involvement and ESR was observed in cluster II (**Table 2**). No differences in gender ($p = 0.393$), age ($p = 0.721$) and treatment usage (**Table 2**) were found. These results were maintained after excluding VERA patients from the analysis (**Supplementary Table 3**), thus suggesting a milder course of RA patients using cluster II, since cluster I patients were hallmarked by a more active disease despite being more intensively treated than their cluster II-counterparts. Although higher ESR and frequency of autoantibodies was found in cluster III RA patients,

TABLE 1 | Association between gene expression signatures and clinical features in SLE patients.

	Cluster I (n = 33)	Cluster III (n = 42)	p-value
DISEASE FEATURES			
Disease duration, years; median (range)	12.12 (0.33–39.00)	14.75 (0.17–32.00)	0.222
Age at diagnosis, years; median (range)	38.10 (18 - 68)	28.50 (19 - 65)	0.023
ESR, mm/h	10.50 (10.25)	14.50 (12.75)	0.071
Disease activity (SLEDAI)	3.50 (5.00)	2.00 (3.58)	0.769
CLINICAL MANIFESTATIONS, *N*(%)			
Malar rash	16 (48.4)	24 (57.1)	0.456
Discoid lesions	10 (31.2)	7 (16.6)	0.161
Photosensitivity	17 (51.1)	24 (57.1)	0.627
Oral ulcers	16 (48.4)	24 (57.1)	0.456
Arthritis	22 (66.6)	29 (69.0)	0.826
Serositis	8 (24.2)	9 (21.4)	0.773
Cytopenia	24 (72.7)	27 (64.2)	0.437
Lupus nephritis	5 (15.1)	17 (40.4)	0.021
Neurological disorder	3 (9.0)	5 (11.9)	0.695
AUTOANTIBODIES, *N*(%)			
ANA	33 (100)	42 (100)	–
Anti-dsDNA	28 (84.4)	32 (76.1)	0.352
Anti-SSA/Ro	12 (39.3)	28 (66.6)	0.009
Anti-SSB/La	4 (12.1)	8 (19.0)	0.417
Anti-Sm	1 (3.0)	5 (11.9)	0.160
Anti-RNP	1 (3.0)	10 (23.8)	0.012
Anti-RibP	3 (9.0)	6 (14.2)	0.522
RF	5 (15.1)	8 (19.0)	0.319
TREATMENTS, *N*(%)			
None	1 (3.0)	2 (4.7)	–
Glucocorticoids	14 (42.4)	15 (35.7)	0.328
Antimalarials	27 (81.1)	39 (92.8)	0.720
Mycophenolate mophetil	0 (0)	1 (2.3)	-

Variables were expressed as median (interquartile range) or n(%), unless otherwise stated. Differences were assessed by Mann-Withney or chi-square tests (or Fisher exact test, when appropriate), according to the distribution of the variables.

the low sample size observed was insufficient to drawn firm conclusions.

In sum, gene expression profiles defined by IRF4 and IRGs expression are associated with clinical features of severity in SLE patients as well as with disease activity and clinical stage in RA. Additional and larger studies are warranted to shed some light into their potential clinical implications as a biomarker.

IRF4 and IRGs Expression Upon TNFα-Blockade

In order to get insight into the IRF4 expression and its association with that of IRGs upon TNFα-blockade, as well as its potential relevance as a biomarker of therapy outcome, the IRF4 and IRGs expression was prospectively analyzed in a subgroup of 13 biological-naïve RA patients at baseline (BL) and after three months upon TNFα-blockade (post-treatment, PT).

No changes in IRF4 expression, neither in IRGs, were detected in the whole group upon TNFα-blockade (**Figure 4A**). IRF4 expression did not correlate DAS28 at BL ($r = -0.088, p = 0.775$) nor PT ($r = 0.306$, $p = 0.310$). No changes in leukocytes, neutrophils, lymphocytes or monocytes counts were observed upon treatment (all $p > 0.050$, data not shown). When patients were stratified by treatment response, increasing IRF4 expression upon treatment was observed in responders compared to their non-responder counterparts (**Figure 4A**). No difference in IRF4 at baseline was observed between groups ($p = 0.464$).

Next, the associations among IRF4 and IRGs upon TNFα-blockade were studied. Correlation plots revealed clear differences among these genes between baseline and post-treatment samples (**Figure 4B**). Additionally, the network analyses (**Figure 4C**) confirmed changes in the correlation profiles among IRF4 and the IRGs. Stronger associations among IFI44L, IFI6, and MX1 were found in the BL samples, with weak or no associations with IRF4. This picture partially mirrored that of observed in SLE patients in the cross-sectional analysis. Interestingly, a more uniform pattern among all genes was observed after treatment, similar to that of the RA patients in the cross-sectional study, hence suggesting distinct gene expression programs before and after TNFα-blockade.

Taken together, these results confirm that changes in IRF4 expression are associated with therapy outcomes upon TNFα-blockade in the short-term (3 months). Moreover, the associations among genes largely differed before and after treatment, hence confirming qualitative changes in the gene expression program in this scenario. These findings warrant further studies to elucidate the relevance of these changes in the long-term.

Validation in Public Microarrays Datasets

Finally, data of IRF4 expression in peripheral blood in autoimmune patients was extracted from publicly available microarray datasets downloaded from the GEO database in order to validate our results. Five datasets containing relevant samples were retrieved: 4 datasets analyzing RA patients (1 in peripheral blood and 3 in synovial tissue) and 1 dataset including multiple sclerosis (MS) patients (peripheral blood).

First, GSE17755 included gene expression data from 45 HC, 22 SLE, and 112 RA patients. IRF4 was found to be differentially expressed by GEO2R (adjusted $p = 3.13{\cdot}10^{-4}$) among groups, increased expression being confirmed in RA (**Figure 5A**). Next, in order to gain additional insight on the IRF4 expression in RA, datasets containing gene expression data from target tissues (synovial membrane) were analyzed. GSE55457 included gene expression data from 10 HC, 10 osteoarthritis (OA) patients and 13 RA patients. IRF4 was observed to be differentially expressed among patients (adjusted $p = 6.40{\cdot}10^{-4}$), being upregulated in RA (**Figure 5B**). An equivalent result was obtained from GSE55235 (10 HC, 10 OA, and 10 RA) (adjusted $p = 1.04{\cdot}10^{-4}$) (**Figure 5C**). Results from GSE36700 containing synovial tissue samples from 5 OA, 4 SLE, 5 microcrystalline arthritis (MA) and 7 RA patients confirmed the differential expression of IRF4 (adjusted $p = 8.4{\cdot}10^{-4}$), again being upregulated in RA (**Figure 5D**). Finally, data on

TABLE 2 | Association among gene expression signatures and clinical features in RA patients.

	Cluster I (*n* = 67)	Cluster II (*n* = 23)	Cluster III (*n* = 8)	*p*-value
DISEASE FEATURES				
Disease duration, years; median (range)	3.80 (0–30.00)	4.91 (0.17–20.00)	5.37 (1.75–16.25)	0.360
Age at diagnosis, years; median (range)	46.29 (23 - 62)	49.16 (19 - 61)	50.33 (18 - 65)	0.968
ESR, mm/h	21.50 (29.50)	10.50 (19.00)	37.50 (36.25)	0.025[a]
Disease activity (DAS28)	4.40 (2.08)	3.10 (1.94)	3.76 (3.02)	<0.001[b]
Tender Joint Count	3.00 (5.00)	1.00 (2.00)	0.00 (5.00)	0.019[c]
Swollen Joint Count	4.00 (9.00)	1.00 (3.50)	2.50 (5.25)	0.004[d]
Patient global assessment (0–100)	50.00 (34.00)	25.00 (40.00)	50.00 (41.25)	0.028[e]
Pain assessment (0–10)	5.00 (3.65)	2.00 (5.00)	4.50 (4.75)	0.020[f]
HAQ (0–3)	1.12 (0.92)	0.50 (1.25)	0.50 (1.41)	0.020[g]
AUTOANTIBODIES, *N*(%)				
RF	41 (61.2)	12 (52.1)	5 (62.5)	0.645
ACPA	40 (59.7)	14 (60.8)	6 (75.0)	0.411
RF or ACPA	44 (65.5)	15 (65.0)	7 (87.5)	0.641
RF and ACPA	31 (46.2)	10 (43.4)	5 (62.5)	0.229
TREATMENTS, *N*(%)				
None (VERA)	16 (23.8)	1 (4.3)	0 (0.0)	0.047
Glucocorticoids	41 (61.2)	9 (39.1)	5 (62.5)	0.286
Methotrexate	41 (61.2)	17 (73.9)	7 (87.5)	0.130
TNFα blockers	24 (35.8)	8 (34.7)	4 (50.0)	0.773

Variables were expressed as median (interquartile range) or n(%), unless otherwise stated. Differences were assessed by Kruskal-Wallis or chi-square tests (or Fisher exact test, when appropriate), according to the distribution of the variables. The p-values in the table correspond to the Kruskal-Wallis or chi-square tests. Multiple comparisons tests (Dunn-Bonferroni correction) were performed when the Kruskal-Wallis test revealed significant differences among groups and p-values were summarized in superscripts. [a]*I vs. II: $p = 0.080$, II vs. III: $p = 0.032$, I vs. III: $p = 0.409$.*

[b]*I vs. II: $p < 0.001$, II vs. III: $p = 0.070$, I vs. III: $p = 0.497$.*

[c]*I vs. II: $p = 0.003$, II vs. III: $p = 0.433$, I vs. III: $p = 0.574$.*

[d]*I vs. II: $p = 0.043$, II vs. III: $p = 0.841$, I vs. III: $p = 0.233$.*

[e]*I vs. II: $p = 0.020$, II vs. III: $p = 0.518$, I vs. III: $p = 0.910$.*

[f]*I vs. II: $p = 0.009$, II vs. III: $p = 0.438$, I vs. III: $p = 0.774$.*

[g]*I vs. II: $p = 0.028$, II vs. III: $p = 0.790$, I vs. III: $p = 0.443$.*

IRF4 expression was analyzed in other autoimmune diseases. GSE41846 contained gene expression data from a cross-sectional study on 54 untreated and 57 IFNβ-treated multiple sclerosis (MS) patients. IRF4 was found to be differentially expressed (adjusted $p = 3.63\cdot10^{-8}$), being upregulated in IFNβ-treated patients (**Figure 5E**). The same dataset contained follow up data (longitudinally collected at 1 year visit) from 42 untreated MS patients and 67 IFNβ-treated MS patients supporting the increased IRF4 expression (adjusted $p = 1.59\cdot10^{-7}$) (**Figure 5F**).

Taken together, these analyses confirmed the differential expression of IRF4 in autoimmune patients, being increased in RA patients both in peripheral blood and in peripheral tissues, as well as in MS after IFNβ treatment.

DISCUSSION

Despite the type I IFN signature being widely recognized as a common mediator in several systemic autoimmune diseases, a precise definition of its components and regulatory mechanisms is still lacking. Indeed, some authors have highlighted that distinct mediators may be differentially associated with the type I IFN signature(s) in different diseases. The findings herein presented shed new light on the role of a new factor, the IRF4, as a new player in this scenario. A differential activation of the IRF4 expression together with distinct associations with IRGs define global expression signatures in SLE and RA patients with clinical relevance. Taken together, our results expand the notion of the IFN signature shaping by IRFs in autoimmune diseases.

A major breakthrough of our study was the characterization of different gene expression signatures driven by IRF4 and IRGs. The differential associations among these genes delineate distinct gene interactions that can provide additional information to better understand the structure of the IFN signature in different diseases. Although early studies only considered the type I IFN signature as a sole measure of IRGs activation, recent studies have stressed the need of more complex approaches. In this sense, Reynier and colleagues (46) demonstrated that the overall state of correlation must be also considered when analyzing genes with similar expression patterns, such as the type I IFN signature in order to account for co-regulation and co-expression phenomena. Using an equivalent approach, we have found that beyond their differential expression, the figures of IRF4 and IRGs differed in terms of their mutual associations among conditions, hence adding another layer of complexity to the analysis of the type I IFN signature. In fact, SLE and RA patients clearly differed in the associations observed between IRF4 and the IRGs, thus

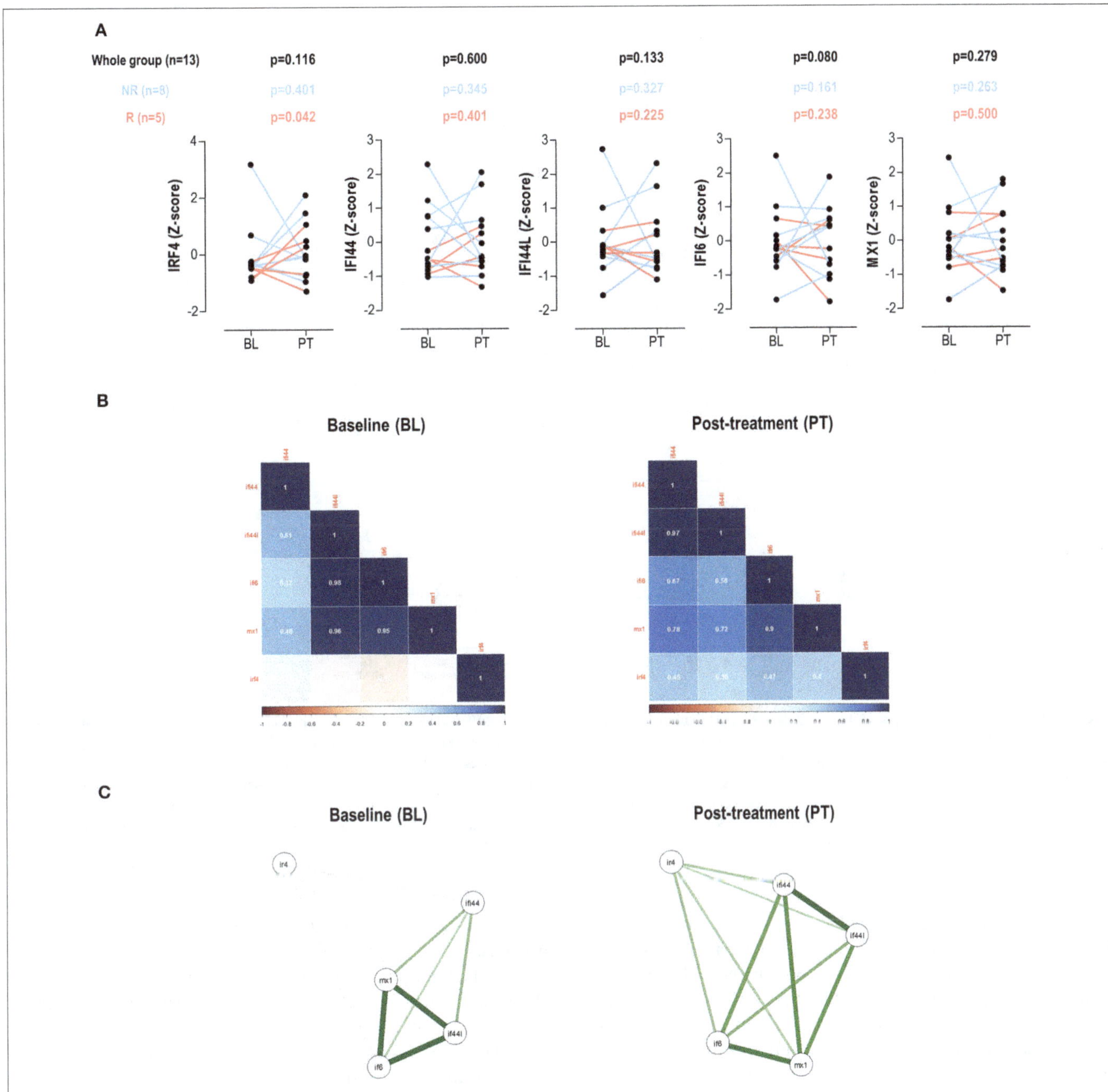

FIGURE 4 | Changes in IRF4 and IRGs expression upon TNFa-blockade. **(A)** Paired analyses (Wilcoxon tests) of the IRF4 and IRGs expression at baseline (BL) and post-treatment (PT) upon TNFα-blockade in a group of 13 biological-naïve RA patients prospectively followed up. Patients were denoted in red (responders) and blue (moderate/non-responders). The *p*-values show on top of the graphs were derived from the analysis of the whole patient population ($n = 13$, black numbers), responders ($n = 5$, red numbers), or non-responders (blue, $n = 8$). **(B)** Correlation plots and network analyses **(C)** of the IRF4 and IRGs expression in BL and PT samples.

pointing to distinct molecular programs hallmarking these two conditions.

The heterogeneity of the type I IFN signature has been largely debated during last years. Data suggest that heterogeneity in the type I IFN signature activation and genetic make-up contribute to the clinical heterogeneity observed in rheumatic conditions (7), thus underlining the need of a better understanding of the IFN signature architecture. Recently, de Jong and colleagues have found that certain diversification of the type I IFN signature can be recognized among different diseases (39). More importantly, this diversification has been suggested to parallel the clinical course of some patients (37, 39, 41). In

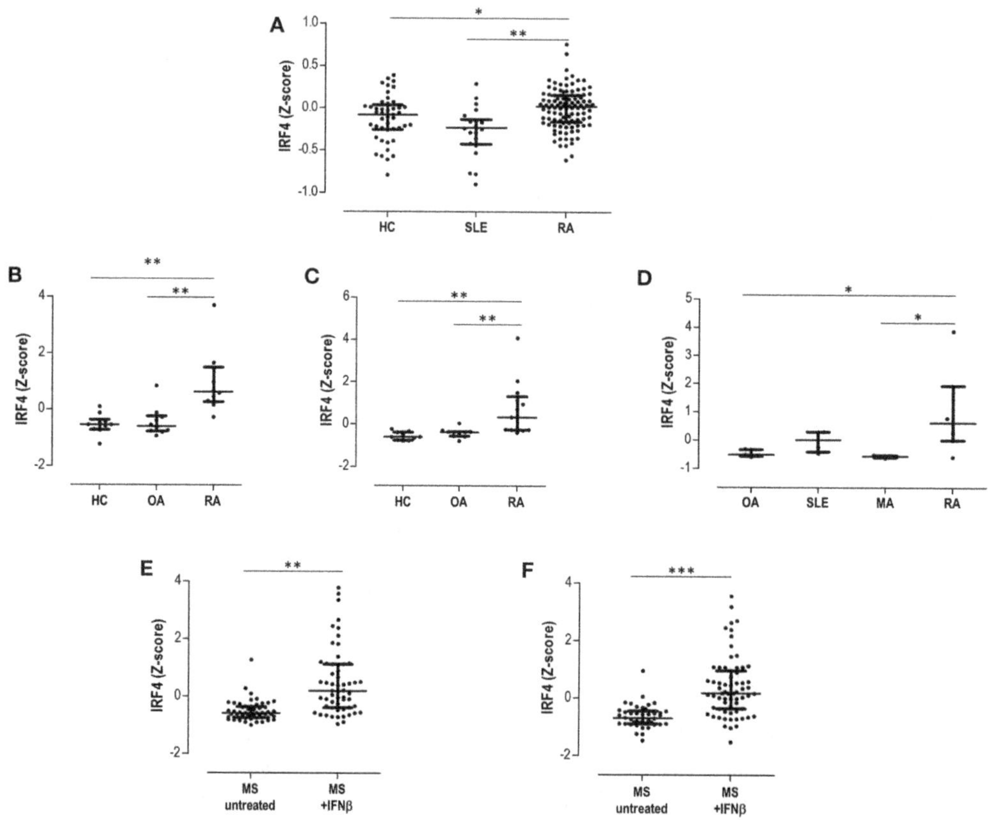

FIGURE 5 | Validation in publicly available GEO datasets. **(A)** Expression of IRF4 in peripheral blood in HC, SLE patients and RA patients extracted from the dataset GSE17755. The differential expression of IRF4 in synovial membranes from RA patients was confirmed in datasets GSE55457 **(B)**, GSE55235 **(C)**, and GSE36700 **(D)**. The expression of IRF4 in MS patients under IFNb treatment was evaluated in the dataset GSE41846 in cross-sectional **(E)** and prospective **(F)** samples. Expression data from each dataset were extracted and Z-scores were calculated and plotted in scatter dot plots. Each dot represents one individual and bars represent median values. Upper and lower whiskers represent the 75th and 25th values, respectively. IRF4 was confirmed to be differentially expressed in each dataset with the GEO2R tool, as indicated in the Results section. Statistical analysis on graphs was performed by conventional tests (Kruskal-Wallis or Mann-Withney *U*-tests, as appropriate). The *p*-values are indicated as follows: $^{*}p < 0.050$, $^{**}p < 0.010$, and $^{***}p < 0.001$.

a similar way, we have reported that different profiles can be distinguished in the type I IFN signature of RA patients according to their clinical stage (36). As a consequence, this body of evidence strongly supports that the type I IFN signature may be more complex than initially thought and its fine structure emerges as a relevant topic. In the present study, we went further by defining gene signatures related to the type I IFN signature and IRF4 expression, which were differentially used by different autoimmune diseases. These gene expression programs identified subsets of patients with distinct clinical features, hence strengthening their clinical relevance. The fact that different gene signatures are linked to specific clinical features within a single disease may account for the controversy observed at the disease level among studies and may help to dissect the molecular complexity of these conditions. Furthermore, these differences were observed to correlate with clinical phenotypes. As a consequence, our findings provide a rationale to include the IRF4 in future studies assessing the type I IFN signature in autoimmune patients to resolve the heterogeneity of the IFN signature as well as to gain additional insight into the differential architecture of the IFN signature in these complex diseases.

The distinct, mutual expression patterns related to IRF4 and IRGs expression in SLE and RA patients support the concept that IRFs could play a role in the regulation and editing of the type I IFN signature in autoimmunity. Although previously restricted to IRF3 and IRF7, our findings expand the notion that IRFs may be associated with the modulation of IRGs toward new family members, the IRF4. IRF4 has been reported to be a negative regulator of the TLR pathway (32, 47), hence leading to a decreased expression of a number of IRGs *in vitro*. Interestingly, IRF4 has been demonstrated to interact with MyD88, a molecular hub for the control of IRGs expression (32). More importantly, IRF4 competes with IRF5 for MyD88 interaction, and IRF4 expression leads to the inhibition of IRF5-dependent genes. Accordingly, gene expression profiles from $Irf4^{-/-}$ macrophages mirrored that of their $Irf5^{-/-}$ counterparts (32). Furthermore, a recent paper by Forero and coworkers has added new clues to the relationship of IRF4 and IRGs (31). Using an inducible expression system, it has been demonstrated that IRF4 acts as a regulator of IRGs induction, different subsets of IRGs being identified: from positively (such as ISG60 or OAS) to negatively regulated IRGs (MX1). Additionally, the IRGs differ in terms of their sensitivity to the IRF4-mediated modulation, which may be caused by a different affinity of IRF4 for Interferon-sensitive response element (ISRE) sites in such IRGs (47). Taken together, these lines of evidence underline the role of IRF4 in shaping the type I IFN signature. However, the clinical relevance of these findings remained unknown. The findings herein presented shed new light into the clinical value of this complex regulation between IRF4 and IRGs in autoimmune patients and prove this field worthy of further research in order to better delineate the effect of IRFs on the IFN signature(s) in autoimmunity.

In addition to deciphering new interactions within the IFN signature in systemic autoimmune conditions, our results are relevant from a translational point of view. First, the global analysis of IRF4 and IRGs allow us to identify a subset of SLE patients with clinical features of disease severity and enhanced autoantibody production (cluster III). Interestingly, RA patients exhibiting the same gene expression signature mirrored such clinical characteristics. Moreover, RA patients showing the gene signature characterized by a high IRF4 expression exhibited a low-grade clinical phenotype, hence pointing to a connection between IRF4 expression and mild disease course and/or a better response to therapies. This notion was supported by our results from the prospective analysis in patients undergoing TNFα-blockade, increasing IRF4 expression being related to a good clinical outcome. Further follow up studies to elucidate the long-term clinical relevance of these findings are warranted.

Despite the fact that clusters defined by IRF4 and IRGs were related to disease activity/severity, the patient populations were overall related to a mild disease activity. This was especially clear in SLE patients, since patients exhibited a good control of the disease despite the scarce use of strong immunosuppressants or biological drugs. However, our experimental approach was able to identify a disease subset with markers of severity and poor prognosis (increased nephritis and autoantibodies), regardless of disease activity. Whether the lack of differences in the SLEDAI score may be attributed to the overall low disease activity of the SLE patients cannot be totally excluded. However, since disease activity fluctuates, the IRF4/IRGs system may be a more reliable marker of severity in these patients. In the case of RA patients, both IRF4 expression level (elevated in cluster II patients and increasing levels in TNFα-blockade responders) and its associations with IRGs was associated with disease activity, hence adding another layer of complexity to the clinical relevance of the IFN signature structure in this condition.

The different pictures observed for the type I IFN signature in SLE and RA, especially regarding IRF4 activation, are relevant to understand unresolved questions from previous studies. On the one hand, Smiljanovic and colleagues demonstrated that the IFN signature observed in RA patients qualitatively differs from that of their SLE counterparts in terms of target genes and transcription factors binding sites, and, remarkably, genomic imprints found in RA patients were more heterogeneous (48). The differential upregulation of IRF4 between these two conditions together with the usage of the 3 gene clusters in RA compared to only 2 being observed in SLE is line with these findings, hence reinforcing the role of IRF4 in this setting. Additionally, IFNβ has been reported to contribute to the global type I IFN signature in RA (49), whereas other systemic conditions, such as SLE, are thought to be mostly IFNα-driven (39). Interestingly, our results support a link between IFNβ and IRF4 upregulation. Hence, IRF4 emerges as a pivotal player to understand the divergences in the IFN signature among conditions from a mechanistic perspective. Additionally, the protective effects of IFNβ in RA (50, 51) align with the mild clinical course of RA patients with elevated IRF4 expression. Consequently, it may be conceivable that IRF4 could be regarded as a pharmacodynamic clinical biomarker for IFNβ treatment in RA patients, a major unmet need that limits the application of this therapy. Recently, increased serum IFN-β/α ratio activity in RA patients has been demonstrated to predict poor clinical outcome upon TNF inhibition (52). Unfortunately, important methodological differences limit the interpretation of our findings in the light of the results reported by Wampler and coworkers. Finally, Gordon and colleagues found that the IFN signature in RA can be also influenced by TNF (53), thus supporting that mediators other than type I IFNs contribute to this expression program in RA patients. Interestingly, IRF4 has been linked to the NFkB pathway (31, 54, 54), which is central for RA pathogenesis. Since the NFkB pathway is activated by TNF signaling, IRF4 could be an important mediator to understand the TNF-related type I IFN signature upregulation in RA. Being associated with a milder course and clinical response to TNFa-blockade, it is tempting to speculate that IRF4 upregulation may be considered as a therapeutic opportunity in RA. However, its functional association with NFkB pathway needs to carefully considered in this setting. As a consequence, the potential conception of IRF4 as a therapeutic target warrants further investigation.

In conclusion, our results revealed that distinct levels of expression and differential associations of IRF4 with IRGs may identify gene expression signatures with clinical relevance in SLE and RA patients. To the best of our knowledge, this is the first study analyzing the IRF4 expression in peripheral blood in autoimmune patients and its association with IRGs expression as well as with clinical features and treatment outcomes. Therefore, this proof-of-concept study sheds new light on the structure of type I IFN signature and support a role for IRF4 as potential modulator with clinical added value. A number of potential limitations of the present study must be acknowledge. First, patient populations were not fully comparable in terms of disease duration, as expected from distinct clinical entities with different age at onset. Moreover, a mild clinical course was observed in the SLE population, whereas an overall low degree of activity was found in RA patients. Although clear associations between IRF4 and activity/severity were retrieved, future studies including patients with very high disease activity would be advisable to further confirm our results. Finally, a partial number of IRGs and only IRF4 (among all IRFs family members) were included in this study. Whether the IFN signature shaping can be extended to other IRFs remains unknown and warrants further studies. Therefore, the findings herein presented pave the ground for future, larger studies involving a higher number of IRFs and IRGs in different autoimmune conditions.

AUTHOR CONTRIBUTIONS

JR-C carried out most of the experimental procedures, performed the statistical analyses and drafted and edited the manuscript. PL performed some experimental procedures. MA-L, LC-M, and FB-G were in charge of patients' recruitment and clinical data management. AS conceived the study, designed the protocols and drafted and edited the manuscript. All authors read and approved the final version of the manuscript.

ACKNOWLEDGMENTS

This work was supported by European Union FEDER funds and Fondo de Investigación Sanitaria (FIS, PI12/00523 and PI16/00113; ISCIII, Spain), and SER/FER funds (Sociedad Española de Reumatología, FER043/2016). JR-C is supported by a postdoctoral contract from the Juan de la Cierva program (FJCI-2015-23849; MINECO, Spain).

REFERENCES

1. Rodriguez-Carrio J, Lopez P, Suarez A. Type I IFNs as biomarkers in rheumatoid arthritis: towards disease profiling and personalized medicine. *Clin Sci.* (2015) 128:449–64. doi: 10.1042/CS20140554
2. Kalliolias GD, Ivashkiv LB. Overview of the biology of type I interferons. *Arthritis Res Ther.* (2010) 12:1–9. doi: 10.1186/ar2881
3. Rönnblom L, Eloranta M-L. The interferon signature in autoimmune diseases. *Curr Opin Rheumatol.* (2013) 25:248–53. doi: 10.1097/BOR.0b013e32835c7e32
4. Higgs BW, Liu Z, White B, Zhu W, White WI, Morehouse C, et al. Patients with systemic lupus erythematosus, myositis, rheumatoid arthritis and scleroderma share activation of a common type I interferon pathway. *Ann Rheum Dis.* (2011) 70:2029–36. doi: 10.1136/ard.2011.150326
5. van der Pouw Kraan TCTM, van Baarsen LGM, Wijbrandts CA, Voskuyl AE, Rustenburg F, Baggen JM, et al. Expression of a pathogen-response program in peripheral blood cells defines a subgroup of rheumatoid arthritis patients. *Genes Immun.* (2008) 9:16–22. doi: 10.1038/sj.gene.6364438
6. van der Pouw Kraan TCTM, Wijbrandts CA, van Baarsen LGM, Voskuyl AE, Rustenburg F, Baggen JM, et al. Rheumatoid arthritis subtypes identified by genomic profiling of peripheral blood cells: assignment of a type I interferon signature in a subpopulation of patients. *Ann Rheum Dis.* (2007) 66:1008–14. doi: 10.1136/ard.2006.063412
7. Muskardin TLW, Niewold TB. Type I interferon in rheumatic diseases. *Nat Rev Rheumatol.* (2018) 14:214–28. doi: 10.1038/nrrheum.2018.31
8. Landolt-Marticorena C. The need for preclinical biomarkers in systemic autoimmune rheumatic diseases. *J Rheumatol.* (2015) 42:152–4. doi: 10.3899/jrheum.141366
9. Tektonidou MG, Ward MM. Validation of new biomarkers in systemic autoimmune diseases. *Nat Rev Rheumatol.* (2011) 7:708–17. doi: 10.1038/nrrheum.2011.157
10. van de Putte LBA, Atkins C, Malaise M, Sany J, Russell AS, van Riel PLCM, et al. Efficacy and safety of adalimumab as monotherapy in patients with rheumatoid arthritis for whom previous disease modifying antirheumatic drug treatment has failed. *Ann Rheum Dis.* (2004) 63:508–16. doi: 10.1136/ard.2003.013052
11. Wijbrandts CA, Tak PP. Prediction of response to targeted treatment in rheumatoid arthritis. *Mayo Clin Proc.* (2017) 92:1129–43. doi: 10.1016/j.mayocp.2017.05.009
12. Burmester GR, Mariette X, Montecucco C, Monteagudo-Sáez I, Malaise M, Tzioufas AG, et al. Adalimumab alone and in combination with disease-modifying antirheumatic drugs for the treatment of rheumatoid arthritis in clinical practice: the research in active rheumatoid arthritis (ReAct) trial. *Ann Rheum Dis.* (2007) 66:732–9. doi: 10.1136/ard.2006.066761
13. Wright HL, Cox T, Moots RJ, Edwards SW. Neutrophil biomarkers predict response to therapy with tumor necrosis factor inhibitors in rheumatoid arthritis. *J Leukoc Biol.* (2017) 101:785–95. doi: 10.1189/jlb.5A0616-258R
14. Honda K, Takaoka A, Taniguchi T. Type I interferon [corrected] gene induction by the interferon regulatory factor family of transcription factors. *Immunity* (2006) 25:349–60. doi: 10.1016/j.immuni.2006.08.009
15. Taniguchi T, Ogasawara K, Takaoka A, Tanaka N. IRF family of transcription factors as regulators of host defense. *Annu Rev Immunol.* (2001) 19:623–55. doi: 10.1146/annurev.immunol.19.1.623
16. Zhang X-J, Jiang D-S, Li H. The interferon regulatory factors as novel potential targets in the treatment of cardiovascular diseases. *Br J Pharmacol.* (2015) 172:5457–76. doi: 10.1111/bph.12881
17. Miyamoto M, Fujita T, Kimura Y, Maruyama M, Harada H, Sudo Y, et al. Regulated expression of a gene encoding a nuclear factor, IRF-1, that specifically binds to IFN-beta gene regulatory elements. *Cell* (1988) 54:903–13.
18. Matsuyama T, Kimura T, Kitagawa M, Pfeffer K, Kawakami T, Watanabe N, et al. Targeted disruption of IRF-1 or IRF-2 results in abnormal type I IFN gene induction and aberrant lymphocyte development. *Cell* (1993) 75:83–97.
19. Niewold TB, Kelly JA, Flesch MH, Espinoza LR, Harley JB, Crow MK. Association of the IRF5 risk haplotype with high serum interferon-alpha activity in systemic lupus erythematosus patients. *Arthritis Rheum.* (2008) 58:2481–7. doi: 10.1002/art.23613
20. Takaoka A, Yanai H, Kondo S, Duncan G, Negishi H, Mizutani T, et al. Integral role of IRF-5 in the gene induction programme activated by Toll-like receptors. *Nature* (2005) 434:243–9. doi: 10.1038/nature03308
21. Honda K, Yanai H, Negishi H, Asagiri M, Sato M, Mizutani T, et al. IRF-7 is the master regulator of type-I interferon-dependent immune responses. *Nature* (2005) 434:772–7. doi: 10.1038/nature03464
22. Wang J, Basagoudanavar SH, Wang X, Hopewell E, Albrecht R, García-Sastre A, et al. NF-kappa B RelA subunit is crucial for early IFN-beta expression and resistance to RNA virus replication. *J Immunol.* (2010) 185:1720–9. doi: 10.4049/jimmunol.1000114
23. Schafer SL, Lin R, Moore PA, Hiscott J, Pitha PM. Regulation of type I interferon gene expression by interferon regulatory factor-3. *J Biol Chem.* (1998) 273:2714–20.
24. Fensterl V, Grotheer D, Berk I, Schlemminger S, Vallbracht A, Dotzauer A. Hepatitis A virus suppresses RIG-I-mediated IRF-3 activation to block induction of beta interferon. *J Virol.* (2005) 79:10968–77. doi: 10.1128/JVI.79.17.10968-10977.2005
25. De Silva NS, Simonetti G, Heise N, Klein U. The diverse roles of IRF4 in late germinal center B-cell differentiation. *Immunol Rev.* (2012) 247:73–92. doi: 10.1111/j.1600-065X.2012.01113.x
26. Huber M, Lohoff M. IRF4 at the crossroads of effector T-cell fate decision. *Eur J Immunol.* (2014) 44:1886–95. doi: 10.1002/eji.201344279
27. Yamamoto M, Kato T, Hotta C, Nishiyama A, Kurotaki D, Yoshinari M, et al. Shared and distinct functions of the transcription factors IRF4 and IRF8 in myeloid cell development. *PLoS ONE* (2011) 6:e25812. doi: 10.1371/journal.pone.0025812
28. de Jong TD, Lübbers J, Turk S, Vosslamber S, Mantel E, Bontkes HJ, et al. The type I interferon signature in leukocyte subsets from peripheral blood of

patients with early arthritis: a major contribution by granulocytes. *Arthritis Res Ther.* (2016) 18:165. doi: 10.1186/s13075-016-1065-3

29. Raj P, Rai E, Song R, Khan S, Wakeland BE, Viswanathan K, et al. Regulatory polymorphisms modulate the expression of HLA class II molecules and promote autoimmunity. *Elife* (2016) 5: e12089. doi: 10.7554/eLife.12089
30. López-Isac E, Martín J-E, Assassi S, Simeón CP, Carreira P, Ortego-Centeno N, et al. Brief report: irf4 newly identified as a common susceptibility locus for systemic sclerosis and rheumatoid arthritis in a cross-disease meta-analysis of genome-wide association studies. *Arthritis Rheumatol.* (2016) 68:2338–44. doi: 10.1002/art.39730
31. Forero A, Moore PS, Sarkar SN. Role of IRF4 in IFN-stimulated gene induction and maintenance of Kaposi sarcoma-associated herpesvirus latency in primary effusion lymphoma cells. *J Immunol.* (2013) 191:1476–85. doi: 10.4049/jimmunol.1202514
32. Negishi H, Ohba Y, Yanai H, Takaoka A, Honma K, Yui K, et al. Negative regulation of Toll-like-receptor signaling by IRF-4. *Proc Natl Acad Sci USA.* (2005) 102:15989–94. doi: 10.1073/pnas.0508327102
33. Hochberg MC. Updating the American college of rheumatology revised criteria for the classification of systemic lupus erythematosus. *Arthritis Rheum.* (1997) 40:1725. doi: 10.1002/1529-0131(199709)40:9<1725::AID-ART29>3.0.CO;2-Y
34. Aletaha D, Neogi T, Silman AJ, Funovits J, Felson DT, Bingham CO, et al. 2010 rheumatoid arthritis classification criteria: an American college of rheumatology/European league against rheumatism collaborative initiative. *Arthritis Rheum.* (2010) 62:2569–81. doi: 10.1002/art.27584
35. Van Gestel AM, Anderson JJ, Van Riel PLCM, Boers M, Haagsma CJ, Rich B, et al. ACR and EULAR improvement criteria have comparable validity in rheumatoid arthritis trials. *J Rheumatol.* (1999) 26:705–11.
36. Rodríguez-Carrio J, Alperi-López M, López P, Ballina-García FJ, Suárez A. heterogeneity of the type i interferon signature in rheumatoid arthritis: a potential limitation for its use as a clinical biomarker. *Front Immunol.* (2017) 8:2007. doi: 10.3389/fimmu.2017.02007
37. de Jong TD, Vosslamber S, Blits M, Wolbink G, Nurmohamed MT, van der Laken CJ, et al. Effect of prednisone on type I interferon signature in rheumatoid arthritis: consequences for response prediction to rituximab. *Arthritis Res Ther.* (2015) 17:78. doi: 10.1186/s13075-015-0564-y
38. De Jong TD, Blits M, De Ridder S, Vosslamber S, Wolbink G, Nurmohamed MT, et al. Type I interferon response gene expression in established rheumatoid arthritis is not associated with clinical parameters. *Arthritis Res Ther.* (2016) 18:290. doi: 10.1186/s13075-016-1191-y
39. de Jong TD, Vosslamber S, Mantel E, de Ridder S, Wesseling JG, van der Pouw Kraan TCTM, et al. Physiological evidence for diversification of IFNα- and IFNβ-mediated response programs in different autoimmune diseases. *Arthritis Res Ther.* (2016) 18:49. doi: 10.1186/s13075-016-0946-9
40. de Jong TD, Sellam J, Agca R, Vosslamber S, Witte BI, Tsang-A-Sjoe M, et al. A multi-parameter response prediction model for rituximab in rheumatoid arthritis. *Joint Bone Spine* (2017) 85:219–26 doi: 10.1016/j.jbspin.2017.02.015
41. Vosslamber S, Raterman HG, van der Pouw Kraan TCTM, Schreurs MWJ, von Blomberg BME, Nurmohamed MT, et al. Pharmacological induction of interferon type I activity following treatment with rituximab determines clinical response in rheumatoid arthritis. *Ann Rheum Dis.* (2011) 70:1153–9. doi: 10.1136/ard.2010.147199
42. El-Sherbiny YM, Psarras A, Md Yusof MY, Hensor EMA, Tooze R, Doody G, et al. A novel two-score system for interferon status segregates autoimmune diseases and correlates with clinical features. *Sci Rep.* (2018) 8:5793. doi: 10.1038/s41598-018-24198-1
43. Md Yusof MY, Psarras A, El-Sherbiny YM, Hensor EMA, Dutton K, Ul-Hassan S, et al. Prediction of autoimmune connective tissue disease in an at-risk cohort: prognostic value of a novel two-score system for interferon status. *Ann Rheum Dis.* (2018) 77:1432–9. doi: 10.1136/annrheumdis-2018-213386
44. Edgar R, Domrachev M, Lash AE. Gene expression omnibus: NCBI gene expression and hybridization array data repository. *Nucleic Acids Res.* (2002) 30:207–10. doi: 10.1093/nar/30.1.207
45. Benjamini Y, Hochberg Y. Controlling the false discovery rate: a practical and powerful approach to multiple testing. *J R Stat Soc Ser B* (1995) 57:289–300. doi: 10.2307/2346101
46. Reynier F, Petit F, Paye M, Turrel-Davin F, Imbert PE, Hot A, et al. Importance of correlation between gene expression levels: application to the type i interferon signature in rheumatoid arthritis. *PLoS ONE* (2011) 6:24828. doi: 10.1371/journal.pone.0024828
47. Rosenbauer F, Waring JF, Foerster J, Wietstruk M, Philipp D, Horak I. Interferon consensus sequence binding protein and interferon regulatory factor-4/Pip form a complex that represses the expression of the interferon-stimulated gene-15 in macrophages. *Blood* (1999) 94:4274–81.
48. Smiljanovic B, Grün JR, Biesen R, Schulte-Wrede U, Baumgrass R, Stuhlmüller B, et al. The multifaceted balance of TNF-α and type I/II interferon responses in SLE and RA: how monocytes manage the impact of cytokines. *J Mol Med.* (2012) 90:1295–309. doi: 10.1007/s00109-012-0907-y
49. Mavragani CP, La DT, Stohl W, Crow MK. Association of the response to tumor necrosis factor antagonists with plasma type I interferon activity and interferon-β/α ratios in rheumatoid arthritis patients: a post hoc analysis of a predominantly hispanic cohort. *Arthritis Rheum.* (2010) 62:392–401. doi: 10.1002/art.27226
50. Tak PP, Hart BA, Kraan MC, Jonker M, Smeets TJ, Breedveld FC. The effects of interferon beta treatment on arthritis. *Rheumatology* (1999) 38:362–9.
51. Smeets TJ, Dayer JM, Kraan MC, Versendaal J, Chicheportiche R, Breedveld FC, et al. The effects of interferon-beta treatment of synovial inflammation and expression of metalloproteinases in patients with rheumatoid arthritis. *Arthritis Rheum.* (2000) 43:270–4. doi: 10.1002/1529-0131(200002)43:2<270::AID-ANR5>3.0.CO;2-H
52. Wampler Muskardin T, Vashisht P, Dorschner JM, Jensen MA, Chrabot BS, Kern M, et al. Increased pretreatment serum IFN-β/α ratio predicts non-response to tumour necrosis factor α inhibition in rheumatoid arthritis. *Ann Rheum Dis.* (2016) 75:1757–62. doi: 10.1136/annrheumdis-2015-208001
53. Gordon RA, Grigoriev G, Lee A, Kalliolias GD, Ivashkiv LB. The interferon signature and STAT1 expression in rheumatoid arthritis synovial fluid macrophages are induced by tumor necrosis factor α and counter-regulated by the synovial fluid microenvironment. *Arthritis Rheum.* (2012) 64:3119–28. doi: 10.1002/art.34544
54. Pfeffer LM, Kim J-G, Pfeffer SR, Carrigan DJ, Baker DP, Wei L, et al. Role of nuclear factor-kappaB in the antiviral action of interferon and interferon-regulated gene expression. *J Biol Chem.* (2004) 279:31304–11. doi: 10.1074/jbc.M308975200

6

The C-Terminal Transactivation Domain of STAT1 has a Gene-Specific Role in Transactivation and Cofactor Recruitment

*Matthias Parrini[1], Katrin Meissl[1], Mojoyinola Joanna Ola[1], Therese Lederer[1], Ana Puga[1], Sebastian Wienerroither[2], Pavel Kovarik[2], Thomas Decker[2], Mathias Müller[1,3] and Birgit Strobl[1]**

[1] *Department of Biomedical Sciences, Institute of Animal Breeding and Genetics, University of Veterinary Medicine Vienna, Vienna, Austria,* [2] *Max F. Perutz Laboratories, University of Vienna, Vienna, Austria,* [3] *University Center Biomodels Austria, University of Veterinary Medicine Vienna, Vienna, Austria*

Correspondence:
Birgit Strobl
birgit.strobl@vetmeduni.ac.at

STAT1 has a key role in the regulation of innate and adaptive immunity by inducing transcriptional changes in response to cytokines, such as all types of interferons (IFN). STAT1 exist as two splice isoforms, which differ in regard to the C-terminal transactivation domain (TAD). STAT1β lacks the C-terminal TAD and has been previously reported to be a weaker transcriptional activator than STAT1α, although this was strongly dependent on the target gene. The mechanism of this context-dependent effects remained unclear. By using macrophages from mice that only express STAT1β, we investigated the role of the C-terminal TAD during the distinct steps of transcriptional activation of selected target genes in response to IFNγ. We show that the STAT1 C-terminal TAD is absolutely required for the recruitment of RNA polymerase II (Pol II) and for the establishment of active histone marks at the class II major histocompatibility complex transactivator (*CIIta*) promoter IV, whereas it is dispensable for histone acetylation at the guanylate binding protein 2 (*Gbp2*) promoter but required for an efficient recruitment of Pol II, which correlated with a strongly reduced, but not absent, transcriptional activity. IFNγ-induced expression of *Irf7*, which is mediated by STAT1 in complex with STAT2 and IRF9, did not rely on the presence of the C-terminal TAD of STAT1. Moreover, we show for the first time that the STAT1 C-terminal TAD is required for an efficient recruitment of components of the core Mediator complex to the IFN regulatory factor (*Irf*) 1 and *Irf8* promoters, which both harbor an open chromatin state under basal conditions. Our study identified novel functions of the STAT1 C-terminal TAD in transcriptional activation and provides mechanistic explanations for the gene-specific transcriptional activity of STAT1β.

Keywords: macrophage, IFNγ, interferon regulatory factor 1 (IRF1), IRF8, transcriptional coactivator, mediator, RNA polymerase II, signal transducer and activator of transcription

INTRODUCTION

Signal-induced reprogramming of gene expression is a crucial part of cellular responses to environmental stimuli. Inducible transcriptional control relies on signal-activated transcription factors (TFs) that bind to DNA regulatory elements distant from the transcriptional start site (TSS) and facilitate the recruitment of transcriptional co-regulators and the general transcriptional machinery, including RNA polymerase II (Pol II). Binding to co-regulatory proteins, such as chromatin remodeling and histone modifying enzymes, occurs through one or more transactivation domains (TADs, also called activation domains) present in TFs (1, 2). Mediator, a large modular protein complex with varying subunit composition, bridges TFs with Pol II and coordinates DNA-loop formation, transcriptional initiation, and post-initiation events (3, 4). Transcription can be induced by *de novo* recruitment of Pol II, which requires assembly of a pre-initiation complex (PIC), or by releasing Pol II from a paused state into productive elongation (5–8). Transcriptional induction is accompanied by phosphorylation of Pol II at serine (S) residues in the heptapeptide repeats within its C-terminal domain (CTD). S5 phosphorylation is triggered by cyclin dependent kinase (CDK) 7, the kinase subunit of the general TF (GTF) complex TFIIH, and allows Pol II to initiate transcription. Typically, after 20–60 nucleotides from the TSS, Pol II is driven into a paused condition by negative elongation factors. S2 phosphorylation of the Pol II CTD is executed by CDK9, the kinase subunit of the positive transcription elongation factor b (p-TEFb), which also phosphorylates negative elongation factors and enables the release of paused Pol II from the promoter (9).

Signal transducer and activator of transcription (STAT) 1 is used for signaling by several cytokines, including all types of IFNs, which are crucial regulators of innate and adaptive immunity. Absence of STAT1 in humans and mice results in severe immunodeficiencies, including high sensitivity to bacterial and viral infections (10, 11). Activation of STAT1 occurs through phosphorylation at tyrosine 701 (Y701) by receptor-associated Janus kinases (JAKs). Type II IFN (IFNγ) mainly activates STAT1 homodimers, which translocate to the nucleus and bind to gamma-IFN activated sequences (GAS) in target gene promoters. Type I and type III IFNs mainly signal through the IFN-stimulated gene factor 3 (ISGF3) TF complex, which consists of STAT1, STAT2, and IFN regulatory factor 9 (IRF9), and binds to IFN-stimulated response elements (ISRE) (11, 12). The STAT1 TAD has been initially identified by the characterization of the naturally occurring splice variants STAT1α and STAT1β. The latter lacks 38 amino acids at the C-terminus and was unable to induce transcription in response to IFNγ when transfected into STAT1-deficient cells and analyzed *in vitro* using chromatin templates (13, 14). Moreover, transactivating activity could be transferred by fusing the 39 C-terminal amino acids to the yeast GAL4 DNA-binding domain (15–17). The STAT1 C-terminal TAD is constitutively active but its function can be modulated by phosphorylation at S727 (18, 19). In the context of IFNγ, S727 phosphorylation occurs within chromatin and is mediated by CDK8 (18). The probably best described function of the C-terminal TAD of STAT1 is its interaction with the histone acetyltransferase CBP/p300 (20, 21). The STAT1 C-terminal TAD also directly interacts with minichromosome maintenance protein 5 (MCM5) and DNA repair-associated tumor suppressor BRCA1 (17, 22, 23). However, the N-terminal region of STAT1 can also bind p300/CBP (24) and it remained unclear whether regions distinct from the C-terminal TAD contribute to the interactions with MCM5 or BRCA1. Our studies with gene-modified mice have shown that the absence of the C-terminal TAD of STAT1 does not abolish transcriptional responses to IFNγ but has modest to severe effects on a subset of target genes (25). Deletion of the C-terminal TAD of STAT1 and mutation of S727 to alanine (S727A) have overlapping but not identical consequences on transcriptional responses to IFNγ (18, 19, 25), indicating that the functions of the C-terminal TAD are not solely exerted through its serine phosphorylation.

In this study we investigated the role of the STAT1 C-terminal TAD in transactivation and cofactor recruitment to paradigmatic IFNγ-inducible genes. The availability of mice that express only the STAT1β isoform (*Stat1*$^{\beta/\beta}$) enabled us to analyze transcriptional activity of STAT1β in primary immune cells under control of the endogenous promoter (25). We report an essential role of the STAT1 C-terminal TAD for an efficient recruitment of distinct Mediator subunits to the *Irf1* and the *Irf8* gene promoters in primary macrophages and for the post-recruitment regulation of Pol II. We furthermore report that the STAT1 C-terminal TAD is absolutely required for the induction of class II major histocompatibility complex transactivator (*CIIta*) through enabling recruitment of Pol II, strongly promotes Pol II recruitment to the guanylate binding protein 2 (*Gbp2*) promoter but is dispensable for the ISRE-driven induction of *Irf7*. Our results shed new light on the communication of STAT1 with the transcriptional machinery and provide mechanistic insights into STAT1 isoform-specific transcriptional activities.

MATERIALS AND METHODS

Mice and Ethics Statement

C57BL/6N (wild-type, *WT*) mice were purchased from Janvier Labs. *Stat1*$^{\beta/\beta}$ (25), *Stat2*$^{-/-}$ (26), *Irf9*$^{-/-}$ (27), and *Irf1*$^{-/-}$ (28) were on C57BL/6 background. *Stat1*$^{\beta/\beta}$*Stat2*$^{-/-}$ and *Stat1*$^{\beta/\beta}$*Irf9*$^{-/-}$ were generated by crossing *Stat1*$^{\beta/\beta}$ with *Stat2*$^{-/-}$ or *Irf9*$^{-/-}$ mice. Mice were housed under specific pathogen-free conditions according to Federation of European Laboratory Animal Science Associations (FELASA) guidelines. Mice were bred at the University of Veterinary Medicine Vienna according to the guidelines of the Federal Ministry of Science, Research and Economy section 8ff of the Animal Science and Experiments Act, Tierversuchsgesetz [TVG], BMWF-68.205/0068-WF/V/3b/2015. The study did not involve animal experiments as defined in the TVG and did not require ethical approval according to the local and national guidelines.

Cell Culture and Cytokines

Bone marrow-derived macrophages (BMDMs) were isolated and differentiated from bone marrow (tibia and femur) of 8–12 weeks old sex-matched mice. BMDMs were differentiated for 7–9 days on Petri dishes (Greiner Bio-One) in DMEM (Sigma-Aldrich) supplemented with 10% FCS (Gibco/Thermo Fisher Scientific), 15% L929 cell-conditioned medium, 2 mM L-glutamine (Sigma-Aldrich), 100 U/ml penicillin, 100 μg/ml streptomycin, (Sigma-Aldrich) and 50 μM β-mercaptoethanol (Gibco/Thermo Fisher Scientific). Cells were treated with recombinant mouse 100 U/ml IFNγ (Millipore, IF005) for the times indicated.

mRNA and Pre-mRNA Expression Analysis

Total RNA was isolated using peqGOLD TriFast™ (VWR) according to manufacturer's instructions. cDNA synthesis and RT-qPCR were performed as described (25, 29). For assays that are located in introns or exon-intron junctions, total RNA was DNase-treated prior to cDNA synthesis. Controls without reverse transcriptase were included for all RT-qPCRs. Primers for pre-mRNA analyses are listed in **Supplementary Table 1**. Sequences of primers and probes for *Ube2d2* (ID 3377) and *Irf1* (ID 3848) mRNA analysis are available at the Real-Time Primer and Probe Database (http://www.rtprimerdb.org/). Primers for *Irf7* (QT00245266) and *Irf8* (QT00174195) mRNA analysis were purchased from Qiagen. qPCRs were done in duplicate on a Bio-Rad CFX96 Touch™ realtime machine.

Whole Cell Extracts and Western Blotting

BMDMs (10^6 cells/well) were stimulated with IFNγ (100 U/ml) for the times indicated, lysed and used for Western blot analysis as described previously (30) with the following adaptations: cells were lysed in 50 mM Tris-HCl (pH 8.0), 150 mM NaCl, 0.5% IGEPAL CA-630 (v/v), 10% glycerol (v/v), 0.1 mM EDTA, 2 mM DTT, 0.2 mM Na-vanadate, 25 mM Na-fluoride, 1 μg/ml leupeptin, 1 μg/ml aprotinin, 0.1 μg pepstatin and 1 mM PMSF. The following antibodies were used: anti-IRF1 (Santa Cruz, SC-640), anti-phospho-Tyr701 STAT1, and anti-STAT1 (Cell Signaling Technology, 9167 and 9172), anti-pan-ERK (BD Transduction Laboratories, 610123; p42 is shown in our experiments). Peroxidase-conjugated secondary antibodies (mouse and rabbit) were from Cell Signaling Technology (7076 and 7074). Blots were scanned with a Chemidoc analyzer (Bio-Rad).

Flow Cytometric Analysis of MHC Class II

BMDMs were stimulated with 100 U/mL of IFNγ for 24 h, washed with PBS, harvested and stained for 15 min at 4°C with anti-MHC Class II (I-A/I-E)-PE (BD Biosciences, BD-557000) or isotype control (rat IgG2bκ-PE, BD Biosciences, BD553989). Data were acquired on a BD FACSCanto II and analyzed with the BD FACSDiva software version 8 (BD Biosciences).

Chromatin Immunoprecipitation (ChIP) Assay and qPCR

The ChIP protocol was adapted from Nissen and Yamamoto (31) and Hauser et al. (32) with the following modifications: 2.5 × 10^7 cells were cross-linked for 10 min at room temperature with 1% formaldehyde in PBS. For H3, H3ac, H4ac, H3K4me3, Pol II, S5pPol II, S2pPol II, STAT1, STAT3, and CDK9 ChIPs, cells were lysed with wash buffer I and II as described (32) and nuclei were lysed in 50 mM Tris-HCl pH 8, 1% SDS, 10 mM EDTA, 1x SIGMAFAST™ Protease Inhibitor (Sigma-Aldrich) and 1 mM PMSF. For STAT2, MED1, MED4, MED18, MED24, MED26, and ERCC3 ChIPs, cells were lysed as described (31) in 10 mM Tris-HCl at pH 8, 1 mM EDTA, 0.5 mM EGTA, 100 mM NaCl, 0.1% Na-deoxycholate, 0.5% N-lauroylsarcosine, 1x SIGMAFAST™ Protease Inhibitor and 1 mM PMSF. For all ChIPs, 25 μg chromatin per IP was used. Antibodies were pulled down with 50 μl of Protein G Dynabeads® (30 mg/ml, Novex, 10009D). qPCRs were done in duplicate on a Stratagene MX3000 or a Bio-Rad CFX96 Touch™ qPCR machine. Primers are listed in **Supplementary Table 2**, primers for the *Irf1* and *Gbp2* gene bodies were as previously described (18). Values are displayed as % input control (for Pol II, S5pPol II, S2pPol II, STAT1, STAT2, MED1, MED4, MED18, MED24, MED26, ERCC3, and CDK9) or relative to H3 (H3ac, H4ac, and H3K4me3). The following antibodies were used: anti-STAT1 (Cell Signaling Technology, 9172, 5 μl/ChIP), anti-Pol2 (Santa Cruz Biotechnology, SC-899-X; 4 μg/ChIP), anti-S5pPol2 (Bethyl, A300-655A; 0.7 μg/ChIP), anti-S2pPol2 (Bethyl, A300-654A; 0.7 μg/ChIP), anti-MED1 (TRAP220, Santa Cruz Biotechnology, SC-5334-X; 4 μg/ChIP, anti-MED4 (Abcam, ab129170; 5 μl/ChIP), anti-MED18 (Bethyl, A300-777A; 0.7 μg/ChIP), anti-MED24 (TRAP100, Bethyl, A300-472A; 0.7 μg/ChIP), anti-MED26 (CRSP70, Santa Cruz Biotechnology, SC-48776-X; 4 μg/ChIP), anti-CDK9 (Santa Cruz Biotechnology, SC-484; 4 μg/ChIP), and anti-ERCC3 (TFIIH subunit, Bethyl, A301-337A; 0.7 μg/ChIP) antibody.

Statistical Analysis

Statistical analyses were done with IBM SPSS Version 22 (univariat mixed model with genotype and stimulation as fixed effects and experiment as random effect) or GraphPad Prism Version 6 (Student's *t*-test; **Figure 1F**).

RESULTS

STAT1β Has Target Gene-Specific Transcriptional Activity

We have shown previously that STAT1β has a differential ability to induce target gene expression in response to IFNγ (25). However, total mRNA analysis is strongly influenced by mRNA decay rates and does not necessarily reflect transcriptional activity. Moreover, STAT1β shows prolonged tyrosine phosphorylation and prolonged *Irf1* and *Gbp2* promoter occupancy in the absence of STAT1α, which may prolong transcriptional activity (25). We thus analyzed pre-mRNA expression of paradigmatic target genes at different time points after IFNγ treatment in $Stat1^{\beta/\beta}$ and *WT* cells. As STAT1 homodimer-driven primary response genes we selected *Irf1* and *Irf8* (33, 34), as secondary response genes that require cooperation of STAT1 dimers with IRF1 we analyzed *CIIta* and *Gbp2* (35–39) and as IFNγ-activated ISGF3-driven gene, we selected *Irf7* (40–42).

Irf1 pre-mRNA expression was rapidly induced in response to IFNγ and was around 2-fold lower in $Stat1^{\beta/\beta}$ compared to *WT* cells at 1 hour (h) and 6 h after treatment (**Figure 1A**). *Irf8* pre-mRNA expression was more transient and around 4-fold lower at 6 h after treatment in $Stat1^{\beta/\beta}$ compared to *WT* cells (**Figure 1B**). Expression of both *Irf1* and *Irf8* pre-mRNAs did not differ between $Stat1^{\beta/\beta}$ and *WT* cells at 24 h after treatment, suggesting that STAT1β does not show increased transcriptional activity at late time points after treatment (**Figures 1A,B**). As expected for secondary response genes, *CIIta* and *Gbp2* pre-mRNA synthesis increased at later time points after IFNγ treatment in *WT* cells (**Figures 1C,D**). *CIIta* pre-mRNA was barely detectable in $Stat1^{\beta/\beta}$ cells (**Figure 1C**), whereas *Gbp2*

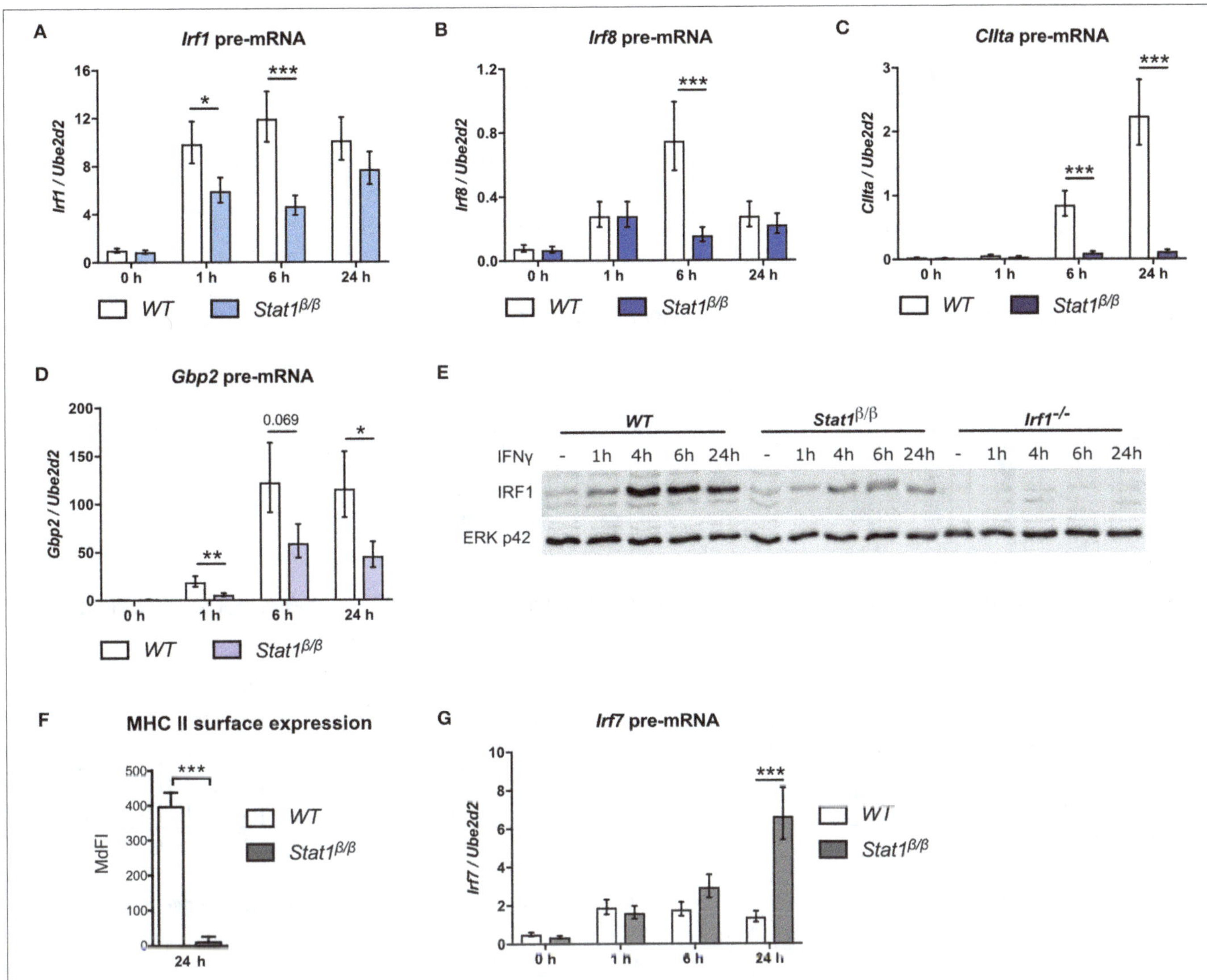

FIGURE 1 | Transcriptional activity of STAT1β at the *Irf1, Irf8, CIlta, Gbp2,* and *Irf7* genes. BMDMs from *WT* and *Stat1*$^{β/β}$ mice were stimulated with IFNγ for the times indicated or left untreated (0 h, -). Total RNA **(A–D, G)** or protein extracts **(E)** were isolated. *Irf1* **(A)**, *Irf8* **(B)**, *CIlta* **(C)**, *Gbp2* **(D)**, and *Irf7* **(G)** pre-mRNA expression was determined by RT-qPCR. Data were normalized to the housekeeping gene *Ube2d2*. Mean values ± SE from three independent experiments are shown. **(E)** IRF1 protein levels were determined by Western blotting. ERK p42 was used as loading control. Data are as representative of two independent experiments. Original uncropped blots are shown in **Supplementary Figure 1**. **(F)** BMDMs from *WT* and *Stat1*$^{β/β}$ mice were stimulated with IFNγ for 24 h. MHC class II surface levels were determined by flow cytometry. Median fluorescence intensities (MdFI) ±standard error (SE) from two independent experiments are shown. **(A–D, F–G)** $^{*}P \leq 0.05$, $^{**}P \leq 0.01$, $^{***}P \leq 0.001$. Significances are only indicated for the comparisons between genotypes.

pre-mRNA was clearly upregulated, albeit to reduced levels compared to *WT* cells (**Figure 1D**). In support of the pre-mRNA data, IFNγ induced considerably lower IRF1protein levels in *Stat1*$^{β/β}$ than in *WT* cells (**Figure 1E**), whereas surface levels of the CIITA-regulated major histocompatibility complex class II (MHC II) proteins remained at basal levels in *Stat1*$^{β/β}$ cells (**Figure 1F**). Surprisingly, *Irf7* pre-mRNA synthesis was profoundly increased 24 h after treatment in *Stat1*$^{β/β}$ compared to *WT* cells, while it did not differ between the genotypes at early time points (**Figure 1G**). Taken together, these data show that STAT1β has gene-specific transcriptional activity which ranges from completely impaired (*CIlta*) or reduced (*Irf1, Irf8, Gbp2*) to an increased activity at late time points after IFNγ treatment (*Irf7*).

Absence of STAT1α Differentially Impairs IFNγ-Induced Histone Modification and the Recruitment of Pol II to the *CIIta* and *Gbp2* Promoters

To test whether differences in *CIIta* and *Gbp2* expression relate to differences in STAT1 or IRF1 binding, we performed site-directed ChIP experiments. Transcriptional induction of *CIIta* in response to IFNγ requires chromatin remodeling by the

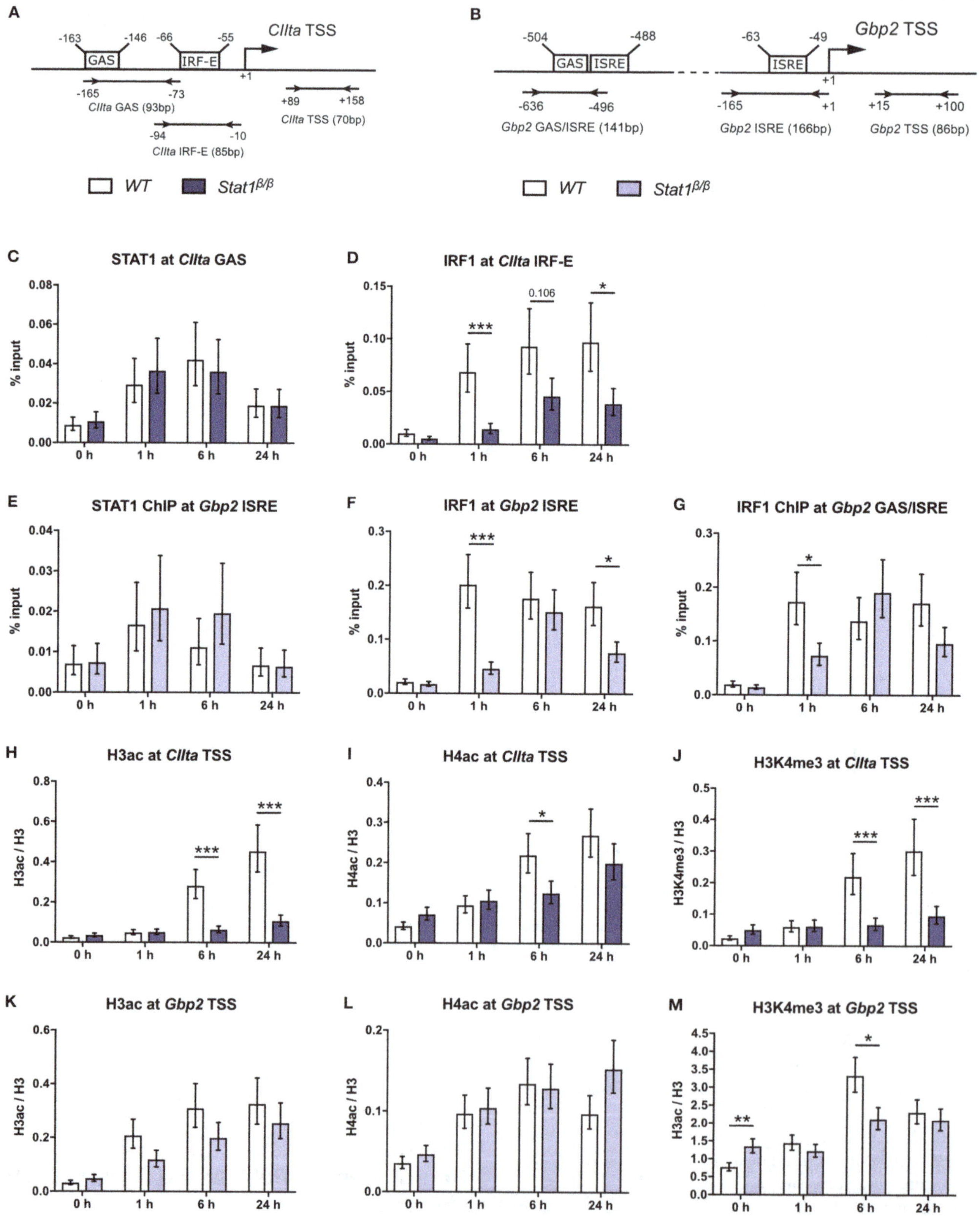

FIGURE 2 | STAT1 and IRF1 binding to the *Cllta* promoter IV (pIV) and the *Gbp2* promoters and IFNγ-induced histone modifications. **(A,B)** Schematic representation of the murine *Cllta* and *Gbp2* promoter regions. STAT1 and IRF1 binding sites, the TSS, and the position of the primers used for the ChIP analyses are depicted.

(Continued)

FIGURE 2 | (C–M) BMDMs from *WT* and *Stat1*$^{\beta/\beta}$ mice were stimulated with IFNγ for the times indicated or left untreated (0 h). STAT1 and IRF1 binding to the *CIIta* **(C, D)** and the *Gbp2* **(E–G)** promoter binding sites was analyzed by ChIP. H3 pan-acetylation (H3ac), H4 pan-acetylation (H4ac), and H3 lysine 4 trimethylation (H3K4me3) around the *CIIta* **(H–J)** and the *Gbp2* **(K–M)** TSS was determined by ChIP. Data were normalized to the input control **(C–G)** and the total levels of H3 **(H–M)**. Mean values ± SE from three **(C–G, H,J,K,M)** or four **(I,L)** independent experiments are shown; $^*P \leq 0.05$, $^{**}P \leq 0.01$, $^{***}P \leq 0.001$. Significances are only indicated for the comparisons between genotypes.

SWI/SNF protein Brahma-related gene 1 (BRG1) (43). The presence of BRG1 is also required for STAT1 binding to the IFNγ-responsive *CIIta* promoter IV (pIV) and the *Gbp2* promoter (37). At the *CIIta* pIV, STAT1 binding additionally relies on cooperation with upstream transcription factor 1 (USF-1), which associates with the adjacent IRF-E box that is also bound by IRF1 (**Figure 2A**). STAT1 occupancy at the GAS site of the *CIIta* pIV was similar between *Stat1*$^{\beta/\beta}$ and WT cells (**Figure 2C**), demonstrating that the STAT1 C-terminal TAD is not required for binding to the *CIIta* promoter and supporting previous studies demonstrating that the STAT1-BRG1 interaction is mediated through the N-terminal and coiled-coil domains of STAT1 (44). Despite the strongly reduced availability of IRF1 in *Stat1*$^{\beta/\beta}$ cells, IRF1 was still detectable at *CIIta* pIV, although its binding was delayed and promoter occupancy was around 2–3-fold lower than in *WT* cells at 6 h after treatment (**Figure 2D**). The *Gbp2* promoter contains two IFNγ-responsive elements: a promoter proximal region containing an ISRE site and a distal region with adjoining GAS and ISRE sites (**Figure 2B**). The distal GAS site binds STAT1 dimers (38) and showed prolonged association with STAT1β in the absence of STAT1α (25). In contrast, the ISRE-containing proximal promoter binds non-canonical STAT1-containing complexes (19) and showed similar STAT1 occupancy in *Stat1*$^{\beta/\beta}$ and *WT* cells (**Figure 2E**). In line with previous studies (45) we found association of IRF1 with the proximal and distal *Gbp2* promoter elements. Association of IRF1 with both promoter elements was delayed and reduced in *Stat1*$^{\beta/\beta}$ compared to *WT* cells (**Figures 2F,G**). Taken together these data support previous studies indicating that the C-terminal TAD of STAT1 is not required for binding to GAS elements (21, 46, 47) and show that the reduced availability of IRF1 delays but does not completely abolish the recruitment of IRF1 to the *Gbp2* and *CIIta* promoters.

Transcriptional induction of *CIIta* and *Gbp2* by IFNγ is accompanied by an increase in acetylation of histones 3 and 4 (19, 37, 45, 48). IFNγ-induced histone 3 acetylation (H3ac) was nearly abolished and histone 4 acetylation (H4ac) strongly reduced around the *CIIta* pIV TSS in *Stat1*$^{\beta/\beta}$ compared to *WT* cells (**Figures 2H,I**), whereas the upregulation of H3ac and H4ac at the *Gbp2* promoter was largely intact (**Figures 2K,L**). In contrast, IFNγ-induced H3 lysine 4 trimethylation (H3K4me3), which marks active promoter regions (49), was lower in *Stat1*$^{\beta/\beta}$ cells at the *CIIta* and the *Gbp2* promoter (**Figures 2J,M**). *Stat1*$^{\beta/\beta}$ cells had modestly higher levels of H3K4me3 at the *Gbp2* promoter than *WT* cells under basal conditions (**Figure 2M**), although this did not correlate with an increase in *Gbp2* pre-mRNA synthesis (**Figure 1D**).

We next analyzed whether the differences in histone acetylation between *CIIta* and *Gbp2* in *Stat1*$^{\beta/\beta}$ cells correlate with differences in the recruitment of Pol II. IFNγ induced a strong increase in Pol II occupancy at the *CIIta* pIV TSS at 6 h after treatment, which was completely absent in *Stat1*$^{\beta/\beta}$ cells (**Figure 3A**). In line with the total Pol II data, promoter occupancy of S5 phosphorylated Pol II (S5pPol II) and S2pPol II did not increase around the *CIIta* TSS in *Stat1*$^{\beta/\beta}$ cells in response to IFNγ (**Figures 3B,C**). Although Pol II recruitment and phosphorylation at the *Gbp2* promoter was also severely impaired in *Stat1*$^{\beta/\beta}$ cells (**Figures 3D–F**), IFNγ still induced an increase in S2pPol II occupancy within the *Gbp2* gene body. In line with the pre-mRNA (**Figure 1D**), S2pPol II occupancy within the *Gbp2* gene body was strongly reduced in *Stat1*$^{\beta/\beta}$ cells compared to *WT* cells (**Figure 3G**).

Taken together, these data indicate a differential requirement for the STAT1 C-terminal TAD for the establishment of active histone marks at the *CIIta* and *Gbp2* promoter and show that STAT1 C-terminal TAD-independent histone acetylation at the *Gbp2* is not sufficient to enable efficient recruitment Pol II.

IRF9 and STAT2 Are Not Required for the Induction of *Irf1* by STAT1β

It is becoming increasingly evident that IFNs not only signal through STAT1 homodimers and ISGF3 but also through non-canonical complexes, such as STAT1-STAT2 heterodimers, STAT1-IRF9, or STAT2-IRF9 (27, 50–52). To exclude that the absence of STAT1α favors the formation of non-canonical STAT1-complexes and to confirm that the induction of *Irf7* but not *Irf1* depends on the presence of STAT2 and IRF9, we crossed *Stat1*$^{\beta/\beta}$ mice with mice lacking either STAT2 (*Stat1*$^{\beta/\beta}$*Stat2*$^{-/-}$) or IRF9 (*Stat1*$^{\beta/\beta}$*Irf9*$^{-/-}$). In line with the importance of type I IFN-ISGF3 signaling in the regulation of basal STAT1 expression (53), STAT1β protein levels were reduced in the absence of STAT2 and, to a lesser extent, in the absence of IRF9 (**Figure 4A**). However, *Irf1* mRNA was still upregulated in response to IFNγ in *Stat1*$^{\beta/\beta}$*Stat2*$^{-/-}$ and *Stat1*$^{\beta/\beta}$*Irf9*$^{-/-}$ cells (**Figure 4B**), confirming that its induction does not rely on the presence of IRF9 or STAT2. IFNγ-triggered *Irf7* mRNA expression was completely abolished in *Stat1*$^{\beta/\beta}$*Stat2*$^{-/-}$ and *Stat1*$^{\beta/\beta}$*Irf9*$^{-/-}$ cells (**Figure 4C**), supporting previous studies demonstrating that the induction of *Irf7* by IFNγ requires the presence of STAT2 and/or IRF9 (41). It is important to note that previous studies have established that other STAT proteins cannot compensate for the loss of STAT1 in upregulating most of the classical ISGs, including *Irf1* and *Irf8* (54–57), further underscoring the notion that STAT1β homodimers are capable of inducing GAS-driven genes, albeit to reduced levels as compared to STAT1α homodimers or STAT1α/STAT1β dimers.

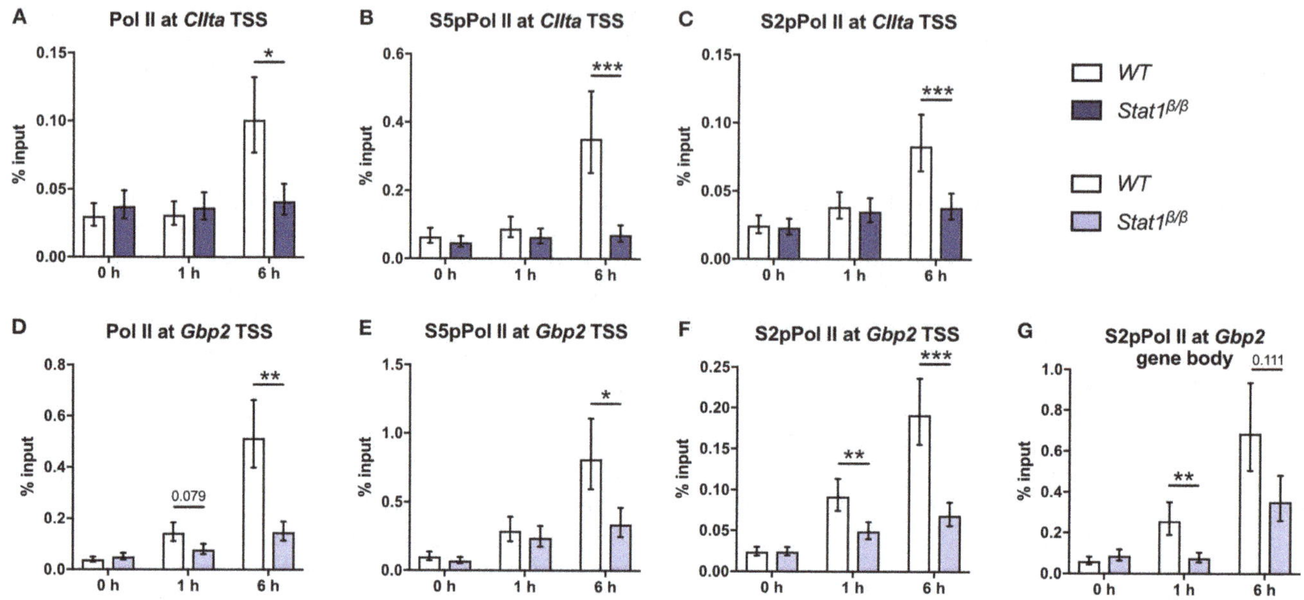

FIGURE 3 | Promoter occupancy of Pol II, S5 phosphorylated Pol II (S5pPol II), and S2 phosphorylated Pol II (S2pPol II) around the *Cllta* and *Gbp2* TSS and of S2pPol II at the *Gbp2* gene body. BMDMs from *WT* and *Stat1*$^{\beta/\beta}$ mice were stimulated with IFNγ for the times indicated or left untreated (0 h). The association of Pol II, S5pPol II, and S2pPol II with the TSS of **(A–C)** *Cllta* pIV and **(D–F)** *Gbp2* TSS, and **(G)** association of S2pPol II with the *Gbp2* gene body was determined by ChIP. Data were normalized to the input control. Mean values ± SE from three **(D,G)**, four **(A,B)** or five **(C,E,F)** independent experiments are shown; $^{*}P \leq 0.05$, $^{**}P \leq 0.01$, $^{***}P \leq 0.001$. Significances are only indicated for the comparisons between genotypes.

Absence of STAT1α Does Not Affect the Establishment of Active Histone Marks at the *Irf1* and *Irf8* Promoters

We next investigated the impact of the STAT1 C-terminal TAD on STAT1 and STAT2 binding kinetics and the establishment of active histone marks at the *Irf1*, *Irf8*, and *Irf7* promoters. The *Irf7* promoter contains two adjoining ISRE sites downstream of its TSS (**Figure 5A**). Consistent with the regulation of *Irf7* by ISGF3 (41), IFNγ induced a rapid association of STAT1 and STAT2 to the *Irf7* promoter (**Figures 5D,E**). STAT1 and STAT2 occupancy was similar at 1 h and 6 h but considerably higher at 24 h after treatment in *Stat1*$^{\beta/\beta}$ as compared to *WT* cells (**Figures 5D,E**). In contrast to our previous observations at the GAS sites of the *Irf1* promoter and the distal *Gbp2* promoter (25), STAT1 occupancy around the GAS site within the *Irf8* promoter was not different between *Stat1*$^{\beta/\beta}$ and *WT* cells (**Figure 5F**), suggesting that the prolonged phosphorylation of STAT1β in the absence of STAT1α (25) prolongs promoter binding in a promoter context-specific manner.

In line with a previous study indicating that the *Irf1* gene harbors a permissive chromatin conformation under basal conditions in bone marrow-derived macrophages (58), we found higher H3ac, H4ac, and H3K4me3 to H3 ratios at the *Irf1* promotor than at the *CIlta* and *Gbp2* promoters in untreated cells, irrespective of the presence of STAT1α (**Figures 5G–I**, compare to **Figures 2H–M**). Except for an around 2-fold higher level of H4ac at 1 h after IFNγ treatment in *Stat1*$^{\beta/\beta}$ cells, we did not observe differences between *Stat1*$^{\beta/\beta}$ and *WT* cells (**Figures 5G–I**). Neither IFNγ treatment nor the absence of STAT1α affected the levels of H3ac, H4ac, or H3K4me3 at the *Irf8* promoter (**Figures 5J–L**). Despite the high basal H3ac and H4ac levels at the *Irf7* promoter, acetylation increased within 1 h of IFNγ treatment, which was again independent of the presence of the STAT1 C-terminal TAD (**Figures 5M,N**). In contrast, H3K4me3 levels did not increase in response to IFNγ treatment but slightly decreased at 24 h after treatment in *Stat1*$^{\beta/\beta}$ and *WT* cells (**Figure 5O**).

The C-Terminal TAD of STAT1 Facilitates an Efficient Recruitment of Mediator Complex Subunits to the *Irf1* Promoter and Promotes Transcription at a Post-Initiation Step

To address the question why STAT1β has reduced transcriptional activity at the *Irf1* gene we next analyzed the recruitment and phosphorylation of Pol II and the recruitment of components of the Mediator complex and GTF complexes TFIIH and p-TEFb (**Figure 6A**). IFNγ-induced an around 3-fold increase in Pol II promoter occupancy at the *Irf1* TSS in *Stat1*$^{\beta/\beta}$ and *WT* cells (**Figure 6B**), indicating that the STAT1 C-terminal TAD is not required to recruit Pol II to the *Irf1* promoter. As shown in **Figure 6C**, the association of S5pPol II with the *Irf1* promoter increased upon IFNγ treatment and was not different between *Stat1*$^{\beta/\beta}$ and *WT* cells at 1 h after treatment. Promoter occupancy of S5pPol II was modestly reduced at 6 h after treatment in *Stat1*$^{\beta/\beta}$ compared to *WT* cells, although this did not reach statistical significance. CDK7, the kinase

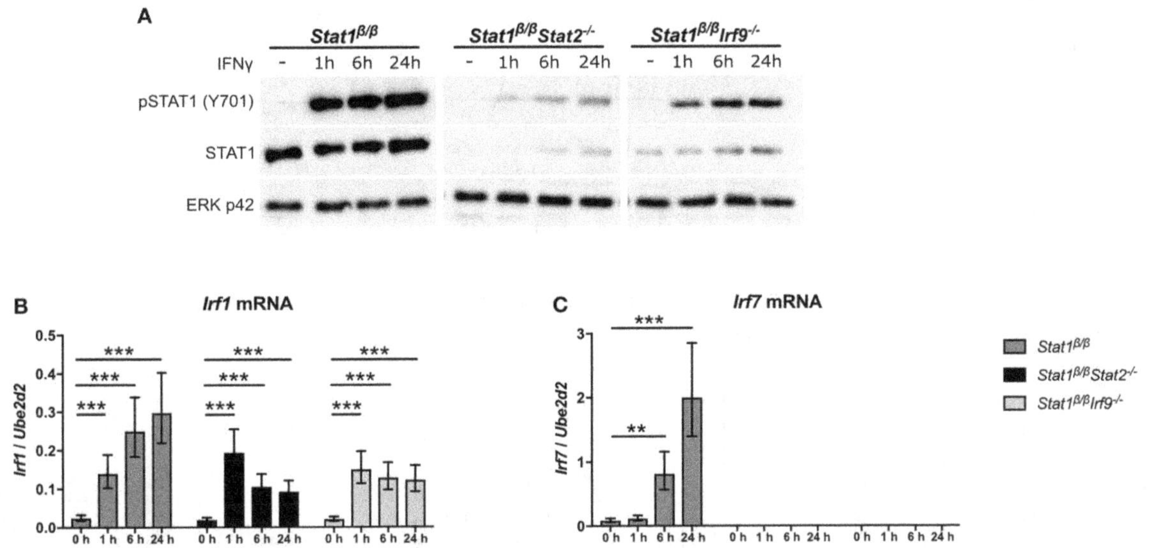

FIGURE 4 | IFNγ induced expression of *Irf1* and *Irf7* in *Stat1*$^{\beta/\beta}$ cells in the absence of STAT2 or IRF9. BMDMs derived from *Stat1*$^{\beta/\beta}$, *Stat1*$^{\beta/\beta}$*Stat2*$^{-/-}$ and *Stat1*$^{\beta/\beta}$*Irf9*$^{-/-}$ mice were stimulated with IFNγ for the times indicated or left untreated (0 h, -). **(A)** Protein was isolated and Tyr701-phosphorylated STAT1 (pSTAT1) and STAT1 protein levels determined by Western blotting. ERK p42 was used as loading control. One representative out of three independent experiments is shown. Original uncropped blots are shown in **Supplementary Figure 2**. **(B,C)** Total RNA was isolated and *Irf1* **(B)** and *Irf7* **(C)** mRNA expression was determined by RT-qPCR. Data were normalized to *Ube2d2*. Mean values ± SE from three **(C)** or four **(B)** independent experiments are shown. $^{*}P \leq 0.05$, $^{**}P \leq 0.01$, $^{***}P \leq 0.001$. Significances are only indicated for the comparisons between genotypes.

that phosphorylates Pol II at S5 in its CTD is a component of the TFIIH complex that also contains ERCC3 [(59) and **Figure 6A**]. Consistent with the S5pPol II data, association of ERCC3 with the *Irf1* promoter was similar in *Stat1*$^{\beta/\beta}$ and *WT* cells at 1 h, whereas it was reduced at 6 h after IFNγ treatment in *Stat1*$^{\beta/\beta}$ compared to *WT* cells (**Figure 6F**). To proceed into productive elongation Pol II requires the recruitment of the p-TEFb complex and the activation of its associated kinase CDK9, which can phosphorylate Pol II at S2 in its CTD [(6) and **Figure 6A**]. CDK9 promoter occupancy (**Figure 6G**) and association of S2pPol II with the *Irf1* promoter (**Figure 6D**) did not significantly differ between *Stat1*$^{\beta/\beta}$ and *WT* cells 1 h after treatment but were strongly reduced at 6 h after treatment (**Figures 6G,D**). In contrast, levels of S2pPol II within the *Irf1* gene body, which is an indicator for productive transcriptional elongation, was already clearly lower at 1 h after treatment in *Stat1*$^{\beta/\beta}$ than in *WT* cells (**Figure 6E**). Thus, during the early phases of the IFNγ response the impaired release of poised Pol II is not due to an impaired recruitment of TFIIH or p-TEFb to the *Irf1* promoter. The Mediator complex is a central transcriptional co-activator that bridges TFs with Pol II and is involved in the regulation of multiple steps of the transcriptional cycle, including the formation of a stable PIC, transcriptional elongation and transcriptional re-initiation (3, 60). Given the high complexity of Mediator, we analyzed the recruitment of selected subunits of the head, middle and tail modules [(61) and **Figure 6A**] to the *Irf1* promoter. We found a profound increase of MED18 (head), MED4 (middle) and MED24 (tail) promoter occupancy around the *Irf1* GAS after IFNγ stimulation in *WT* macrophages (**Figures 6H–J**). Recruitment of MED18 did not differ between *Stat1*$^{\beta/\beta}$ and *WT* cells, whereas recruitment of MED4 and MED24 was reduced in *Stat1*$^{\beta/\beta}$ cells (**Figures 6H–J**). The MED1 and MED26 subunits are not always associated with the Mediator complex but, dependent on the target gene, can be central to its functionality. MED1 has been described important for nuclear receptor interaction (62, 63) and MED26 to interact with the super elongation complex, which contains p-TEFb (64). Similar to MED4 and MED24, MED26 and MED1 were recruited less efficiently to the *Irf1* promoter in *Stat1*$^{\beta/\beta}$ than in *WT* cells (**Figures 6K,L**). *Stat1*$^{\beta/\beta}$ cells already showed reduced association of Mediator components at the time point when promoter occupancy of ERCC3 and CDK9 did not differ from *WT* cells (i.e., 1 h after treatment, **Figures 6F,G**), indicating that the recruitment of TFIIH and p-TEFb to the *Irf1* promoter is independent of an increase in promoter association of MED1, MED4, MED24, and MED26 at the *Irf1* gene at early time points after stimulation.

The Importance of the C-Terminal TAD of STAT1 for an Efficient Recruitment of Mediator Components and the Release of Poised Pol II Extends to the *Irf8* Promoter

Next, we analyzed the recruitment and phosphorylation of Pol II and the recruitment of Mediator components to the *Irf8* gene. IFNγ induced an around 2-fold increase in Pol II promoter occupancy at the *Irf8* TSS in *Stat1*$^{\beta/\beta}$ and *WT* cells (**Figure 7A**). S5pPol II and S2pPol II occupancy at the *Irf8* promoter followed a similar pattern as at the *Irf1* promoter, although association of S2pPol II with the TSS was not significantly different between

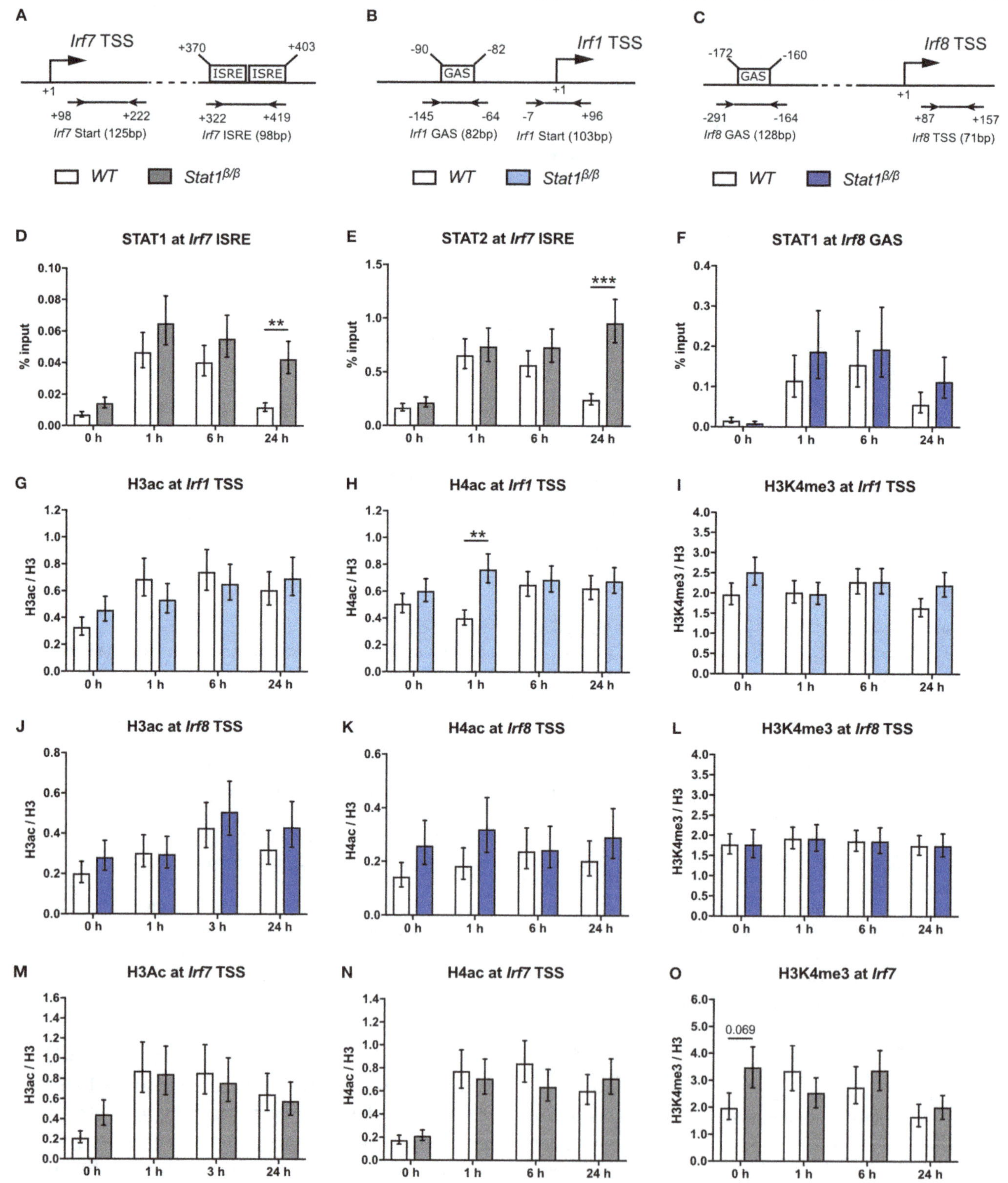

FIGURE 5 | STAT1 and IRF1 binding to the *Irf7* and *Irf8* promoters and H3ac and H4ac and H3K4me3 around the *Irf1*, *Irf8*, and *Irf7* TSS before and after IFNγ treatment. **(A–C)** Schematic representation of the murine *Irf7* **(A)**, *Irf1* **(B)**, and *Irf8* **(C)** promoter regions. GAS and ISRE sites, the TSS and the position of the primers used for the ChIP analyses are depicted. **(D–O)** BMDMs from *WT* and *Stat1*$^{\beta/\beta}$ mice were stimulated with IFNγ for the times indicated or left untreated (0 h). STAT1 and STAT2 binding at the *Irf7* ISRE **(D,E)** and STAT1 binding at the *Irf8* **(F)** GAS element was analyzed by ChIP. H3 pan-acetylation (H3ac), H4 pan-acetylation (H4ac), and H3 lysine 4 trimethylation (H3K4me3) around the *Irf1* **(G–I)**, the *Irf8* **(J–L)**, and the *Irf7* **(M–O)** TSS was determined by ChIP. Data were normalized to the input control **(D–F)** or the total levels of H3 **(G–O)**. Mean values ± SE from three to four independent experiments are shown; $^{**}P \leq 0.01$, $^{***}P \leq 0.001$. Significances are only indicated for the comparisons between genotypes.

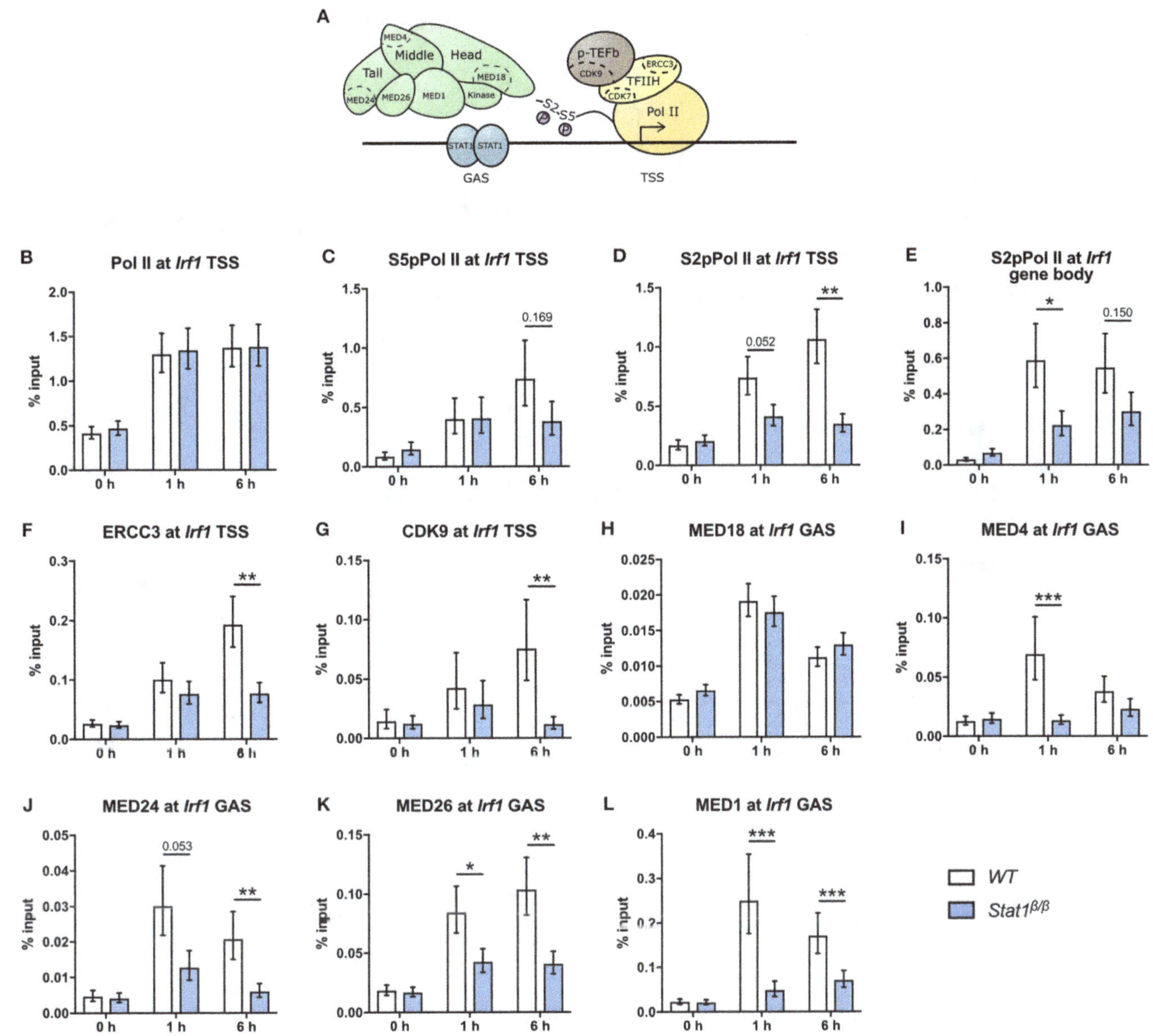

FIGURE 6 | Recruitment and phosphorylation of Pol II at *Irf1* gene and occupancy of TFIIH, p-TEFb, and Mediator components at the *Irf1* TSS. **(A)** Schematic representation of Pol II, GTFs, and the Mediator complex at a GAS-driven gene promoter. Components of the Mediator, TFIIH, and p-TEFb complexes analyzed by ChIP are indicated. **(B–L)** BMDMs from *WT* and *Stat1*$^{\beta/\beta}$ mice were stimulated with IFNγ for the times indicated or left untreated (0 h). Association of Pol II, S5pPol II, and S2pPol II with the *Irf1* promoter around the TSS **(B–D)** and of S2pPol II within the *Irf1* gene body **(E)**. Association of ERCC3 **(F)** and CDK9 **(G)** at the *Irf1* TSS and of MED18 **(H)**, MED4 **(I)**, MED24 **(J)**, MED26 **(K)**, and MED1 **(L)** at the *Irf1* GAS. Data were normalized to the input control. Mean values ± SE from two **(H)** or three (all others) independent experiments are shown; *$P \leq 0.05$, **$P \leq 0.01$, ***$P \leq 0.001$.

Stat1$^{\beta/\beta}$ and *WT* cells after 6 h stimulation (**Figures 7B,C**). S2pPol II occupancy within the *Irf8* gene body was even higher in *Stat1*$^{\beta/\beta}$ than in *WT* cells under basal conditions (**Figure 7D**), although this did not correlate with increased *Irf8* pre-mRNA levels (**Figure 1B**). In line with the pre-mRNA data, S2pPol II occupancy within the *Irf8* gene body was lower in *Stat1*$^{\beta/\beta}$ than in *WT* cells at 1 and 6 h after treatment (**Figure 7D**). Taken together these data suggest that the STAT1 C-terminal TAD facilitates the release of Pol II into productive elongation also at the *Irf8* promoter. Although we were unable to reliably detect *Irf8* promoter sequences in MED4 and MED18 ChIPs under our experimental conditions, we observed reduced recruitment of MED1 and MED24, but not MED26, to the *Irf8* promoter in *Stat1*$^{\beta/\beta}$ compared to *WT* cells (**Figures 7E–G**), indicating that the requirement for the C-terminal TAD of STAT1 for an efficient recruitment of subunits of the Mediator complex extends to other GAS-driven genes, such as *Irf8*, but may affect distinct Mediator subunits depending on the target gene.

In line with the unimpaired transcriptional induction of *Irf7* (**Figure 1G**), *Stat1*$^{\beta/\beta}$ cells did not differ from *WT* cells with

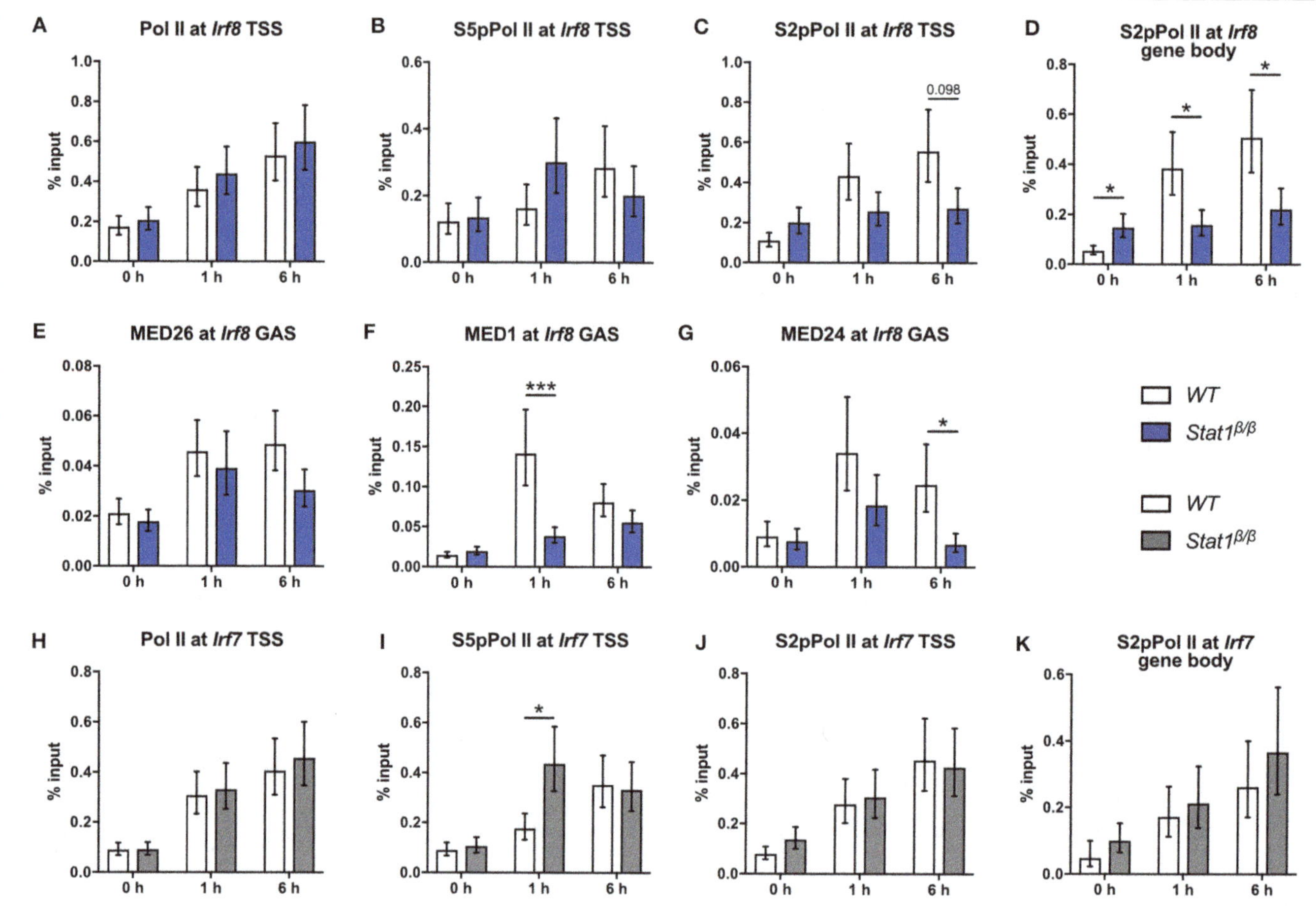

FIGURE 7 | Recruitment and phosphorylation of Pol II at the *Irf8* and *Irf7* genes and occupancy of Mediator components at the *Irf8* promoter. **(A–K)** BMDMs from WT and $Stat1^{\beta/\beta}$ mice were stimulated with IFNγ for the times indicated or left untreated (0 h). Association of Pol II, S5pPol II, and S2pPol II with the *Irf8* **(A–C)** and the *Irf7* promoters **(H–J)** around the TSS and of S2pPol II within the respective gene bodies **(D,K)** was determined by ChIP. The promoter occupancy of MED26 **(E)**, MED1 **(F)**, and MED24 **(G)** at the *Irf8* GAS. Data were normalized to the input control. Mean values ± SE from two **(K)**, three **(A–I)** or four **(J)** independent experiments are shown; $^*P \leq 0.05$, $^{**}P \leq 0.01$, $^{***}P \leq 0.001$.

respect to the association of Pol II and S2pPol II at the *Irf7* TSS and S2pPol II within the *Irf7* gene body at 1 h and 6 h after IFNγ treatment (**Figures 7H–K**). Promoter occupancy of S5pPol II at the *Irf7* TSS was transiently higher in $Stat1^{\beta/\beta}$ than in *WT* cells (**Figure 7I**) but this did not translate into higher levels of S2pPol II at the TSS or within the gene body or an increased transcriptional activity (**Figures 7J,K and Figure 1G**) at this time point. The finding that the induction of *Irf7* does not require the presence of the STAT1 C-terminal TAD is consistent with earlier studies indicating and that in the context of ISGF3 the TAD is provided by STAT2 (65).

DISCUSSION

In this study we used primary macrophages from mice that only express the STAT1β isoform to investigate the role of the C-terminal TAD of STAT1 in the IFNγ-induced transcriptional activation of the *Irf1, Irf7, Irf8, Gbp2,* and *CIIta* genes under physiologic conditions. Using pre-mRNA and ChIP analyses, we show for the first time that STAT1β has gene-specific transcriptional activity that correlates with a gene-specific requirement for the C-terminal TAD for IFNγ-induced histone modification, recruitment of Pol II and association of components of the Mediator complex to target gene promoters (**Table 1**).

The most important finding of our study is that the STAT1 C-terminal TAD is required for an efficient association of components of the Mediator complex to the *Irf1* and *Irf8* promoters and an efficient release of poised Pol II. Many TFs interact directly with the Mediator complex, although TFs target distinct Mediator subunits (66). With the exception of STAT2, it is unclear how STAT proteins interact with the Mediator complex. STAT2 binding to MED14 increases ISGF3-induced transcription but it remained undetermined whether the contact to MED14 is through the C-terminal TAD of STAT2 (65). Our data indicate that the STAT1 C-terminal TAD is involved in the recruitment of components of the Mediator tail (MED24), middle (MED4) and flexible (MED1, MED26) submodules to the

TABLE 1 | Summary of ChIP results at 1 and 6 h after IFNγ treatment.

Gene		*Ciita*		*Gbp2*		*Irf1*		*Irf8*		*Irf7*	
Time of IFNγ treatment		1 h	6 h	1 h	6 h	1 h	6 h	1 h	6 h	1 h	6 h
ChIP	site of PCR										
STAT1	GAS	=	=	↓[a]	=[a]	↓[a]	=[a]	=	=	NA	
STAT1	ISRE	NA		=	=	NA		NA		=	=[b]
STAT2	ISRE	NA		NA		NA		NA		=	=[b]
IRF1	ISRE/IRF-E	↓↓	=	↓↓	=	NA		NA		NA	
IRF1	GAS-ISRE	NA		↓↓	=	NA		NA		NA	
H3ac	TSS	–	↓↓	=	=	–	–	–	–	=	=
H4ac	TSS	–	↓	=	=	↑	–	–	–	=	=
H3K4me3	TSS	–	↓↓	–	↓	–	–	–	–	–	–
Pol II	TSS	–	↓↓	(↓)	↓↓	=	=	=	=	=	=
S5pPol II	TSS	–	↓↓	=	↓↓	=	=	–	=	↑	=
S2pPol II	TSS	–	↓↓	↓	↓↓	(↓)	↓↓	=	(↓)	=	=
S2pPol II	gene body	ND		↓↓	=	↓↓	=	↓↓	↓↓	=	=
ERCC3	GAS	ND		ND		=	↓↓	ND		ND	
CDK9	GAS	ND		ND		=	↓↓	ND		ND	
MED18	GAS	ND		ND		=	=	ND		ND	
MED4	GAS	ND		ND		↓↓	=	ND		ND	
MED24	GAS	ND		ND		(↓)	↓↓	=	↓↓	ND	
MED26	GAS	ND		ND		↓	↓↓	=	=	ND	
MED1	GAS	ND		ND		↓↓	↓↓	↓↓	=	ND	

Changes between $Stat1^{\beta/\beta}$ *and WT cells are indicated by symbols: =, no change; –, not induced by IFNγ and no change; ↑, increased; ↓, decreased; ↓↓, strongly decreased (i.e., more than 2-fold) with* $p \leq 0.05$*; (↓), decreased with a p value between 0.05 and 0.1 in* $Stat1^{\beta/\beta}$ *compared to WT cells; NA, not applicable; ND, not determined*

[a]*previously published data (25)*

[b]*increased at 24 h after treatment.*

STAT1 homodimer-driven *Irf1* gene. Pol II recruitment was not affected by the absence of the STAT1 C-terminal TAD indicating that Pol II binding to the *Irf1* promoter is independent of the core Mediator complex which, according to the definition as the minimal set of Mediator subunits required to reconstitute a functional Mediator complex *in vitro,* consists of head and middle modules held together by MED14 (67). Interestingly, we show that the recruitment of MED18, a component of the Mediator head submodule, to the *Irf1* promoter does not require the presence of the STAT1 C-terminal TAD. This is in line with the current concept that the head module of the Mediator complex interacts with Pol II (67) and suggests that this does not require input from the STAT1 C-terminal TAD. Our data are also consistent with a previous study that indicated impaired recruitment of MED1 to the *Irf1* promoter in the absence of STAT1α (18). Notably, the STAT1 S727A mutation did not affect *Irf1* transcription (18), arguing against the requirement for S727 phosphorylation for the recruitment of the Mediator core complex to the *Irf1* gene.

Another interesting finding of our study is that the STAT1 C-terminal TAD facilitates the association of TFIIH and p-TEFb to the *Irf1* promoter in a time-dependent manner, as evidenced by the promoter occupancy of the TFIIH component ERCC3 and the p-TEFb kinase CDK9. Within the first hour of IFNγ treatment, promoter occupancy of ERCC3 and CDK9 did not differ between $Stat1^{\beta/\beta}$ and *WT* cells, suggesting that the recruitment of these GTFs to the *Irf1* promoter is independent of the STAT1 C-terminal TAD and the Mediator core complex. In contrast, promoter occupancy of ERCC3 and CDK9 was strongly reduced in $Stat1^{\beta/\beta}$ compared to WT cells at 6 h after treatment. While the reduced promoter occupancy of ERCC3 did not correlate with significant differences in the levels of S5 phosphorylated Pol II, promoter occupancy of S2 phosphorylated Pol II at the *Irf1* TSS was clearly lower in $Stat1^{\beta/\beta}$ than in *WT* cells, which is consistent with a role of CDK9 in the phosphorylation of S2 of Pol II. It has to be taken into consideration that *Irf1* transcription is induced within 30–60 min after IFNγ treatment (35, 45) and thus data at the 6 h time point may reflect effects on transcriptional re-initiation. Transcriptional re-initiation is facilitated by scaffold PICs that remain after Pol II escape, contain most of the pre-initiation factors, including TFIIH and Mediator, and are stabilized by TFs (3, 68). It thus seems reasonable to speculate that the STAT1 C-terminal TAD may be required to stabilize re-initiation scaffolds at the *Irf1* promoter. The STAT1 C-terminal TAD is also required for the recruitment of CDK8, a component of the Mediator kinase module, which has been implicated in multiple aspects of the transcriptional cycle, including transcriptional re-initiation (3). The recent finding that STAT1 requires processive transcription for its dephosphorylation and promoter dissociation (69) prompts the hypothesis that transcriptionally compromised STAT1β homodimers accumulate at the promoters and prevent transcriptional re-initiation. However, it is also possible that the time-dependent effects observed relate to the heterogeneity of the cell population and reflect an increase in the number of cells responding to IFNγ over time. Further studies are required to distinguish between these possibilities and to test a potential involvement of the STAT1 C-terminal TAD in the regulation of transcriptional re-initiation.

It also remains to be investigated how the STAT1 C-terminal TAD mediates the transition of poised Pol II at the *Irf1* promoter into productive elongation within the first hour of stimulation. TFIIH and S5 phosphorylation of Pol II were not affected by the absence of the STAT C-terminal TAD, indicating unimpaired early elongation. The release of paused Pol II into productive elongation requires phosphorylation of negative elongation factors by p-TEFb. The association of the p-TEFb kinase CDK9 with the *Irf1* promoter was not affected by the absence of the STAT1 C-terminal TAD at 1 h after stimulation, arguing against an impaired recruitment of p-TEFb as underlying mechanism. However, different p-TEFb-containing complexes may be recruited in the absence or presence of the C-terminal TAD (67, 70). Another interesting possibility is that the absence of the C-terminal TAD might result in premature transcriptional termination due to a failure to recruit MCM5-containing complexes. This hypothesis is supported by previous studies that demonstrated interactions of MCM5 with the STAT1 C-terminal TAD (17) and IFNγ-induced association of MCM5 and MCM3 with the promoter and intergenic regions of *Irf1* (71), suggesting that MCM2-MCM7 complexes move along with Pol II during *Irf1* transcript elongation possibly unwinding DNA through their helicase activity (71).

Importantly, the STAT1 C-terminal TAD facilitates, but is not absolutely required, for the recruitment of Mediator components to the *Irf1* and *Irf8* promoters and for its transcriptional activity at these genes. This is in line with earlier studies demonstrating that STAT1β is capable of inducing transcription of naked DNA in transcription assays *in vitro* (21). In contrast to our study, cell transfection experiments indicated an absolute requirement for the STAT1 C-terminal TAD for the induction of *Irf1* (13, 21). The reason for this discrepancy is unclear, but may relate to the presence of paused Pol II and active histone marks at the *Irf1* locus in primary macrophages (58). In the fibrosarcoma cell line 2fTGH, the *Irf1* gene requires STAT1-dependent histone methylation, including H3K4me3, for its transcriptional induction by IFNγ (72) whereas we and others (58) show that H3K4me3 is already high under basal conditions and does not further increase upon IFNγ or lipopolysaccharide treatment in primary macrophages. Notably, the *Irf1* promoter also has active chromatin marks in many primary human cell types, including cells of the myeloid lineage (73).

In contrast to *Irf1* and *Irf8*, induction of the *CIIta* gene was completely abolished in *Stat1*$^{\beta/\beta}$ cells. Unresponsiveness to STAT1β correlated with an impaired IFNγ-induced histone acetylation (H3ac and H4ac) and H3K4me3 at the *CIIta* promoter and a failure to recruit Pol II. In line with the ChIP data, IFNγ-induced *CIIta* pre-mRNA synthesis and up-regulation of MHC class II proteins at the cell surface were completely abolished in the absence of the STAT1 C-terminal TAD. As *Stat1*$^{\beta/\beta}$ cells show a considerably reduced upregulation of IRF1, we cannot distinguish whether the impaired induction of *CIIta* is due to a role of the STAT1 C-terminal TAD at the *CIIta* promoter or to the reduced availability and promoter occupancy of IRF1.

In contrast to *CIIta* pIV, H3, and H4 acetylation at the *Gbp2* promoter was not dependent on the C-terminal TAD of STAT1. This is surprising, as previous studies using *Stat1*$^{-/-}$ and *Irf1*$^{-/-}$ cells suggested that H4 acetylation at the *Gbp2* promoter is mediated through STAT1, although these studies are complicated by the fact that *Irf1*$^{-/-}$ cells have reduced STAT1 protein levels and *Stat1*$^{-/-}$ cells fail to upregulate IRF1 (45). Further support for an involvement of STAT1 in the recruitment of histone acetyltransferases (HATs) to the *Gbp2* promoter came from the analysis of cells harboring a point mutation of S727 within the C-terminal TAD (*Stat1*^{S727A}), which have strongly reduced H4 acetylation and fail to recruit CBP to the *Gbp2* promoter (19, 45). The reason for the discrepancy between *Stat1*$^{\beta/\beta}$ and *Stat1*^{S727A} remains unclear. It seems possible that STAT1 recruits HATs directly or indirectly through regions distinct from the C-terminal TAD (24) and that this is inhibited by S727 phosphorylation of the TAD. Alternatively, the absence of the C-terminal TAD and mutation of S727 may differentially affect recruitment of HATs and histone deacetylases (HDACs). Further studies are required to delineate the exact role of the STAT1 C-terminal TAD and its serine phosphorylation in the recruitment of HATs and HDACs and acetylation of H3 and H4 at specific lysine residues. Despite the unimpaired histone acetylation, recruitment of Pol II and transcriptional induction of *Gbp2* were severely impaired in the absence of the STAT1 C-terminal TAD, indicating that histone acetylation is not sufficient to recruit Pol II and induce gene expression. However, low-level of Pol II recruitment still occurred in *Stat1*$^{\beta/\beta}$ cells which correlated with impaired, but not absent, transcriptional activity and may relate to the interaction of IRF1 with Pol II (45).

Collectively, our data provide the first evidence that the STAT1 C-terminal TAD facilitates transcription through the recruitment of the Mediator complex to GAS-driven genes that harbor an open chromatin state. Our study also provides further evidence for the hypothesis that regions distinct from the C-terminal TAD contribute to the transactivating activity of STAT1. It remains to be investigated whether the gene-specific requirement for the STAT1 C-terminal TAD for histone acetylation at GAS-driven genes reflects gene-specific functional cooperativity with other TFs or co-factors or the recruitment of distinct HATs or HDACs. It also has to be taken into consideration that STAT1 activity at distal enhancers may contribute to the gene-specific transactivating activity of STAT1β (48, 74–76). Many aspects of innate and adaptive immunity are regulated by STAT1. Thus, a better understanding of its interaction with the transcriptional machinery and of the function of its individual isoforms may help to fine-tune therapeutic and diagnostic strategies that interfere with STAT1 functions.

AUTHOR CONTRIBUTIONS

MP performed most of the experiments. KM did the laboratory work related to the FACS experiments, contributed to data interpretation, performed the statistical analysis, helped with data presentation, and edited the manuscript. MO and TL performed qPCR analyses, AP performed some of the ChIP experiments and SW provided help with the ChIP technology. PK, TD, and MM were involved in the study design, provided crucial input throughout the project, and edited the manuscript. BS designed the study and wrote the manuscript. MM critically reviewed the manuscript. BS and MM obtained funding. All the authors approved the manuscript.

ACKNOWLEDGMENTS

We thank Claus Vogl for help with the statistical analysis and Joanna Bancerek and Ekaterini Platanitis for technical help with the ChIP experiments. We are grateful to Wilfried Ellmeier for critical input and valuable discussions.

REFERENCES

1. Frietze S, Farnham PJ. Transcription factor effector domains. *Subcell Biochem.* (2011) 52:261–77. doi: 10.1007/978-90-481-9069-0_12
2. Latchman DS. Transcription factors: an overview. *Int J Biochem Cell Biol.* (1997) 29:1305–12. doi: 10.1016/S1357-2725(97)00085-X
3. Allen BL, Taatjes DJ. The mediator complex: a central integrator of transcription. *Nat Rev Mol Cell Biol.* (2015) 16:155–66. doi: 10.1038/nrm3951
4. Kornberg RD. The molecular basis of eukaryotic transcription. *Proc Natl Acad Sci USA.* (2007) 104:12955–61. doi: 10.1073/pnas.0704138104
5. Nechaev S, Adelman K. Pol II waiting in the starting gates: regulating the transition from transcription initiation into productive elongation. *Biochim Biophys Acta* (2011) 1809:34–45. doi: 10.1016/j.bbagrm.2010.11.001
6. Chen FX, Smith ER, Shilatifard A. Born to run: control of transcription elongation by RNA polymerase II. *Nat Rev Mol Cell Biol.* (2018) 19:464–78. doi: 10.1038/s41580-018-0010-5
7. Medzhitov R, Horng T. Transcriptional control of the inflammatory response. *Nat Rev Immunol.* (2009) 9:692–703. doi: 10.1038/nri2634
8. Shandilya J, Roberts SG. The transcription cycle in eukaryotes: from productive initiation to RNA polymerase II recycling. *Biochim Biophys Acta* (2012) 1819:391–400. doi: 10.1016/j.bbagrm.2012.01.010
9. Sims RJ III, Belotserkovskaya R, Reinberg, D. Elongation by RNA polymerase II: the short and long of it. *Genes Dev.* (2004) 18:2437–68. doi: 10.1101/gad.1235904
10. Boisson-Dupuis S, Kong XF, Okada S, Cypowyj S, Puel A, Abel L, et al. Inborn errors of human STAT1: allelic heterogeneity governs the diversity of immunological and infectious phenotypes. *Curr Opin Immunol.* (2012) 24:364–78. doi: 10.1016/j.coi.2012.04.011
11. Levy DE, Darnell JE Jr. Stats: transcriptional control and biological impact. *Nat Rev Mol Cell Biol.* (2002) 3:651–62. doi: 10.1038/nrm909
12. Ramana CV, Chatterjee-Kishore M, Nguyen H, Stark GR. Complex roles of Stat1 in regulating gene expression. *Oncogene* (2000) 19:2619–27. doi: 10.1038/sj.onc.1203525
13. Muller M, Laxton C, Briscoe J, Schindler C, Improta T, Darnell JE Jr, et al. Complementation of a mutant cell line: central role of the 91 kDa polypeptide of ISGF3 in the interferon-alpha and -gamma signal transduction pathways. *EMBO J.* (1993) 12:4221–8. doi: 10.1002/j.1460-2075.1993.tb06106.x
14. Schindler C, Fu XY, Improta T, Aebersold R, Darnell JE Jr. Proteins of transcription factor ISGF-3: one gene encodes the 91-and 84-kDa ISGF-3 proteins that are activated by interferon alpha. *Proc Natl Acad Sci USA.* (1992) 89:7836–9. doi: 10.1073/pnas.89.16.7836
15. Paulson M, Pisharody S, Pan L, Guadagno S, Mui AL, Levy DE. Stat protein transactivation domains recruit p300/CBP through widely divergent sequences. *J Biol Chem.* (1999) 274:25343–9. doi: 10.1074/jbc.274.36.25343
16. Shen Y, Darnell JE Jr. Antiviral response in cells containing Stat1 with heterologous transactivation domains. *J Virol.* (2001) 75:2627–33. doi: 10.1128/JVI.75.6.2627-2633.2001
17. Zhang JJ, Zhao Y, Chait BT, Lathem WW, Ritzi M, Knippers R, et al. Ser727-dependent recruitment of MCM5 by Stat1alpha in IFN-gamma-induced transcriptional activation. *EMBO J.* (1998) 17:6963–71. doi: 10.1093/emboj/17.23.6963
18. Bancerek J, Poss ZC, Steinparzer I, Sedlyarov V, Pfaffenwimmer T, Mikulic I, et al. CDK8 kinase phosphorylates transcription factor STAT1 to selectively regulate the interferon response. *Immunity* (2013) 38:250–62. doi: 10.1016/j.immuni.2012.10.017
19. Varinou L, Ramsauer K, Karaghiosoff M, Kolbe T, Pfeffer K, Muller M, et al. Phosphorylation of the Stat1 transactivation domain is required for full-fledged IFN-gamma-dependent innate immunity. *Immunity* (2003) 19:793–802. doi: 10.1016/S1074-7613(03)00322-4
20. Wojciak JM, Martinez-Yamout MA, Dyson HJ, Wright PE. Structural basis for recruitment of CBP/p300 coactivators by STAT1 and STAT2 transactivation domains. *EMBO J.* (2009) 28:948–58. doi: 10.1038/emboj.2009.30
21. Zakharova N, Lymar ES, Yang E, Malik S, Zhang JJ, Roeder RG, et al. Distinct transcriptional activation functions of STAT1alpha and STAT1beta on DNA and chromatin templates. *J Biol Chem.* (2003) 278:43067–73. doi: 10.1074/jbc.M308166200
22. DaFonseca CJ, Shu F, Zhang JJ. Identification of two residues in MCM5 critical for the assembly of MCM complexes and Stat1-mediated transcription activation in response to IFN-gamma. *Proc Natl Acad Sci USA.* (2001) 98:3034–9. doi: 10.1073/pnas.061487598
23. Ouchi T, Lee SW, Ouchi M, Aaronson SA, Horvath CM. Collaboration of signal transducer and activator of transcription 1 (STAT1) and BRCA1 in differential regulation of IFN-gamma target genes. *Proc Natl Acad Sci USA.* (2000) 97:5208–13. doi: 10.1073/pnas.080469697
24. Zhang JJ, Vinkemeier U, Gu W, Chakravarti D, Horvath CM, Darnell JE Jr. Two contact regions between Stat1 and CBP/p300 in interferon gamma signaling. *Proc Natl Acad Sci USA.* (1996) 93:15092–6. doi: 10.1073/pnas.93.26.15092
25. Semper C, Leitner NR, Lassnig C, Parrini M, Mahlakoiv T, Rammerstorfer M, et al. STAT1beta is not dominant negative and is capable of contributing to gamma interferon-dependent innate immunity. *Mol Cell Biol.* (2014) 34:2235–48. doi: 10.1128/MCB.00295-14
26. Park C, Li S, Cha E, Schindler C. Immune response in Stat2 knockout mice. *Immunity* (2000) 13:795–804. doi: 10.1016/S1074-7613(00)00077-7
27. Kimura T, Kadokawa Y, Harada H, Matsumoto M, Sato M, Kashiwazaki Y, et al. Essential and non-redundant roles of p48 (ISGF3 gamma) and IRF-1 in both type I and type II interferon responses, as revealed by gene targeting studies. *Genes Cells* (1996) 1:115–24. doi: 10.1046/j.1365-2443.1996.08008.x
28. Reis LF, Ruffner H, Stark G, Aguet M, Weissmann C. Mice devoid of interferon regulatory factor 1 (IRF-1) show normal expression of type I interferon genes. *EMBO J.* (1994) 13:4798–806. doi: 10.1002/j.1460-2075.1994.tb06805.x
29. Leitner NR, Strobl B, Bokor M, Painz R, Kolbe T, Rulicke T, et al. A time- and dose-dependent STAT1 expression system. *BMC Biotechnol.* (2006) 6:48. doi: 10.1186/1472-6750-6-48
30. Strobl B, Bubic I, Bruns U, Steinborn R, Lajko R, Kolbe T, et al. Novel functions of tyrosine kinase 2 in the antiviral defense against murine cytomegalovirus. *J Immunol.* (2005) 175:4000–8. doi: 10.4049/jimmunol.175.6.4000
31. Nissen RM, Yamamoto KR. The glucocorticoid receptor inhibits NFkappaB by interfering with serine-2 phosphorylation of the RNA polymerase II carboxy-terminal domain. *Genes Dev.* (2000) 14:2314–29. doi: 10.1101/gad.827900
32. Hauser C, Schuettengruber B, Bartl S, Lagger G, Seiser C. Activation of the mouse histone deacetylase 1 gene by cooperative histone phosphorylation and acetylation. *Mol Cell Biol.* (2002) 22:7820–30. doi: 10.1128/MCB.22.22.7820-7830.2002
33. Kanno Y, Kozak CA, Schindler C, Driggers PH, Ennist DL, Gleason SL, et al. The genomic structure of the murine ICSBP gene reveals the presence of the gamma interferon-responsive element, to which an ISGF3 alpha subunit (or similar) molecule binds. *Mol Cell Biol.* (1993) 13:3951–63. doi: 10.1128/MCB.13.7.3951

34. Pine R, Canova A, Schindler C. Tyrosine phosphorylated p91 binds to a single element in the ISGF2/IRF-1 promoter to mediate induction by IFN alpha and IFN gamma, and is likely to autoregulate the p91 gene. *EMBO J.* (1994) 13:158–67. doi: 10.1002/j.1460-2075.1994.tb06245.x
35. Morris AC, Beresford GW, Mooney MR, Boss JM. Kinetics of a gamma interferon response: expression and assembly of CIITA promoter IV and inhibition by methylation. *Mol Cell Biol.* (2002) 22:4781–91. doi: 10.1128/MCB.22.13.4781-4791.2002
36. Muhlethaler-Mottet A, Otten LA, Steimle V, Mach B. Expression of MHC class II molecules in different cellular and functional compartments is controlled by differential usage of multiple promoters of the transactivator CIITA. *EMBO J.* (1997) 16:2851–60. doi: 10.1093/emboj/16.10.2851
37. Ni Z, Karaskov E, Yu T, Callaghan SM, Der S, Park DS, et al. Apical role for BRG1 in cytokine-induced promoter assembly. *Proc Natl Acad Sci USA.* (2005) 102:14611–6. doi: 10.1073/pnas.0503070102
38. Briken V, Ruffner H, Schultz U, Schwarz A, Reis LF, Strehlow I, et al. Interferon regulatory factor 1 is required for mouse Gbp gene activation by gamma interferon. *Mol Cell Biol.* (1995) 15:975–82. doi: 10.1128/MCB.15.2.975
39. Lew DJ, Decker T, Strehlow I, Darnell JE. Overlapping elements in the guanylate-binding protein gene promoter mediate transcriptional induction by alpha and gamma interferons. *Mol Cell Biol.* (1991) 11:182–91. doi: 10.1128/MCB.11.1.182
40. Lu R, Au WC, Yeow WS, Hageman N, Pitha PM. Regulation of the promoter activity of interferon regulatory factor-7 gene. Activation by interferon snd silencing by hypermethylation. *J Biol Chem.* (2000) 275:31805–12. doi: 10.1074/jbc.M005288200
41. Rauch I, Rosebrock F, Hainzl E, Heider S, Majoros A, Wienerroither S, et al. Noncanonical effects of IRF9 in intestinal inflammation: more than type I and type III interferons. *Mol Cell Biol.* (2015) 35:2332–43. doi: 10.1128/MCB.01498-14
42. Zhang L, Pagano JS. IRF-7, a new interferon regulatory factor associated with Epstein-Barr virus latency. *Mol Cell Biol.* (1997) 17:5748–57. doi: 10.1128/MCB.17.10.5748
43. Pattenden SG, Klose R, Karaskov E, Bremner R. Interferon-gamma-induced chromatin remodeling at the CIITA locus is BRG1 dependent. *EMBO J.* (2002) 21:1978–86. doi: 10.1093/emboj/21.8.1978
44. Zhang Y, Cheng MB, Zhang YJ, Zhong X, Dai H, Yan L, et al. A switch from hBrm to Brg1 at IFNgamma-activated sequences mediates the activation of human genes. *Cell Res.* (2010) 20:1345–60. doi: 10.1038/cr.2010.155
45. Ramsauer K, Farlik M, Zupkovitz G, Seiser C, Kroger A, Hauser H, et al. Distinct modes of action applied by transcription factors STAT1 and IRF1 to initiate transcription of the IFN-gamma-inducible gbp2 gene. *Proc Natl Acad Sci USA.* (2007) 104:2849–54. doi: 10.1073/pnas.0610944104
46. Shuai K, Stark GR, Kerr IM, Darnell JE Jr. A single phosphotyrosine residue of Stat91 required for gene activation by interferon-gamma. *Science* (1993) 261:1744–6. doi: 10.1126/science.7690989
47. Vinkemeier U, Cohen SL, Moarefi I, Chait BT, Kuriyan J, Darnell JE Jr. DNA binding of *in vitro* activated Stat1 alpha, Stat1 beta and truncated Stat1: interaction between NH2-terminal domains stabilizes binding of two dimers to tandem DNA sites. *EMBO J.* (1996) 15:5616–26. doi: 10.1002/j.1460-2075.1996.tb00946.x
48. Ni Z, Abou El Hassan M, Xu Z, Yu T, Bremner R. The chromatin-remodeling enzyme BRG1 coordinates CIITA induction through many interdependent distal enhancers. *Nat Immunol.* (2008) 9:785–93. doi: 10.1038/ni.1619
49. Justin N, De Marco V, Aasland R, Gamblin SJ. Reading, writing and editing methylated lysines on histone tails: new insights from recent structural studies. *Curr Opin Struct Biol.* (2010) 20:730–8. doi: 10.1016/j.sbi.2010.09.012
50. Bluyssen HA, Muzaffar R, Vlieststra RJ, van der Made AC, Leung S, Stark GR, et al. Combinatorial association and abundance of components of interferon-stimulated gene factor 3 dictate the selectivity of interferon responses. *Proc Natl Acad Sci USA.* (1995) 92:5645–9. doi: 10.1073/pnas.92.12.5645
51. Fink K, Grandvaux N. STAT2 and IRF9: Beyond ISGF3. *JAKSTAT* (2013) 2:e27521. doi: 10.4161/jkst.27521
52. Majoros A, Platanitis E, Kernbauer-Holzl E, Rosebrock F, Muller M, Decker T. Canonical and non-canonical aspects of JAK-STAT signaling: lessons from interferons for cytokine responses. *Front Immunol.* (2017) 8:29.
53. Gough DJ, Messina NL, Clarke CJ, Johnstone RW, Levy DE. Constitutive type I interferon modulates homeostatic balance through tonic signaling. *Immunity* (2012) 36:166–74. doi: 10.1016/j.immuni.2012.01.011
54. Durbin JE, Hackenmiller R, Simon MC, Levy DE. Targeted disruption of the mouse Stat1 gene results in compromised innate immunity to viral disease. *Cell* (1996) 84:443–50. doi: 10.1016/S0092-8674(00)81289-1
55. Gil MP, Bohn E, O'Guin AK, Ramana CV, Levine B, Stark GR, et al. Biologic consequences of Stat1-independent IFN signaling. *Proc Natl Acad Sci USA.* (2001) 98:6680–5. doi: 10.1073/pnas.111163898
56. Meraz MA, White JM, Sheehan KC, Bach EA, Rodig SJ, Dighe AS, et al. Targeted disruption of the Stat1 gene in mice reveals unexpected physiologic specificity in the JAK-STAT signaling pathway. *Cell* (1996) 84:431–42. doi: 10.1016/S0092-8674(00)81288-X
57. Ramana CV, Gil MP, Han Y, Ransohoff RM, Schreiber RD, Stark GR. Stat1-independent regulation of gene expression in response to IFN-gamma. *Proc Natl Acad Sci USA.* (2001) 98:6674–9. doi: 10.1073/pnas.111164198
58. Hargreaves DC, Horng T, Medzhitov R. Control of inducible gene expression by signal-dependent transcriptional elongation. *Cell* (2009) 138:129–45. doi: 10.1016/j.cell.2009.05.047
59. Thomas MC, Chiang CM. The general transcription machinery and general cofactors. *Crit Rev Biochem Mol Biol.* (2006) 41:105–78. doi: 10.1080/10409230600648736
60. Eychenne T, Werner M, Soutourina J. Toward understanding of the mechanisms of Mediator function *in vivo*: focus on the preinitiation complex assembly. *Transcription* (2017) 8:328–42. doi: 10.1080/21541264.2017.1329000
61. Malik S, Roeder RG. The metazoan Mediator co-activator complex as an integrative hub for transcriptional regulation. *Nat Rev Genet.* (2010) 11:761–72. doi: 10.1038/nrg2901
62. Belakavadi M, Pandey PK, Vijayvargia R, Fondell JD. MED1 phosphorylation promotes its association with mediator: implications for nuclear receptor signaling. *Mol Cell Biol.* (2008) 28:3932–42. doi: 10.1128/MCB.02191-07
63. Malik S, Guermah M, Yuan CX, Wu W, Yamamura S, Roeder RG. Structural and functional organization of TRAP220, the TRAP/mediator subunit that is targeted by nuclear receptors. *Mol Cell Biol.* (2004) 24:8244–54. doi: 10.1128/MCB.24.18.8244-8254.2004
64. Takahashi H, Parmely TJ, Sato S, Tomomori-Sato C, Banks CA, Kong SE, et al. Human mediator subunit MED26 functions as a docking site for transcription elongation factors. *Cell* (2011) 146:92–104. doi: 10.1016/j.cell.2011.06.005
65. Lau JF, Nusinzon I, Burakov D, Freedman LP, Horvath CM. Role of metazoan mediator proteins in interferon-responsive transcription. *Mol Cell Biol.* (2003) 23:620–8. doi: 10.1128/MCB.23.2.620-628.2003
66. Borggrefe T, Yue X. Interactions between subunits of the Mediator complex with gene-specific transcription factors. *Semin Cell Dev Biol.* (2011) 22:759–68. doi: 10.1016/j.semcdb.2011.07.022
67. Jeronimo C, Robert F. The mediator complex: at the nexus of RNA polymerase II transcription. *Trends Cell Biol.* (2017) 27:765–83. doi: 10.1016/j.tcb.2017.07.001
68. Reid G, Hubner MR, Metivier R, Brand H, Denger S, Manu D, et al. Cyclic, proteasome-mediated turnover of unliganded and liganded ERalpha on responsive promoters is an integral feature of estrogen signaling. *Mol Cell* (2003) 11:695–707. doi: 10.1016/S1097-2765(03)00090-X
69. Wiesauer I, Gaumannmuller C, Steinparzer I, Strobl B, Kovarik P. Promoter occupancy of STAT1 in interferon responses is regulated by processive transcription. *Mol Cell Biol.* (2015) 35:716–27. doi: 10.1128/MCB.01097-14
70. Knuesel MT, Taatjes DJ. Mediator and post-recruitment regulation of RNA polymerase II. *Transcription* (2011) 2:28–31. doi: 10.4161/trns.2.1.13950
71. Snyder M, He W, Zhang JJ. The DNA replication factor MCM5 is essential for Stat1-mediated transcriptional activation. *Proc Natl Acad Sci USA.* (2005) 102:14539–44. doi: 10.1073/pnas.0507479102
72. Buro LJ, Chipumuro E, Henriksen MA. Menin and RNF20 recruitment is associated with dynamic histone modifications that regulate signal transducer and activator of transcription 1 (STAT1)-activated transcription of the interferon regulatory factor 1 gene (IRF1). *Epigenet Chrom.* (2010) 3:16. doi: 10.1186/1756-8935-3-16

73. Bachu M, Dey A, Ozato K. Chromatin landscape of the IRF genes and role of the epigenetic reader BRD4. *J Interferon Cytokine Res.* (2016) 36:470–5. doi: 10.1089/jir.2015.0179
74. Qiao Y, Giannopoulou EG, Chan, CH, Park SH, Gong S, Chen J, et al. Synergistic activation of inflammatory cytokine genes by interferon-γ-induced chromatin remodeling and toll-like receptor signaling. *Immunity* (2013) 39:454–69. doi: 10.1016/j.immuni.2013.08.009
75. Satoh J, Tabunoki HA. Comprehensive profile of ChIP-Seq-based STAT1 target genes suggests the complexity of STAT1-mediated gene regulatory mechanisms. *Gene Regul Syst Biol.* (2013) 7:41–56. doi: 10.4137/GRSB.S11433
76. Abou El Hassan M, Huang K, Eswara MB, Xu Z, Yu T, et al. Properties of STAT1 and IRF1 enhancers and the influence of SNPs. *BMC Mol Biol.* (2017) 18:6. doi: 10.1186/s12867-017-0084-1

7

The Molecular Basis of Viral Inhibition of IRF- and STAT-Dependent Immune Responses

Hao-Sen Chiang[1,2*] *and Helene Minyi Liu*[3*]

[1] Department of Life Science, National Taiwan University, Taipei, Taiwan, [2] Genome and Systems Biology Degree Program, National Taiwan University, Taipei, Taiwan, [3] Graduate Institute of Biochemistry and Molecular Biology, College of Medicine, National Taiwan University, Taipei, Taiwan

Correspondence:
Hao-Sen Chiang
hschiang@ntu.edu.tw
Helene Minyi Liu
mliu@ntu.edu.tw

The antiviral innate immunity is the first line of host defense against virus infections. In mammalian cells, viral infections initiate the expression of interferons (IFNs) in the host that in turn activate an antiviral defense program to restrict viral replications by induction of IFN stimulated genes (ISGs), which are largely regulated by the IFN-regulatory factor (IRF) family and signal transducer and activator of transcription (STAT) family transcription factors. The mechanisms of action of IRFs and STATs involve several post-translational modifications, complex formation, and nuclear translocation of these transcription factors. However, many viruses, including human immunodeficiency virus (HIV), Zika virus (ZIKV), and herpes simplex virus (HSV), have evolved strategies to evade host defense, including alteration in IRF and STAT post-translational modifications, disturbing the formation and nuclear translocation of the transcription complexes as well as proteolysis/degradation of IRFs and STATs. In this review, we discuss and summarize the molecular mechanisms by which how viral components may target IRFs and STATs to antagonize the establishment of antiviral host defense. The underlying host-viral interactions determine the outcome of viral infection. Gaining mechanistic insight into these processes will be crucial in understanding how viral replication can be more effectively controlled and in developing approaches to improve virus infection outcomes.

Keywords: interferon, interferon-regulatory factor, signal transducer and activator of transcription signaling, interferon-stimulated gene, antiviral response, viral attenuation, viral antagonism

INTRODUCTION

Interferons (IFNs) were originally discovered in 1957 as proteins that interfere with virus replication (1, 2). Since then, IFNs are now divided into three sub-families: type I, II, and III with broad functions not limited to host defense against microbial infection (3–5). These secreted IFNs initiate signaling by binding distinct cell surface receptors to mount proper immune responses. Type I IFNs comprise the largest IFN family including IFN-α, IFN-β, and other subtypes. All type I IFNs bind a ubiquitously expressed heterodimeric transmembrane receptor, which is known as the IFN-α receptor (IFNAR) complex to mediate antiviral effects of type I IFNs (3). IFN-γ is the sole type II IFN largely secreted by innate lymphocytes and T cells that binds to IFN-γ receptor (IFNGR) complex and activates several immune responses to intracellular pathogens (5). Distinct from type I and type II IFNs, type III IFNs are recently discovered and consist of IFN-λ1 (interleukin-29 [IL-29]), IFN-λ2 (IL-29A), IFN-λ3 (IL-28B), and IFN-λ4 (6). They engage the mucosal surface-abundant receptor complex, IFN-λ receptor (IFNLR, also known as IL-28R) that consists of two subunits: IFNLR1 and IL10R2 in the initiation of protection against viral infection at mucosal barriers (4).

Upon virus infection, IFNs are immediately induced by the recognition of pathogen-associated molecular patterns (PAMPs) through cytoplasmic and endosomal pattern-recognition receptors (PRRs) or by cytokine-receptor binding (7). The IFN-regulatory factor (IRF) family proteins are transcription factors with critical and diverse roles that connect the sensing of microbial signatures to the expression of IFNs and pro-inflammatory cytokines as well as innate immune responses (8–10). After IFN binding and receptor dimerization, all IFNs induce IFN-stimulated gene (ISG) expression for effective antiviral responses through the activation of IFN receptor-associated Janus kinase-signal transducer and activator of transcription (JAK-STAT) pathway (11). As obligate intracellular microbes, viruses must engage with the host throughout their replication; it is therefore unsurprised that pathogenic viruses often antagonize IFN responses to establish successful infections by targeting the aforementioned pathways.

In this review, we critically explore the current understanding of IRF and STAT family proteins in host antiviral immune responses activated by IFNs; we also examine how pathogenic viruses have evolved various mechanisms to suppress IRF- and STAT-mediated signaling.

IRFS IN THE PRODUCTION OF IFNS DURING VIRUS INFECTION

The mammalian IRF family proteins are structurally related transcription factors consisting of nine members: IRF1, IRF2, IRF3, IRF4 (also called ICSAT [IFN consensus sequence-binding protein for activated T-cells], LSIRF [lymphocyte-specific IRF], PIP [PU.1-interacting protein]), IRF5, IRF6, IRF7, IRF8 (also referred to ICSBP [IFN consensus sequence-binding protein]), and IRF9 (also known as ISGF3γ [IFN-stimulated gene factor 3γ]) (9). Among nine IRFs, IRF1, IRF3, IRF5, and IRF7 play a pivotal role in the induction of IFN gene transcription during viral infection (12, 13). IRF2 and IRF4 have been implicated in the suppression of type I IFN signaling (14–16). All IRF family proteins possess two conserved functional domains: an amino (N)-terminal DNA-binding domain (DBD) and a carboxy (C)-terminal IRF-associated domain (IAD) (17). DBD is characterized by five conserved tryptophan residues that forms a helix-turn-helix structure and recognizes consensus DNA sequence known as IFN-stimulated response element (ISRE) (18). In contrast to N-terminal regions, the C-terminal regions of IRFs display a broad diversity. Two types of IAD have been identified: IAD1 and IAD2 (19). While IAD1 is conserved in all IRFs except IRF1 and IRF2, IAD2 is shared only by IRF1 and IRF2 (20). The C-terminal regions of IRFs are also involved in the interactions with other IRF family proteins or transcription factors/co-activators that are critical for the induction of IFN (21, 22). For example, IRF3 forms a complex with CREB binding protein (CBP)/p300 histone acetyltransferase (HAT) through the IAD1 domain for the induction of *Ifnb1* transcription in response to virus infection (21). In the following sections, we discuss the distinct contribution of IRFs to type I IFN induction through cytoplasmic and endosomal PRR signaling cascades (**Figure 1**).

IRF3 and IRF7 Are the Master Regulators of Type I IFN Expression in RLR Signaling

During virus infection, type I IFNs are produced in infected cells via the recognition of viral PAMPs by binding to specific PRRs, such as cytosolic retinoic acid-inducible gene I (RIG-I)-like receptors (RLRs) and transmembrane Toll-like receptors (TLRs) resulting in the activation of downstream IRF3 and IRF7 pathways (7, 23). Several RNA viruses directly enter the cytoplasm where they are detected by RLR family members: RIG-I and melanoma differentiation-associated gene 5 (MDA5) (24). Ligand recognition results in the recruitment of RIG-I and MDA5 to the mitochondria where they interact with mitochondria antiviral signaling protein (MAVS) through the N-terminal caspase recruitment domain (CARD) domains in RLRs and MAVS. This association relays signals to the downstream TANK-binding kinase 1 (TBK1) and IκB kinase-ε (IKKε) that phosphorylate IRF3 and IRF7 (24).

IRF3 is a constitutively expressed but tightly regulated transcription factor in the cytoplasm. It presents in an inactive form due to its auto-inhibitory mechanisms (25). Virus infections induce specific IRF3 phosphorylation that leads to its dimerization with itself or with IRF7 and forms a complex containing CBP/p300 and other coactivators followed by translocation into the nucleus for the expression of IFN-β (26). The activation process of IRF7 is similar to that of IRF3 in response to viral PAMPs. However, in contrast to constitutively expressed IRF3, the basal expression level of IRF7 is minimum but is strongly induced by type I IFN-mediated responses in an autocrine feedback loop after virus infection (discussed in detail below) (9). Moreover, a recent study from IRF3/IRF5/IRF7 triple knockout mice suggests that in addition to IRF3 and IRF7, IRF5 is also a key transcriptional factor responsible for RLR- and MAVS-mediated type I IFN expression (27).

Contributions of IRFs to the Induction of Cytosolic DNA-Mediated and TLR3/7/8/9-Mediated Type I IFN

Similar to the involvement of RLR-mediated type I IFN expression, IRF3 and IRF7 also contribute to the signaling pathways downstream of cytosolic DNA sensing and endosomal DNA/RNA recognition for the inductions of IFN-α and IFN-β during virus infection (7). Among several known cytosolic DNA sensors for the detection of viral infection, cyclic-GMP-AMP (cGAMP) synthase (cGAS) is the most recently identified (28). Upon viral DNA binding, cGAS catalyzes the production of cGAMP from ATP and GTP, a second messenger that binds and activates the endoplasmic reticulum membrane protein stimulator of IFN genes (STING) for the production of type I IFN (28, 29). STING functions as an adaptor protein that promotes TBK1-dependent IRF3/7 phosphorylation (30–33).

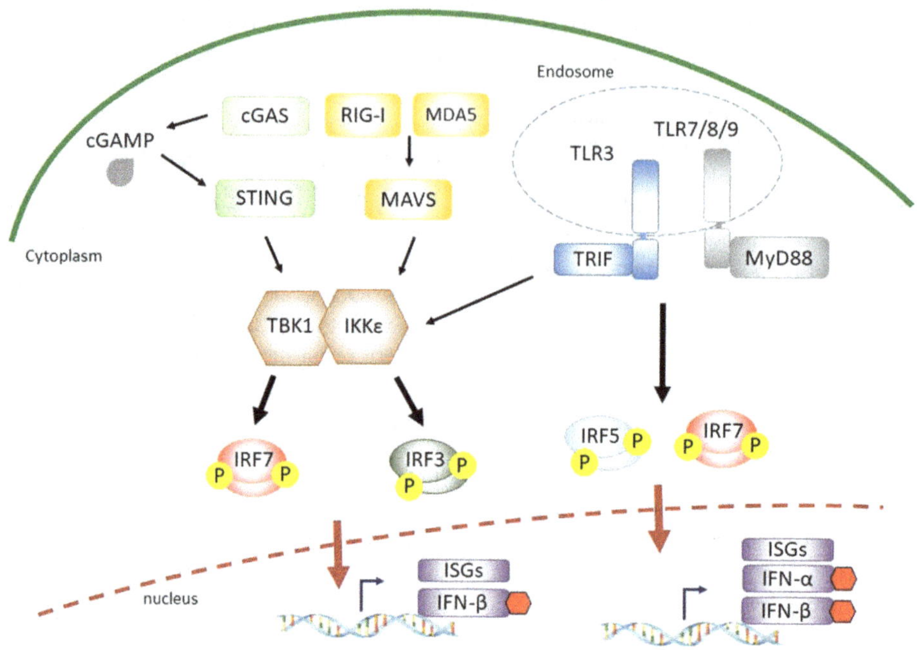

FIGURE 1 | Interferon (IFN)-regulatory factors (IRFs) involved in cytosolic nucleic acid sensing and endosomal Toll-like receptor (TLR) signaling. During virus infection, retinoic acid-inducible gene I (RIG-I) or melanoma differentiation-associated gene 5 (MDA5) recognize cytosolic double-stranded RNA and recruit the adaptor protein mitochondria antiviral signaling protein (MAVS), which leads to the activation of TANK-binding kinase 1 (TBK1)/IκB kinase-ε (IKKε). Cytosolic double-stranded DNA is detected by cyclic-GMP-AMP (cGAMP) synthase (cGAS) or other receptors (such as DEAD-box helicase 41 (DDX41), gamma-IFN-inducible protein 16 (IFI16), not shown) to induce stimulator of IFN genes (STING)-mediated TBK1 and IKKε activation. Activated TBK1/IKKε then phosphorylate IRF3 and IRF7 that translocate into the nucleus for the induction of IFN-β. The sensing of viral pathogen-associated molecular patterns (PAMPs) by endosomal TLR3 or TLR7/8/9 leads to the phosphorylation and activation of IRF5 and IRF7 through adaptor proteins TIR-domain-containing adapter-inducing IFN (TRIF) or myeloid differentiation primary response 88 (MyD88), respectively, for the expression of type I IFNs.

Transmembrane TLR3, TLR7/8, and TLR9 are the most well characterized PRRs for the recognition of viral PAMPs located in the endosomal compartments (34). TLRs initiate shared and distinct signaling pathways by recruiting different adaptor molecules for type I IFN expression. TLR3 recognizes viral dsRNA and utilizes TIR-domain-containing adapter-inducing IFN (TRIF) as an adaptor to recruit downstream TBK1, resulting in IRF3/7 phosphorylation and type I IFN production. Upon the engagements with viral ssRNA and unmethylated CpG DNA motifs by TLR7/8 and TLR9, respectively, these TLRs signal through myeloid differentiation primary response 88 (MyD88) to activate IKKα- or IKKβ-dependent phosphorylation and activation of IRF7 or IRF5, allowing the production of type I IFNs (35–37). Taken together, these studies highlight the importance of IRF3/5/7 phosphorylation and activation in the downstream of cytoplasmic/endosomal PRR signaling leading to type I IFN expression during virus infection.

IRFS AND STATS IN IFN-MEDIATED INNATE IMMUNE RESPONSES

Mammalian immune systems utilize IRFs, STATs and IFNs to integrate and process distinct signals to orchestrate host antiviral immunity. This has been proven in several studies utilizing genetically-modified mice that lack IFNAR, IFNGR, IFNLR, STAT1, or STAT2, respectively. These gene-knockout mice are highly susceptible to virus infections due to the impaired IFN signaling and responses (38–42). In the following sections, we examine the current understandings of how IFNs initiate antiviral immune responses via binding to their cognate heterodimeric receptors through downstream canonical JAK-STAT signaling (**Figure 2**).

Canonical IFN-Activated JAK-STAT Pathway

Almost all cell types respond to type I and type II IFNs for effective antiviral immunity (43, 44). However, the specific type III IFN receptor subunit IFNLR1 is mainly expressed on epithelial cells and immune cells, such as neutrophils that provides the first line of antiviral defense at the mucosal surfaces of gastrointestinal and respiratory tracts (42, 45). The ligation between IFN and IFNR results in receptor dimerization or oligomerization that allows the transphosphorylation of receptor-associated JAK on tyrosine residues. Subsequently, activated JAKs induce tyrosine phosphorylation of IFNR cytoplasmic tails where provides the binding sites for C-terminal Src-homology-2 (SH2) domains of STAT proteins. The STATs are then recruited to

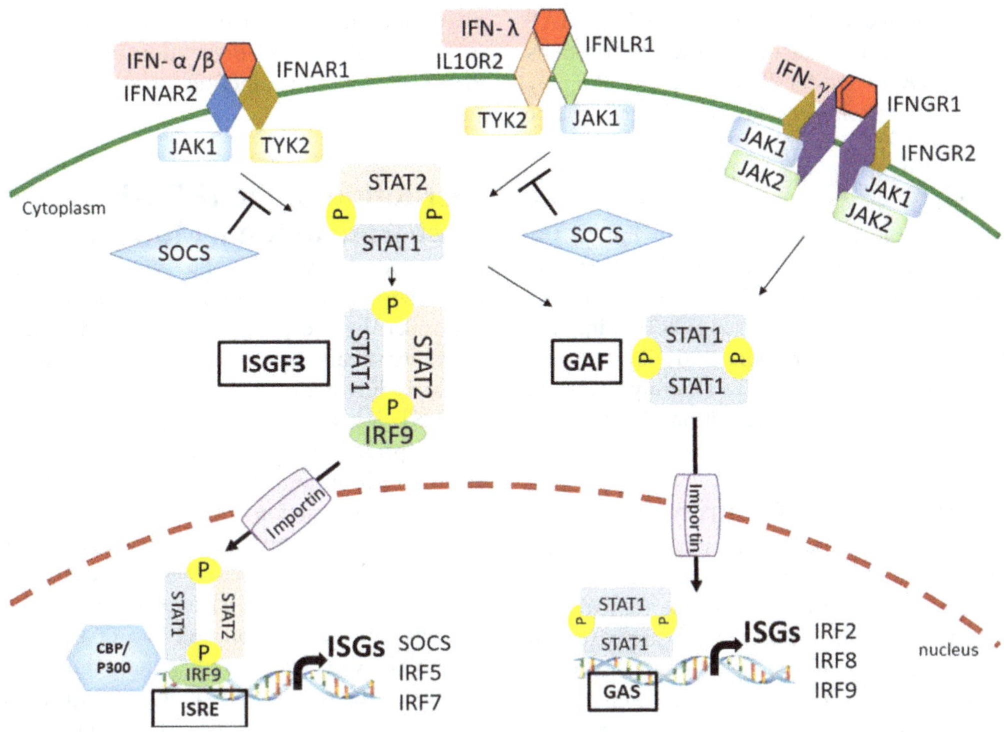

FIGURE 2 | Interferon (IFN)-dependent IFN stimulated gene (ISG) transcription through the Janus kinase-signal transducer and activator of transcription (JAK-STAT) signaling. By binding to the IFN-α receptor (IFNAR) or IFN-λ receptor (IFNLR), type I/III IFNs activate the JAK-STAT pathway leading to the formation of IFN-stimulated gene factor 3 (ISGF3) and gamma-IFN activation factor (GAF) complexes. The ligation between IFN-γ and IFN-γ receptor (IFNGR) also activate the GAF complex. ISGF3 and GAF complexes then translocate into the nucleus mediated by importins and recruit additional coactivators, such as CREB binding protein (CBP)/p300 on the IFN-stimulated response element (ISRE)- or gamma IFN activated sequence (GAS)-containing promoters to stimulate expression of a distinct group of ISGs. Eventually, a set of ISGs are produced and amplify the IFN response. IFN-induced suppressor of cytokine signaling (SOCS) proteins inhibit JAK-STAT signaling by binding to phosphorylated tyrosine residues on either JAK1 or tyrosine kinase 2 (TYK2).

the JAKs followed by phosphorylation at a tyrosine residue (46). In the canonical pathway of type I IFN-mediated and type III IFN-mediated signaling, the phosphorylation of STAT1 on tyrosine 701 and STAT2 on tyrosine 690 leads to the formation of STAT1/STAT2 heterodimer that interacts with IRF9 to form the IFN-stimulated gene factor 3 (ISGF3) complex. ISGF3 complex then redirects and translocates into the nucleus to trigger ISG expressions by binding to ISRE and recruiting additional coactivators, such as CBP/p300 on the promoters of a distinct group of target genes (44, 47–49). In addition to forming the ISGF3 complex, all types of IFNs are able to induce a STAT1/STAT1 homodimer, known as gamma IFN–activation factor (GAF) that activates ISG transcription by direct binding to the gamma IFN activated sequence (GAS)-containing genes (4, 44). Besides the STAT1/STAT2 heterodimer and STAT1/STAT1 homodimer, type I IFNs can also activate STAT3/STAT3, STAT4/STAT4, STAT5/STAT5, and STAT6/STAT6 homodimers as well as STAT1/STAT3, STAT1/STAT4, STAT1/STAT5, STAT2/STAT3, and STAT5/STAT6 heterodimers. All of these homodimers and heterodimers can bind to GAS and drive the expression of GAS-containing ISGs (44).

ISGs and Regulation of JAK-STAT Family Proteins

ISGs are proteins present at baseline but are enhanced upon virus infection in JAK-STAT dependent pathways. A subset of ISGs are well-characterized for their direct antiviral activities. For example, IFN-induced proteins with tetratricopeptide repeat 1–3 (IFIT1–3), viperin, and myxovirus resistance 1 (Mx1) can all inhibit virus replication (50). JAK2, STAT1, STAT2, and IRF9 belong to another subset of ISGs that amplify JAK-STAT signaling to reinforce IFN responses (3). Moreover, ISGs, such as RIG-I, cGAS, IRF5, and IRF7 can further prime cells for increased detection of viral PAMPs and upregulated IFN expressions (51). Interestingly, the expression of subsets of ISGs can also be induced directly by IRFs in a pathway that is independent of JAK-STAT signaling (52). For example, IRF3 initiates the expressions of IFN-stimulated gene 15 (ISG15) and sterile alpha motif and HD domain containing protein 1 (SAMHD1) as the first responders in antiviral immunity (53, 54). Similar to IRF3, IRF1 mediates a rapid IFN-independent antiviral response downstream of RLR adaptor protein MAVS localized specifically on peroxisome (55–57). IRF7 can regulate ISG expression in the absence of IFN signaling as well (50, 58).

In addition to JAK2. STAT1, STAT2, IRF9 themselves, several other ISGs are also implicated in the regulation of JAK-STAT signaling. Suppressor of cytokine signaling (SOCS) proteins including SOCS1 and SOCS3 inhibit JAK-STAT signaling by binding to phosphorylated tyrosine residues on either JAK1 or tyrosine kinase 2 (TYK2) (59). Another ISG: the ubiquitin-specific peptidase 18 (USP18) suppresses JAK-STAT signaling induced by type I IFN at the level of IFN receptor. USP18 specifically interacts with the IFNAR2 subunit to inhibit the interaction between JAK and the IFN receptor (60). Furthermore, recent findings indicate that type I IFN-induced STAT3 cooperates with phospholipid scramblase 2 (PLSCR2) to interact with STAT2 and suppress type I IFN response (61, 62). It would be critical to further determine whether STAT family members also interact with other proteins for the regulation of JAK-STAT pathways.

Protein Regulators of STAT Family Proteins

As STAT family proteins are essential signaling mediators, their activation are tightly-regulated by several mechanisms in order to downregulate IFN-mediated antiviral response (63). STATs reside in an inactive form in the cytoplasm but are activated and translocate into the nucleus in response to IFN signaling. Several nucleocytoplasmic transport factors are essential for the nuclear import of phosphorylated STATs. For example, importin-α5 (also called karyopherin α1[KPNA1]) regulates nuclear import of STAT1 (64, 65). Moreover, STAT3 nuclear import is mediated by importin-α3 (66). Interestingly, the presence of phosphorylated STATs in the nucleus is transient. STAT1 can be dephosphorylated in the nucleus and actively export to the cytoplasm by the chromosome region maintenance 1 (CRM1) export receptor in a nuclear export signal (NES)-dependent manner (67). Recently, a metheyltransferase SET domain-containing protein 2 (SETD2) has been identified as a critical type I IFN signaling amplifier. Although the expression of SETD2 itself is not upregulated by type I IFN, SETD2 enhances the methylation of STAT1 on K525 as well as ISG expressions for antiviral immunity (68). However, the detail mechanism underlying the regulation and selectivity of SETD2-mediated ISG expression has not been fully explored.

VIRAL REGULATION AND EVASION OF THE IRF- AND STAT-DEPENDENT ANTI-VIRAL PATHWAYS

In order to establish successful infections, viruses have evolved a variety of strategies to counteract host antiviral innate immunity. The infection outcome is determined by the race between the kinetics of virus replications and the competence of antiviral gene expression levels at the early-onset of the infection. Studies of virus-host interactions have revealed infection-induced signaling pathways that result in IRF and STAT activations as the major targets of regulation and evasion of the host anti-viral responses. The molecular mechanisms by which viruses target IRFs and STATs are highly diverse, including inhibition of IRF/STAT expressions, disruption of the post-translational modifications, alterations in the localizations, prevention of transcriptional complex formation, and promoting the degradation of IRFs and STATs.

Disruption of the IRF/STAT Post-translational Modifications

For rapid response to the viral infections, the activation of antiviral innate immunity in mammalian cells is largely controlled by the post-translational modifications of the PRR, the downstream signaling adaptor proteins, as well as the key transcription factors, IRFs and STATs. Phosphorylation of IRF3, IRF7, STAT1, and STAT2 are highly critical for their downstream transcriptional activation, and therefore these phosphorylation events are commonly targeted by viruses. By directly promoting the dephosphorylation of IRFs and STATs or indirectly inhibiting upstream kinase activities, the activation of these transcription factors are then controlled by the invading viruses.

Vaccinia virus (VACV) encodes a late gene VH1, which is packaged into the virion and is a dual-specificity phosphatase (69). VH1 was later found to have immediate effects against host antiviral activities by directly dephosphorylating STAT1 at Tyr701 and Ser727 to reduce STAT1 activation (70, 71). Besides, VACV encodes another virulence factor, C6, which binds to the IRF3/7 kinase TBK-1 and interferes the phosphorylation and activation of IRF3 and IRF7 (72). Several other DNA viruses also have similar mechanisms to target TBK1 and/or IKKε to inhibit the phosphorylation of IRF3. It has been recently reported that the VP24 of herpes simplex virus (HSV) can target TBK1/IKKε to inhibit the phosphorylation of IRF3 (73, 74). Also, several viruses have evolved viral products that may interfere the interaction between STAT1 and JAK/TyK, e.g., the NS5A protein of Hepatitis C virus can physically interact with STAT1 to interfere the phosphorylation of STAT1 at Tyr701 (75, 76). Another example is the NSP1 protein encoded by Rotavirus, of which the expression alone may block STAT1 phosphorylation and activation (77). Ebola virus VP35 prevents the TBK1-dependent phosphorylation of IRF3 (78, 79). Marburg virus, which is closely related to Ebola virus, encodes a matrix protein VP40 to antagonize the phosphorylation of both STAT1 and STAT2 (80).

In addition, viruses may regulate IRF/STAT phosphorylation indirectly by promoting the expression of the negative regulators of IRF/STAT kinases, such as suppressor of cytokine signaling (SOCS) family, to minimize the induction of ISGs. It has been reported that Hepatitis B virus (HBV) infection as well as Hepatitis C virus (HCV) core protein may induce the expression of suppressor of cytokine signaling 3 (SOCS3) (81, 82). The e antigen of HBV, HBeAg, also stimulates the expression of suppressor of cytokine signaling 2 (SOCS2) (83). The induction of SOCS family subsequently impairs IFN/JAK/STAT signaling and therefore attenuating the activation of STAT1, which may contribute to the establishment of persistent infections of HBV and HCV.

Virus-Induced Proteolysis or Degradation of IRF/STAT Proteins

Many viruses, such as picornaviruses and flaviviruses, encode viral proteases for viral replications. In addition to their essential roles in the virus life cycles, the viral proteases often target host proteins involved in IFN induction and response pathways to escape the host antiviral innate immunity (84). The 3C proteases (3Cpro) encoded by enterovirus (EV) 71 and EV68 disturb the expression of type I IFN and ISGs by directly cleaving IRF7 (85, 86). Porcine deltacoronavirus nsp5 cleaves STAT2 to antagonize type I IFN responses (19). These proteolytic events of IRFs and STATs often lead to the degradation of these transcription factors. For example, besides cleaving IRF7, the 3Cpro of enterovirus 71 also targets IRF9 for proteolytic degradation (87).

Conversely, a variety of viral proteins may also promote the proteasome-dependent or lysosome-dependent protein degradation of IRFs and STATs. It has been shown that the Vpu accessory protein of human immunodeficiency virus (HIV) mediates the depletion of IRF3 through lysosomal degradation or caspase-dependent cleavage (88, 89). HIV YU2 mutant which lacks the expression of Vpu could not control the activation of IRF3 upon infection (89). The NSP1 of rotavirus, a putative E3 ubiquitin ligase, mediates the degradation of cellular factors, including IRF3, IRF5, IRF7, and IRF9 but not IRF1, through recognizing the common IAD1 domain of these IRFs (90, 91).

Several members of the *Paramyxoviridae*, such as parainfluenza viruses, have developed strategies to target either STAT1 or STAT2 for degradation. The expression of a single viral protein, human parainfluenza virus type 2 (hPIV-2) V protein, may inhibit the type I IFN response by inducing the proteolytic degradation of STAT2 (92), and Newcastle disease virus (NDV) also encodes a V protein which can target STAT1 for degradation. The V protein of canine parainfluenza virus 5 (also known as *simian virus 5*) degrades both STAT1 and STAT2 in a proteasome-dependent manner (93). The NS5 proteins of flaviviruses, including dengue virus (DENV) and Zika virus (ZIKV), also share the common characteristics to target STAT2 for proteasome-dependent degradation (94–97).

Re-localization of IRF/STATs by Viral Proteins

After phosphorylated, the nuclear translocation of the activated IRFs and STATs is another key step to induce the transcription of downstream genes, and this process is largely dependent on the cellular nuclear import and export machineries, including importin and CRM-1 proteins. Hence, viruses have developed various strategies to negatively regulate IFN induction and response pathways by altering the localizations of activated IRFs and STATs. Ebola virus VP24 binds to the α5 and α6 subunits of importin, which are the essential components of the nuclear transporter, to block the nuclear translocation of phosphorylated STAT1 (98, 99). EV71 suppresses IFN responses by blocking STAT1 signaling through inducing importin-α5 degradation in a caspase-3-dependent manner (100). As described previously, nuclear STAT1, STAT2, and IRF9 cycle back to the cytoplasm in a CRM1-dependent nuclear export manner. Certain viral proteins, such as the nsp2 of chikungunya virus, can promote the nuclear export of STATs (101, 102). During Nipah virus infection, the V protein can directly bind to STAT1 and STAT2 in the cytoplasm, and the N protein of Nipah virus restricts the complex formation of STAT1/STAT2, which along with the CRM1-dependent nuclear export of STAT1 and STAT2 additively result in the accumulation of STAT1 and STAT2 in the cytoplasm (103–105).

Viruses may also encode proteins which can directly bind to IRFs and STATs and maintain their cytoplasmic distribution. The C proteins of hPIV-1, which belongs to the *Paramyxoviridae*, blocks IFN signaling by interacting and retaining STAT1 and STAT2 in the perinuclear region in the infected cells (106). Similarly, the C protein of Sendai virus, also known as murine paramyxovirus, binds p-STAT1 to inhibit STAT1 dimerization and nuclear translocation (107, 108). Measles virus, which also belongs to the *Paramyxoviridae*, does not inhibit the tyrosine phosphorylation of STAT1 and STAT2 but encodes a viral protein, V protein, which directly interacts with STAT1, STAT2, and IRF9 in the cytoplasm to prevent their nuclear translocation (109). In addition to the *Paramyxoviridae*, the monkey rotavirus and human rotavirus Wa strain also do not restrict the activation phosphorylation of STAT1 and STAT2 but retain these transcription factors in the cytoplasm (110). HSV-1 encodes several IFN antagonists, including ICP0, which inhibits IRF3 nuclear accumulation but not IRF3 phosphorylation (111). Human papilloma virus (HPV) E7 protein interacts with IRF9 in the cytoplasm and subsequently inhibits the nuclear translocation of IRF9 as well as the formation of ISGF3 (112).

Interference of the Transcriptional Complex Formation of IRFs and STATs

After translocation into the nucleus, the activated IRFs and STATs will then bind to the promoter region on the chromosomal DNA and recruit other transcription activators to initiate the transcription of downstream genes. A distinct group of viral proteins, viral homologs to cellular IRFs, known as vIRFs, are reported to be encoded by Kaposi's sarcoma-associated herpesvirus (KSHV) and the rhesus macaque rhadinovirus (RRV). KHSV vIRF3 interacts with host IRF5 and IRF7, and vIRF3 can suppress IRF7 DNA binding activity to inhibit IFN-α production (113, 114). Furthermore, KHSV vIRF1 binds to p300 and interferes with CBP/p300-IRF3 complex formation as well as the HAT activity of p300, and thus prevents IRF3-mediated transcriptional activation (115). HSV-1 also utilizes a similar strategy to abrogate CBP recruitment by IRF3 through the viral protein VP16 (116). RRV-encoded R6 is a virion-associated vIRF, which is capable to prevent IRF3/CBP complex docking to the IFNβ promoter region to minimize the induction of type I IFN expression upon RRV infection (117).

Besides vIRFs, other viral proteins have also been reported to regulate the DNA-binding activities and transcriptional complex formation. For example, Porcine bocavirus (PBoV) NP1 protein inhibits the DNA-binding activity of IRF3 and the DNA-binding activity ISGF3 through interactions with the DNA-binding domain of IRF9 (118, 119). The nsp1 of porcine epidemic diarrhea virus (PEDV) and the nsp1 α subunit of porcine reproductive and respiratory syndrome virus (PRRSV) both suppress the type I IFN production by promoting the proteasome dependent degradation of CBP (120, 121).

Inhibition of IRF and STAT Protein Expression

As described in ISGs and Regulation of JAK/STAT Family Proteins, the protein expression levels of various of the IRFs and STATs are upregulated in response to viral infections and IFN signaling, such as IRF7 and STAT1 (51), to form a positive feedback loop for the enhancement of antiviral activities. Therefore, disturbing the activation of basally expressed endogenous IRFs and STATs not only directly impairs the induction of the initial round of antiviral gene expressions but also prohibits the magnification of the antiviral responses against virus replication. Without sufficient and efficient antiviral gene expression in the infected cells, the viruses may competently replicate and produce viral progenies to infect neighboring cells and therefore establish a successful infection.

Some viruses directly inhibit the expression of IRFs at the transcriptional level, e.g., Epstein-Barr virus (EBV) BRLF1 inhibits the transcription of IRF3 and IRF7 (122). Another major mechanism for herpes viruses to curtail the expression of IRFs and STATs is virion host shut-off (VHS), which is mediated by the tegument protein UL41 (123). It has been shown that through its own endoribonuclease activity, HSV VHS selectively promotes the degradation of host mRNAs made before infection, including the mRNA of ISGs (124, 125). Many of the RNA viruses, including *Caliciviridae*, *Coronaviridae*, *Picornaviridae*, O*orthomyxoviridae*, *Reoviridae*, and many others, have strategies to induce host translational shut-off and thus prevent the infected cells to synthesize new peptides and proteins, including those IFN-stimulated IRFs and STATs. Viruses may also upregulate certain miRNA to tune the expression of factors involved in the activation of IRFs and STATs. A recent report showed that miR-373, which reduces the expression of both JAK1 and IRF9, is upregulated by HCV infection to suppress the response to IFNs in the infected cells (126).

CONCLUSION AND PERSPECTIVES

In the past decades, the inductions and responses of IFNs have been much revealed. The regulatory network of antiviral innate immunity including IFNs and many other cytokines is extremely complex in the mammalian cells. Since viruses carry much less genetic information than the eukaryotic cells, analyses of which cellular factors are targeted by viral products to dampen the innate immunity pathway provide us with great means to identify the crucial signaling molecules for mammalian antiviral activities. The critical role STAT1 in antiviral immunity is well-pronounced since viruses have developed numerous strategies to target STAT1 as a result of evolution. Notably, the development of STAT1 KO mice as *in vivo* animal models for viral infections has provided valuable tools for future virology and immunology studies (127–129).

As we reviewed in this article, all pathogenic viruses have multiple strategies to antagonize the host antiviral innate immunity. Intriguingly, several viruses selectively inhibit the type I IFN-induced but not type II IFN-induced STAT1 phosphorylation, such as ZIKV (130, 131). How this is beneficial to the virus life cycle remains to be further investigated. With better understanding the molecular mechanisms behind, future developments of antiviral agents and vaccines will be accelerated.

AUTHOR CONTRIBUTIONS

All authors contributed equally to this work. H-SC and HL conceptualized, wrote, and edited the manuscript.

ACKNOWLEDGMENTS

The authors apologize to colleagues whose work could not be cited due to space constraints. We appreciate all the members of H-SC Laboratory and HL Laboratory for interactive discussions.

REFERENCES

1. Isaacs A, Lindenmann J. Virus interference. I. The interferon. *Proc R Soc Lond B Biol Sci.* (1957) 147:258–67. doi: 10.1098/rspb.1957.0048
2. Lindenmann J, Burke DC, Isaacs A. Studies on the production, mode of action and properties of interferon. *Br J Exp Pathol.* (1957) 38:551–62.
3. Ivashkiv LB, Donlin LT. Regulation of type I interferon responses. *Nat Rev Immunol.* (2014) 14:36–49. doi: 10.1038/nri3581
4. Wack A, Terczynska-Dyla E, Hartmann R. Guarding the frontiers: the biology of type III interferons. *Nat Immunol.* (2015) 16:802–9. doi: 10.1038/ni.3212
5. Ivashkiv LB. IFNgamma: signalling, epigenetics and roles in immunity, metabolism, disease and cancer immunotherapy. *Nat Rev Immunol.* (2018) 18:545–58. doi: 10.1038/s41577-018-0029-z
6. Prokunina-Olsson L, Muchmore B, Tang W, Pfeiffer RM, Park H, Dickensheets H, et al. A variant upstream of IFNL3 (IL28B) creating a new interferon gene IFNL4 is associated with impaired clearance of hepatitis C virus. *Nat Genet.* (2013) 45:164–71. doi: 10.1038/ng.2521
7. Thompson MR, Kaminski JJ, Kurt-Jones EA, Fitzgerald KA. Pattern recognition receptors and the innate immune response to viral infection. *Viruses* (2011) 3:920–40. doi: 10.3390/v3060920

8. Honda K, Taniguchi T. IRFs: master regulators of signalling by Toll-like receptors and cytosolic pattern-recognition receptors. *Nat Rev Immunol.* (2006) 6:644–58. doi: 10.1038/nri1900
9. Ikushima H, Negishi H, Taniguchi T. The IRF family transcription factors at the interface of innate and adaptive immune responses. *Cold Spring Harb Symp Quant Biol.* (2013) 78:105–16. doi: 10.1101/sqb.2013.78.020321
10. Tamura T, Yanai H, Savitsky D, Taniguchi T. The IRF family transcription factors in immunity and oncogenesis. *Annu Rev Immunol.* (2008) 26:535–84. doi: 10.1146/annurev.immunol.26.021607.090400
11. Schindler C, Levy DE, Decker T. JAK-STAT signaling: from interferons to cytokines. *J Biol Chem.* (2007) 282:20059–63. doi: 10.1074/jbc.R700016200
12. Honda K, Takaoka A, Taniguchi T. Type I interferon [corrected] gene induction by the interferon regulatory factor family of transcription factors. *Immunity* (2006) 25:349–60. doi: 10.1016/j.immuni.2006.08.009
13. Odendall C, Kagan JC. The unique regulation and functions of type III interferons in antiviral immunity. *Curr Opin Virol.* (2015) 12:47–52. doi: 10.1016/j.coviro.2015.02.003
14. Hida S, Ogasawara K, Sato K, Abe M, Takayanagi H, Yokochi T, et al. CD8(+) T cell-mediated skin disease in mice lacking IRF-2, the transcriptional attenuator of interferon-alpha/beta signaling. *Immunity* (2000) 13:643–55. doi: 10.1016/S1074-7613(00)00064-9
15. Honda K, Mizutani T, Taniguchi T. Negative regulation of IFN-alpha/beta signaling by IFN regulatory factor 2 for homeostatic development of dendritic cells. *Proc Natl Acad Sci USA.* (2004) 101:2416–21. doi: 10.1073/pnas.0307336101
16. Negishi H, Ohba Y, Yanai H, Takaoka A, Honma K, Yui K, et al. Negative regulation of Toll-like-receptor signaling by IRF-4. *Proc Natl Acad Sci USA.* (2005) 102:15989–94. doi: 10.1073/pnas.0508327102
17. Takaoka A, Tamura T, Taniguchi T. Interferon regulatory factor family of transcription factors and regulation of oncogenesis. *Cancer Sci.* (2008) 99:467–78. doi: 10.1111/j.1349-7006.2007.00720.x
18. Darnell JE Jr, Kerr IM, Stark GR. Jak-STAT pathways and transcriptional activation in response to IFNs and other extracellular signaling proteins. *Science* (1994) 264:1415–21. doi: 10.1126/science.8197455
19. Meraro D, Hashmueli S, Koren B, Azriel A, Oumard A, Kirchhoff S, et al. Protein-protein and DNA-protein interactions affect the activity of lymphoid-specific IFN regulatory factors. *J Immunol.* (1999) 163:6468–78.
20. Yanai H, Negishi H, Taniguchi T. The IRF family of transcription factors: Inception, impact and implications in oncogenesis. *Oncoimmunology* (2012) 1:1376–86. doi: 10.4161/onci.22475
21. Yoneyama M, Suhara W, Fukuhara Y, Fukuda M, Nishida E, Fujita T. Direct triggering of the type I interferon system by virus infection: activation of a transcription factor complex containing IRF-3 and CBP/p300. *EMBO J.* (1998) 17:1087–95. doi: 10.1093/emboj/17.4.1087
22. Yang H, Ma G, Lin CH, Orr M, Wathelet MG. Mechanism for transcriptional synergy between interferon regulatory factor (IRF)-3 and IRF-7 in activation of the interferon-beta gene promoter. *Eur J Biochem.* (2004) 271:3693–703. doi: 10.1111/j.1432-1033.2004.04310.x
23. Loo YM, Gale M Jr. Immune signaling by RIG-I-like receptors. *Immunity* (2011) 34:680–92. doi: 10.1016/j.immuni.2011.05.003
24. Reikine S, Nguyen JB, Modis Y. pattern recognition and signaling mechanisms of RIG-I and MDA5. *Front Immunol.* (2014) 5:342. doi: 10.3389/fimmu.2014.00342
25. Qin BY, Liu C, Lam SS, Srinath H, Delston R, Correia JJ, et al. Crystal structure of IRF-3 reveals mechanism of autoinhibition and virus-induced phosphoactivation. *Nat Struct Biol.* (2003) 10:913–21. doi: 10.1038/nsb1002
26. Wathelet MG, Lin CH, Parekh BS, Ronco LV, Howley PM, Maniatis T. Virus infection induces the assembly of coordinately activated transcription factors on the IFN-beta enhancer *in vivo*. *Mol Cell* (1998) 1:507–18. doi: 10.1016/S1097-2765(00)80051-9
27. Lazear HM, Lancaster A, Wilkins C, Suthar MS, Huang A, Vick SC, et al. IRF-3, IRF-5, and IRF-7 coordinately regulate the type I IFN response in myeloid dendritic cells downstream of MAVS signaling. *PLoS Pathog.* (2013) 9:e1003118. doi: 10.1371/annotation/4de7ddfd-52df-4f87-8ca4-d48afe646ca8
28. Sun L, Wu J, Du F, Chen X, Chen ZJ. Cyclic GMP-AMP synthase is a cytosolic DNA sensor that activates the type I interferon pathway. *Science* (2013) 339:786–91. doi: 10.1126/science.1232458
29. Ma Z, Damania B. The cGAS-STING defense pathway and its counteraction by viruses. *Cell Host Microbe* (2016) 19:150–8. doi: 10.1016/j.chom.2016.01.010
30. Ishikawa H, Barber GN. STING is an endoplasmic reticulum adaptor that facilitates innate immune signalling. *Nature* (2008) 455:674–8. doi: 10.1038/nature07317
31. Ishikawa H, Ma Z, Barber GN. STING regulates intracellular DNA-mediated, type I interferon-dependent innate immunity. *Nature* (2009) 461:788–92. doi: 10.1038/nature08476
32. Zhao W. Negative regulation of TBK1-mediated antiviral immunity. *FEBS Lett.* (2013) 587:542–8. doi: 10.1016/j.febslet.2013.01.052
33. Cai X, Chiu YH, Chen ZJ. The cGAS-cGAMP-STING pathway of cytosolic DNA sensing and signaling. *Mol Cell* (2014) 54:289–96. doi: 10.1016/j.molcel.2014.03.040
34. Carty M, Bowie AG. Recent insights into the role of Toll-like receptors in viral infection. *Clin Exp Immunol.* (2010) 161:397–406. doi: 10.1111/j.1365-2249.2010.04196.x
35. Hoshino K, Sugiyama T, Matsumoto M, Tanaka T, Saito M, Hemmi H, et al. IkappaB kinase-alpha is critical for interferon-alpha production induced by Toll-like receptors 7 and 9. *Nature* (2006) 440:949–53. doi: 10.1038/nature04641
36. Lopez-Pelaez M, Lamont DJ, Peggie M, Shpiro N, Gray NS, Cohen P. Protein kinase IKKbeta-catalyzed phosphorylation of IRF5 at Ser462 induces its dimerization and nuclear translocation in myeloid cells. *Proc Natl Acad Sci USA.* (2014) 111:17432–7. doi: 10.1073/pnas.1418399111
37. Ren J, Chen X, Chen ZJ. IKKbeta is an IRF5 kinase that instigates inflammation. *Proc Natl Acad Sci USA.* (2014) 111:17438–43. doi: 10.1073/pnas.1418516111
38. Huang S, Hendriks W, Althage A, Hemmi S, Bluethmann H, Kamijo R, et al. Immune response in mice that lack the interferon-gamma receptor. *Science* (1993) 259:1742–5. doi: 10.1126/science.8456301
39. Meraz MA, White JM, Sheehan KC, Bach EA, Rodig SJ, Dighe AS, et al. Targeted disruption of the Stat1 gene in mice reveals unexpected physiologic specificity in the JAK-STAT signaling pathway. *Cell* (1996) 84:431–42. doi: 10.1016/S0092-8674(00)81288-X
40. Park C, Li S, Cha E, Schindler C. Immune response in Stat2 knockout mice. *Immunity* (2000) 13:795–804. doi: 10.1016/S1074-7613(00)00077-7
41. de Weerd NA, Samarajiwa SA, Hertzog PJ. Type I interferon receptors: biochemistry and biological functions. *J Biol Chem.* (2007) 282:20053–7. doi: 10.1074/jbc.R700006200
42. Mahlakõiv T, Hernandez P, Gronke K, Diefenbach A, Staeheli P. Leukocyte-derived IFN-alpha/beta and epithelial IFN-lambda constitute a compartmentalized mucosal defense system that restricts enteric virus infections. *PLoS Pathog.* (2015) 11:e1004782. doi: 10.1371/journal.ppat.1004782
43. Müller U, Steinhoff U, Reis LF, Hemmi S, Pavlovic J, Zinkernagel RM, et al. Functional role of type I and type II interferons in antiviral defense. *Science* (1994) 264:1918–21. doi: 10.1126/science.8009221
44. Platanias LC. Mechanisms of type-I- and type-II-interferon-mediated signalling. *Nat Rev Immunol.* (2005) 5:375–86. doi: 10.1038/nri1604
45. Zanoni I, Granucci F, Broggi A. Interferon (IFN)-lambda takes the Helm: immunomodulatory roles of type III IFNs. *Front Immunol.* (2017) 8:1661. doi: 10.3389/fimmu.2017.01661
46. Levy DE, Darnell JE Jr. Stats: transcriptional control and biological impact. *Nat Rev Mol Cell Biol.* (2002) 3:651–62. doi: 10.1038/nrm909
47. Schindler C, Fu XY, Improta T, Aebersold R, Darnell JE. Proteins of transcription factor ISGF-3: one gene encodes the 91-and 84-kDa ISGF-3 proteins that are activated by interferon alpha. *Proc Natl Acad Sci USA.* (1992) 89:7836–9. doi: 10.1073/pnas.89.16.7836
48. Bhattacharya S, Eckner R, Grossman S, Oldread E, Arany Z, D'Andrea A, et al. Cooperation of Stat2 and p300/CBP in signalling induced by interferon-alpha. *Nature* (1996) 383:344–7. doi: 10.1038/383344a0
49. Zhang JJ, Vinkemeier U, Gu W, Chakravarti D, Horvath CM, Darnell JE. Two contact regions between Stat1 and CBP/p300 in interferon gamma signaling. *Proc Natl Acad Sci USA.* (1996) 93:15092–6. doi: 10.1073/pnas.93.26.15092
50. Schoggins JW, Rice CM. Interferon-stimulated genes and their antiviral effector functions. *Curr Opin Virol.* (2011) 1:519–25. doi: 10.1016/j.coviro.2011.10.008

51. Schneider WM, Chevillotte MD, Rice CM. Interferon-stimulated genes: a complex web of host defenses. *Annu Rev Immunol.* (2014) 32:513–45. doi: 10.1146/annurev-immunol-032713-120231
52. Wu J, Chen ZJ. Innate immune sensing and signaling of cytosolic nucleic acids. *Annu Rev Immunol.* (2014) 32:461–88. doi: 10.1146/annurev-immunol-032713-120156
53. Morales DJ, Lenschow DJ. The antiviral activities of ISG15. *J Mol Biol.* (2013) 425:4995–5008. doi: 10.1016/j.jmb.2013.09.041
54. Maelfait J, Bridgeman A, Benlahrech A, Cursi C, Rehwinkel J. Restriction by SAMHD1 limits cGAS/STING-dependent innate and adaptive immune responses to HIV-1. *Cell Rep.* (2016) 16:1492–1501. doi: 10.1016/j.celrep.2016.07.002
55. Schmid S, Mordstein M, Kochs G, García-Sastre A, Tenoever BR. Transcription factor redundancy ensures induction of the antiviral state. *J Biol Chem.* (2010) 285:42013–22. doi: 10.1074/jbc.M110.165936
56. Schoggins JW, Wilson SJ, Panis M, Murphy MY, Jones CT, Bieniasz P, et al. A diverse range of gene products are effectors of the type I interferon antiviral response. *Nature* (2011) 472:481–5. doi: 10.1038/nature09907
57. Dixit E, Boulant S, Zhang Y, Lee AS, Odendall C, Shum B, et al. Peroxisomes are signaling platforms for antiviral innate immunity. *Cell* (2010) 141:668–81. doi: 10.1016/j.cell.2010.04.018
58. Daffis S, Samuel MA, Suthar MS, Keller BC, Gale M, Diamond MS. Interferon regulatory factor IRF-7 induces the antiviral alpha interferon response and protects against lethal West Nile virus infection. *J Virol.* (2008) 82:8465–75. doi: 10.1128/JVI.00918-08
59. Croker BA, Kiu H, Nicholson SE. SOCS regulation of the JAK/STAT signalling pathway. *Semin Cell Dev Biol.* (2008) 19:414–22. doi: 10.1016/j.semcdb.2008.07.010
60. Malakhova OA, Kim KI, Luo JK, Zou W, Kumar KG, Fuchs SY, et al. UBP43 is a novel regulator of interferon signaling independent of its ISG15 isopeptidase activity. *EMBO J.* (2006) 25:2358–67. doi: 10.1038/sj.emboj.7601149
61. Wang WB, Levy DE, Lee CK. STAT3 negatively regulates type I IFN-mediated antiviral response. *J Immunol.* (2011) 187:2578–85. doi: 10.4049/jimmunol.1004128
62. Tsai MH, Lee CK. STAT3 cooperates with phospholipid scramblase 2 to suppress type I interferon response. *Front Immunol.* (2018) 9:1886. doi: 10.3389/fimmu.2018.01886
63. Chen W, Daines MO, Khurana Hershey GK. Turning off signal transducer and activator of transcription (STAT): the negative regulation of STAT signaling. *J Allergy Clin Immunol.* (2004) 114:476–89; quiz 490. doi: 10.1016/j.jaci.2004.06.042
64. McBride KM, Banninger G, McDonald C, Reich NC. Regulated nuclear import of the STAT1 transcription factor by direct binding of importin-alpha. *EMBO J.* (2002) 21:1754–63. doi: 10.1093/emboj/21.7.1754
65. Fagerlund R, Mélen K, Kinnunen L, Julkunen I. Arginine/lysine-rich nuclear localization signals mediate interactions between dimeric STATs and importin alpha 5. *J Biol Chem.* (2002) 277:30072–8. doi: 10.1074/jbc.M202943200
66. Liu L, McBride KM, Reich NC. STAT3 nuclear import is independent of tyrosine phosphorylation and mediated by importin-alpha3. *Proc Natl Acad Sci USA.* (2005) 102:8150–5. doi: 10.1073/pnas.05010 643102
67. McBride KM, McDonald C, Reich NC. Nuclear export signal located within theDNA-binding domain of the STAT1transcription factor. *EMBO J.* (2000) 19:6196–206. doi: 10.1093/emboj/19.22.6196
68. Chen K, Liu J, Liu S, Xia M, Zhang X, Han D, et al. Methyltransferase SETD2-mediated methylation of STAT1 is critical for interferon antiviral activity. *Cell* (2017) 170:492–506 e14. doi: 10.1016/j.cell.2017.06.042
69. Liu K, Lemon B, Traktman P. The dual-specificity phosphatase encoded by vaccinia virus, VH1, is essential for viral transcription *in vivo* and *in vitro*. *J Virol.* (1995) 69:7823–34.
70. Koksal AC, Cingolani G. Dimerization of Vaccinia virus VH1 is essential for dephosphorylation of STAT1 at tyrosine 701. *J Biol Chem.* (2011) 286:14373–82. doi: 10.1074/jbc.M111.226357
71. Najarro P, Traktman P, Lewis JA. Vaccinia virus blocks gamma interferon signal transduction: viral VH1 phosphatase reverses Stat1 activation. *J Virol.* (2001) 75:3185–96. doi: 10.1128/JVI.75.7.3185-3196.2001
72. Unterholzner L, Sumner RP, Baran M, Ren H, Mansur DS, Bourke NM, et al. Vaccinia virus protein C6 is a virulence factor that binds TBK-1 adaptor proteins and inhibits activation of IRF3 and IRF7. *PLoS Pathog.* (2011) 7:e1002247. doi: 10.1371/journal.ppat.1002247
73. Christensen MH, Jensen SB, Miettinen JJ, Luecke S, Prabakaran T, Reinert LS, et al. HSV-1 ICP27 targets the TBK1-activated STING signalsome to inhibit virus-induced type I IFN expression. *EMBO J.* (2016) 35:1385–99. doi: 10.15252/embj.201593458
74. Zhang D, Su C, Zheng C. Herpes simplex virus 1 serine protease VP24 blocks the DNA-sensing signal pathway by abrogating activation of interferon regulatory factor 3. *J Virol.* (2016) 90:5824–5829. doi: 10.1128/JVI.00186-16
75. Cao J, Zhou Y, Gong GZ. Effect of HCV NS5A on STAT1 phosphorylation and nuclear translocation induced by IFN alpha-2b. *Zhonghua Gan Zang Bing Za Zhi* (2006) 14:894–7.
76. Kumthip K, Chusri P, Jilg N, Zhao L, Fusco DN, Zhao H, et al. Hepatitis C virus NS5A disrupts STAT1 phosphorylation and suppresses type I interferon signaling. *J Virol.* (2012) 86:8581–91. doi: 10.1128/JVI.00533-12
77. Sen A, Rott L, Phan N, Mukherjee G, Greenberg HB. Rotavirus NSP1 protein inhibits interferon-mediated STAT1 activation. *J Virol.* (2014) 88:41–53. doi: 10.1128/JVI.01501-13
78. Hartman AL, Bird BH, Towner JS, Antoniadou ZA, Zaki SR, Nichol ST. Inhibition of IRF-3 activation by VP35 is critical for the high level of virulence of ebola virus. *J Virol.* (2008) 82:2699–704. doi: 10.1128/JVI.02344-07
79. Basler CF, Mikulasova A, Martinez-Sobrido L, Paragas J, Mühlberger E, Bray M, et al. The Ebola virus VP35 protein inhibits activation of interferon regulatory factor 3. *J Virol.* (2003) 77:7945–56. doi: 10.1128/JVI.77.14.7945-7956.2003
80. Valmas C, Grosch MN, Schümann M, Olejnik J, Martinez O, Best SM, et al. Marburg virus evades interferon responses by a mechanism distinct from ebola virus. *PLoS Pathog.* (2010) 6:e1000721. doi: 10.1371/journal.ppat.1000721
81. Koeberlein B, zur Hausen A, Bektas N, Zentgraf H, Chin R, Nguyen LT, et al. Hepatitis B virus overexpresses suppressor of cytokine signaling-3 (SOCS3) thereby contributing to severity of inflammation in the liver. *Virus Res.* (2010) 148:51–9. doi: 10.1016/j.virusres.2009.12.003
82. Collins AS, Ahmed S, Napoletano S, Schroeder M, Johnston JA, Hegarty JE, et al. Hepatitis C virus (HCV)-induced suppressor of cytokine signaling (SOCS) 3 regulates proinflammatory TNF-alpha responses. *J Leukoc Biol.* (2014) 96:255–63. doi: 10.1189/jlb.2A1211-608RRRR
83. Kim K, Kim KH, Cheong J. Hepatitis B virus X protein impairs hepatic insulin signaling through degradation of IRS1 and induction of SOCS3. *PLoS ONE* (2010) 5:e8649. doi: 10.1371/journal.pone.0008649
84. Gupta SP. Viral proteases and their inhibitors. London: Elsevier; Academic Press (2017). xv, 499 pages.
85. Lei X, Xiao X, Xue Q, Jin Q, He B, Wang J. Cleavage of interferon regulatory factor 7 by enterovirus 71 3C suppresses cellular responses. *J Virol.* (2013) 87:1690–8. doi: 10.1128/JVI.01855-12
86. Xiang Z, Liu L, Lei X, Zhou Z, He B, Wang J. 3C Protease of enterovirus D68 inhibits cellular defense mediated by interferon regulatory factor 7. *J Virol.* (2016) 90:1613–21. doi: 10.1128/JVI.02395-15
87. Hung HC, Wang HC, Shih SR, Teng IF, Tseng CP, Hsu JT. Synergistic inhibition of enterovirus 71 replication by interferon and rupintrivir. *J Infect Dis.* (2011) 203:1784–90. doi: 10.1093/infdis/jir174
88. Park SY, Waheed AA, Zhang ZR, Freed EO, Bonifacino JS. HIV-1 Vpu accessory protein induces caspase-mediated cleavage of IRF3 transcription factor. *J Biol Chem.* (2014) 289:35102–10. doi: 10.1074/jbc.M114.50 97062
89. Doehle BP, Chang K, Rustagi A, McNevin J, McElrath MJ, Gale M. Vpu mediates depletion of interferon regulatory factor 3 during HIV infection by a lysosome-dependent mechanism. *J Virol.* (2012) 86:8367–74. doi: 10.1128/JVI.00423-12
90. Barro M, Patton JT. Rotavirus NSP1 inhibits expression of type I interferon by antagonizing the function of interferon regulatory factors IRF3, IRF5, and IRF7. *J Virol.* (2007) 81:4473–81. doi: 10.1128/JVI.02498-06
91. Arnold MM, Barro M, Patton JT. Rotavirus NSP1 mediates degradation of interferon regulatory factors through targeting of the dimerization domain. *J Virol.* (2013) 87:9813–21. doi: 10.1128/JVI.01146-13

92. Parisien JP, Lau JF, Rodriguez JJ, Sullivan BM, Moscona A, Parks GD, et al. The V protein of human parainfluenza virus 2 antagonizes type I interferon responses by destabilizing signal transducer and activator of transcription 2. *Virology* (2001) 283:230–9. doi: 10.1006/viro.2001.0856
93. Andrejeva J, Young DF, Goodbourn S, Randall RE. Degradation of STAT1 and STAT2 by the V proteins of simian virus 5 and human parainfluenza virus type 2, respectively: consequences for virus replication in the presence of alpha/beta and gamma interferons. *J Virol.* (2002) 76:2159–67. doi: 10.1128/jvi.76.5.2159-2167.2002
94. Ashour J, Laurent-Rolle M, Shi PY, García-Sastre A. NS5 of dengue virus mediates STAT2 binding and degradation. *J Virol.* (2009) 83:5408–18. doi: 10.1128/JVI.02188-08
95. Jones M, Davidson A, Hibbert L, Gruenwald P, Schlaak J, Ball S, et al. Dengue virus inhibits alpha interferon signaling by reducing STAT2 expression. *J Virol.* (2005) 79:5414–20. doi: 10.1128/JVI.79.9.5414-5420.2005
96. Dar HA, Zaheer T, Paracha RZ, Ali A. Structural analysis and insight into Zika virus NS5 mediated interferon inhibition. *Infect Genet Evol.* (2017) 51:143–152. doi: 10.1016/j.meegid.2017.03.027
97. Grant A, Ponia SS, Tripathi S, Balasubramaniam V, Miorin L, Sourisseau M, et al. Zika Virus Targets Human STAT2 to Inhibit Type I Interferon Signaling. *Cell Host Microbe* (2016) 19:882–90. doi: 10.1016/j.chom.2016.05.009
98. Xu W, Edwards MR, Borek DM, Feagins AR, Mittal A, Alinger JB, et al. Ebola virus VP24 targets a unique NLS binding site on karyopherin alpha 5 to selectively compete with nuclear import of phosphorylated STAT1. *Cell Host Microbe* (2014) 16:187–200. doi: 10.1016/j.chom.2014.07.008
99. Shabman RS, Gulcicek EE, Stone KL, Basler CF. The Ebola virus VP24 protein prevents hnRNP C1/C2 binding to karyopherin alpha1 and partially alters its nuclear import. *J Infect Dis.* (2011) 204 Suppl. 3:S904–10. doi: 10.1093/infdis/jir323
100. Wang C, Sun M, Yuan X, Ji L, Jin Y, Cardona CJ, et al. Enterovirus 71 suppresses interferon responses by blocking Janus kinase (JAK)/signal transducer and activator of transcription (STAT) signaling through inducing karyopherin-alpha1 degradation. *J Biol Chem.* (2017) 292:10262–74. doi: 10.1074/jbc.M116.745729
101. Göertz GP, McNally KL, Robertson SJ, Best SM, Pijlman GP, Fros JJ. The methyltransferase-like domain of chikungunya virus nsP2 inhibits the interferon response by promoting the nuclear export of STAT1. *J Virol.* (2018) 92:e01008-18. doi: 10.1128/JVI.01008-18
102. Fros JJ, Liu WJ, Prow NA, Geertsema C, Ligtenberg M, Vanlandingham DL, et al. Chikungunya virus nonstructural protein 2 inhibits type I/II interferon-stimulated JAK-STAT signaling. *J Virol.* (2010) 84:10877–87. doi: 10.1128/JVI.00949-10
103. Sugai A, Sato H, Takayama I, Yoneda M, Kai C. Nipah and hendra virus nucleoproteins inhibit nuclear accumulation of signal transducer and activator of transcription 1 (STAT1) and STAT2 by interfering with their complex formation. *J Virol.* (2017) 91:e01136-17. doi: 10.1128/JVI.00 1136-17
104. Rodriguez JJ, Cruz CD, Horvath CM. Identification of the nuclear export signal and STAT-binding domains of the Nipah virus V protein reveals mechanisms underlying interferon evasion. *J Virol.* (2004) 78:5358–67. doi: 10.1128/JVI.78.10.5358-5367.2004
105. Rodriguez JJ, Parisien JP, Horvath CM. Nipah virus V protein evades alpha and gamma interferons by preventing STAT1 and STAT2 activation and nuclear accumulation. *J Virol.* (2002) 76:11476–83. doi: 10.1128/JVI.76.22.11476-11483.2002
106. Schomacker H, Hebner RM, Boonyaratanakornkit J, Surman S, Amaro-Carambot E, Collins PL, et al. The C proteins of human parainfluenza virus type 1 block IFN signaling by binding and retaining Stat1 in perinuclear aggregates at the late endosome. *PLoS ONE* (2012) 7:e28382. doi: 10.1371/journal.pone.0028382
107. Oda K, Oda T, Matoba Y, Sato M, Irie T, Sakaguchi T. Structural analysis of the STAT1:STAT2 heterodimer revealed the mechanism of Sendai virus C protein-mediated blockade of type 1 interferon signaling. *J Biol Chem.* (2017) 292:19752–66. doi: 10.1074/jbc.M117.786285
108. Oda K, Matoba Y, Irie T, Kawabata R, Fukushi M, Sugiyama M, et al. Structural basis of the inhibition of STAT1 activity by sendai virus C protein. *J Virol.* (2015) 89:11487–99. doi: 10.1128/JVI.01887-15
109. Palosaari H, Parisien JP, Rodriguez JJ, Ulane CM, Horvath CM. STAT protein interference and suppression of cytokine signal transduction by measles virus V protein. *J Virol.* (2003) 77:7635–44. doi: 10.1128/JVI.77.13.7635-7644.2003
110. Holloway G, Truong TT, Coulson BS. Rotavirus antagonizes cellular antiviral responses by inhibiting the nuclear accumulation of STAT1, STAT2, and NF-kappaB. *J Virol.* (2009) 83:4942–51. doi: 10.1128/JVI.01450-08
111. Paladino P, Collins SE, Mossman KL. Cellular localization of the herpes simplex virus ICP0 protein dictates its ability to block IRF3-mediated innate immune responses. *PLoS ONE* (2010) 5:e10428. doi: 10.1371/journal.pone.0010428
112. Melroe GT, DeLuca NA, Knipe DM. Herpes simplex virus 1 has multiple mechanisms for blocking virus-induced interferon production. *J Virol.* (2004) 78:8411–20. doi: 10.1128/JVI.78.16.8411-8420.2004
113. Bi X, Yang L, Mancl ME, Barnes BJ. Modulation of interferon regulatory factor 5 activities by the Kaposi sarcoma-associated herpesvirus-encoded viral interferon regulatory factor 3 contributes to immune evasion and lytic induction. *J Interferon Cytokine Res.* (2011) 31:373–82. doi: 10.1089/jir.2010.0084
114. Joo CH, Shin YC, Gack M, Wu L, Levy D, Jung JU. Inhibition of interferon regulatory factor 7 (IRF7)-mediated interferon signal transduction by the Kaposi's sarcoma-associated herpesvirus viral IRF homolog vIRF3. *J Virol.* (2007) 81:8282–92. doi: 10.1128/JVI.00235-07
115. Seo T, Lee D, Lee B, Chung JH, Choe J. Viral interferon regulatory factor 1 of Kaposi's sarcoma-associated herpesvirus (human herpesvirus 8) binds to, and inhibits transactivation of, CREB-binding protein. *Biochem Biophys Res Commun.* (2000) 270:23–7. doi: 10.1006/bbrc.2000.2393
116. Xing J, Ni L, Wang S, Wang K, Lin R, Zheng C. Herpes simplex virus 1-encoded tegument protein VP16 abrogates the production of beta interferon (IFN) by inhibiting NF-kappaB activation and blocking IFN regulatory factor 3 to recruit its coactivator CBP. *J Virol.* (2013) 87:9788–801. doi: 10.1128/JVI.01440-13
117. Morin G, Robinson BA, Rogers KS, Wong SW. A Rhesus Rhadinovirus Viral Interferon (IFN) Regulatory factor is virion associated and inhibits the early IFN antiviral response. *J Virol.* (2015) 89:7707–21. doi: 10.1128/JVI.01175-15
118. Zhang R, Fang L, Wang D, Cai K, Zhang H, Xie L, et al. Porcine bocavirus NP1 negatively regulates interferon signaling pathway by targeting the DNA-binding domain of IRF9. *Virology* (2015) 485:414–21. doi: 10.1016/j.virol.2015.08.005
119. Zhang R, Fang L, Wu W, Zhao F, Song T, Xie L, et al. Porcine bocavirus NP1 protein suppresses type I IFN production by interfering with IRF3 DNA-binding activity. *Virus Genes* (2016) 52:797–805. doi: 10.1007/s11262-016-1377-z
120. Zhang Q, Shi K, Yoo D. Suppression of type I interferon production by porcine epidemic diarrhea virus and degradation of CREB-binding protein by nsp1. *Virology* (2016) 489:252–68. doi: 10.1016/j.virol.2015.12.010
121. Han M, Du Y, Song C, Yoo D. Degradation of CREB-binding protein and modulation of type I interferon induction by the zinc finger motif of the porcine reproductive and respiratory syndrome virus nsp1alpha subunit. *Virus Res.* (2013) 172:54–65. doi: 10.1016/j.virusres.2012.12.012
122. Bentz GL, Liu R, Hahn AM, Shackelford J, Pagano JS. Epstein-Barr virus BRLF1 inhibits transcription of IRF3 and IRF7 and suppresses induction of interferon-beta. *Virology* (2010) 402:121–8. doi: 10.1016/j.virol.2010.0 03.014
123. Read GS, Karr BM, Knight K. Isolation of a herpes simplex virus type 1 mutant with a deletion in the virion host shutoff gene and identification of multiple forms of the vhs (UL41) polypeptide. *J Virol.* (1993) 67:7149–60.
124. Chee AV, Roizman B. Herpes simplex virus 1 gene products occlude the interferon signaling pathway at multiple sites. *J Virol.* (2004) 78:4185–96. doi: 10.1128/JVI.78.8.4185-4196.2004
125. Taddeo B, Zhang W, Roizman B. The herpes simplex virus host shutoff RNase degrades cellular and viral mRNAs made before infection but not viral mRNA made after infection. *J Virol.* (2013) 87:4516–22. doi: 10.1128/JVI.00005-13
126. Mukherjee A, Di Bisceglie AM, Ray RB. Hepatitis C virus-mediated enhancement of microRNA miR-373 impairs the JAK/STAT signaling pathway. *J Virol.* (2015) 89:3356–65. doi: 10.1128/JVI. 03085-14

127. Kuo YP, Tsai KN, Luo YC, Chung PJ, Su YW, Teng Y, et al. Establishment of a mouse model for the complete mosquito-mediated transmission cycle of Zika virus. *PLoS Negl Trop Dis.* (2018) 12:e0006417. doi: 10.1371/journal.pntd.0006417
128. Bradfute SB, Stuthman KS, Shurtleff AC, Bavari S. A STAT-1 knockout mouse model for Machupo virus pathogenesis. *Virol J.* (2011) 8:300. doi: 10.1186/1743-422X-8-300
129. Wan SW, Chen PW, Chen CY, Lai YC, Chu YT, Hung CY, et al. Therapeutic effects of monoclonal antibody against dengue virus NS1 in a STAT1 knockout mouse model of dengue infection. *J Immunol.* (2017) 199:2834–44. doi: 10.4049/jimmunol.1601523
130. Chaudhary V, Yuen KS, Chan JF, Chan CP, Wang PH, Cai JP, et al. Selective activation of type II interferon signaling by zika virus NS5 protein. *J Virol.* (2017) 91:e00163-17. doi: 10.1128/JVI.00163-17
131. Bowen JR, Quicke KM, Maddur MS, O'Neal JT, McDonald CE, Fedorova NB, et al. Zika virusantagonizes type I interferon responses during infection of human dendritic cells. *PLoS Pathog.* (2017) 13:e1006164. doi: 10.1371/journal.ppat.1006164

8

Signal Integration of IFN-I and IFN-II with TLR4 Involves Sequential Recruitment of STAT1-Complexes and NFκB to Enhance Pro-Inflammatory Transcription

Anna Piaszyk-Borychowska[1]*, Lajos Széles*[2]*, Attila Csermely*[2]*, Hsin-Chien Chiang*[3]*, Joanna Wesoły*[4]*, Chien-Kuo Lee*[3]*, Laszlo Nagy*[2,5*] *and Hans A. R. Bluyssen*[1*]

[1] *Department of Human Molecular Genetics, Adam Mickiewicz University, Poznan, Poland,* [2] *Department of Biochemistry and Molecular Biology, University of Debrecen, Debrecen, Hungary,* [3] *Graduate Institute of Immunology, National Taiwan University College of Medicine, Taipei, Taiwan,* [4] *Laboratory of High Throughput Technologies, Adam Mickiewicz University, Poznan, Poland,* [5] *Departments of Medicine and Biological Chemistry, Johns Hopkins All Children's Hospital, Johns Hopkins University School of Medicine, St. Petersburg, FL, United States*

Correspondence:
Hans A. R. Bluyssen
h.bluyss@amu.edu.pl
Laszlo Nagy
lnagy@jhmi.edu

Atherosclerosis is a chronic inflammatory disease of the blood vessels, characterized by atherosclerotic lesion formation. Vascular Smooth Muscle Cells (VSMC), macrophages (MΦ), and dendritic cells (DC) play a crucial role in vascular inflammation and atherosclerosis. Interferon (IFN)α, IFNγ, and Toll-like receptor (TLR)4 activate pro-inflammatory gene expression and are pro-atherogenic. Gene expression regulation of many pro-inflammatory genes has shown to rely on Signal Integration (SI) between IFNs and TLR4 through combinatorial actions of the Signal Transducer and Activator of Transcription (STAT)1 complexes ISGF3 and γ-activated factor (GAF), and Nuclear Factor-κB (NFκB). Thus, IFN pre-treatment ("priming") followed by LPS stimulation leads to enhanced transcriptional responses as compared to the individual stimuli. To characterize the mechanism of priming-induced IFNα + LPS- and IFNγ + LPS-dependent SI in vascular cells as compared to immune cells, we performed a comprehensive genome-wide analysis of mouse VSMC, MΦ, and DC in response to IFNα, IFNγ, and/or LPS. Thus, we identified IFNα + LPS or IFNγ + LPS induced genes commonly expressed in these cell types that bound STAT1 and p65 at comparable γ-activated sequence (GAS), Interferon-stimulated response element (ISRE), or NFκB sites in promoter proximal and distal regions. Comparison of the relatively high number of overlapping ISRE sites in these genes unraveled a novel role of ISGF3 and possibly STAT1/IRF9 in IFNγ responses. In addition, similar STAT1-p65 co-binding modes were detected for IFNα + LPS and IFNγ + LPS up-regulated genes, which involved recruitment of STAT1 complexes preceding p65 to closely located GAS/NFκB or ISRE/NFκB composite sites already upon IFNα or IFNγ treatment. This STAT1-p65 co-binding significantly increased after subsequent LPS exposure and correlated with histone acetylation, PolII recruitment, and amplified target gene transcription in a STAT1-p65 co-bound dependent manner.

Thus, co-binding of STAT1-containing transcription factor complexes and NFκB, activated by IFN-I or IFN-II together with LPS, provides a platform for robust transcriptional activation of pro-inflammatory genes. Moreover, our data offer an explanation for the comparable effects of IFNα or IFNγ priming on TLR4-induced activation in vascular and immune cells, with important implications in atherosclerosis.

Keywords: inflammation, interferons, TLR4, signal integration, atherosclerosis, JAK-STAT, STAT1 and NFκB

INTRODUCTION

Atherosclerosis is a chronic inflammatory disease of the blood vessels, characterized by atherosclerotic lesion formation. Early onset of atherosclerosis is represented by recruitment of blood leukocytes to the injured vascular endothelium and altered contractility of Vascular Smooth Muscle Cells (VSMC) modulated by multiple inflammatory mediators (1). Accordingly, pro-inflammatory pathways activated by Toll-like receptors (TLRs), and Interferons (IFNs) have been identified as key components of atherogenesis (2–4). Type I (IFN-I; IFNα), and II (IFN-II; IFNγ) IFNs both induce IFN-stimulated gene (ISG) expression through Janus kinase (JAK)-dependent phosphorylation of Signal Transducer and Activator of Transcription (STAT)1. STAT1 homodimers, known as γ-activated factor (GAF), activate transcription in response to both IFN types by direct binding to IFN-II activation site γ-activated sequence (GAS)-containing genes. Association of Interferon Regulatory Factor (IRF)9 with STAT1-STAT2 heterodimers [known as Interferon-stimulated gene factor 3 (ISGF3)] in response to IFN-I, redirects these complexes to a distinct group of target genes harboring the Interferon-stimulated response element (ISRE) (5, 6). Limited evidence exists for a role of ISGF3 in IFN-II responses of ISRE-containing genes. Likewise, for a restricted number of ISGs, a non-canonical STAT1/IRF9 complex was shown to control IFNγ-responsiveness (7–9). The partially overlapping and differential activation of transcription factor complexes and regulation of target gene expression by IFN-I and IFN-II, may be a consequence of the biological similarities and differences of these two IFN types.

TLR4 ligation results in the prompt activation of multiple transcription factors, including members of the Nuclear Factor-κB (NFκB) and IRF families (10, 11). These factors rapidly induce the expression of hundreds of genes that amplify the initial inflammatory response, exert antimicrobial activities and initiate the development of acquired immunity. Several of the cytokines that are up-regulated in the initial wave of immediate early gene expression function in feed forward transcriptional loops—particularly important examples being IFN-I, which induce a secondary wave of STAT1- and STAT2-dependent gene expression, and Tumor necrosis factor (TNF) which sustains NFκB signaling.

Gene expression regulation of many pro-inflammatory genes has shown to rely on Signal Integration (SI) between IFNs and TLR4 through combinatorial actions of the STAT1-containing complexes ISGF3 and GAF with NFκB. For example, previous analyses of the murine *Nos2* promoter revealed an IFN response region (containing GAS and ISRE sites) and binding sites for NFκB (12). Indeed, sequential and cooperative contributions of NFκB preceding ISGF3 were shown to be involved in the transcriptional induction of the *Nos2* gene in macrophages (MΦ) infected with the intracellular bacterial pathogen *Listeria monocytogenes* (13). The *Nos2* gene reflects a larger group of genes, co-regulated by TLR4 and IFNs (14, 15). On the other hand, the profound effects of IFNγ pre-treatment ("priming") on TLR4-induced MΦ activation have also long been recognized. In this respect, SI between IFNγ and lipopolysaccharide (LPS) relies on combinatorial actions of STAT1 with NFκB and IRFs on ISRE/NFκB or GAS/NFκB binding sites, which leads to enhanced transcriptional regulation of many pro-inflammatory genes. Together, this coordinates the antimicrobial and inflammatory responses in MΦ, but also in dendritic cells (DC) (16–19). Recently, we characterized the role of STAT1 in the transcriptional response pathways involved in the interaction between IFN-II and TLR4 signaling in endothelial cells (EC) and VSMC (20). Promoter analysis of the genes encoding multiple chemokines, adhesion molecules and antiviral and antibacterial response proteins, predicted that cooperation between NFκB and STAT1 is involved in the amplified transcriptional regulation of responses to IFN-II and LPS. The synergistic interactions between IFNγ and TLR4 also resulted in increased T-cell migration and impaired aortic contractility in a STAT1-dependent manner (20). Interestingly, expression of the *Nos2* gene in MΦ in response to IFNα/LPS behaved similar as after IFNγ/LPS (21), reflecting the existing overlap in activation mechanisms between the different types of IFN. However, the mechanistic role of SI between IFN-I and TLR4, in the context of "priming," in vascular and immune cell has not been studied in much detail.

To characterize the mechanism of priming-induced IFNα + LPS- and IFNγ + LPS-dependent SI in vascular cells as compared to immune cells, we performed a comprehensive genome-wide analysis of VSMC, MΦ, and DC in response to IFNα, IFNγ, and/or LPS. Thus, through increased histone acetylation and RNA polymerase II (PolII) recruitment co-binding of transcription factor complexes activated by IFN-I or IFN-II

Abbreviations: ChIP, Chromatin Immunoprecipitation; Co-IP, Co-immunoprecipitation; DC, Dendritic cells; EC, Endothelial cells; GAF, γ-activated factor; GO, Gene ontology; IFN, Interferon; IRF, Interferon Regulatory Factor; ISG, IFN-stimulated gene; ISGF3, Interferon-stimulated gene factor 3; ISRE, Interferon-stimulated response element; JAK, Janus kinase; LPS, Lipopolysaccharide; MΦ, Macrophages; NFκB, Nuclear Factor-κB; PolII, RNA polymerase II; ROS, Reactive oxygen species; SI, Signal Integration; STAT, Signal Transducer and Activator of Transcription; TNF, Tumor necrosis factor; TLR, Toll-like receptor; VSMC, Vascular Smooth Muscle Cells.

together with LPS, including GAF, ISGF3, STAT1/IRF9, and p65-p50 heterodimers provide a platform for robust transcriptional activation of pro-inflammatory genes. Moreover, our data offer an explanation for the comparable effects of IFNα or IFNγ priming on TLR4-induced activation in vascular and immune cells, with important implications in atherosclerosis.

MATERIALS AND METHODS

VSMC, MΦ, and DC Isolation

WT mice (strain background C57BL/6) were obtained from Charles River Laboratories. STAT1$^{-/-}$ mice (strain background C57BL/6) (22) were kindly provided by Thomas Decker (Department of Microbiology, Immunobiology and Genetics, University of Vienna). Before any manipulations, animals were euthanized by cervical dislocation under isoflurane anesthesia. Primary VSMC were isolated from WT and STAT1$^{-/-}$ mice aortas by enzymatic digestion (23). Briefly, aortas were dissected out and carefully cleaned from remnant fat and connecting tissue and cut into rings. Next, tissue was incubated with digestion mix consisting of DMEM [Thermo Fisher Scientific (TFS), 11960044] supplemented with 0.744 U/ml Elastase I (Sigma Aldrich, E1250), 1 mg/ml Collagenase II (Sigma Aldrich, 1148090) and 1 mg/ml soybean trypsin inhibitor (TFS, 17075029) for 1 h at 37°C. After digestion the cell suspension was passed through 100 μm cell strainer and left undisturbed for 1 week. Examination of marker gene (α-actin, smoothelin, calponin) expression by RT-PCR was used to assess VSMC cell phenotype. Freshly isolated femur and tibia form WT mice were cleaned from remnant muscle tissue by scrapping. Both ends of the bones were cut and bone-marrow was flushed and centrifuged for 5 min, 1,500 rpm. The cell pellet was incubated in ACK buffer (pH 7.2–7.4) in order to lyse red blood cells. Monocytes were purified through a Ficoll-Paque gradient (GE Healthcare, 17-1440). Afterwards primary MΦ were differentiated in DMEM medium [Thermo Fisher Scientific (TFS), 11960044] supplemented with 30% L929 conditioned medium (containing M-CSF), 15% FBS (Sigma-Aldrich, F7524) and 1:100 antibiotic/antimycotic solution (Sigma-Aldrich, A5955) for 5 days (24). Similarly, primary DC were differentiated from bone-marrow using a solution containing RPMI1640 medium (Sigma-Aldrich, R5886), 200 U/ml rmGM-CSF (PeproTech, 315-03), 10% FBS (Sigma-Aldrich, F7524), 1:100 antibiotic/antimycotic solution (Sigma-Aldrich, A5955), 2 mM L-glutamine (Sigma-Aldrich, 67513), and 50 μM β-ME (TFS, 31350-010) for 6 days according to a modified Lutz et al. protocol (25). Purity of MΦ and DC populations was assessed by flow cytometry, with F4/80 and CD11b, CD11c markers, respectively. Experimental procedures performed in this study, encompassing sacrificing mice for bone marrow or tissue isolation, did not require any medical ethical approval in accordance with the local legislation and institutional requirements.

Cell Culture and Treatment

WT and STAT1$^{-/-}$ VSMC were cultured in DMEM complete medium (TFS, 11960044) supplemented with 10% FBS (TFS, 10500-064), 1:100 L-glutamine (BioWest, X0550), and 1:100 antibiotic/antimycotic solution (Sigma-Aldrich, A5955). On the day before treatment, complete medium was exchanged onto 2% FBS containing starving medium. Differentiated MΦ and DC were immediately placed in serum free medium (TFS, 12065074) or 2% FBS (Sigma-Aldrich, F7524) containing RMPI1640 (Sigma-Aldrich, R5886) supplemented with 1:100 antibiotic/antimycotic solution (Sigma-Aldrich, A5955) and 50 μM β-ME (TFS, 31350-010), respectively, for 24 h. Afterwards, cells were treated with single stimulus as follows: 1,000 U/ml of IFNα (Merck Millipore, IF009) or 10 ng/ml of IFNγ (TFS, PMC4031) for 8 h; 10 ng/ml (MΦ and DC)/1 μg/ml (VSMC) of LPS (Sigma-Aldrich, L4391) for 4 h. To further study the effect of IFNs pre-treatment on LPS signaling the cells were first treated with IFNα or IFNγ, after 4 h LPS was added to the same cell culture plates for an additional 4 h, what resulted in a total of 8 h treatment with IFNs and 4 h treatment with LPS, at concentrations listed above. Described treatment strategy was applied in both RNA-seq and ChIP-seq experiments performed in this study.

Gene Ontology (GO)

Protein ANalysis THrough Evolutionary Relationships (PANTHER) resource (26) was applied to identify statistically overrepresented GO terms for mapped lists of commonly up-regulated [Fold Change (FC) > 2] genes in VSMC, MΦ, and DC after combined treatment with IFNα + LPS (579 genes) and IFNγ + LPS (536 genes), using GO Biological Process Complete annotation data set. GO terms subjected for further comparison between the gene lists were selected as representative terms related to biological functions involved in immune, inflammatory, defense and stress response. Only GO terms with p-value of <0.05 were considered as significantly enriched.

Promoter Analysis

Over-represented conserved Transcription Factor Binding Sites (TFBS) for STAT1 and NFκB were screened in the regulatory regions of commonly up-regulated (FC > 2) genes in VSMC, MΦ and DC after combined treatment with IFNα + LPS (579 genes) and IFNγ + LPS (536 genes) using pSCAN webserver (27). JASPAR Profiles for: GAS—MA0137.2, MA0137.3, ISRE—MA0652.1, MA0137.1, MA0.517.1, and NFκB—MA0105.1, MA0105.3. TFBS were analyzed in the region of −950/+50 bp to the nearest gene transcription start site. Applied threshold of matrix similarity score for potential GAS/ISRE and NFκB binding site was ≥0.85 and ≥0.90, respectively.

Western Blot

Protein extracts from primary WT VSMC were prepared using Radio Immuno Precipitation Assay (RIPA) buffer (50 mM Tris-HCl, pH = 8.0 (Invitrogen, 15568025), 150 mM NaCl (Sigma-Aldrich, S9888), 1% Nonidet-40 (Bio-Shop, NON505), 0.5% sodium deoxycholate (Bio-Shop, DCA333), 0.1% SDS (Bio-Shop, SDS001), 1% protease inhibitor cocktail (Sigma-Aldrich, P8340), 1% EDTA (TFS, 15575-038), 0.1% PMSF (Sigma-Aldrich, 93482), and stored at −80°C. Protein concentrations were quantified using Bicinchoninic Acid (BCA) kit (Pierce, 23227). Sixty microgram of protein was heated in Bolt LDS buffer (Invitrogen, B0008) in 70°C for 10 min and loaded on Blot 4–12% Bis-Tris Plus Gels (Invitrogen, NW04120BOX), electrophoresed and transferred to PVDF membrane (GVS Nort America, 1231325). Western blot experiments were performed using SNAP ID Protein Detection System (Merck Millipore). Membranes were blocked either with 0.125% non-fat dry milk or with 1% BSA in TBS-Tween (TBS-T) and incubated with primary antibodies: tSTAT1 (CST, 14994, D1K9Y) 1:500, pSTAT1 (CST, 7649, D4A7) 1:500, tSTAT2 (CST, 72604, D9J7L) 1:400, pSTAT2 (Merck Millipore, 07-224) 1:500, IRF1 (CST, 8478, D5E4) 1:300, IRF9 (CST, 28845, D9I5H) 1:500, tp65 (CST, 6956, L8F6) 1:500, tubulin (Merck Millipore, 04-1117, EP1332Y) 1:2,000 and next with secondary HRP-conjugated antibodies: anti-rabbit (Sigma-Aldrich, A9169) 1:20,000, anti-mouse (Sigma-Aldrich, A9044) 1:20,000. Antibody-antigen complexes were visualized by enhanced chemiluminescence (ECL) using Luminata Forte HRP Substrate (Merck Millipore, WBLUF0500) and detected with G:Box System (Syngene). Image Studio Lite software (LI-COR Biosciences) was used for western blot quantification.

Co-immunoprecipitation (Co-IP)

VSMC WT cells were lysed for 30 min in co-IP buffer [1% NP-40 (Bio-Shop, NON505), 150 mM NaCl (Sigma-Aldrich, S9888), 1 mM EDTA (TFS, 15575-038), 50 mM Tris HCl pH 7.5 (Invitrogen, 15567027) 10% Glycerol (Bio-Shop, GLY001)] supplemented with protease inhibitors. Cell lysates were immunoprecipitated with IRF1 (CST, 8478, D5E4) and IRF9 (CST, 28845, D9I5H) antibodies overnight at 4°C. Immunocomplexes were isolated with Dynabeads Protein A/G [TFS, 10008D(A), 10009D(G)] saturated with 1% BSA (Sigma-Aldrich, A3059), by gentle rocking for 3 h at . Beads were washed 3 times with ice-cold co-IP buffer and once with Tris-EDTA buffer. Next bound proteins were retrieved by boiling in Bolt LDS buffer (Invitrogen, B0008) for 10 min. Immunocomplexes were analyzed by Western blot (described in Materials and Methods section, Western blot) with tSTAT1 (CST, 14994, D1K9Y) 1:500 and tSTAT2 (CST, 72604, D9J7L) 1:400.

RNA-seq Experimental Procedure

Total RNA from primary WT VSMC, WT MΦ, and WT DC treated as described above was isolated using GeneMATRIX Universal RNA Purification Kit (EURx, E3598). RNA-seq libraries were prepared from at least three biological replicates using a TruSeq RNA Library Preparation kit (Illumina, RS-122) according to the manufacturer's protocol. Libraries were quantified by Qubit fluorometer (TFS) and the quality was assessed with Agilent High Sensitivity DNA kit (Agilent Technologies, 5067-4626). Libraries were sequenced with Illumina HiScanSQ sequencer. To validate the quality of RNA-seq dataset, primary WT VSMC, WT MΦ, and WT DC were treated as described previously and 1 μg of RNA was used to synthetize complementary DNA with RevertAid Reverse Transcriptase (TFS, EP0441). *Cxcl9, Cxcl10, Ccl5, Nos2, Gbp6* transcripts were quantified using Maxima SYBR Green/ROX qPCR Master Mix (TFS, K0223) and CFX Connect Thermal Cycler System (Bio-Rad). Target gene levels were normalized to β-actin (ACTB) and quantified as described elsewhere (28) (described in Results section; data not shown).

Chromatin Immunoprecipitation (ChIP)-seq Experimental Procedure

ChIP was carried out as previously described (29), with minor modifications. Briefly, primary WT and STAT1$^{-/-}$ VSMC treated as described above were double-cross-linked with 0.5 M DSG (Sigma-Aldrich, 80424) for 45 min followed by 1% formaldehyde (TFS, 28906) for 10 min. Glycine (Sigma-Aldrich, G7126) was added for 10 min in 125 mM final concentration to stop cross-linking process. After fixation, nuclei were isolated by addition of ChIP Lysis Buffer (1% Triton X-100 (Bio-Shop, TRX777), 0.1% SDS (Bio-Shop, SDS001), 150 mM NaCl (Sigma-Aldrich, S9888), 1 mM EDTA (TFS, 15575-038), and 20 mM Tris, pH 8.0 (TFS, 15568-025). Chromatin was sonicated with Diagenode Bioruptor to generate fragments of 100–2,000 bp and immunoprecipitated with tSTAT1 (Santa Cruz, sc-346), pSTAT1 (CST, 7649, D4A7), tSTAT2 (CST, 72604, D9J7L), pSTAT2 (Merck Millipore, 07-224), IRF1 (CST, 8478, D5E4), IRF9 (CST, 28845, D9I5H), tp65 (CST, 6956, L8F6), RNA Polymerase II (Merck Millipore, 05-623, CTD4H8), Acetyl-Histone H3 (Lys27) (CST, 8173, D5E4), and Tri-Methyl-Histone H3 (Lys27) (CST, 9733, C36B11) antibodies. Following overnight incubation at 4°C, Dynabeads Protein A/G [TFS, 10008D(A), 10009D(G)] were added and incubated for 6 h at 4°C with rotation. Beads were washed at 4°C. DNA-protein complexes were eluted with Elution Buffer (1%SDS (Bio-Shop, SDS001), 0.1 M NaHCO3 (Sigma-Aldrich, S5761), and de-cross-linked with 0.2 M NaCl (Sigma-Aldrich, S9888) at 65°C. DNA was purified with MinElute PCR Purification kit (Qiagen, 28006) and quantified with Qubit fluorometer (TFS). ChIP-seq libraries were prepared from two biological replicates (for tSTAT1 and tp65 IPs) using TruSeq ChIP Library Preparation kit (Illumina, IP-202) according to the manufacturer's instructions. Libraries were quantified by Qubit fluorometer (TFS) and the quality was assessed with Agilent High Sensitivity DNA kit (Agilent Technologies, 5067-4626). Libraries were sequenced with Illumina HiSeq 2500 sequencer. Quality of ChIP-seq dataset was validated by ChIP-PCR experiments for selected STAT1 and p65 target genes (described in Results section; data not shown). All presented ChIP-PCR assays were performed using biological duplicates with primers listed in **Table S2** (Supplementary Material). Statistical significance was estimated by two-way ANOVA and unpaired two-tailed student T-test.

RNA-seq Data Analysis

RNA-seq raw sequence reads analysis was performed using Strand NGS software. After pre-alignment quality control (QC), alignment to the mouse mm10 (GRCm38) genome assembly was carried out using internal Strand NGS aligner which follows the Burrows-Wheeler Alignment (BWA) approach. All aligned reads were normalized using DESeq package. The data of the RNA-seq can be found at the NCBI GEO DataSets, with the accession number GSE120807. To determine differentially expressed genes (FC $\geq$ 2: up-regulated) gene lists were first filtered based on their normalized signal intensity values, with lower cut-off value>8.

FC was calculated for these genes across different conditions and the resulting lists of up-regulated genes were used for the further downstream analysis. 18 lists (3 cell types × 6 conditions: control, IFNα, IFNγ, LPS, IFNα + LPS, IFNγ + LPS) of differentially expressed genes were compared and visualized using BioVenn diagram tool (30). Heatmaps presenting log2 transformed FC values for commonly up-regulated genes in VSMC, MΦ and DC after combined treatment with IFNα+LPS (579 genes) and IFNγ + LPS (536 genes) across control, IFNα, IFNγ, LPS, IFNα + LPS and IFNγ + LPS treatment conditions were generated using GraphPad Prism v.7 software.

ChIP-seq Data Analysis

The primary analysis of ChIP-seq raw sequence reads was carried out using ChIP-seq analysis command line pipeline (31). Sequence reads were aligned to the mouse mm10 (GRCm38) genome assembly using the BWA tool (v0.7.10) (32), and bam files were created by SAMTools (v0.1.19) (32). Following converting mapped reads (bam files) by makeTagDirectory (HOMER v4.2 Hypergeometric Optimization of Motif EnRichment (33) to become accessible by the further HOMER tools, genome coverage (bedgraph) files were created by makeUCSCfile.pl (HOMER) (33) and converted to tiled data files (tdfs) by IGVtools (34). Peaks were predicted by MACS2 (v2.0.10) (q-value $\leq$ 0.01) (35), and artifacts were removed according to the blacklist of ENCODE (36). Intersections, subtractions, and merging of the predicted peaks (bed files) were made with BedTools (v2.23.0) (37). Tdf and bed files were visualized and genomic snapshots were taken with IGV2.3 (38). The closest gene for each peak was identified by annotatePeaks.pl (HOMER). The identification of DNA motifs was carried out in two steps. First, scanMotifGenomeWide.pl (HOMER) was used to identify all of the motifs genome-wide, specified by the publicly available motif files. Second, we determined the intersection between the identified motifs and peaks using intersectBed (bedtools). Sequencing data were submitted to NCBI GEO DataSets under accession number GSE120806.

RD (Read Distribution) Plot Preparation

For clustering, occupancy values (expressed as Reads Per Kilobase Million, RPKM) were calculated for all STAT1 and p65 peaks. The peaks were clustered using k-means clustering (n = 10) based on the binding pattern of STAT1 and p65 in 6 samples (12 ChIP-seq data sets in total). Normalized tag counts for RD histograms were generated by HOMER and then visualized by Java TreeView.

Peak Distribution Plot (Histogram) Preparation

Distances between summits of STAT1 and the closest p65 peaks summits were calculated using Phyton. Histograms were generated by annotatePeaks.pl from HOMER (with option-size 2,000 and -hist 25) and visualized by R using package ggplot2.

Integrative RNA-seq and ChIP-seq Analysis

GAS, ISRE and NFκB-p65 consensus motifs from HOMER database (GAS—motif273, ISRE—motif140, NFκB—motif208; motif logos in Supplementary Material, **Figure S1**) were re-mapped to the called peak regions in STAT1 and p65 ChIP-seq experiments, after treatment with IFNα + LPS and IFNγ + LPS in VSMC. Next, list of 579 and 536 up-regulated commonly expressed genes in vascular and immune cells treated with IFNα + LPS and IFNγ + LPS, respectively, identified from RNA-seq experiment, were overlapped with the lists of re-mapped motifs regions. The lists of annotated genes containing re-mapped GAS, ISRE and NFκB motifs were initially filtered according to motif distance from the closest annotated gene TSS (–/+100 kb) and according to Motif Score Threshold (MST) (GAS—MST 6, ISRE—MST 6, NFκB—MST 7). Distribution of consensus GAS, ISRE, and NFκB binding sites occupied by STAT1 and p65 across the genome was classified into seven categories of genomic locations: promoter/TSS (−1 kb to +100 bp), introns, intergenic, exon, 5′ UTR, 3′ UTR, and TTS. Re-mapped motifs distribution was plotted by the percentage of total number of occupied GAS, ISRE and NFκB binding sites under treatment with IFNα + LPS or IFNγ + LPS.

RESULTS

Commonly IFNα + LPS and IFNγ + LPS Regulated Genes Unravel Mechanistic and Functional Overlap of Priming-induced SI

To characterize the mechanism of priming-induced IFNα + LPS- and IFNγ + LPS-dependent SI in vascular cells as compared to immune cells, we compared genome-wide transcriptional responses of VSMC, MΦ, and DC in response to IFNα (8 h), IFNγ (8 h), or LPS (4 h) alone, or after combined treatment (IFNα 8 h + LPS 4 h; IFNγ 8 h + LPS 4 h) using RNA-seq. Consequently, 579 genes were commonly up-regulated in VSMC, MΦ, and DC after combined treatment with IFNα + LPS (**Figure 1A**). Likewise, 536 genes were commonly expressed after combined treatment with IFNγ +L PS (**Figure 1A**). The complete lists of up-regulated genes in response to IFNα, IFNγ, or LPS alone, or after combined treatments in each cell type are shown in **Table S1**. To validate the quality of our RNA-seq dataset, the expression of a number of these genes, including *Cxcl9, Cxcl10, Ccl5, Nos2, Gbp6* was additionally confirmed by RT-PCR (data not shown).

Heatmaps presenting the expression pattern of the commonly 579 IFNα + LPS and 536 IFNγ + LPS regulated genes in VSMC, illustrate the potential effect of SI after combined treatment with IFNα + LPS or IFNγ + LPS as compared to the single stimuli (**Figure 1B**). Increasing brightness of red color in the heatmap reflects increasing gene expression levels, which in general are visibly higher after combined treatment with IFNα + LPS and IFNγ + LPS in comparison to single stimuli. After comparing the overall range and distribution of the common gene expression after single or combined stimulation (**Figure 1C**), in VSMC the effect of SI was clearly visible in the presented box plot. The median gene expression after combined treatment with IFNα + LPS and IFNγ + LPS was higher in comparison to single treatments with IFNs or LPS (**Figure 1C**). **Tables 1A,B** offer insight in the top-30

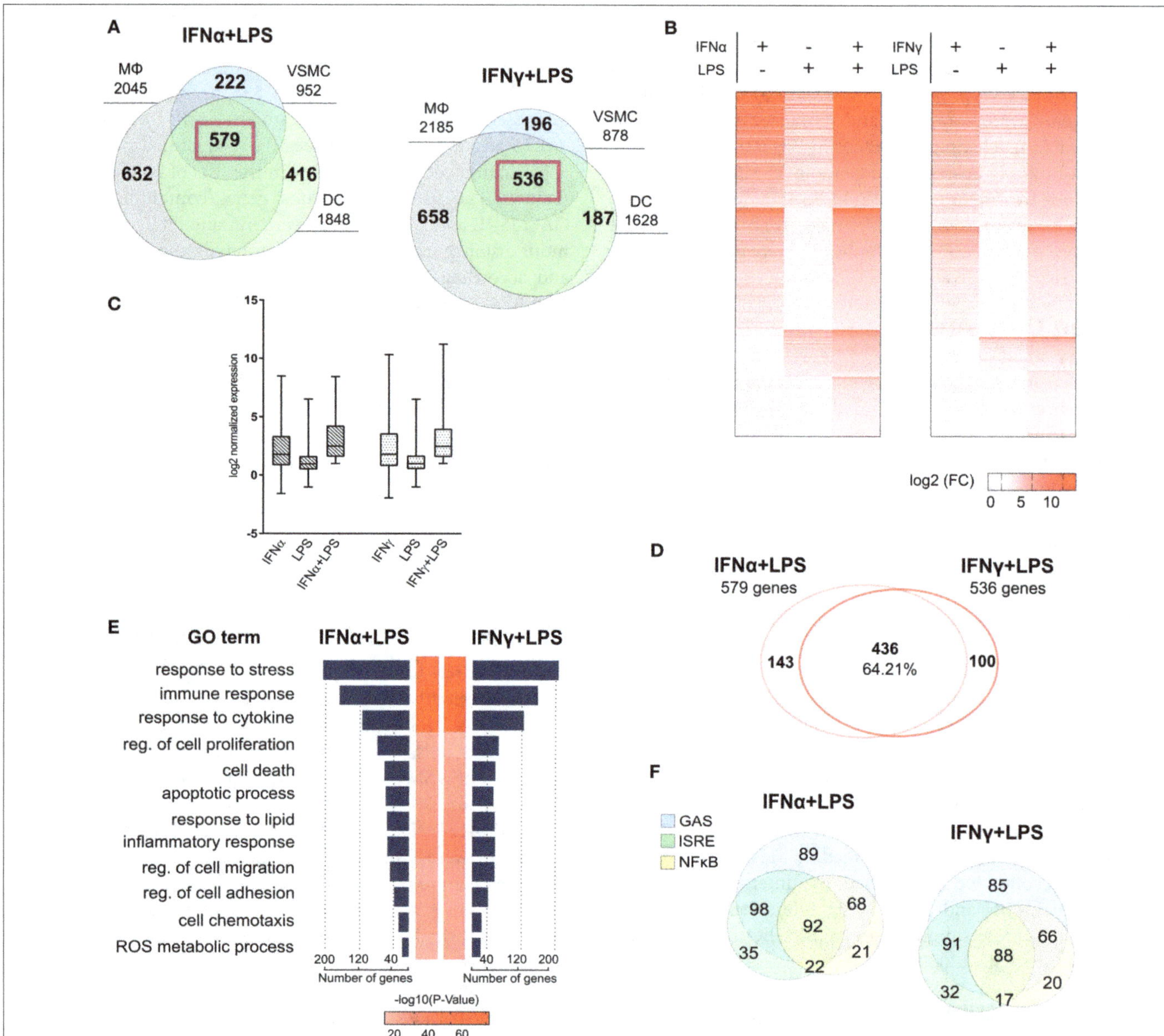

FIGURE 1 | Mechanistic and functional characteristics of common gene expression between VSMC and MΦ, DC in response to IFNα + LPS and IFNγ + LPS. **(A)** Venn diagrams based on RNA-seq results showing intersection between lists of up-regulated (FC > 2) genes in VSMC, MΦ, and DC after combined stimulation with IFNα (8 h) + LPS (4 h) and IFNγ (8 h) + LPS (4 h). The gene lists for these Venn diagrams are shown in **Table S1**. Common 579 IFNα + LPS and 536 IFNγ + LPS-induced genes between three cell types were highlighted by violet frames. **(B)** Heatmap plots depicting expression pattern of commonly up-regulated, 579 IFNα (8 h) +LPS (4 h)- and 536 IFNγ (8 h) + LPS (4 h)-induced genes in VSMC, resulting from RNA-seq. Three main columns on each heatmap represent one particular treatment condition [IFNα (8 h), IFNγ (8h), LPS (4 h), IFNα (8 h) + LPS (4 h), or IFNγ (8 h) + LPS (4 h)]. Increasing brightness of red color indicates a higher gene expression level (gene expression is presented as log2 FC in comparison to control). **(C)** Box-plot representation of gene expression distribution for commonly up-regulated genes by IFNα (8 h) + LPS (4 h) and IFNγ (8 h) + LPS (4 h) resulting from RNA-seq (gene expression is presented as log2 FC in comparison to control) in VSMC. The line within each box represents the median and the lower and upper boundaries of each box indicate first and third quartiles, respectively. **(D)** Comparison of commonly up-regulated genes by IFNα (8h) + LPS (4 h) and IFNγ (8 h) + LPS (4 h) from RNA-seq, showing 64.21% overlap between the gene lists. **(E)** GO analysis of commonly up-regulated genes by IFNα (8 h) + LPS (4 h) and IFNγ (8 h) + LPS (4 h) (RNA-seq) revealed a strong enrichment for terms reflecting pro-inflammatory and pro-atherogenic biological functions. *P*-value < 0.05. **(F)** Venn diagram distribution of promoter located (−950/+50 bp) GAS, ISRE, and NFκB binding sites among commonly up-regulated genes by IFNα (8 h) + LPS (4 h) and IFNγ (8 h) + LPS(4 h) from RNA-seq experiment.

of these commonly up-regulated genes and illustrate the way they respond to IFNα + LPS and IFNγ + LPS in VSMC as compared to the single stimuli. The genes affected by SI (reflected by increased gene expression after combined treatment with IFNα + LPS or IFNγ + LPS vs. the sum of the single treatments; see Materials and Methods) are marked with an

TABLE 1A | Representative top-30 genes commonly up-regulated (FC > 2) by IFNα + LPS in VSMC, MΦ, and DC, reflecting SI between IFNα and LPS in VSMC.

No.	IFNα + LPS induced common genes	VSMC			Binding site		
		IFNα	LPS	IFNα + LPS	GAS	ISRE	NFκB
1	F830016B08Rik*	196.8	6.4	345.9	•	•	–
2	Ifi44	356.3	4.4	343.7	–	•	–
3	Cxcl10*	75.9	4.6	312.1	•	•	•
4	BC023105*	187.1	19.9	289.2	–	–	–
5	Nos2*	4.9	90.9	287.1	•	•	•
6	Gm4955*	209.5	5.4	260.2	–	–	–
7	Gm15725	294.6	2.9	259.8	–	–	–
8	Iigp1*	179.7	9.2	242.3	•	•	–
9	Gm4951*	178.6	6.9	233.4	•	•	–
10	Gbp9*	78.8	22.9	215.9	–	•	•
11	Gbp11*	62.1	13.6	196.5	•	•	–
12	Apod	213.7	2.2	194.9	–	•	•
13	Gm4841*	99.8	9.0	181.4	•	•	–
14	Gbp4*	36.4	16.4	162.0	•	•	•
15	Gm14446	164.5	1.8	157.8	–	–	–
16	Mx1*	128.8	3.3	155.9	–	•	•
17	Ifit1*	113.3	11.1	153.6	–	•	–
18	Gm12250*	94.8	3.6	142.3	•	•	–
19	Gm4902*	126.5	3.8	139.3	–	–	–
20	Tnfsf10*	35.8	3.2	128.9	•	•	•
21	Usp18*	96.3	8.9	127.5	–	•	•
22	Gbp1*	91.7	17.5	125.5	–	•	–
23	Gbp6*	36.9	23.5	117.2	•	•	•
24	Gbp10*	35.6	21.1	115.2	–	•	•
25	Ch25h*	3.5	19.6	112.6	•	•	•
26	Tgtp2	114.2	2.6	110.7	•	•	–
27	Gm6904*	94.9	2.6	107.8	–	•	–
28	Zbp1*	95.5	5.8	106.3	•	•	•
29	Saa3*	5.1	66.6	105.7	•	–	•
30	Phf11*	100.2	3.2	105.7	–	–	–

*Gene expression levels were presented as FC relative to control in VSMCs. Signal Integrated genes (FC IFNα + LPS > FC IFNα + FC LPS) were marked by an asterisk (*). Overlapping genes between IFNα + LPS- and IFNγ + LPS-induced commonly up-regulated genes (**Table 1B**) were color-coded by blue. Presence of GAS, ISRE, or NFκB binding sites in the promoters of listed genes was indicated by a dot (•).*

asterisk (**Tables 1A,B**). Strikingly, significant overlap could be observed between commonly up-regulated genes in response to IFNα + LPS and IFNγ + LPS. Indeed, the Venn diagram in **Figure 1D** shows 64.21% overlap between the 579 IFNα +LPS and 536 IFNγ + LPS commonly up-regulated genes (**Figure 1D**). Moreover, GO analysis of these 579 IFNα + LPS and 536 IFNγ + LPS commonly up-regulated genes revealed significant enrichment in overlapping terms connected to stress, immune and inflammatory response, response to cytokine, regulation of cell proliferation and migration, regulation of cell adhesion and chemotaxis, cell death and apoptotic process, response to lipid, and reactive oxygen species (ROS) metabolic process, all reflecting pro-inflammatory and pro-atherogenic biological functions. This also confirms the existence of functional overlap between vascular and immune cells, mediated by the interaction of both IFNs with LPS, which results in the execution of cell type-common biological responses (**Figure 1E**).

On the same lists of IFNα + LPS and IFNγ + LPS commonly up-regulated genes we also performed *in silico* promoter analysis, for the presence of ISRE, STAT, or NFκB binding sites in the proximal promoter (−950 to +100 bp). The predicted representation of individual or combined GAS, ISRE, or NFκB binding sites is depicted in **Figure 1F**. Most of the genes contained either single GAS sites (89 IFNα + LPS genes and 85 IFNγ + LPS genes) or rather combinations of potential GAS-ISRE (98 IFNα + LPS genes and 91 IFNγ + LPS genes), GAS-NFκB (68 IFNα + LPS genes and 66 IFNγ + LPS genes), ISRE-NFκB (22 IFNα + LPS genes and 17 IFNγ+LPS genes), or GAS-ISRE-NFκB (92 IFNα + LPS genes and 88 IFNγ + LPS genes) binding sites. Together this suggested that a common SI

TABLE 1B | Representative top-30 genes commonly up-regulated (FC > 2) by IFNγ + LPS in VSMC, MΦ, and DC, reflecting SI between IFNγ and LPS in VSMC.

No.	IFNγ + LPS induced common genes	VSMC			Binding site		
		IFNγ	LPS	IFNγ + LPS	GAS	ISRE	NFκB
1	Cxcl9*	82.2	4.0	2380.5	•	–	•
2	F830016B08Rik*	1272.1	6.4	2306.6	•	•	•
3	Gm4841*	1087.3	9.0	1650.3	•	•	•
4	Nos2*	1.8	90.9	933.3	•	•	•
5	BC023105*	600.8	19.9	909.4	–	–	–
6	Gbp4*	304.3	16.4	795.8	•	•	•
7	Iigp1*	687.7	9.2	779.3	•	•	–
8	Ubd*	95.6	5.8	655.1	•	•	•
9	Gbp10*	315.9	21.1	588.2	•	•	•
10	Gbp9*	304.8	22.9	586.1	–	•	•
11	Gbp6*	266.1	23.5	555.3	•	•	•
12	Serpina3f*	200.1	13.0	529.6	•	•	•
13	Gbp11*	302.3	13.6	482.7	•	•	–
14	Gm12250	502.9	3.6	477.8	•	•	–
15	Gbp8*	215.5	12.9	405.2	•	•	•
16	Ciita	704.4	2.0	376.5	•	•	•
17	Cxcl10*	49.8	4.6	364.9	•	•	•
18	Gbp1*	295.0	17.5	364.8	–	•	–
19	Gja4*	82.3	1.6	329.9	•	•	•
20	Gm4951*	300.1	6.9	327.2	•	–	–
21	Batf2*	191.4	3.1	298.4	•	•	–
22	Lcn2*	3.8	36.5	289.2	–	–	•
23	Gbp2*	219.7	13.4	284.4	–	•	•
24	Igtp	328.8	5.3	274.1	•	•	–
25	Tgtp2	261.9	2.6	262.5	•	•	–
26	Gm5970*	183.1	2.3	236.1	–	–	–
27	Ccl8*	115.8	18.6	231.4	•	•	•
28	Tgtp1*	216.7	2.4	222.4	•	•	•
29	Gbp5*	67.7	9.2	211.5	•	•	•
30	Saa3*	4.2	66.6	196.1	•	–	•

*Gene expression levels were presented as FC relative to control in VSMCs. Signal Integrated genes (FC IFNγ + LPS > FC IFNγ + FC LPS) were marked by an asterisk (*). Overlapping genes between IFNγ + LPS- and IFNα + LPS-induced commonly up-regulated genes (**Table 1A**) were color-coded by blue. Presence of GAS, ISRE, or NFκB binding sites in the promoters of listed genes was indicated by a dot (•).*

mechanism is involved in the interaction between IFNα and LPS or IFNγ and LPS in VSMC, in analogy to MΦ and DC.

Genome-wide Binding of STAT1 and p65 to IFNα + LPS and IFNγ + LPS Regulated Genes Is Mediated Through Comparable Single and Co-binding Modes

To obtain further insight in the mechanism of priming-induced SI between IFNs and LPS in VSMC, we characterized the genome-wide binding of STAT1 and NFκB (p65) to the regulatory regions of IFNα + LPS and IFNγ + LPS commonly up-regulated genes. Thus, we performed ChIP-seq on chromatin from VSMC exposed to IFNα (8 h), IFNγ (8 h), or LPS (4 h) alone, or combined treatment (IFNα 8 h + LPS 4 h; IFNγ 8 h + LPS 4 h).

Clustering analysis of the genomic regions occupied by STAT1 and/or p65 in response to single or combined treatments (**Figure 2A**) are visualized as tag counts (blue signals) in the RD plot. This analysis revealed that a subset of STAT1 and p65 binding regions (i.e., Cluster 7) were clearly co-occupied by these transcription factors when combined treatments (IFNα + LPS or IFNγ + LPS) were used, reflected by increased blue color intensity on the graph (**Figure 2A**). However, other genomic regions correlated with binding of STAT1 or p65 alone [i.e., Cluster C1, C9 (p65 only), Cluster C2 and C8 (STAT1 only)]. Subsequently, using HOMER software, GAS, ISRE, and NFκB consensus motifs (**Figures S1A–C**) were re-mapped to STAT1 and p65 binding regions and compared to the lists of 579 IFNα + LPS and 536 IFNγ + LPS commonly up-regulated genes (**Figure 2B**). Genomic binding analysis indicated that the STAT1 (GAS or ISRE) and p65 (NFκB) binding sites were primarily located in distant intergenic regions and intronic regions, while to a lesser extent in promoters, of IFNα + LPS- and IFNγ + LPS-responsive genes (**Figure 2B**). A similar

A
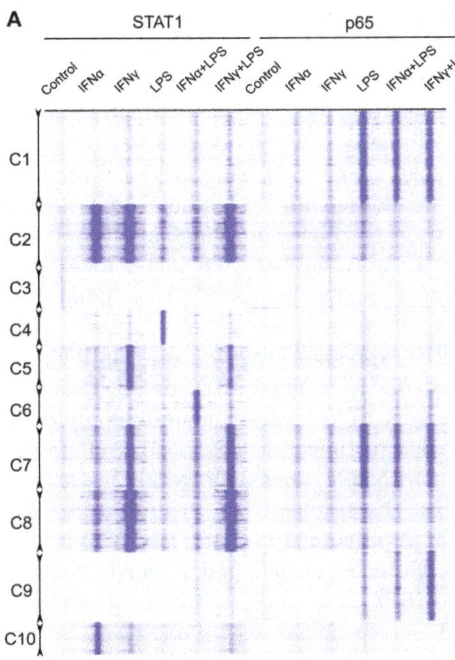

B
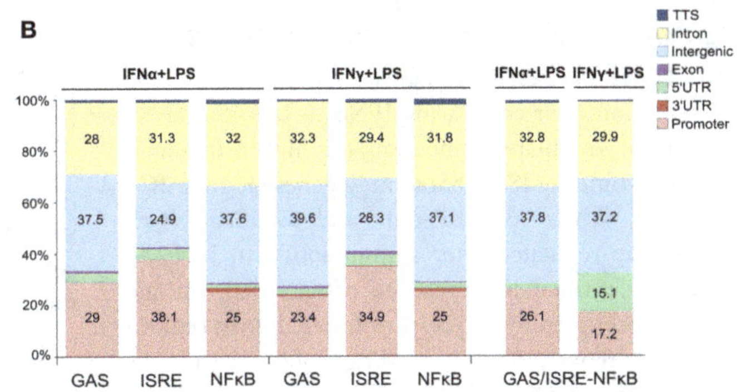

C

Binding mode	IFNα+LPS	IFNγ+LPS	Overlap [%]
GAS	6	17	13,0
ISRE	81	45	29,4
NFκB	85	28	15,9
GAS-ISRE	51	53	32,7
GAS-NFκB	23	40	11,1
ISRE-NFκB	94	59	21,6
GAS-ISRE-NFκB	99	178	29,6

FIGURE 2 | Genome-wide role of STAT1 and p65 in transcriptional regulation of commonly up-regulated IFNα + LPS- and IFNγ + LPS-induced genes. **(A)** RD heatmaps for ChIP-seq peaks clustered (*k*-means clustering) based on STAT1 and p65 binding pattern across control, IFNα (8 h), IFNγ (8 h), LPS (4 h), IFNα (8 h) + LPS (4 h), IFNγ (8 h) + LPS (4 h) treatment conditions in VSMC. Identified clusters are marked as Cluster (C) 1–10. **(B)** Global distribution of STAT1 (GAS and ISRE) and p65 (NFκB) occupied binding sites (from ChIP-seq) in 7 genomic locations (color-coded with the mapping provided in the legend): promoter/TSS (−1 kb to +100 bp), introns, intergenic, exon, 5′ UTR, 3′ UTR, and TTS. Re-mapped motifs distribution was plotted by the percentage of total number of occupied GAS, ISRE, and NFκB binding sites present in the regulatory regions of commonly up-regulated IFNα (8 h) + LPS (4 h)- and IFNγ (8 h) + LPS (4 h)-induced genes. **(C)** Representation of STAT1 and p65 occupied binding sites identified by ChIP-seq, representing "single" modes (STAT1 binding to GAS and/or ISRE; p65 binding to NFκB) or "co-binding" modes (STAT1 binding to GAS and/or ISRE together with p65 to NFκB). Table depict number of the genes within each STAT1/p65 binding mode among IFNα (8 h) + LPS (4 h)- and IFNγ (8 h) + LPS (4 h)-induced genes together with percentage overlap between the two treatment conditions.

distribution could be observed for the location of STAT1-NFκB co-binding sites (**Figure 2B**), which is in agreement with the above presented promoter analysis (**Figure 1F**), and predict the presence of multiple STAT1 and NFκB binding sites in the promoters of the IFNα + LPS and IFNγ + LPS commonly up-regulated genes.

By next comparing genome-wide binding results for STAT1 and p65 after VSMC stimulation with IFNα + LPS and IFNγ + LPS, we could identify different groups of genes, where STAT1 bound to consensus ISRE and/or GAS sites and p65 to NFκB sites. These binding sites were present in gene regulatory regions and existed in different combinations. As such we could distinguish genes which contained solitary ISRE, GAS, or NFκB sites, but also GAS-ISRE, ISRE-NFκB, GAS-NFκB, or GAS-ISRE-NFκB sites. Based on these gene groups we further defined STAT1 and p65 binding modes, including "single" (STAT1 binding to GAS and/or ISRE; p65 to NFκB) or "co-binding" (STAT1 binding to GAS and/or ISRE + p65 to NFκB) (**Figure 2C**). Among IFNα + LPS-induced genes, 6 GAS-only, 81 ISRE-only, 85 NFκB-only, and 51 GAS-ISRE containing genes, were identified. In case of IFNγ + LPS stimulation, we could distinguish 17 GAS-only, 45 ISRE-only, 28 NFκB-only, and 53 GAS-ISRE containing genes. Together they reflect the "single" binding mode. In addition, IFNα + LPS- and IFNγ + LPS-induced genes also included STAT1-p65 "co-binding" genes, which could be divided in GAS-NFκB: 23 and 40 genes, ISRE-NFκB: 94 and 59 genes and GAS-ISRE-NFκB genes: 99 and 178 genes, respectively.

Comparison of the different binding modes between IFNα + LPS- and IFNγ + LPS-induced conditions, identified a substantial overlap for NFκB-only (15.9%), GAS-only (13%), and ISRE-only (29.4%) containing genes from the "single" mode (**Figure 2C**). As reported previously, both IFN-I and IFN-II direct GAF complexes to GAS motifs, what is reflected by 13% overlap between the two conditions within GAS-only mode in our study. Yet 29.4% overlap found between IFNα- and IFNγ-activated genes within ISRE-only mode was very surprising, since limited evidence exists for a role of ISGF3 in IFN-II-driven gene expression. Likewise, this overlap could be observed for GAS-ISRE (32.7%), GAS-NFκB (11.1%), ISRE-NFκB (21.6%), and GAS-ISRE-NFκB genes (29.6%) from the "co-binding" mode (**Figure 2C**).

Collectively, this suggests that a common genome-wide SI mechanism exists, which involves combinatorial actions of ISGF3 or GAF with NFκB on ISRE/NFκB or GAS/NFκB binding sites, in the interaction of IFNα and LPS or IFNγ and LPS in VSMC.

STAT1 as Part of ISGF3 Regulates Transcription of ISRE-containing Genes in Response to IFN-I and IFN-II

A striking observation after comparing IFNα + LPS and IFNγ + LPS commonly up-regulated genes was the high number of overlapping STAT1-binding ISRE-containing genes (**Figure 2C**). Close examination of the 45 ISRE-only and 59 ISRE-NFκB containing genes, up-regulated after stimulation with IFNγ + LPS (**Figure 2C**), identified the presence of an ISRE, but no GAS binding site, occupied by STAT1 in the regulatory regions of these genes. Moreover, STAT1 binding could already be observed after treatment of VSMC with IFNγ alone (data not shown), correlating with their transcriptional activity. Among these genes were classical ISRE-containing genes, from which we selected *Ifit1, Mx2, Oas2, Cxcl10,* and *Irf7* (**Figure 3A**) to further characterize the nature of this STAT1-dependent mechanism in several experiments. All 5 genes were highly responsive to IFNα and to a lesser extent to IFNγ, with *Ifit1, Mx2,* and *Cxcl10* being effected by SI after combined treatment with IFNα + LPS and IFNγ + LPS (**Figure 3A**). This correlated with the slight increase in STAT1 and STAT2 phosphorylation in response to both stimuli as compared to the individual ones (**Figure 3B**). *Ifit1, Mx2, Oas2,* and *Irf7* are examples of ISRE-only genes, which is in agreement with a single STAT1-binding peak (**Figure 3D**). In case of *Cxcl10* two STAT1-binding peaks were previously identified by Rauch et al., distal and proximal, corresponding to a known ISRE-GAS composite site and a single ISRE motif, respectively (9). Therefore, in this part of our study, the single ISRE site present in the proximal region of the *Cxcl10* promoter was chosen to further validate IFN-dependent STAT1 recruitment (**Figure 3D**). IGV genome browser views exhibited binding of STAT1 to ISRE-containing regions of all of these genes in VSMC, treated with IFNα, IFNγ, LPS, IFNα + LPS, and IFNγ + LPS (**Figure 3D**). STAT1 ChIP-seq results were further verified by quantitative ChIP-PCR, which demonstrated a significant enrichment of tSTAT1 recruitment to ISRE motifs present in the promoters of *Ifit1, Mx2, Oas2, Cxcl10,* and *Irf7* after stimulation with both IFNα and IFNγ (**Figure 3E**). This coincided with the binding of pSTAT1, which was significantly higher after IFNγ treatment than after IFNα treatment and reflected STAT1 phosphorylation levels under these conditions (**Figure 3E**). Similarly, we examined the potential binding of pSTAT2, tSTAT2, and IRF9 under these conditions (**Figures 3F,G**, respectively). It demonstrated increased recruitment of pSTAT2 to the ISRE-containing promoters of *Ifit1, Mx2, Oas2, Cxcl10,* and *Irf7* genes, after stimulation with IFNα and surprisingly with IFNγ (**Figure 3F**). Like pSTAT1, the level of pSTAT2 enrichment was in line with the STAT2 phosphorylation levels, which unexpectedly could also be detected after IFNγ and IFNγ + LPS treatment (**Figure 3B**). The binding of IRF9 showed a similar pattern as that of pSTAT2 and corresponded to IRF9 expression levels present in IFNα, IFNγ, and/or LPS treated cells (**Figure 3B**). The simultaneous recruitment of pSTAT1, pSTAT2, and IRF9 after IFNα and IFNγ treatment, clearly correlated with the involvement of ISGF3 in the transcriptional regulation of these ISRE-containing genes in response to both types of IFN. Indeed, co-IP of IRF9 with STAT1 and STAT2 in IFNα and IFNγ-treated VSMC corroborated this observation (**Figure 3C**). The expression pattern of these genes closely mirrored the binding pattern of pSTAT2 and IRF9, being higher after IFNα treatment in comparison to IFNγ treatment. Interestingly, the binding of STAT1 displayed an opposite pattern (higher after IFNγ treatment than after IFNα). This suggested the participation of STAT1 in an additional ISRE-binding complex in IFNγ-treated cells. Based on the high phosphorylation levels of STAT1 and the increased expression of IRF9 under these conditions, this complex could possibly consist of STAT1 homodimers together with IRF9 (39).

Since IRF1 expression levels increased in IFNα, IFNγ, and/or LPS treated VSMC (**Figure 3B**), we also tested the possible involvement of a STAT1-IRF1 containing complex. Interestingly, IRF1 was also recruited to these ISRE-containing genes after stimulation with IFNγ, but only weakly upon IFNα treatment (**Figure 3H**). The strongest IRF1 recruitment was noticed for *Ifit1* and *Mx2*, in comparison to *Oas2, Cxcl10,* and *Irf7* gene promoters. However, no interaction could be detected between STAT1 and IRF1 under these conditions (**Figure 3C**), pointing to a STAT1-independent role of IRF1 in the transcriptional regulation of a selective group of ISRE-containing genes.

Our results are in agreement with the existence of a more general mechanism in mouse primary VSMC, in which the IFNα response of ISRE-containing genes is mainly driven by ISGF3. In contrast, their IFNγ response is mediated by ISGF3 and potentially by STAT1/IRF9.

Recruitment of STAT1 and p65 in Response to IFNα + LPS or IFNγ + LPS Is Restricted to GAS/NFκB or ISRE/NFκB Composite Sites

Subsequently, we concentrated on the overlap of STAT1-p65 "co-binding" modes between IFNα + LPS- and IFNγ + LPS-induced conditions. Interestingly, genome-wide these co-binding sites occurred at a similar distance of not more than ~200 bp (**Figure 4A**). First, we determined how many of the genes which were assigned either to GAS-NFκB, ISRE-NFκB, or GAS-ISRE-NFκB modes (**Figure 2C**) were affected by SI under these conditions. We identified 170 of such genes up-regulated by IFNα + LPS and 211 by IFNγ + LPS, of which 106 were in common (**Figure 4B**). From this list of genes, we selected several examples representing the three STAT1-p65 "co-binding" modes: *Serpina3i, Steap4, Irf1* (GAS-NFκB mode), *Ccl5, Ifit1, Gbp6* (ISRE-NFκB mode), *Cxcl10, Gbp7* (GAS-ISRE-NFκB mode). The RNA-seq FC values, representing gene expression changes upon treatment with IFNα, IFNγ, LPS, and IFNα + LPS, IFNγ + LPS, are presented in **Figure 4C**. Indeed, all of these genes were responsive to at least two single stimuli and affected by SI, reflected by increased gene expression after combined treatment with IFNα + LPS or IFNγ + LPS in comparison to the sum of the single treatments (**Figure 4C**).

STAT1 and p65 ChIP-seq IGV genome browser views of these pre-selected genes in response to IFNα + LPS and IFNγ + LPS, encompass the different STAT1-p65 "co-binding" modes

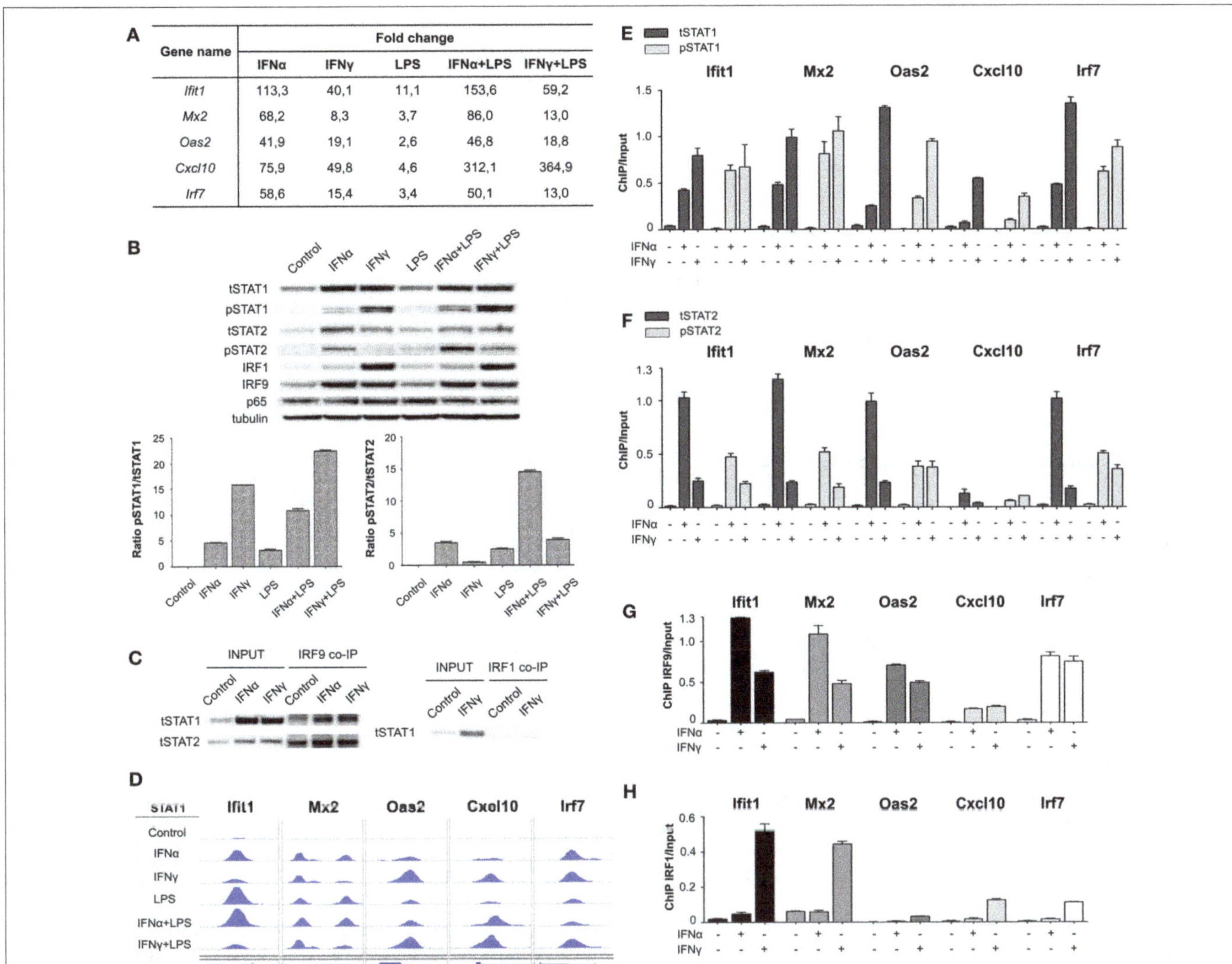

Gene name	Fold change				
	IFNα	IFNγ	LPS	IFNα+LPS	IFNγ+LPS
Ifit1	113,3	40,1	11,1	153,6	59,2
Mx2	68,2	8,3	3,7	86,0	13,0
Oas2	41,9	19,1	2,6	46,8	18,8
Cxcl10	75,9	49,8	4,6	312,1	364,9
Irf7	58,6	15,4	3,4	50,1	13,0

FIGURE 3 | STAT1, STAT2, IRF9, and IRF1 in transcriptional regulation of ISRE-containing genes under stimulation with IFN-I and IFN-II. **(A)** Gene expression values (FC in comparison to control) for *Ifit1*, *Mx2*, *Oas2*, *Cxcl10,* and *Irf7* genes, resulting from RNA-seq: VSMC untreated or treated with IFNα (8 h), IFNγ (8 h), LPS (4 h), IFNα (8 h) + LPS (4 h), IFNγ (8 h) + LPS (4 h). **(B)** Western blot. Protein extracts were isolated from VSMC untreated or treated with IFNα (8 h), IFNγ (8 h), LPS (4 h), IFNα (8 h) + LPS (4 h), IFNγ (8 h) + LPS (4 h). Levels of tSTAT1, pSTAT1, tSTAT2, pSTAT2, IRF1, IRF9, p65, and tubulin were assessed by Western blot. $n = 3$, one representative blot is presented; Western blot quantification. Bars represent mean quantification of pSTAT1/tSTAT1 and pSTAT2/tSTAT2 ratio (normalized to tubulin). Mean ± s.e.m., $n = 3$; **(C)** Co-IP. Protein extracts were isolated from VSMC untreated or treated with IFNα (8 h) and IFNγ (8 h), immunoprecipitated with IRF9 or IRF1 antibodies and analyzed by tSTAT1 and/or tSTAT2 Western blot. $n = 3$, one representative blot is presented. **(D)** Representative views of STAT1 ChIP-seq peaks detected in the ISRE-containing promoters of *Ifit1*, *Mx2*, *Oas2*, *Cxcl10,* and *Irf7* genes, in untreated or IFNα (8 h), IFNγ (8 h), LPS (4 h), IFNα (8 h) + LPS (4 h), IFNγ (8 h) + LPS (4 h)-stimulated VSMC. STAT1 peaks were mapped onto the mouse reference genome mm10 and visualized using the IGV genome browser. **(E)** VSMC were untreated or treated with IFNα (8 h) and IFNγ (8 h) and ChIP-PCR validation of tSTAT1 and pSTAT1 binding to ISRE motif present in the promoters at *Ifit1*, *Mx2*, *Oas2*, *Cxcl10,* and *Irf7* genes was performed. Mean ± s.e.m., $n = 2$. Primers are listed in **Table S2**. ChIP-PCR. VSMC were untreated or treated with IFNα (8 h) and IFNγ (8 h), chromatin was isolated and immunoprecipitated with **(F)** tSTAT2, pSTAT2, **(G)** IRF9 and **(H)** IRF1 antibodies, followed by ChIP-PCR analysis. Mean ± s.e.m., $n = 2$. Primers are listed in **Table S2**.

(**Figure 4D**). IGV tracks reveal the binding pattern of STAT1 and p65 to the promoters of *Serpina3i, Steap4, Irf1* (GAS-NFκB sites), *Ccl5, Ifit1, Gbp6* (ISRE-NFκB sites), *Cxcl10, Gbp7* (GAS-ISRE-NFκB sites) genes, after stimulation with IFNα, IFNγ, LPS, and combined treatments with IFNα + LPS or IFNγ + LPS (**Figure 4D**). In case of *Cxcl10* two STAT1-p65 co-binding peaks could be observed (**Figure 4D**), distal and proximal, corresponding to a known GAS-ISRE-NFκB composite site and a combined ISRE-NFκB motif (9, 40). In this second part of our study, the GAS-ISRE-NFκB composite site present in the distal region of the *Cxcl10* promoter was chosen to further validate IFN-dependent STAT1 and p65 recruitment.

In conclusion, for the majority of these genes STAT1 and p65 binding peaks were closely aligned in the co-bound gene promoters, what further correlated with the close proximity of GAS and NFκB or ISRE and NFκB binding sites. This close

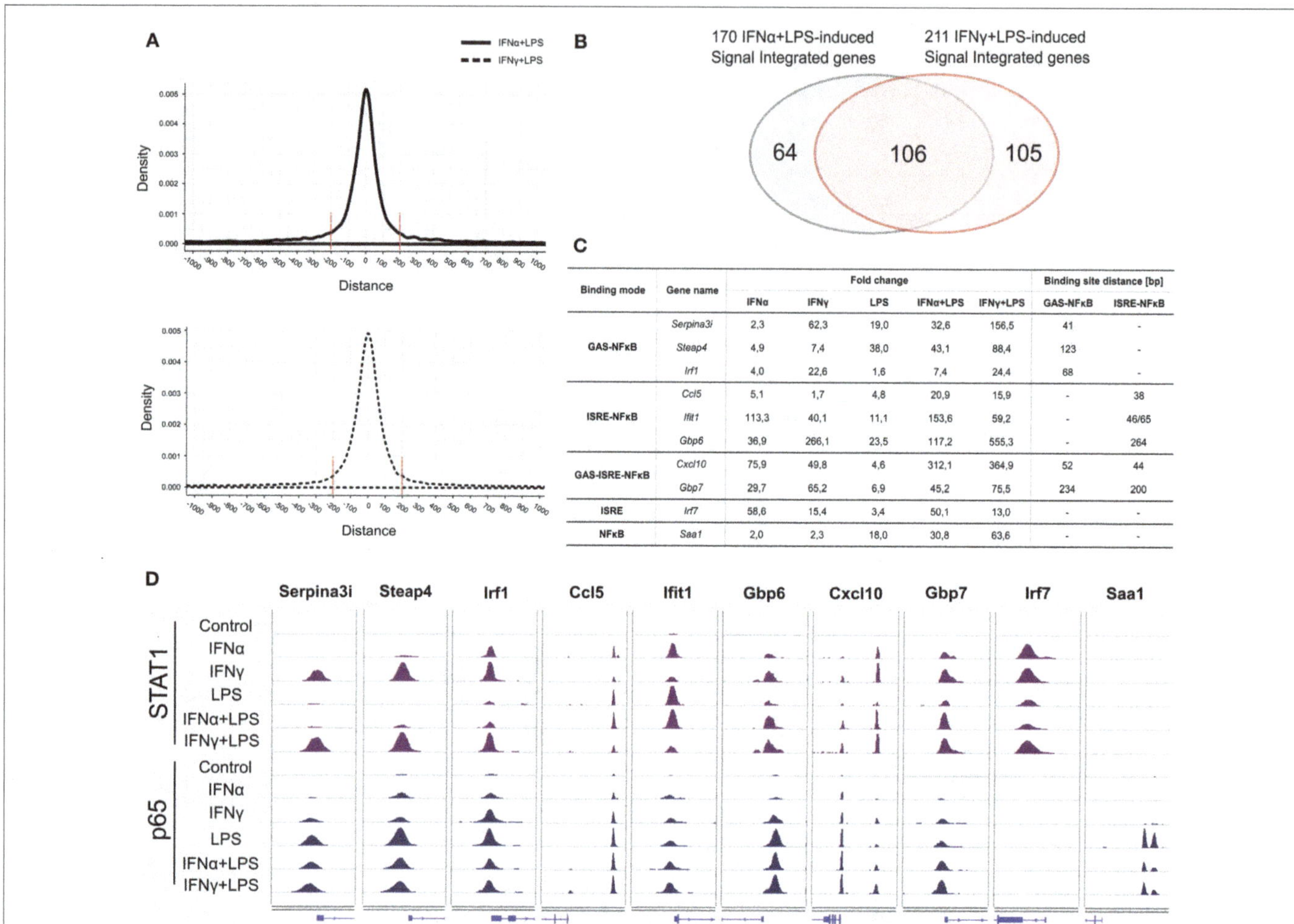

Binding mode	Gene name	Fold change					Binding site distance [bp]	
		IFNα	IFNγ	LPS	IFNα+LPS	IFNγ+LPS	GAS-NFκB	ISRE-NFκB
GAS-NFκB	*Serpina3i*	2,3	62,3	19,0	32,6	156,5	41	-
	Steap4	4,9	7,4	38,0	43,1	88,4	123	-
	Irf1	4,0	22,6	1,6	7,4	24,4	68	-
ISRE-NFκB	*Ccl5*	5,1	1,7	4,8	20,9	15,9	-	38
	Ifit1	113,3	40,1	11,1	153,6	59,2	-	46/65
	Gbp6	36,9	266,1	23,5	117,2	555,3	-	264
GAS-ISRE-NFκB	*Cxcl10*	75,9	49,8	4,6	312,1	364,9	52	44
	Gbp7	29,7	65,2	6,9	45,2	75,5	234	200
ISRE	*Irf7*	58,6	15,4	3,4	50,1	13,0	-	-
NFκB	*Saa1*	2,0	2,3	18,0	30,8	63,6	-	-

FIGURE 4 | Representatives of STAT1 and p65 "single" and "co-binding" modes. **(A)** Peak distribution plots showing distances between summits of STAT1 and the closest p65 peak summits resulted from ChIP-seq in VSMC under IFNα (8 h) + LPS (4 h) and IFNγ (8 h) + LPS (4 h) treatment conditions. **(B)** Venn diagram showing the intersection of 170 IFNα (8 h) + LPS (4 h)- and 211 IFNγ (8 h) + LPS (4 h)-activated SI genes resulting from RNA-seq. **(C)** Table presents gene expression values (FC in comparison to control), resulting from RNA-seq experiment: VSMC treated with IFNα (8 h), IFNγ (8 h), LPS (4 h), IFNα (8 h) + LPS (4 h), IFNγ (8 h) + LPS (4 h) and GAS-NFκB and ISRE-NFκB binding sites distance (bp) for selected genes representing identified STAT1 and p65 'co-binding' modes: GAS-NFκB: *Serpina3i*, *Steap4*, *Irf1*; ISRE-NFκB: *Ccl5*, *Ifit1*, *Gbp6*; GAS-ISRE-NFκB: *Cxcl10* and *Gbp7*; ISRE: *Irf7*; NFκB: *Saa1*. **(D)** Representative views of STAT1 and p65 ChIP-seq peaks (STAT1: violet peaks, p65: dark blue peaks) identified in the regulatory regions of *Serpina3i*, *Steap4*, *Irf1*, *Ccl5*, *Ifit1*, *Gbp6*, *Cxcl10*, *Gbp7*, *Irf7,* and *Saa1* genes, in untreated or IFNα (8 h), IFNγ (8 h), LPS (4 h), IFNα (8 h) + LPS (4 h), IFNγ (8 h) + LPS (4 h)-stimulated VSMC. STAT1- and p65-binding peaks were mapped onto the mouse reference genome mm10 and visualized using the IGV genome browser.

binding sites distribution may be a pre-requisite for effective STAT1 and p65 collaboration.

STAT1 Recruitment to GAS/NFκB or ISRE/NFκB Composite Sites Precedes p65 and Correlates With Elevated Transcription of IFNα + LPS and IFNγ + LPS Regulated Genes in VSMC

Validation experiments for STAT1 and p65 by quantitative ChIP-PCR, using freshly isolated material (**Figures 5A,B**) confirmed the binding pattern of both STAT1 and p65 as presented in **Figure 4D**. It also supported the following conclusions. First, for all genes, STAT1 and p65 binding peaks were closely aligned in the promoters. This correlated with the close proximity of GAS and NFκB or ISRE and NFκB binding sites (~200 bp; **Figure 4C**), which may be a pre-requisite for effective STAT1 and p65 collaboration. Moreover, **Tables 1A,B** confirm the presence of GAS, ISRE, and NFκB binding sites [indicated by a dot (•)] in the promoters of 30 of the highest commonly up-regulated genes by IFNγ + LPS and IFNα + LPS in VSMC. This additionally emphasizes the observation that the availability of multiple binding sites for these transcription factors within the gene promoters may play a role in coordination of immediate and robust gene transcriptional activation.

Second, although stimulation with both IFN-I and IFN-II resulted in elevated levels of total STAT1 protein, but not for total p65 (**Figure 3B**), for the majority of the genes the potency

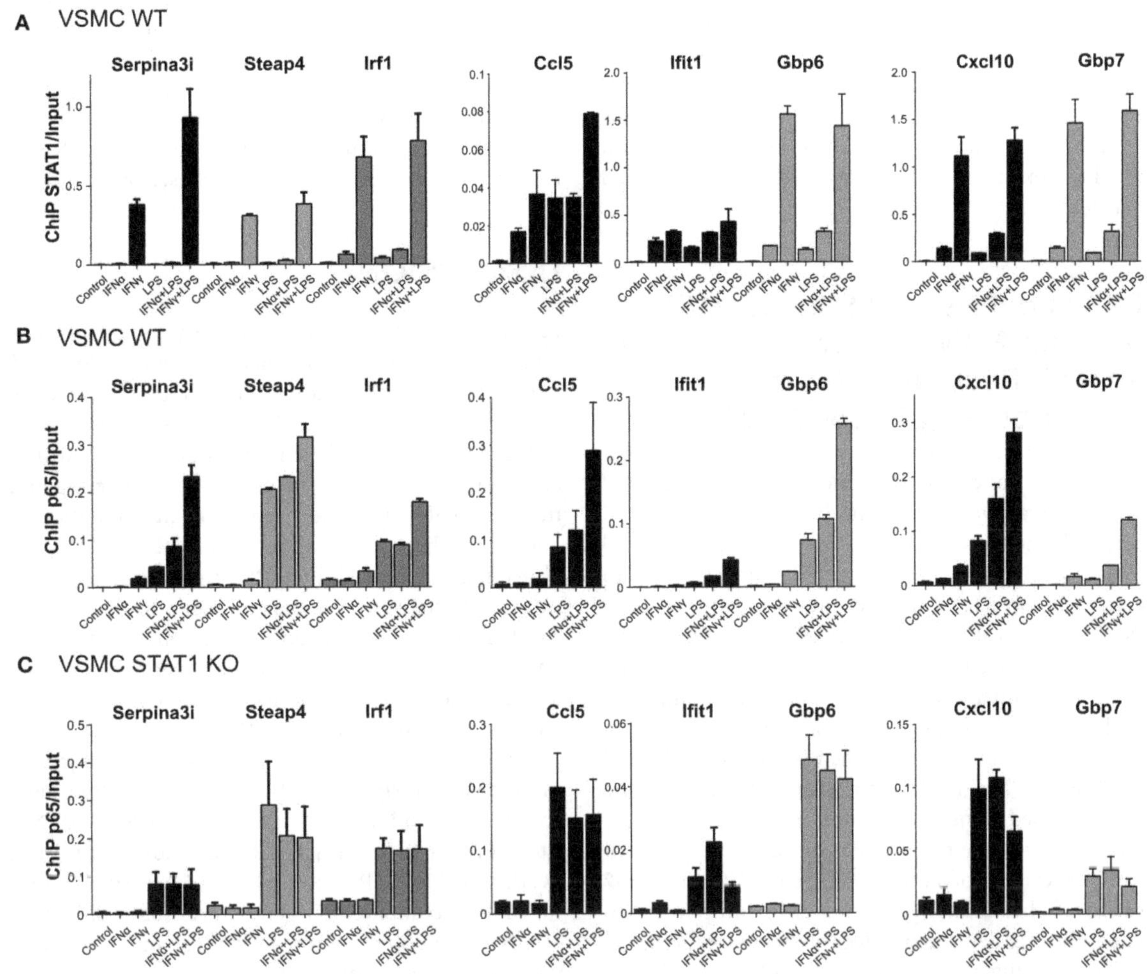

FIGURE 5 | STAT1 modulates increased p65 recruitment to GAS/NFκB or ISRE/NFκB composite sites. **(A)** ChIP-PCR of STAT1 at *Serpina3i*, *Steap4*, *Irf1*, *Ccl5*, *Ifit1*, *Gbp6*, *Cxcl10*, and *Gbp7* gene promoters (primers are listed in **Table S2**) in VSMC WT treated with IFNα (8 h), IFNγ (8 h), LPS (4 h), IFNα (8 h) + LPS (4 h), IFNγ (8 h) + LPS (4 h). Mean ± s.e.m., $n = 2$. **(B)** ChIP-PCR of p65 at *Serpina3i*, *Steap4*, *Irf1*, *Ccl5*, *Ifit1*, *Gbp6*, *Cxcl10*, and *Gbp7* gene promoters in VSMC WT treated with IFNα (8 h), IFNγ (8 h), LPS (4 h), IFNα (8 h) + LPS (4 h), IFNγ (8 h) + LPS (4 h). Mean ± s.e.m., $n = 2$. **(C)** ChIP-PCR of p65 at *Serpina3i*, *Steap4*, *Irf1*, *Ccl5*, *Ifit1*, *Gbp6*, *Cxcl10*, and *Gbp7* gene promoters in VSMC STAT1 KO treated with IFNα (8 h), IFNγ (8 h), LPS (4 h), IFNα (8 h) + LPS (4 h), IFNγ (8 h) + LPS (4 h). Mean ± s.e.m., $n = 2$.

of STAT1 recruitment correlated with that of p65 binding. Interestingly, this was not restricted to IFNα + LPS and IFNγ + LPS treatments, but also clearly visible after single treatments with IFNα or IFNγ. In general, STAT1 and p65 binding after IFNγ and IFNγ + LPS was stronger than after IFNα and IFNα + LPS (**Figures 5A,B**). Third, increased p65 binding after single treatments with IFNα or IFNγ could only be detected at GAS/NFκB or ISRE/NFκB composite sites (**Figure 4D**), but not at genes with solitary NFκB binding sequences (exemplified by *Saa1*; **Figure 4D**).

Fourth, for all STAT1-p65 co-bound gene promoters except *Gbp6*, we observed a moderate increase in the recruitment of STAT1 after combined treatment with IFNγ + LPS in comparison to IFNγ alone. Likewise, combined treatment with IFNα + LPS resulted in slightly increased STAT1 binding in comparison to IFNα single treatment (**Figure 5A**). Notably, binding of STAT1 after IFNα treatment was significantly weaker in comparison to IFNγ-induced STAT1 recruitment, likewise to increased STAT1 recruitment after combined treatment. This observation correlated with FC expression values of examined STAT1-p65 "co-bound" genes (**Figure 4C**), which in general were more responsive to IFNγ + LPS than to IFNα + LPS. The same was true for p65, which recruitment, similar to STAT1 was increased after IFNα + LPS or IFNγ + LPS treatment in comparison to single LPS stimulation yet to a much higher extent (**Figure 5B**). In contrast, ChIP-PCR for p65 on chromatin isolated from untreated, IFNα, IFNγ, LPS, IFNα + LPS, IFNγ + LPS-treated STAT1 KO VSMC, for all genes resulted in abrogated recruitment of p65 after single treatments with IFNα or IFNγ (**Figure 5C**). Moreover, p65 binding remained unaltered after combined treatments with IFNα + LPS or IFNγ + LPS in comparison to LPS alone (**Figure 5C**).

Together, these observations could point to a STAT1-dependent role in the nearby recruitment of p65 upon single IFNα or IFNγ treatment, via closely located GAS and NFκB or ISRE and NFκB binding sites in the promoters of SI genes. More important, this STAT1-p65 co-binding was significantly increased upon subsequent LPS exposure and resulted in amplified transcriptional activity.

IFNα + LPS and IFNγ + LPS Induced SI Correlates With Active Histone Marks and Increased PolII Recruitment in a STAT1-p65 Co-binding Dependent Manner

To understand in more detail the epigenetic changes that coincide with STAT1 and p65 co-binding we investigated the establishment of active histone marks at the *Cxcl10* and *Gbp7* "co-binding" mode promoters. We observed increased enrichment of H3K27Ac at these promoters in response to IFNα, IFNγ, and LPS, which was further increased after IFNα + LPS and IFNγ + LPS treatment (**Figure 6A**). As expected, the binding pattern of the negative H3K27me3 mark was opposite to that of H3K27Ac under the different treatment conditions (**Figure 6A**). This could indicate that these genes harbor a permissive chromatin conformation, which is positively affected by IFNα + LPS and IFNγ + LPS stimulation. To address the mechanism of increased transcription after STAT1 and p65 co-binding we also analyzed the recruitment of PolII. As shown in **Figure 6A**, the association of PolII with the *Cxcl10* and *Gbp7* promoters mirrored that of the H3K27Ac mark and pointed to a STAT1-p65 co-binding dependent effect on histone acetylation and transcriptional activity upon IFNα + LPS and IFNγ + LPS treatment.

To further prove this, we analyzed the enrichment pattern of these two histone marks and PolII at the promoters of the "single" binding mode genes *Irf7* (STAT1 only) and *Saa1* (NFκB only) (**Figures 4D**, **6B**). Indeed, H3K27Ac and PolII binding to the *Irf7* promoter showed an increase after IFNα, IFNγ, and LPS treatment. The opposite was true for H3K27me3 binding (**Figure 6C**), whereas the binding patterns for H3K27Ac, H3K27me3 and PolII did not significantly change after IFNα + LPS or IFNγ + LPS induction (**Figure 6C**). This was in line with STAT1 only binding, and no NFκB (**Figures 4D**, **6B**), and the lack of SI on transcriptional activity (**Figure 4C**). For the *Saa1* promoter H3K27Ac association was not affected by IFNα or IFNγ treatment, but increased to a similar extent after LPS, IFNα + LPS, and IFNγ + LPS stimulation (**Figure 6C**). This coincided with NFκB only binding, and no STAT1 (**Figures 4D**, **6B**). A similar, but only marginal LPS-mediated effect on abrogated H3K27me3 binding could be observed for the *Saa1* promoter (**Figure 6C**). PolII recruitment to the *Saa1* promoter exhibited a similar LPS-dependent pattern as that of H3K27Ac, although a slight increase was observed in response to IFNγ + LPS. This correlated with transcriptional activity of *Saa1*, which was substantially increased upon IFNα + LPS and IFNγ + LPS stimulation as compared to single stimuli (**Figure 4C**).

Our results suggest that STAT1 and p65 bind to DNA independently, yet in a sequential manner, directed by IFN-I or IFN-II treatment followed by LPS stimulation. As such, stimulation with IFNs results in robust STAT1 recruitment to ISRE and/or GAS motifs in gene promoters and potentially introduces chromatin modifications to increase NFκB binding to closely located sites and enhance transcription.

DISCUSSION

Excessive immune and inflammatory responses, communicated by immune, and vascular cells contribute to local inflammation and vascular dysfunction, followed by atherosclerotic plaque formation within the intima of the arterial wall. Priming-induced SI of IFN-II, and possibly IFN-I, with TLR4 is a common phenomenon in atheroma interacting immune cells that modulates important aspects of inflammation, with STAT1 and NFκB being central mediators. Thus, IFN pre-treatment ("priming") followed by LPS stimulation leads to enhanced transcriptional responses as compared to the individual stimuli. To characterize the mechanism of priming-induced IFNα + LPS- and IFNγ + LPS-dependent SI in vascular cells as compared to immune cells, we performed a comprehensive genome-wide analysis of mouse VSMC, MΦ, and DC in response to IFNα, IFNγ, and/or LPS. Specifically, we aimed at providing mechanistic insight in the cooperative binding of STAT1 complexes with NFκB to ISRE/NFκB and/or GAS/NFκB binding sites in relation to transcription and how this is involved in the overlap of IFN-I/LPS and IFN-II/LPS activated SI in VSMC.

First, we compared the gene expression profiles of the different cell types exposed to the individual or combined stimuli, to identify the commonly up-regulated genes as a result of the interaction between IFNα and LPS or between IFNγ and LPS. Generally, in all three cell types combined treatment with IFNα + LPS or IFNγ + LPS resulted in a synergistic increase in gene expression as compared to single treatments, pointing to a common effect of SI mediated by the different IFNs (**Figure 1**). In agreement with the similar effect of SI mediated by the different IFNs and LPS, we observed >64% overlap between commonly up-regulated genes in response to IFNα + LPS and IFNγ + LPS. GO analysis revealed functional overlap of these genes connected to stress, immune and inflammatory response, response to cytokine, regulation of cell proliferation and migration, regulation of cell adhesion and chemotaxis, cell death and apoptotic process, response to lipid, and ROS metabolic process, all reflecting pro-inflammatory and pro-atherogenic biological functions (**Figure 1**). Together this may be a reflection of the partial overlap in activation of transcription factor complexes and regulation of target gene expression by IFN-I and IFN-II, which results in the execution of cell type-common biological responses. Subsequent promoter analysis of these genes indeed predicted the presence of either single GAS sites or rather combinations of potential GAS-ISRE, GAS-NFκB, or GAS-ISRE-NFκB binding motifs, with a similar binding site distribution between IFNα + LPS and IFNγ + LPS treatment conditions (**Figure 1**). In general, under these conditions ISRE

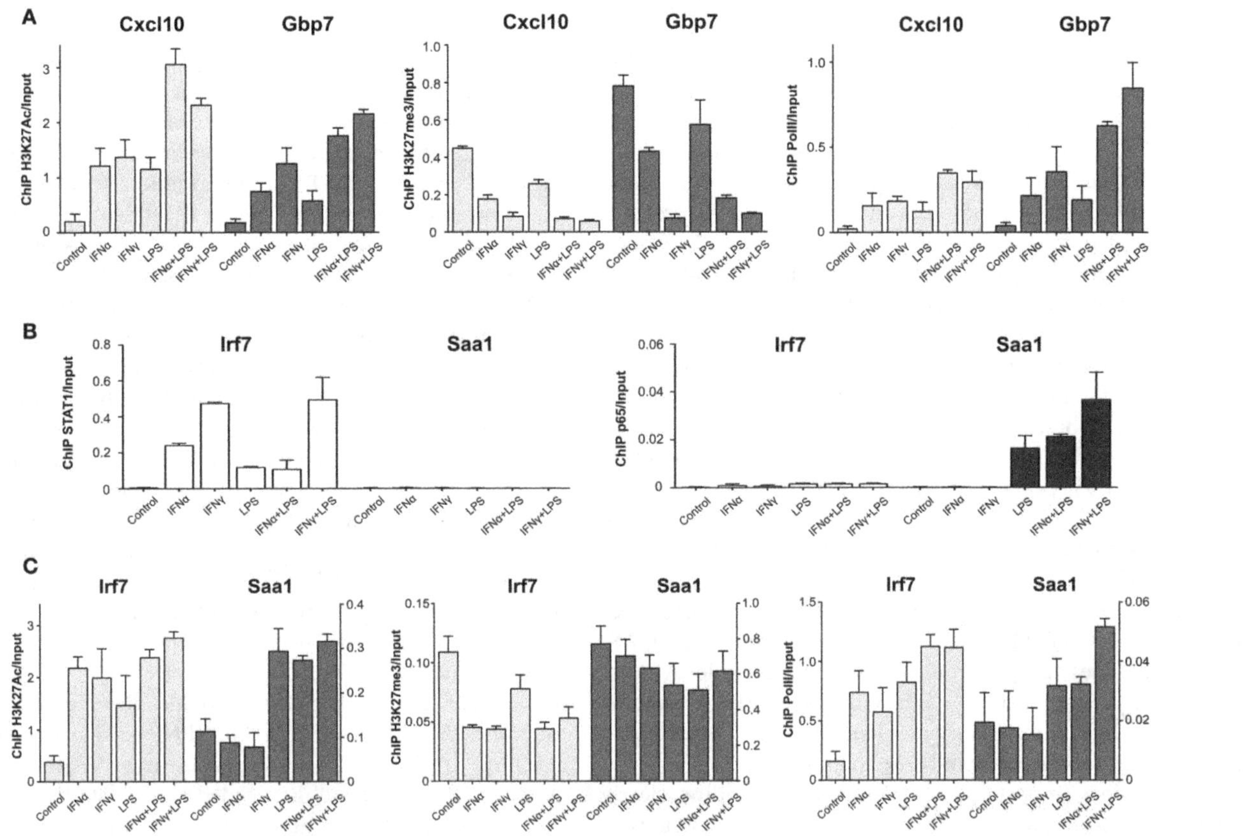

FIGURE 6 | PolII and histone modification changes upon stimulation with IFNs and LPS at promoters of STAT1 and p65 "co-binding" and "single" modes representatives. **(A)** ChIP-PCR of H3K27Ac, H3K27me3, and PolII at *Cxcl10* and *Gbp7* gene promoters (primers are listed in **Table S2**) in VSMC treated with IFNα (8 h), IFNγ (8 h), LPS (4 h), IFNα (8 h) + LPS (4 h), IFNγ (8 h) + LPS (4 h). Mean ± s.e.m., $n = 2$. **(B)** ChIP-PCR of STAT1 and p65 at *Irf7* and *Saa1* gene promoters (primers are listed in **Table S2**) in VSMC treated with IFNα (8 h), IFNγ (8 h), LPS (4 h), IFNα (8 h) + LPS (4 h), IFNγ (8 h) + LPS (4 h). Mean ± s.e.m., $n = 2$. **(C)** ChIP-PCR of H3K27Ac, H3K27me3 and PolII at *Irf7* and *Saa1* gene promoters (primers are listed in **Table S2**) in VSMC treated with IFNα (8 h), IFNγ (8 h), LPS (4 h), IFNα (8 h) + LPS (4 h), IFNγ (8 h) + LPS (4 h). Mean ± s.e.m., $n = 2$.

motifs correspond to binding of STAT1 and STAT2 (in the form of ISGF3) and possibly different IRFs (IRF1, IRF7, IRF8, IRF9), GAS motifs to that of STAT1 binding and NFκB motifs to binding of p65 and p50. Previously we revealed, that the promoters of genes affected by the SI between IFNγ and LPS, like *Cxcl9, Cxcl10,* and *Nos2,* which are also present among the highest expressed common genes in the current study, contain STAT-NFκB and IRF-NFκB modules or combinations of separate ISRE, GAS or NFκB binding sites (20, 41). Together this suggested that a common SI mechanism is involved in the interaction between IFNα and LPS or IFNγ and LPS in VSMC, MΦ, and DC. Together this suggested that although VSMC, MΦ, and DC perform cell type specific functions in a healthy vessel, stimulation with pro-inflammatory stimuli results in activation of a common SI mechanism in the interaction between IFNα and LPS or IFNγ and LPS.

To understand this mechanism of SI in more detail, we characterized the genome-wide binding of STAT1 and NFκB (p65) to the IFNα + LPS- and IFNγ + LPS commonly up-regulated genes. Using ChIP-seq on chromatin from VSMC, STAT1 and p65 bound IFNα + LPS and IFNγ + LPS up-regulated genes were identified, containing GAS, ISRE, or NFκB binding motifs located in promoter regions, but also to up- and downstream genomic regions. Obviously, the interaction between IFNα + LPS and IFNγ + LPS increased the genome-wide number of STAT1 and p65 binding sites (as compared to individual treatments), correlating with the observed SI effect on transcription under these conditions (data not shown). The vast majority of STAT1 and p65 binding events localized outside gene promoters (**Figure 2**). This correlates with the general view of genome-wide occupancy of individual transcription factors, which regulate gene expression through integrated action of proximal and distal *cis*-regulatory elements [reviewed in (42)], the latter being functionally related with cell type-specific gene expression (43). This binding site distribution coincided with other studies. For example, in IFNγ stimulated HeLa S3 cells, Satoh et al. provided evidence for the presence of STAT1 binding GAS motifs in intronic regions (44), while others observed that ~50% of the total STAT1-occupied binding sites were intragenic and 25% intergenic (45). Similar observations have been reported for NFκB. As shown for LPS-treated THP1 cells, a significant proportion of genome-wide NFκB binding sites are located in proximal upstream promoter regions (26%), whereas an even greater proportion of p65 binding sites were found to be located within introns (38%) (46). On the other hand, in TNFα-treated HeLa cells, location analysis revealed that the p65-binding sites are mainly intragenic (46%) and only 7% are located in promoters, in agreement with previous studies (47). The function of the majority of distal STAT1 and p65 binding sites remains largely unknown. Nevertheless, it predicts the presence of a common regulatory mechanism of ISG transcriptional regulation.

Focusing on binding motifs in gene promoters, we could distinguish different STAT1 and p65 binding modes, including "single" (STAT1 binding to GAS and/or ISRE; p65 to NFκB) or "co-binding" (STAT1 binding to GAS and/or ISRE + p65 to NFκB) (**Figure 2**). Comparison of the different binding modes between IFNα + LPS and IFNγ + LPS induced conditions, identified a substantial overlap for NFκB-only (15.9%), GAS-only (13%), and ISRE-only (29.4%) containing genes from the single mode. Likewise, this overlap could be observed for GAS-ISRE (32.7%), GAS-NFκB (11.1%), ISRE-NFκB (21.6%), and GAS-ISRE-NFκB genes (29.6%) from the co-binding mode. A more detailed comparison of IFNα + LPS and IFNγ + LPS commonly up-regulated ISRE-containing genes identified STAT1 binding to these ISRE sites in response to IFNα and, unexpectedly to IFNγ (**Figure 2**). More important, this STAT1 DNA binding clearly corresponded to transcriptional activity in VSMC, as well as in MΦ and DC. Among these genes were many classical ISRE-containing genes, including *Ifit1, Mx2, Oas2, Irf7,* and *Cxcl10,* which were highly responsive to IFNα and to a lesser extent to IFNγ (**Figure 3A**). All five genes were highly responsive to IFNα and to a lesser extent to IFNγ, with *Ifit1, Mx2,* and *Cxcl10* being effected by SI after combined treatment with IFNα + LPS and IFNγ + LPS (**Figure 3A**). This correlated with the slight increase in STAT1 and STAT2 phosphorylation in response to both stimuli as compared to the individual ones (**Figure 3B**). The simultaneous recruitment of pSTAT1, pSTAT2, and IRF9 after IFNα and IFNγ treatment, clearly was in agreement with the involvement of ISGF3 in the transcriptional regulation of these ISRE-containing genes in response to both types of IFN. The expression pattern of these genes closely mirrored the binding pattern of pSTAT2 and IRF9 and reflected the phosphorylation level of STAT2 and expression of IRF9, being higher after IFNα treatment than after IFNγ treatment.

In support of a direct role for STAT2 in the IFNγ response, its tyrosine phosphorylation was reported in a study using IFNγ-treated wild-type mouse primary embryonic fibroblasts that caused the formation of ISGF3 (8). This was in agreement with observations made from the same group, in which mice lacking IRF9 are impaired not only in their type I IFN response, but also in their IFNγ-induced ISRE-dependent gene expression (48). Similar observations were made by others in MEFs, in which STAT2 phosphorylation was essential for the antiviral potency of IFNγ (49). Together, this revealed the existence of an ISGF3-dependent mechanism by which IFN-I and IFN-II can commonly elicit antiviral activities.

The opposite binding pattern of pSTAT1 (higher after IFNγ treatment than after IFNα; **Figure 3**), as compared to pSTAT2 and IRF9, suggested the participation of STAT1 in an additional ISRE-binding complex in IFNγ-treated cells. Based on the high phosphorylation levels of STAT1 and the increased expression of IRF9 under these conditions, we propose that this complex consists of STAT1 homodimers together with IRF9. The first evidence for STAT1- and IRF9-dependent and STAT2-independent transcriptional regulation of IFNγ-induced gene expression was reported for *Ifit2*, a classical ISRE-regulated gene (39) and CXCL10 (50). More recently a role for STAT1/IRF9 in the regulation of the latter gene was studied in the context of a murine colitis model. Molecular analysis in MΦ confirmed that STAT1/IRF9 complexes form in response to IFNγ and associate with ISRE sequences of enhancer regions 1 and 2 of the *Cxcl10* gene promoter (9). In the same study, the authors observed that the expression of IRF7 and DDX58, two other known ISRE-containing genes, depended on STAT1 and IRF9 as well as on STAT2 for their response to IFNγ pointing to a role of ISGF3 instead of STAT1/IRF9. As such they suggested that ISRE-containing promoters could potentially select STAT1/IRF9 complexes either with or without the STAT2 subunit for the cellular response to IFNγ. However, in the VSMC that we use in our study we cannot provide direct proof for a role of the STAT1/IRF9 complex in IFNγ-mediated responses in addition to ISGF3. Further experiments in VSMC from STAT2 and IRF9 KO mice will be needed to validate this assumption. Interestingly, IRF1 was also recruited to these ISRE-containing genes after stimulation with IFNγ, but only weakly upon IFNα treatment (**Figure 3**). Since no interaction could be detected between STAT1 and IRF1 under these conditions (**Figure 3**), a STAT1-independent role of IRF1 in the transcriptional regulation of a selective group of ISRE-containing genes can be proposed. This was in contrast to the direct interaction between unphosphorylated STAT1 and IRF1, which was detected in U3A cells overexpressing STAT1 tyrosine 701 mutant and proposed to mediate constitutive LMP2 gene expression (51).

Our results are in agreement with the existence of a more general mechanism in mouse primary VSMC, in which ISGF3 and possibly STAT1/IRF9 regulate expression of IFNγ-responsive ISRE-containing genes. Together with STAT1 homodimers binding GAS, this provides an additional twist to the canonical IFNγ signaling pathway, which could explain some of the overlapping responses to IFNα and IFNy in these cells (**Figure 7**). Based on the overlapping expression patterns of these genes in VSMC, MΦ, and DC and the above described findings in MΦ, it is tempting to speculate that the IFNα response of ISRE-containing genes in all three cell types is mainly driven by ISGF3. In contrast, their IFNγ response is mediated by ISGF3 and potentially by STAT1/IRF9 (**Figure 7**). In the latter case a mechanism of competition could be envisioned or selective binding, depending on the ISRE sequence.

To further understand the mechanism of cooperative involvement of STAT1 with NFκB in SI mediated by the interaction of IFNα and LPS or IFNγ and LPS, we next concentrated on the overlap of STAT1-p65 co-binding modes. Therefore, we analyzed in more detail STAT1 and p65 binding

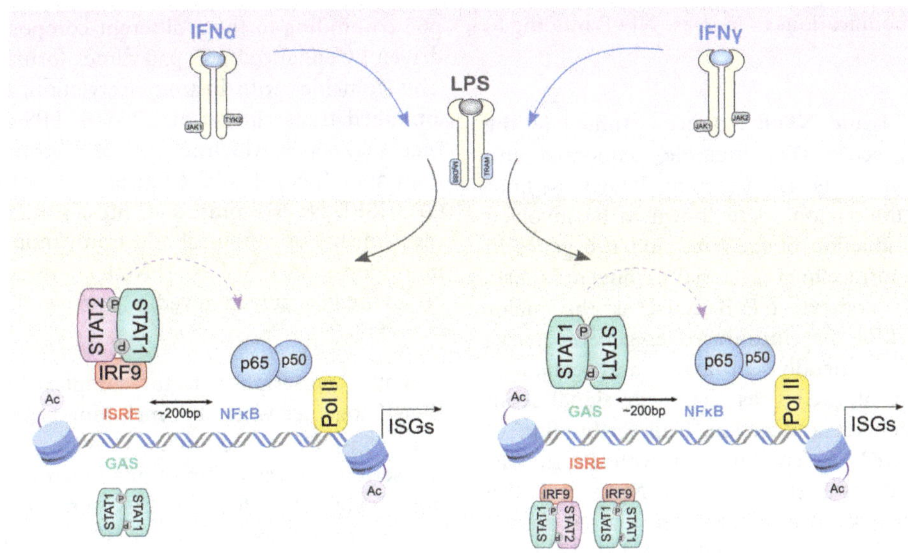

FIGURE 7 | Model describing transcriptional regulation of Signal Integrated genes by STAT1-mediated preceding of p65 and PolII to acetylated GAS/NFκB or ISRE/NFκB composite sites. 1st wave of stimulation: After initial cell exposure to IFNα or IFNγ, receptors dimerize, and facilitate transphosphorylation of receptor-bound JAK1/TYK2 kinases for IFNα and JAK1/JAK2 kinases for IFNγ. Next STAT proteins are recruited, phosphorylated and dimerized, either in a form of ISGF3 complex (STAT1-STAT2 together with IRF9), GAF (STAT1 homodimers) or STAT1/IRF9 complex. Activated transcription factors supply a platform for 2nd wave of stimulation: LPS stimulates TLR4 receptor associated with adapter molecules MyD88 and TRAM and activates NFκB, as well as STAT1-containing transcriptional complexes. IFNα stimulation results in recruitment of ISGF3 to ISRE sites and GAF to GAS sites present in ISGs promoters. IFNγ initiates binding of GAF to GAS sites as well as ISGF3 and possibly STAT1/IRF9 to ISRE elements. Initial binding of STAT1-containing complexes followed by subsequent p65-p50 heterodimers binding (indicated by a violet curved arrow) to NFκB sites closely spaced to ISRE and GAS sites (~200 bp), together results in histone acetylation enrichment and PolII recruitment to ISG promoters. For a detailed explanation, see the text.

patterns in 170 IFNα + LPS and 211 IFNγ + LPS up-regulated genes which were commonly affected by SI in the three cell types (**Figure 4**). Strikingly, for the majority of these genes STAT1 and p65 binding peaks were closely aligned in the co-bound gene promoters, what further correlated with the close proximity of GAS and NFκB (41–234 bp) or ISRE and NFκB (38–264 bp) binding sites (**Figure 4**). This close binding sites distribution may be a pre-requisite for effective STAT1 and p65 collaboration. A similar organization of closely located ISRE and NFκB sites, within ~50 bp proximity, was reported for IRF3 and NFκB co-occupancy to control Sendai virus-induced gene activation (52). Also in IFNγ-treated cells in genome-wide studies co-binding of STAT1 and IRF1 occurred at closely located GAS and ISRE sites (6, 53).

Stimuli-induced binding of two different transcription factors to closely spaced DNA motifs, could assume occurrence of direct protein-protein interactions, which if exceeding >20 bp would have to involve DNA looping (54). Indeed, STAT1 and NFκB have been shown to directly cooperate in several studies (55, 56). On the other hand, although combined action of STAT1 and NFκB was reported to be pivotal for *Cxcl9*, *IP-10*, *Becn1*, and NOS2 gene expression regulation, no direct protein-protein interaction of these transcription factors was observed (40, 57–59). Similarly, by performing co-IP experiments on protein extracts isolated from IFNα + LPS and IFNγ + LPS-treated VSMC, we were not able to detect direct interaction between STAT1 and p65 protein (data not shown). Further examination of the STAT1-p65 co-binding modes unraveled the involvement of a STAT1-dependent role in the nearby recruitment of p65 via closely located GAS-NFκB or ISRE-NFκB binding sites. IFNγ and to a lesser extent IFNα induced STAT1 binding to gene promoters containing either GAS-NFκB (*Serpina3i*, *Steap4*, *Irf1*), ISRE-NFκB (*Ccl5*, *Ifit1*, *Gbp6*), or GAS-ISRE-NFκB (*Cxcl10*, *Gbp7*) motifs. Much weaker STAT1 recruitment was also detected upon LPS stimulation, which correlated with the fact that transcriptional activation of SI genes under these conditions is primarily driven by IFNs (**Tables 1A,B**; **Figures 4, 5**). Interestingly, STAT1 recruitment to these different genes coincided with that of p65 binding, already upon IFNα or IFNγ treatment. This elevated p65 binding after single treatments with IFNα or IFNγ could not be detected at genes with solitary NFκB binding sequences (**Figure 4**). More important, subsequent LPS exposure resulted in increased STAT1-p65 co-binding, mainly driven by enhanced p65 recruitment, which correlated with histone acetylation, PolII recruitment and amplified target gene transcription in a STAT1-p65 co-bound dependent manner. In general, STAT1 and p65 binding after IFNγ and IFNγ + LPS was stronger than after IFNα and IFNα + LPS (**Figure 5**). The fact that we were not able to detect direct STAT1-p65 protein-protein interaction under studied treatment conditions in VSMC (data not shown), we postulate that STAT1 and p65 bind to DNA independently, yet in a sequential manner, directed by IFN-I or IFN-II treatment followed by LPS stimulation. As such, stimulation with IFNs results in robust STAT1 recruitment to

ISRE and/or GAS motifs in gene promoters and potentially introduces chromatin modifications to increase NFκB binding to closely located sites.

Co-binding of STAT1 and NFκB has been studied in the context of bacterial infection. For example, sequential and cooperative contributions of NFκB preceding ISGF3, without direct protein-protein interaction, were shown to be involved in the transcriptional induction of the *Nos2* and *Il-6* genes in MΦ infected with the intracellular bacterial pathogen *Listeria monocytogenes*. In this context, NFκB acted as the major signal stimulated by TLR4 that introduced epigenetic marks to produce transcription friendly chromatin and enhanced subsequent recruitment of ISGF3, as the main signal from subsequent IFNβ production and action. This co-binding of NFκB followed by ISGF3, in combination with PolII, was a prerequisite for productive elongation of Nos2 and Il-6 mRNA (13, 60). Likewise, Wort et al. observed that combined stimulation of primary HPASM cells with TNFα and IFNγ correlated with both increased histone H4 acetylation at distinct NFκB sites and PolII recruitment to the PreproET-1 promoter region (61). Others showed that in IL-10 and LPS-treated phagocytes, STAT3 favored NFκB recruitment to the IL-1ra gene promoter due to its increased acetylation (62). A more comprehensive genome-wide co-binding study of IRF3 and NFκB revealed a mechanism of virus-induced transcriptional activation, in which IRF3 was able to organize promoter-specific recruitment of PolII and NFκB provided the ability to stimulate its efficient and processive elongation (52). On the other hand, Giorgetti et al. demonstrated p65 ability to additively recruit PolII to multiple κB sites containing gene promoters, resulting in elevated gene transcriptional activation (63). In case of IFNγ priming, a synergy mechanism was described, whereby IFNγ created a primed chromatin environment that sustained occupancy of STAT1, IRF1 and associated histone acetylation at pre-selected target genes. This greatly increased and prolonged recruitment of subsequent TLR4-induced transcription factors, including NFκB, and PolII to gene promoters and enhancers (64).

Based on these models our results are predictive of the following mechanism of STAT1-NFκB co-binding involved in the SI of IFN-I and IFN-II with TLR4 in VSMC, MΦ, and DC (**Figure 7**). In the first step, IFN-I activated STAT1 is recruited to closely located ISRE-NFκB or GAS-NFκB binding sites in the form of ISGF3 or GAF, respectively. Likewise, IFNγ stimulates the binding of the STAT1-complexes ISGF3 (and possibly STAT1/IRF9) and GAF to these respective sites. This first wave of STAT1 binding introduces chromatin modifications and initiates subsequent p65-p50 recruitment to adjacent (~200 bp) NFκB sites in response to IFNγ and to a lesser extent after IFNα treatment, which correlates with STAT1-binding potency and levels of transcription. The second step, which is mediated by subsequent LPS stimulation, increases STAT1-p65 co-binding to these different composite sites and is mainly driven by enhanced p65-p50 dimer formation and recruitment. This coincides with histone acetylation, PolII recruitment and amplified transcription of IFNα + LPS and IFNγ + LPS up-regulated genes, which in general is stronger after IFNγ + LPS than after IFNα + LPS (**Figure 7**). In case of genes harboring GAS-ISRE-NFκB composite sites, similar but more complex mechanisms of canonical and non-canonical STAT1 complexes in response to IFN-I or IFN-II combined with LPS-activated NFκB are probably involved.

Thus, transcription factor complexes activated by IFN-I or IFN-II together with LPS, including GAF, ISGF3, STAT1/IRF9, and p65-p50 heterodimers provide a platform for robust transcriptional activation of pro-inflammatory genes. Moreover, our model offer for the first time an explanation for the comparable effects of IFNα or IFNγ priming on TLR4-induced activation in vascular and immune cells, which correlates with the important roles of both IFN types in vascular inflammation and atherosclerosis progression. However, we realize that this is just a predictive model and we cannot rule out the involvement of other STAT1-containing transcription factor complexes or IRFs. Moreover, further investigation will be required to obtain insight in the mechanism of STAT1-dependent NFκB recruitment and subsequent transcriptional regulation under SI, involved in gene-specific scenarios.

AUTHOR CONTRIBUTIONS

AP-B performed ChIP-seq, ChIP-PCR, Western blot and Co-IP experiments, RNA-seq/ChIP-seq downstream *in silico* analysis and was involved in concept development, writing, figures and tables preparation, and editing manuscript. LS and AC performed *in silico* ChIP-seq analysis. H-CC isolated RNA from DC for further RNA-seq experiment and performed RT-PCR validation. C-KL and LN were involved in concept development related to DC and MΦ experimentation. JW critically assessed the manuscript. HB developed the research study concept and was involved in data interpretation, writing and editing the manuscript, and coordinated input from all co-authors.

ACKNOWLEDGMENTS

We thank Thomas Decker for STAT1 KO mice and Adam Olejnik for RNA-seq libraries preparation.

REFERENCES

1. Dzau VJ, Braun-Dullaeus RC, Sedding DG. Vascular proliferation and atherosclerosis: new perspectives and therapeutic strategies. *Nat Med.* (2002) 8:1249–56. doi: 10.1038/nm1102-1249
2. Whitman SC, Ravisankar P, Elam H, Daugherty A. Exogenous interferon-gamma enhances atherosclerosis in apolipoprotein E-/- mice. *Am J Pathol.* (2000) 157:1819–24. doi: 10.1016/S0002-9440(10)64820-1
3. Thacker SG, Zhao W, Smith CK, Luo W, Wang H, Vivekanandan-Giri A, et al. Type I interferons modulate vascular function, repair, thrombosis, and plaque progression in murine models of lupus and atherosclerosis. *Arthritis Rheum.* (2012) 64:2975–85. doi: 10.1002/art.34504
4. Lu Z, Zhang X, Li Y, Jin J, Huang Y. TLR4 antagonist reduces early-stage atherosclerosis in diabetic apolipoprotein E-deficient mice. *J Endocrinol.* (2013) 216:61–71. doi: 10.1530/JOE-12-0338
5. Blaszczyk K, Nowicka H, Kostyrko K, Antonczyk A, Wesoly J, Bluyssen HA. The unique role of STAT2 in constitutive and IFN-induced transcription and antiviral responses. *Cytokine Growth Factor Rev.* (2016) 29:71–81. doi: 10.1016/j.cytogfr.2016.02.010
6. Michalska A, Blaszczyk K, Wesoly J, Bluyssen HAR. A positive feedback amplifier circuit that regulates Interferon (IFN)-stimulated gene expression and controls Type I and Type II IFN responses. *Front Immunol.* (2018) 9:1135. doi: 10.3389/fimmu.2018.01135
7. Bluyssen AR, Durbin JE, Levy DE. ISGF3 gamma p48, a specificity switch for interferon activated transcription factors. *Cytokine Growth Factor Rev.* (1996) 7:11–7. doi: 10.1016/1359-6101(96)00005-6
8. Matsumoto M, Tanaka N, Harada H, Kimura T, Yokochi T, Kitagawa M, et al. Activation of the transcription factor ISGF3 by interferon-gamma. *Biol Chem.* (1999) 380:699–703. doi: 10.1515/BC.1999.087
9. Rauch I, Rosebrock F, Hainzl E, Heider S, Majoros A, Wienerroither S, et al. Noncanonical effects of IRF9 in intestinal inflammation: more than Type I and Type III interferons. *Mol Cell Biol.* (2015) 35:2332–43. doi: 10.1128/MCB.01498-14
10. Hertzog PJ, O'Neill LA, Hamilton JA. The interferon in TLR signaling: more than just antiviral. *Trends Immunol.* (2003) 24:534–9. doi: 10.1016/j.it.2003.08.006
11. Kawai T, Akira S. The role of pattern-recognition receptors in innate immunity: update on Toll-like receptors. *Nat Immunol.* (2010) 11:373–84. doi: 10.1038/ni.1863
12. Kleinert H, Schwarz PM, Forstermann U. Regulation of the expression of inducible nitric oxide synthase. *Biol Chem.* (2003) 384:1343–64. doi: 10.1515/BC.2003.152
13. Farlik M, Reutterer B, Schindler C, Greten F, Vogl C, Muller M, et al. Nonconventional initiation complex assembly by STAT and NF-kappaB transcription factors regulates nitric oxide synthase expression. *Immunity.* (2010) 33:25–34. doi: 10.1016/j.immuni.2010.07.001
14. Proost P, Verpoest S, Van de Borne K, Schutyser E, Struyf S, Put W, et al. Synergistic induction of CXCL9 and CXCL11 by Toll-like receptor ligands and interferon-gamma in fibroblasts correlates with elevated levels of CXCR3 ligands in septic arthritis synovial fluids. *J Leukoc Biol.* (2004) 75:777–84. doi: 10.1189/jlb.1003524
15. Tamassia N, Calzetti F, Ear T, Cloutier A, Gasperini S, Bazzoni F, et al. Molecular mechanisms underlying the synergistic induction of CXCL10 by LPS and IFN-gamma in human neutrophils. *Eur J Immunol.* (2007) 37:2627–34. doi: 10.1002/eji.200737340
16. Schroder K, Sweet MJ, Hume DA. Signal integration between IFNgamma and TLR signalling pathways in macrophages. *Immunobiology.* (2006) 211:511–24. doi: 10.1016/j.imbio.2006.05.007
17. Hu X, Chen J, Wang L, Ivashkiv LB. Crosstalk among Jak-STAT, Toll-like receptor, and ITAM-dependent pathways in macrophage activation. *J Leukoc Biol.* (2007) 82:237–43. doi: 10.1189/jlb.1206763
18. Hu X, Chakravarty SD, Ivashkiv LB. Regulation of interferon and Toll-like receptor signaling during macrophage activation by opposing feedforward and feedback inhibition mechanisms. *Immunol Rev.* (2008) 226:41–56. doi: 10.1111/j.1600-065X.2008.00707.x
19. Hu X, Ivashkiv LB. Cross-regulation of signaling pathways by interferon-gamma: implications for immune responses and autoimmune diseases. *Immunity.* (2009) 31:539–50. doi: 10.1016/j.immuni.2009.09.002
20. Chmielewski S, Olejnik A, Sikorski K, Pelisek J, Blaszczyk K, Aoqui C, et al. STAT1-dependent signal integration between IFNgamma and TLR4 in vascular cells reflect pro-atherogenic responses in human atherosclerosis. *PLoS ONE.* (2014) 9:e113318. doi: 10.1371/journal.pone.0113318
21. Meraz MA, White JM, Sheehan KC, Bach EA, Rodig SJ, Dighe AS, et al. Targeted disruption of the Stat1 gene in mice reveals unexpected physiologic specificity in the JAK-STAT signaling pathway. *Cell.* (1996) 84:431–42. doi: 10.1016/S0092-8674(00)81288-X
22. Durbin JE, Hackenmiller R, Simon MC, Levy DE. Targeted disruption of the mouse Stat1 gene results in compromised innate immunity to viral disease. *Cell.* (1996) 84:443–50. doi: 10.1016/S0092-8674(00)81289-1
23. Kobayashi M, Inoue K, Warabi E, Minami T, Kodama T. A simple method of isolating mouse aortic endothelial cells. *J Atheroscler Thromb.* (2005) 12:138–42. doi: 10.5551/jat.12.138
24. Barish GD, Downes M, Alaynick WA, Yu RT, Ocampo CB, Bookout AL, et al. A Nuclear Receptor Atlas: macrophage activation. *Mol Endocrinol.* (2005) 19:2466–77. doi: 10.1210/me.2004-0529
25. Lutz MB, Kukutsch N, Ogilvie AL, Rossner S, Koch F, Romani N, et al. An advanced culture method for generating large quantities of highly pure dendritic cells from mouse bone marrow. *J Immunol Methods.* (1999) 223:77–92. doi: 10.1016/S0022-1759(98)00204-X
26. Mi H, Huang X, Muruganujan A, Tang H, Mills C, Kang D, et al. PANTHER version 11: expanded annotation data from Gene Ontology and Reactome pathways, and data analysis tool enhancements. *Nucleic Acids Res.* (2017) 45:D183–9. doi: 10.1093/nar/gkw1138
27. Zambelli F, Pesole G, Pavesi G. Pscan: finding over-represented transcription factor binding site motifs in sequences from co-regulated or co-expressed genes. *Nucleic Acids Res.* (2009) 37:W247–52. doi: 10.1093/nar/gkp464
28. Willems E, Leyns L, Vandesompele J. Standardization of real-time PCR gene expression data from independent biological replicates. *Anal Biochem.* (2008) 379:127–9. doi: 10.1016/j.ab.2008.04.036
29. Siersbaek MS, Loft A, Aagaard MM, Nielsen R, Schmidt SF, Petrovic N, et al. Genome-wide profiling of peroxisome proliferator-activated receptor gamma in primary epididymal, inguinal, and brown adipocytes reveals depot-selective binding correlated with gene expression. *Mol Cell Biol.* (2012) 32:3452–63. doi: 10.1128/MCB.00526-12
30. Hulsen T, de Vlieg J, Alkema W. BioVenn - a web application for the comparison and visualization of biological lists using area-proportional Venn diagrams. *BMC Genomics.* (2008) 9:488. doi: 10.1186/1471-2164-9-488
31. Barta E. Command line analysis of ChIP-seq results. *EMBnet J.* (2011) 17:13–7. doi: 10.14806/ej.17.1.209
32. Li H, Durbin R. Fast and accurate short read alignment with Burrows-Wheeler transform. *Bioinformatics.* (2009) 25:1754–60. doi: 10.1093/bioinformatics/btp324
33. Heinz S, Benner C, Spann N, Bertolino E, Lin YC, Laslo P, et al. Simple combinations of lineage-determining transcription factors prime cis-regulatory elements required for macrophage and B cell identities. *Mol Cell.* (2010) 38:576–89. doi: 10.1016/j.molcel.2010.05.004
34. Thorvaldsdottir H, Robinson JT, Mesirov JP. Integrative Genomics Viewer (IGV): high-performance genomics data visualization and exploration. *Brief Bioinform.* (2013) 14:178–92. doi: 10.1093/bib/bbs017
35. Zhang Y, Liu T, Meyer CA, Eeckhoute J, Johnson DS, Bernstein BE, et al. Model-based analysis of ChIP-Seq (MACS). *Genome Biol.* (2008) 9:R137. doi: 10.1186/gb-2008-9-9-r137
36. Consortium EP. An integrated encyclopedia of DNA elements in the human genome. *Nature.* (2012) 489:57–74. doi: 10.1038/nature11247
37. Quinlan AR, Hall IM. BEDTools: a flexible suite of utilities for comparing genomic features. *Bioinformatics.* (2010) 26:841–2. doi: 10.1093/bioinformatics/btq033
38. Robinson JT, Thorvaldsdottir H, Winckler W, Guttman M, Lander ES, Getz G, et al. Integrative genomics viewer. *Nat Biotechnol.* (2011) 29:24–6. doi: 10.1038/nbt.1754
39. Bluyssen HA, Muzaffar R, Vlieststra RJ, van der Made AC, Leung S, Stark GR, et al. Combinatorial association and abundance of components of interferon-stimulated gene factor 3 dictate the selectivity of interferon responses. *Proc Natl Acad Sci USA.* (1995) 92:5645–9. doi: 10.1073/pnas.92.12.5645
40. Ohmori Y, Hamilton TA. Cooperative interaction between interferon (IFN) stimulus response element and kappa B sequence motifs controls IFN

gamma- and lipopolysaccharide-stimulated transcription from the murine IP-10 promoter. *J Biol Chem.* (1993) 268:6677–88.

41. Sikorski K, Wesoly J, Bluyssen HA. Data mining of atherosclerotic plaque transcriptomes predicts STAT1-dependent inflammatory signal integration in vascular disease. *Int J Mol Sci.* (2014) 15:14313–31. doi: 10.3390/ijms150814313
42. Spitz F, Furlong EE. Transcription factors: from enhancer binding to developmental control. *Nat Rev Genet.* (2012) 13:613–26. doi: 10.1038/nrg3207
43. Heinz S, Romanoski CE, Benner C, Glass CK. The selection and function of cell type-specific enhancers. *Nat Rev Mol Cell Biol.* (2015) 16:144–54. doi: 10.1038/nrm3949
44. Satoh J, Tabunoki H. A comprehensive profile of ChIP-Seq-based STAT1 target genes suggests the complexity of STAT1-mediated gene regulatory mechanisms. *Gene Regul Syst Bio.* (2013) 7:41–56. doi: 10.4137/GRSB.S11433
45. Robertson G, Hirst M, Bainbridge M, Bilenky M, Zhao Y, Zeng T, et al. Genome-wide profiles of STAT1 DNA association using chromatin immunoprecipitation and massively parallel sequencing. *Nat Methods.* (2007) 4:651–7. doi: 10.1038/nmeth1068
46. Rao NA, McCalman MT, Moulos P, Francoijs KJ, Chatziioannou A, Kolisis FN, et al. Coactivation of GR and NFKB alters the repertoire of their binding sites and target genes. *Genome Res.* (2011) 21:1404–16. doi: 10.1101/gr.118042.110
47. Lim CA, Yao F, Wong JJ, George J, Xu H, Chiu KP, et al. Genome-wide mapping of RELA(p65) binding identifies E2F1 as a transcriptional activator recruited by NF-kappaB upon TLR4 activation. *Mol Cell.* (2007) 27:622–35. doi: 10.1016/j.molcel.2007.06.038
48. Kimura T, Kadokawa Y, Harada H, Matsumoto M, Sato M, Kashiwazaki Y, et al. Essential and non-redundant roles of p48 (ISGF3 gamma) and IRF-1 in both type I and type II interferon responses, as revealed by gene targeting studies. *Genes Cells.* (1996) 1:115–24. doi: 10.1046/j.1365-2443.1996.08008.x
49. Zimmermann A, Trilling M, Wagner M, Wilborn M, Bubic I, Jonjic S, et al. A cytomegaloviral protein reveals a dual role for STAT2 in IFN-{gamma} signaling and antiviral responses. *J Exp Med.* (2005) 201:1543–53. doi: 10.1084/jem.20041401
50. Majumder S, Zhou LZ, Chaturvedi P, Babcock G, Aras S, Ransohoff RM. p48/STAT-1alpha-containing complexes play a predominant role in induction of IFN-gamma-inducible protein, 10 kDa (IP-10) by IFN-gamma alone or in synergy with TNF-alpha. *J Immunol.* (1998) 161:4736–44.
51. Chatterjee-Kishore M, Wright KL, Ting JP, Stark GR. How Stat1 mediates constitutive gene expression: a complex of unphosphorylated Stat1 and IRF1 supports transcription of the LMP2 gene. *EMBO J.* (2000) 19:4111–22. doi: 10.1093/emboj/19.15.4111
52. Freaney JE, Kim R, Mandhana R, Horvath CM. Extensive cooperation of immune master regulators IRF3 and NFkappaB in RNA Pol II recruitment and pause release in human innate antiviral transcription. *Cell Rep.* (2013) 4:959–73. doi: 10.1016/j.celrep.2013.07.043
53. Abou El Hassan M, Huang K, Eswara MB, Xu Z, Yu T, Aubry A, et al. Properties of STAT1 and IRF1 enhancers and the influence of SNPs. *BMC Mol Biol.* (2017) 18:6. doi: 10.1186/s12867-017-0084-1
54. Heinz S, Glass CK. Roles of lineage-determining transcription factors in establishing open chromatin: lessons from high-throughput studies. *Curr Top Microbiol Immunol.* (2012) 356:1–15. doi: 10.1007/82_2011_142
55. Ganster RW, Guo Z, Shao L, Geller DA. Differential effects of TNF-alpha and IFN-gamma on gene transcription mediated by NF-kappaB-Stat1 interactions. *J Interferon Cytokine Res.* (2005) 25:707–19. doi: 10.1089/jir.2005.25.707
56. Kramer OH, Baus D, Knauer SK, Stein S, Jager E, Stauber RH, et al. Acetylation of Stat1 modulates NF-kappaB activity. *Genes Dev.* (2006) 20:473–85. doi: 10.1101/gad.364306
57. Ganster RW, Taylor BS, Shao L, Geller DA. Complex regulation of human inducible nitric oxide synthase gene transcription by Stat 1 and NF-kappa B. *Proc Natl Acad Sci USA.* (2001) 98:8638–43. doi: 10.1073/pnas.151239498
58. Hiroi M, Ohmori Y. The transcriptional coactivator CREB-binding protein cooperates with STAT1 and NF-kappa B for synergistic transcriptional activation of the CXC ligand 9/monokine induced by interferon-gamma gene. *J Biol Chem.* (2003) 278:651–60. doi: 10.1074/jbc.M204544200
59. Zhu S, Cao L, Yu Y, Yang L, Yang M, Liu K, et al. Inhibiting autophagy potentiates the anticancer activity of IFN1@/IFNalpha in chronic myeloid leukemia cells. *Autophagy.* (2013) 9:317–27. doi: 10.4161/auto.22923
60. Wienerroither S, Shukla P, Farlik M, Majoros A, Stych B, Vogl C, et al. Cooperative transcriptional activation of antimicrobial genes by STAT and NF-kappaB pathways by concerted recruitment of the mediator complex. *Cell Rep.* (2015) 12:300–12. doi: 10.1016/j.celrep.2015.06.021
61. Wort SJ, Ito M, Chou PC, Mc Master SK, Badiger R, Jazrawi E, et al. Synergistic induction of endothelin-1 by tumor necrosis factor alpha and interferon gamma is due to enhanced NF-kappaB binding and histone acetylation at specific kappaB sites. *J Biol Chem.* (2009) 284:24297–305. doi: 10.1074/jbc.M109.032524
62. Tamassia N, Castellucci M, Rossato M, Gasperini S, Bosisio D, Giacomelli M, et al. Uncovering an IL-10-dependent NF-kappaB recruitment to the IL-1ra promoter that is impaired in STAT3 functionally defective patients. *FASEB J.* (2010) 24:1365–75. doi: 10.1096/fj.09-145573
63. Giorgetti L, Siggers T, Tiana G, Caprara G, Notarbartolo S, Corona T, et al. Noncooperative interactions between transcription factors and clustered DNA binding sites enable graded transcriptional responses to environmental inputs. *Mol Cell.* (2010) 37:418–28. doi: 10.1016/j.molcel.2010.01.016
64. Ramsauer K, Farlik M, Zupkovitz G, Seiser C, Kroger A, Hauser H, et al. Distinct modes of action applied by transcription factors STAT1 and IRF1 to initiate transcription of the IFN-gamma-inducible gbp2 gene. *Proc Natl Acad Sci USA.* (2007) 104:2849–54. doi: 10.1073/pnas.0610944104

9

How Dengue Virus Circumvents Innate Immunity

Yu-Ting Kao [1], *Michael M. C. Lai* [2,3] *and Chia-Yi Yu* [1*]

[1] *National Institute of Infectious Diseases and Vaccinology, National Health Research Institutes, Tainan, Taiwan,* [2] *Research Center for Emerging Viruses, China Medical University Hospital, Taichung, Taiwan,* [3] *Institute of Molecular Biology, Academia Sinica, Taipei, Taiwan*

***Correspondence:**
Chia-Yi Yu
epitope@nhri.org.tw

In the battle between a virus and its host, innate immunity serves as the first line of defense protecting the host against pathogens. The antiviral actions start with the recognition of pathogen-associated molecular patterns derived from the virus, then ultimately turning on particular transcription factors to generate antiviral interferons (IFNs) or proinflammatory cytokines via fine-tuned signaling cascades. With dengue virus (DENV) infection, its viral RNA is recognized by the host RNA sensors, mainly retinoic acid inducible gene-I (RIG-I)-like receptors (RLRs) and toll-like receptors. DENV infection also activates the cyclic GMP-AMP synthase–stimulator of interferon genes (cGAS–STING)-mediated DNA-sensing pathway despite the absence of a DNA stage in the DENV lifecycle. In the last decade, DENV has been considered a weak IFN-inducing pathogen with the evidence that DENV has evolved multiple strategies antagonizing the host IFN system. DENV passively escapes from innate immunity surveillance and also actively subverts the innate immune system at multiple steps. DENV targets both RNA-triggered RLR–mitochondrial antiviral signaling protein (RLR–MAVS) and DNA-triggered cGAS–STING signaling to reduce IFN production in infected cells. It also blocks IFN action by inhibiting IFN regulatory factor- and signal transducer and activator of transcription-mediated signaling. This review explores the current understanding of how DENV escapes the control of the innate immune system by modifying viral RNA and viral protein and by post-translational modification of cellular factors. The roles of the DNA-sensing pathway in DENV infection, and how mitochondrial dynamics participates in innate immunity are also discussed.

Keywords: dengue virus, interferon, RLR–MAVS, cGAS–STING, mitochondrial dynamics

Dengue virus (DENV) hijacks the host's cellular machinery and accesses cell resources in multiple ways to accomplish its lifecycle. Cellular immune signaling then turns on various cascades to fight back when the host cell senses this invading pathogen. Therefore, DENV confronts a series of challenges at each step of its lifecycle from virus entry to the release of mature virion. To counteract, DENV not only passively hides to escape the immune surveillance but also directly targets immune mediators to block the antiviral signaling transduction (1–3).

In this review, we discuss how the host cell activates innate immunity in response to DENV infection and the strategies DENV uses to evade the innate immune system. We illustrate the main theme of this article in **Figure 1** and summarize the DENV antagonism (**Table 1**) described in the text.

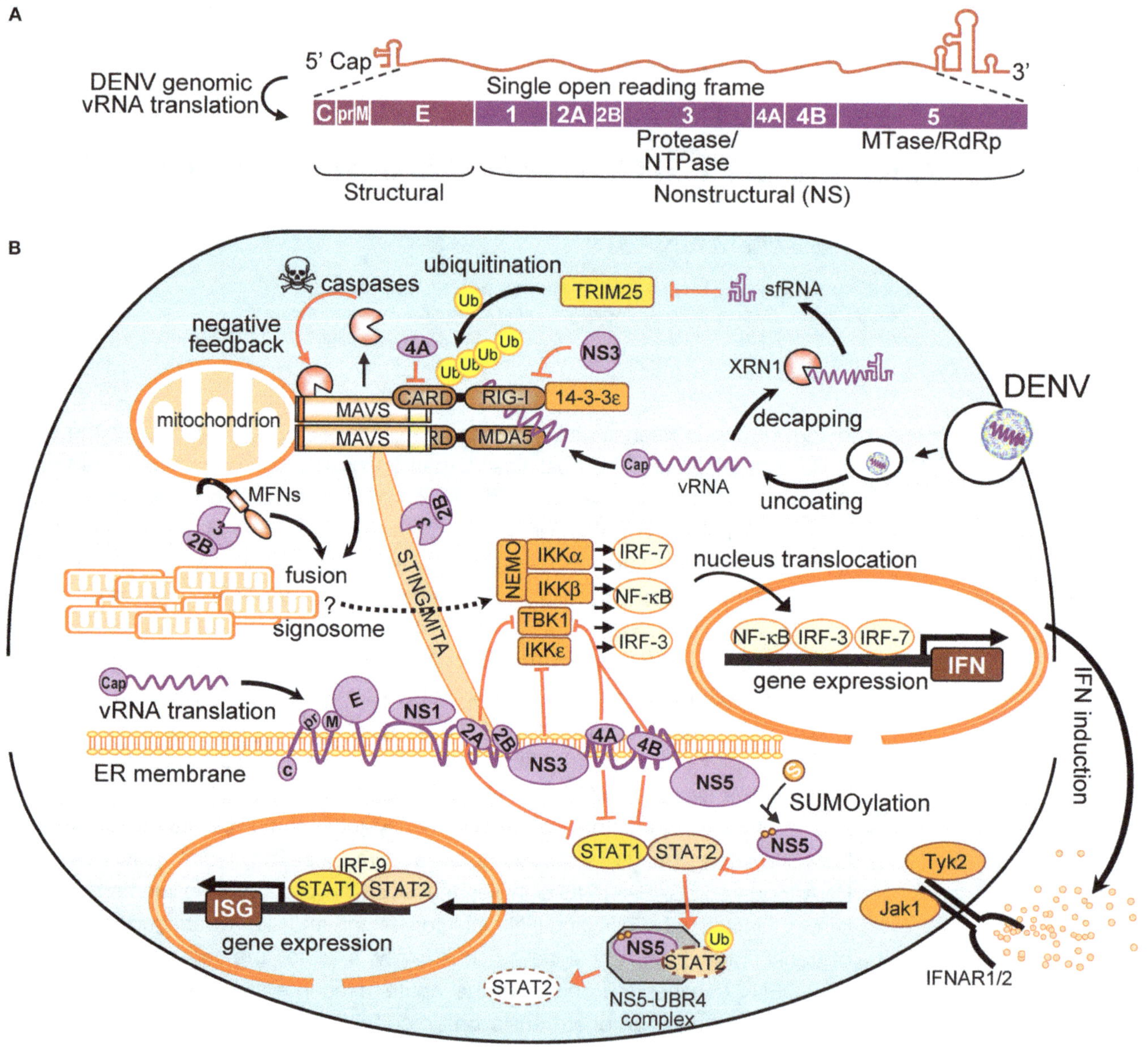

FIGURE 1 | The interplay between dengue virus (DENV) and the interferon (IFN) system. **(A)** The viral proteins encoded by DENV genome are shown. **(B)** The positive signalings/pathways are illustrated with black arrows, and the antagonistic pathways are in red. Refer to the main text for details. vRNA, viral RNA; NTPase, nucleoside triphosphatases; MTase, methyltransferase; RdRp, RNA-dependent RNA polymerase; RIG-I, retinoic acid-inducible gene I; MDA5, melanoma differentiation-associated protein 5; CARD, caspase activation and recruitment domain; Ub, ubiquitin; MAVS, mitochondrial antiviral signaling protein; sfRNA, subgenomic flavivirus RNA; TRIM25, tripartite motif protein 25; MFN, mitofusin; STING, stimulator of interferon genes; MITA, mediator of IRF3 activation; NF-κB, nuclear factor kappa B; NEMO, NF-κB essential modulator; TBK1, TANK binding kinase-1; IKKα/β/ε, IκB kinase alpha/beta/epsilon; IRF, interferon regulatory factor; IFN, interferon; IFNAR, IFN-α/β receptor; STAT, signal transducer and activator of transcription; ISG, IFN-stimulated gene; Jak1, Janus kinase 1; Tyk2, tyrosine kinase 2; UBR4, ubiquitin protein ligase E3 component n-recognin 4; XRN1, 5′-3′ exoribonuclease 1.

BRIEF MOLECULAR VIROLOGY OF DENV

DENV belongs to the genus *Flavivirus* of *Flaviviridae* and is the leading cause of mosquito-borne viral diseases. The DENV virion harbors a messenger-sense, single-stranded RNA (ssRNA) genome that contains a 5′ cap but lacks a 3′ poly-A tail. The DENV invasion starts with cell-surface attachment and receptor binding. After internalization, the nucleocapsid is uncoated, and the virus genome then releases to the cytoplasm. The DENV RNA genome is similar to cellular mRNA, translating a polyprotein precursor in a cap-dependent manner. Viral and cellular proteases then process the polyprotein into three structural proteins (capsid [C], precursor membrane [prM], and envelope [E]) and seven non-structural (NS) proteins

TABLE 1 | Summary of dengue virus (DENV) factors antagonizing the interferon (IFN) system.

DENV factors	Target pathway	Actions	References
sfRNA	RNA-sensing	Binds to TRIM25 to inhibit viral RNA recognition by RIG-I	(4, 5)
NS2A	IFN induction	Antagonizes the phosphorylation of TBK1 and RIG-I-induced IRF3	(6)
	IFN signaling	Inhibits IFN-triggered antiviral actions	(7)
NS2B	DNA-sensing	Targets cGAS for degradation	(8)
NS2B3	DNA-sensing	Cleaves STING through protease-dependent manner	(9, 10)
	IFN induction	Interacts with IKKε to mask part of its kinase domain to prevent the phosphorylation of IRF3	(11)
	Mitochondrial dynamics	Cleaves MFN1 and MFN2 to modulate the MFN-mediated host antiviral defense	(12)
NS3	RNA-sensing	Competes with RIG-I for 14-3-3ε binding to block RIG-I activation	(13)
NS4A	RNA-sensing	Translocates to mitochondrion-associated endoplasmic reticulum membranes to prevent the binding between RIG-I and MAVS.	(14)
	IFN induction	Blocks TBK1 activation	(6)
	IFN signaling	Inhibits of IFN-triggered gene expressions	(7)
NS4B	IFN induction	Antagonizes the phosphorylation of TBK1 and RIG-I-induced IRF3	(6)
	IFN signaling	Inhibits STAT1 phosphorylation and transcriptional activation	(7)
NS5	RNA-sensing	Catalyzes DENV genomic RNA 2'-O methylation mimicking cellular mRNA	(15)
	IFN signaling	Binds and degrades STAT2	(16–18)

sfRNA, subgenomic flaviviral RNA; TRIM25, tripartite motif protein 25; RIG-I, retinoic acid-inducible gene-I; TBK1, TANK binding kinase-1; IRF, interferon regulatory factor; STAT, signal transducer and activator of transcription; cGAS, cyclic GMP-AMP synthase; STING, stimulator of interferon genes; IKKε, IκB kinase epsilon; MFN, mitofusin; MAVS, mitochondrial antiviral signaling protein.

(NS1, NS2A, NS2B, NS3, NS4A, NS4B, and NS5). After that, viral RNA is replicated by the viral RNA-dependent RNA polymerase NS5 in the replication complex. Structural proteins are assembled with the DENV RNA genome in the endoplasmic reticulum (ER) and then transmitted to the Golgi apparatus. Ultimately, the mature and infectious virions are secreted into the extracellular space and await the next round of infection (19, 20).

DENV has evolved many strategies to minimize its exposure *in vitro* because the virus is membrane-enveloped and is liable to dysfunction *in vitro*. Thus, DENV uses the mosquito, the natural syringe, as the vector to preserve, replicate, and transmit itself. Natural feeding of human blood containing DENV viral RNA more than 5 log10-copies/ml seems sufficient to transmit all serotypes of DENV from human to the primary mosquito vector *Aedes aegypti* (21). Therefore, the period of human DENV infectiousness to the *A. aegypti* mosquitoes may vary between viral serotypes but concentrates on the days when a patient develops illness/fever (22). Despite the presence of a protein D7 capable of inhibiting DENV in mosquito saliva (23), the bites with mosquito saliva increase DENV dissemination into the mammalian host (24, 25).

DENV takes advantage of the mammalian host machinery for replication, but the immune system can detect and attack this invading pathogen. In the last decade, DENV has been considered a weak interferon (IFN)-inducing pathogen (26, 27), with the knowledge that DENV has evolved multiple strategies to antagonize the host IFN system (1–3, 28). Understanding how DENV escapes the control of innate immunity may shed some light on the complicated pathogenesis of DENV infection.

THE CONCEPT OF IFN SYSTEM IN INNATE IMMUNITY

Innate immunity specifies particular pattern recognition receptors (PRRs) to distinguish pathogen-associated molecular patterns (PAMPs) of invading pathogens, including both RNA and DNA viruses. The aberrant nucleic acid species in the cytoplasm, such as double-stranded RNA (dsRNA) in the endosome, cytoplasmic DNA and 5′-triphosphorylated RNA, are the unique viral PAMPs that activate corresponding PRRs (29, 30). Once activated, the sensor hands over the signal to its adaptor proteins, which then recruit kinases to phosphorylate transcription factors and ultimately turn on the production of antiviral IFNs and proinflammatory cytokines. The secreted type-I/III IFNs bind to their receptors IFNAR1/2, which activates Janus kinase (Jak)–Signal transducer and activator of transcription (STAT)-mediated signaling and leads to generation of antiviral proteins encoded in IFN-stimulated genes (ISGs) (31, 32). Various antiviral proteins interfere with steps of the viral lifecycle. For example, ribonuclease L (RNase L) is encoded by an ISG that degrades viral RNA to inhibit DENV replication (33). To counteract the host antiviral actions, DENV evolves strategies targeting various steps of the whole defense system, from sensing of the foreign DNA/RNA to the induction, signaling, and manipulation of IFN system. We categorized these various strategies by the stages of IFN system and discussed them below.

THE RNA SENSING PATHWAY

Camouflage is the first strategy to keep DENV away from the alarm bell of innate immunity. Similar to cellular mRNAs,

DENV genomic RNA is capped at the 5′-end. Cellular mRNA is posttranscriptionally capped at the 5′-end comprising a N-7 methylguanosine and one or two 2'-O methylnucleotides (34, 35). Thus, viral RNA lacking 2′-O methylation will be recognized as non-self RNA that elicits innate immunity (35–38). DENV NS5 contains methyltransferase activity that catalyzes both N-7 and 2′-O methylations sequentially (39–41). The DENV lacking 2′-O-methyltransferase activity elicits a significant early innate immune response in host cells and thus replicates with a lower viral load than the wild-type (15). Therefore, DENV hides and stays under the radar in host cells.

DENV enters host cells by receptor-mediated endocytosis, and its RNA is released to the cytosol for translation and replication. The localization of DENV-derived dsRNA is important for recognition by PRRs. By electron tomography analysis, the cytosolic DENV dsRNA was detected in DENV-induced vesicles derived from ER membrane (42). These vesicles quarantine DENV dsRNA from the cytosolic RNA sensors in a digitonin-resistant membrane structure until 72 h postinfection (43). However, these viral RNA species, when leaked to the cytosol, also become targets for several PRRs, including melanoma differentiation-associated protein 5 (MDA5) and retinoic acid-inducible gene-I (RIG-I) in the cytoplasm and toll-like receptor (TLR)-3 in the endosome. These PRRs are essential for host defense surveillance, which synergistically recognizes DENV RNA and then initiates IFN induction (44–46). MDA5 and RIG-I are similar RNA helicases expressed in most cell types. Both contain two caspase activation and recruitment domains (CARDs) at the N-terminus for antiviral signaling initiation. After viral RNA binds to the C-terminal helicase domain, the CARD domain of RIG-I/MDA5 then interacts with the CARD domain of their downstream adaptor, mitochondrial antiviral signaling protein (MAVS) (a.k.a. IPS-1/VISA/Cardif) (47–50). This CARD–CARD interaction clusters MAVS for a signaling cascade, which is required for inducing IFN to establish an antiviral state (49). Actually, RIG-I and MDA5 recognize different RNA structures even though they share a high degree of functional and structural homology. MDA5 mainly recognizes long dsRNA or web-like RNA aggregates, whereas RIG-I preferentially senses short dsRNA and single-stranded uncapped RNA with a tri- or di-phosphate at the 5′-end (51–53). These species/forms of RNA differ from self-RNA in the cytoplasm and can be detected in DENV-infected cells (44, 54). Even though RIG-I or MDA5 alone is sufficient to potentiate DENV-induced IFN-induction signaling, RIG-I and MDA5 together trigger a higher level of IFN induction. Therefore, overexpressing RIG-I or MDA5 can suppress DENV replication; silencing of RIG-I and MDA5 contributes to DENV RNA replication and virus production (44). Because RIG-I and MDA5 share the same adaptor MAVS, lack of MAVS impairs IFN induction in DENV-infected cells (54–56).

The protein level of both RIG-I and MDA5 can be further enhanced by IFN (57), so activation of the RIG-I-MAVS pathway forms a positive feedback loop against DENV infection. In the context of RIG-I activation, the ubiquitin ligase tripartite motif protein 25 (TRIM25) binds to and adds lysine-63 (K63)-linked polyubiquitin at the CARD domain of RIG-I (58–60). The mitochondrial-targeting chaperone protein 14-3-3ε stabilizes the interaction between TRIM25 and RIG-I, thus facilitating K63-linked ubiquitination of RIG-I, which results in MAVS activation (61).

Because ubiquitination and translocation of RIG-I are both required for MAVS activation, DENV evolves strategies to antagonize this step and thus prevents RIG-I-mediated IFN responses. In DENV-infected cells, the uncapped DENV genomic RNA can be digested from the 5′- to 3′-end by the cellular exoribonuclease 1 (XRN1) leaving the incomplete degradation product subgenomic flaviviral RNA (sfRNA) (62). The DENV sfRNA binds to TRIM25, whose binding capacity depends on the sfRNA sequence, thus dampening ubiquitination-mediated RIG-I activation (4, 5). Moreover, DENV NS3 protease contains a 14-3-3ε protein-binding motif RxEP; the binding of these proteins prevents the activated RIG-I from moving from cytosol to mitochondria. Thus, infection of a recombinant DENV, with the RxEP motif replaced by KIKP, triggered a high IFN response that inhibited DENV replication (13). Also, DENV NS4A colocalizes and interacts with MAVS in mitochondrion-associated ER membranes where RIG-I relays the signal to MAVS. The TM3 domain of DENV NS4A is responsible for binding MAVS and thus prevents the association of RIG-I and MAVS (14). Therefore, DENV can disrupt the RIG-I–MAVS interaction directly to suppress IFN production.

In addition to the RIG-I–MAVS pathway, TLR3 and TLR7 are important for recognizing DENV RNA in the endosome. TLR7 senses ssRNA with G- and U-rich sequences (63), whereas TLR3 recognizes dsRNA derived from DENV replication (64). Although, both TLRs are involved in producing a type I IFN response during DENV infection, TLR3 is more effective than TLR7 in IFN induction and DENV inhibition (64). TLR7 also mediates a virus-specific humoral immune response for DENV clearance: administration of combined TLR3 and TLR7 agonists could decrease DENV replication and increase the anti-DENV humoral response in macaques (65). Even though, the direct modulation of TLRs by DENV infection remains to be seen, DENV has been shown to block TLR-mediated antiviral signaling by targeting downstream immune mediators, IκB kinase epsilon (IKKε) and TANK-binding kinase-1 (TBK1) (6, 11).

THE DNA SENSING PATHWAY

Despite the absence of a DNA stage in the DENV lifecycle, DENV infection still activates the DNA-sensing pathway. The cellular DNA should be located in the nucleus or mitochondria. Presence of a DNA molecule in the cytoplasm is thus expected to trigger innate immune responses, such as inflammation and IFN production (66). Cyclic GMP-AMP synthase (cGAS) is a cytosolic DNA sensor that synthesizes cGAMP, a non-canonical cyclic dinucleotide, in response to DNA stimuli (67, 68). cGAMP is a second messenger that binds and activates the adaptor protein encoded in the gene *tmem173*, namely, stimulator of IFN genes (STING) [a.k.a. mediator of IRF3 activation (MITA), or ER IFN stimulator (ERIS)] (69–71). Human STING is a transmembrane protein located on ER membrane and shares 81% similarity (68%

identity) with its murine ortholog MPYS (72). After stimulation, STING is dimerized and then translocated to a perinuclear site where it forms a punctate structure and interacts with TBK1 for activating IFN regulatory factors (IRFs) (70, 71). In addition to activating IRFs and producing IFN, STING activation also triggers NF-κB signaling that leads to the production of pro-inflammatory cytokines (73, 74).

Because DENV is an RNA virus without a DNA stage in its lifecycle, the roles of the DNA-sensing pathway in DENV infection were ignored until DENV protease NS2B3 was found to cleave human STING but not its murine ortholog MPYS (9, 10). Thus, murine MPYS is more competent than human STING in suppressing DENV replication. Even though STING is not essential for IFN production stimulated by a dsRNA analog (73), STING is involved in both DNA and RNA pathogen-sensing pathways. STING can interact with RIG-I and MAVS to enhance the antiviral response (69, 70), which may suggest a crosstalk between viral RNA- and DNA-sensing pathways (75). Therefore, the possibility that DENV may target the DNA-sensing pathway to subvert innate immunity seems logical.

Stimulation of double-stranded DNA but not dsRNA analog enhances the interaction between DENV protease and STING, which then contributes to DENV protease-mediated STING cleavage (10). Therefore, the presence of DNA in cytosol upon DENV infection may contribute to DENV pathogenesis. The release of both genomic and mitochondrial DNA (mtDNA) has been proposed to activate the STING signaling pathway in DENV-infected cells (10). Indeed, aberrant DNA signal appears in cytosol and co-localizes with cGAS upon DENV infection, with the DNA signal resulting from the release of mtDNA rather than genomic DNA (8). Moreover, DENV NS2B mediates cGAS degradation dependent on autophagy–lysosome pathway to avoid IFN production (8). Even though the requirement of mtDNA in the DENV-activated cGAS–STING pathway remains unclear, the roles of mtDNA in DENV pathogenesis are of interest.

THE IFN INDUCTION PATHWAY

After RNA/DNA recognition, both RIG-I–MAVS and cGAS–STING pathways recruit and activate the IKKε/TBK1 and IKKα/β/γ complexes (3). These kinases activate transcription factors, such as NF-κB and IRFs, to turn on IFN mRNA expression (29). Regardless of the multiple strategies used to antagonize RNA/DNA recognition, DENV also subverts this IFN induction step to minimize the antiviral response in infected cells (27, 76).

Although DENV protease activity is required to cleave and block STING signaling, the protease structure itself is able to inhibit IKKε kinase activity. By interacting with the N-terminus of IKKε, NS2B3 masks part of the kinase domain of IKKε to prevent the S386-phosphorylation of IRF3 (11). Despite the presence of two NS2B3-putative cleavage sites within IKKε, neither catalytic nor inactivated NS2B3 protease affects the protein level of IKKε (11). Therefore, DENV protease is able to counteract IFN induction via both catalysis-dependent and -independent mechanisms, with the wild-type DENV protease more competent than the protease-dead mutant. Moreover, DENV NS2A and NS4B regulate innate immune responses by inhibiting TBK1/IKKε-directed downstream signaling instead of targeting MAVS or STING directly (6). Thus, both NS2A and NS4B antagonize IRF3 phosphorylation resulting from the activation of RIG-I, MDA5, MAVS, TBK1 ,or IKKε. Only NS4A of DENV1 but not those of DENV2 or DENV4 blocks TBK1 activation (6), which suggests that DENV1 contains an additional regulatory mechanism against innate immunity.

THE IFN SIGNALING PATHWAY

DENV uses various strategies as described above to prevent the production of IFN by infected cells. Nevertheless, the secreted IFN actively binds to the heterodimeric IFN receptor, IFNAR1/2, which ultimately turns on the expression of many antiviral proteins against DENV infection. After IFN binding, the IFNAR-associated tyrosine kinases Jak1 and tyrosine kinase 2 (Tyk2) undergo autophosphorylation, which then activates downstream transcription factors, mainly STAT1 and STAT2, by phosphorylation. The phosphorylated STATs form a heterotrimeric complex with IRF9, called IFN-stimulated gene factor 3 (ISGF3), which translocates to the nucleus and awakens ISGs to fight against the virus (32, 77, 78). Meanwhile, STAT1 is also modified by the K48-linked conjugation of ubiquitins (79), which tags STAT1 for degradation and shuts off an antiviral response. Accordingly, removing these ubiquitins by the deubiquitinating enzyme USP13 increases the stability of STAT1 proteins and potentiates a stronger IFN-mediated antiviral response against DENV infection (80).

Several viral proteins of DENV are involved in suppressing the IFN-induced signaling. In the presence of IFN, the DENV NS2A, NS4A, and NS4B proteins were found to enhance the replication of an IFN-sensitive recombinant reporter Newcastle disease virus, whereas only DENV NS4A and NS4B significantly reduced the expression of a reporter gene driven by IFN-sensitive response element (7). The NS4B was found to inhibit IFN-induced STAT1 phosphorylation and nuclear translocation, which impairs the transcriptional activity of ISGF3 to turn on antiviral genes (7). Moreover, DENV NS5 can bind to and inhibit the transcription factor STAT2 activated by IFN treatment (16, 17). DENV NS5 recruits the host factor UBR4 to suppress human but not murine STAT2 via the proteasomal degradation pathway (18). Because conjugation of small ubiquitin-like modifier (SUMO) stabilizes DENV NS5 protein to maintain its biological functions, SUMOylation is required for NS5-mediated antagonism of IFN signaling (81).

MANIPULATION OF IFN SYSTEM BY MITOCHONDRIAL DYNAMICS

The roles of mitochondria in innate immunity were largely unknown until strong antiviral activity was detected by overexpressing the mitochondrial protein MAVS (47–50).

Mitochondria move along the cytoskeleton and continuously undergo fusion and fission, which results in the diverse morphology of each mitochondrion (82, 83). MAVS forms prion-like aggregates upon activation (84), which also leads mitochondria to become aggregated in cells overexpressing MAVS (55). Therefore, manipulation of mitochondrial dynamics may regulate antiviral activity in response to virus infection. Indeed, overexpression of the mitochondrial fusion mediator mitofusin 1 (MFN1) rather than MFN2 resulted in a higher-order aggregation of mitochondria that facilitated IFN-induction signaling (12). In contrast, MAVS-mediated IFN-induction signaling was dampened in cells harboring highly fragmented mitochondrial morphology, either by overexpressing a dominant-negative MFN1 (12, 85) or by administration of a chemical disrupting mitochondrial membrane potential (MMP) (86). To manipulate mitochondria toward fragmentation, the virus may suppress fusion or enhance fission. Even though DENV infection triggers MMP disruption (55), which may result in fragmentation of mitochondria (87), the DENV protease NS2B3 alone is sufficient to cleave both MFNs and manipulate mitochondrial morphology (12). Cleavage of both MFN1 and MFN2 suppresses MFN-mediated mitochondrial fusion processes and interferes in MAVS-mediated signalings, such as IFN and cell death induction (12). Hence, mitochondria may serve as platforms transmitting the IFN-induction signal, so that aggregated mitochondria help form a more operative signosome by tethering related molecules with each other. A seemingly conflicting report showed that DENV NS4B induces mitochondria elongation and thus restricts the RIG-dependent IFN response (88). This notion is also consistent with the scenario that disrupted mitochondrial fusion or misassembled signosome leads to disturbed IFN-induction signaling in DENV-infected cells.

CONCLUSIONS

With DENV infection, disease symptoms range from asymptomatic, classical dengue fever to life-threatening dengue hemorrhagic fever and severe dengue shock syndrome. The diverse disease symptoms result from a complicated interaction between DENV and the host. Innate immunity helps the host fight against infection by eliminating DENV and regulating follow-up immune responses. The non-canonical functions of DENV proteins and DENV-derived sfRNA in antagonizing the IFN system further damage infected cells in the battle between DENV and its host. DENV may defeat the host immunity at first line of defense. The seesaw of DENV-inducing and -antagonizing innate immunity in the initial state of infection may contribute to the DENV pathogenesis at some later time. Recent evidence shows that both viral and cellular factors are involved in the host responses upon DENV infection. Therefore, we highlight critical regulatory mechanisms of innate immunity by showing how DENV manipulates it. Notwithstanding unfinished puzzles, antiviral applications derived from all these studies are anticipated.

AUTHOR CONTRIBUTIONS

Y-TK and C-YY conceived and wrote the draft. Y-TK, ML, and C-YY wrote and proofread the manuscript.

REFERENCES

1. Morrison J, Aguirre S, Fernandez-Sesma A. Innate immunity evasion by dengue virus. *Viruses* (2012) 4:397–413. doi: 10.3390/v4030397
2. Green AM, Beatty PR, Hadjilaou A, Harris E. Innate immunity to dengue virus infection and subversion of antiviral responses. *J Mol Biol.* (2014) 426:1148–60. doi: 10.1016/j.jmb.2013.11.023
3. Gack MU, Diamond MS. Innate immune escape by dengue and West Nile viruses. *Curr Opin Virol.* (2016) 20:119–28. doi: 10.1016/j.coviro.2016.09.013
4. Goertz GP, Pijlman GP. Dengue non-coding RNA: TRIMmed for transmission. *Cell Host Microbe* (2015) 18:133–4. doi: 10.1016/j.chom.2015.07.009
5. Manokaran G, Finol E, Wang C, Gunaratne J, Bahl J, Ong EZ, et al. Dengue subgenomic RNA binds TRIM25 to inhibit interferon expression for epidemiological fitness. *Science* (2015) 350:217–21. doi: 10.1126/science.aab3369
6. Dalrymple NA, Cimica V, Mackow ER. Dengue virus ns proteins inhibit RIG-I/MAVS signaling by blocking TBK1/IRF3 phosphorylation: dengue virus serotype 1 NS4A is a unique interferon-regulating virulence determinant. *mBio* (2015) 6:e00553–15. doi: 10.1128/mBio.00553-15
7. Munoz-Jordan JL, Sanchez-Burgos GG, Laurent-Rolle M, Garcia-Sastre A. Inhibition of interferon signaling by dengue virus. *Pro Nat Acad Sci USA.* (2003) 100:14333–8. doi: 10.1073/pnas.2335168100
8. Aguirre S, Luthra P, Sanchez-Aparicio MT, Maestre AM, Patel J, Lamothe F, et al. Dengue virus NS2B protein targets cGAS for degradation and prevents mitochondrial DNA sensing during infection. *Nat Microbiol.* (2017) 2:17037. doi: 10.1038/nmicrobiol.2017.37
9. Aguirre S, Maestre AM, Pagni S, Patel JR, Savage T, Gutman D, et al. DENV inhibits type I IFN production in infected cells by cleaving human STING. *PLoS Pathog.* (2012) 8:e1002934. doi: 10.1371/journal.ppat.1002934
10. Yu CY, Chang TH, Liang JJ, Chiang RL, Lee YL, Liao CL, et al. Dengue virus targets the adaptor protein MITA to subvert host innate immunity. *PLoS Pathog.* (2012) 8:e1002780. doi: 10.1371/journal.ppat.1002780
11. Anglero-Rodriguez YI, Pantoja P, Sariol CA. Dengue virus subverts the interferon induction pathway via NS2B/3 protease-IkappaB kinase epsilon interaction. *Clin Vaccine Immunol.* (2014) 21:29–38. doi: 10.1128/CVI.00500-13
12. Yu CY, Liang JJ, Li JK, Lee YL, Chang BL, Su CI, et al. Dengue virus impairs mitochondrial fusion by cleaving mitofusins. *PLoS Pathog.* (2015) 11:e1005350. doi: 10.1371/journal.ppat.1005350
13. Chan YK, Gack MU. A phosphomimetic-based mechanism of dengue virus to antagonize innate immunity. *Nat Immunol.* (2016) 17:523–30. doi: 10.1038/ni.3393
14. He Z, Zhu X, Wen W, Yuan J, Hu Y, Chen J, et al. Dengue virus subverts host innate immunity by targeting adaptor protein MAVS. *J Virol.* (2016) 90:7219–30. doi: 10.1128/JVI.00221-16
15. Chang DC, Hoang LT, Mohamed Naim AN, Dong H, Schreiber MJ, Hibberd ML, et al. Evasion of early innate immune response by 2'-O-methylation of dengue genomic RNA. *Virology* (2016) 499:259–66. doi: 10.1016/j.virol.2016.09.022

16. Ashour J, Laurent-Rolle M, Shi PY, Garcia-Sastre A. NS5 of dengue virus mediates STAT2 binding and degradation. *J Virol.* (2009) 83:5408–18. doi: 10.1128/JVI.02188-08
17. Mazzon M, Jones M, Davidson A, Chain B, Jacobs M. Dengue virus NS5 inhibits interferon-alpha signaling by blocking signal transducer and activator of transcription 2 phosphorylation. *J Infect. Dis.* (2009) 200:1261–70. doi: 10.1086/605847
18. Morrison J, Laurent-Rolle M, Maestre AM, Rajsbaum R, Pisanelli G, Simon V, et al. Dengue virus co-opts UBR4 to degrade STAT2 and antagonize type I interferon signaling. *PLoS Pathog.* (2013) 9:e1003265. doi: 10.1371/journal.ppat.1003265
19. Apte-Sengupta S, Sirohi D, Kuhn RJ. Coupling of replication and assembly in flaviviruses. *Curr Opin Virol.* (2014) 9:134–42. doi: 10.1016/j.coviro.2014.09.020
20. Guzman MG, Harris E. Dengue. *Lancet* (2015) 385:453–65. doi: 10.1016/S0140-6736(14)60572-9
21. Nguyet MN, Duong TH, Trung VT, Nguyen TH, Tran CN, Long VT, et al. Host and viral features of human dengue cases shape the population of infected and infectious Aedes aegypti mosquitoes. *Proc Nat Acad Sci USA.* (2013) 110:9072–7. doi: 10.1073/pnas.1303395110
22. Carrington LB, Simmons CP. Human to mosquito transmission of dengue viruses. *Front Immunol.* (2014) 5:290. doi: 10.3389/fimmu.2014.00290
23. Conway MJ, Londono-Renteria B, Troupin A, Watson AM, Klimstra WB, Fikrig E, et al. Aedes aegypti D7 saliva protein inhibits dengue virus infection. *PLoS Negl Trop Dis.* (2016) 10:e0004941. doi: 10.1371/journal.pntd.0004941
24. Conway MJ, Watson AM, Colpitts TM, Dragovic SM, Li Z, Wang P, et al. Mosquito saliva serine protease enhances dissemination of dengue virus into the mammalian host. *J Virol.* (2014) 88:164–75. doi: 10.1128/JVI.02235-13
25. Schmid MA, Glasner DR, Shah S, Michlmayr D, Kramer LD, Harris E. Mosquito saliva increases endothelial permeability in the skin, immune cell migration, and dengue pathogenesis during antibody-dependent enhancement. *PLoS Pathog.* (2016) 12:e1005676. doi: 10.1371/journal.ppat.1005676
26. Chang TH, Liao CL, Lin YL. Flavivirus induces interferon-beta gene expression through a pathway involving RIG-I-dependent IRF-3 and PI3K-dependent NF-kappaB activation. *Microbes Infect.* (2006) 8:157–71. doi: 10.1016/j.micinf.2005.06.014
27. Rodriguez-Madoz JR, Bernal-Rubio D, Kaminski D, Boyd K, Fernandez-Sesma A. Dengue virus inhibits the production of type I interferon in primary human dendritic cells. *J Virol.* (2010) 84:4845–50. doi: 10.1128/JVI.02514-09
28. Castillo Ramirez JA, Urcuqui-Inchima S. Dengue virus control of type I IFN responses: a history of manipulation and control. *J Interferon Cytokine Res.* (2015) 35:421–30. doi: 10.1089/jir.2014.0129
29. Takeuchi O, Akira S. Pattern recognition receptors and inflammation. *Cell* (2010) 140:805–20. doi: 10.1016/j.cell.2010.01.022
30. Jensen S, Thomsen AR. Sensing of RNA viruses: a review of innate immune receptors involved in recognizing RNA virus invasion. *J Virol.* (2012) 86:2900–10. doi: 10.1128/JVI.05738-11
31. Doly J, Civas A, Navarro S, Uze G. Type I interferons: expression and signalization. *Cell Mol Life sci.* (1998) 54:1109–21. doi: 10.1007/s000180050240
32. Haller O, Kochs G, Weber F. The interferon response circuit: induction and suppression by pathogenic viruses. *Virology* (2006) 344:119–30. doi: 10.1016/j.virol.2005.09.024
33. Lin RJ, Yu HP, Chang BL, Tang WC, Liao CL, Lin YL. Distinct antiviral roles for human 2',5'-oligoadenylate synthetase family members against dengue virus infection. *J Immunol.* (2009) 183:8035–43. doi: 10.4049/jimmunol.0902728
34. Furuichi Y, LaFiandra A, Shatkin AJ. 5'-Terminal structure and mRNA stability. *Nature* (1977) 266:235–9.
35. Hyde JL, Diamond MS. Innate immune restriction and antagonism of viral RNA lacking 2-O methylation. *Virology* (2015) 479–480:66–74. doi: 10.1016/j.virol.2015.01.019
36. Daffis S, Szretter KJ, Schriewer J, Li J, Youn S, Errett J, et al. 2'-O methylation of the viral mRNA cap evades host restriction by IFIT family members. *Nature* (2010) 468:452–6. doi: 10.1038/nature09489
37. Zust R, Cervantes-Barragan L, Habjan M, Maier R, Neuman BW, Ziebuhr J, et al. Ribose 2'-O-methylation provides a molecular signature for the distinction of self and non-self mRNA dependent on the RNA sensor Mda5. *Nat Immunol.* (2011) 12:137–43. doi: 10.1038/ni.1979
38. Hyde JL, Gardner CL, Kimura T, White JP, Liu G, Trobaugh DW, et al. A viral RNA structural element alters host recognition of nonself RNA. *Science* (2014) 343:783–7. doi: 10.1126/science.1248465
39. Egloff MP, Decroly E, Malet H, Selisko B, Benarroch D, Ferron F, et al. Structural and functional analysis of methylation and 5'-RNA sequence requirements of short capped RNAs by the methyltransferase domain of dengue virus NS5. *J Mol Biol.* (2007) 372:723–36. doi: 10.1016/j.jmb.2007.07.005
40. Liu L, Dong H, Chen H, Zhang J, Ling H, Li Z, et al. Flavivirus RNA cap methyltransferase: structure, function, and inhibition. *Front Biol.* (2010) 5:286–303. doi: 10.1007/s11515-010-0660-y
41. Dong H, Fink K, Zust R, Lim SP, Qin CF, Shi PY. Flavivirus RNA methylation. *J Gen Virol.* (2014) 95(Pt 4):763–78. doi: 10.1099/vir.0.062208-0
42. Welsch S, Miller S, Romero-Brey I, Merz A, Bleck CK, Walther P, et al. Composition and three-dimensional architecture of the dengue virus replication and assembly sites. *Cell Host Microbe* (2009) 5:365–75. doi: 10.1016/j.chom.2009.03.007
43. Uchida L, Espada-Murao LA, Takamatsu Y, Okamoto K, Hayasaka D, Yu F, et al. The dengue virus conceals double-stranded RNA in the intracellular membrane to escape from an interferon response. *Sci Rep.* (2014) 4:7395. doi: 10.1038/srep07395
44. Nasirudeen AM, Wong HH, Thien P, Xu S, Lam KP, Liu DX. RIG-I, MDA5 and TLR3 synergistically play an important role in restriction of dengue virus infection. *PLoS Negl Trop Dis.* (2011) 5:e926. doi: 10.1371/journal.pntd.0000926
45. Surasombatpattana P, Hamel R, Patramool S, Luplertlop N, Thomas F, Despres P, et al. Dengue virus replication in infected human keratinocytes leads to activation of antiviral innate immune responses. *Infect Genet Evol.* (2011) 11:1664–73. doi: 10.1016/j.meegid.2011.06.009
46. Urcuqui-Inchima S, Cabrera J, Haenni AL. Interplay between dengue virus and Toll-like receptors, RIG-I/MDA5 and microRNAs: implications for pathogenesis. *Antiviral Res.* (2017) 147:47–57. doi: 10.1016/j.antiviral.2017.09.017
47. Meylan E, Curran J, Hofmann K, Moradpour D, Binder M, Bartenschlager R, et al. Cardif is an adaptor protein in the RIG-I antiviral pathway and is targeted by hepatitis C virus. *Nature* (2005) 437:1167–72. doi: 10.1038/nature04193
48. Kawai T, Takahashi K, Sato S, Coban C, Kumar H, Kato H, et al. IPS-1, an adaptor triggering RIG-I- and Mda5-mediated type I interferon induction. *Nat. Immunol.* (2005) 6:981–8. doi: 10.1038/ni1243
49. Seth RB, Sun L, Ea CK, Chen ZJ. Identification and characterization of MAVS, a mitochondrial antiviral signaling protein that activates NF-kappaB and IRF 3. *Cell* (2005) 122:669-82. doi: 10.1016/j.cell.2005.08.012
50. Xu LG, Wang YY, Han KJ, Li LY, Zhai Z, Shu HB. VISA is an adapter protein required for virus-triggered IFN-beta signaling. *Mol Cell* (2005) 19:727-40. doi: 10.1016/j.molcel.2005.08.014
51. Kato H, Takeuchi O, Mikamo-Satoh E, Hirai R, Kawai T, Matsushita K, et al. Length-dependent recognition of double-stranded ribonucleic acids by retinoic acid-inducible gene-I and melanoma differentiation-associated gene 5. *J Exp Med.* (2008) 205:1601–10. doi: 10.1084/jem.20080091
52. Takahasi K, Yoneyama M, Nishihori T, Hirai R, Kumeta H, Narita R, et al. Nonself RNA-sensing mechanism of RIG-I helicase and activation of antiviral immune responses. *Mol Cell* (2008) 29:428–40. doi: 10.1016/j.molcel.2007.11.028
53. Weber M, Gawanbacht A, Habjan M, Rang A, Borner C, Schmidt AM, et al. Incoming RNA virus nucleocapsids containing a 5'-triphosphorylated genome activate RIG-I and antiviral signaling. *Cell Host Microbe* (2013) 13:336–46. doi: 10.1016/j.chom.2013.01.012
54. Loo YM, Fornek J, Crochet N, Bajwa G, Perwitasari O, Martinez-Sobrido L, et al. Distinct RIG-I and MDA5 signaling by RNA viruses in innate immunity. *J Virol.* (2008) 82:335–45. doi: 10.1128/JVI.01080-07
55. Yu CY, Chiang RL, Chang TH, Liao CL, Lin YL. The interferon stimulator mitochondrial antiviral signaling protein facilitates cell death by disrupting the mitochondrial membrane potential and by activating caspases. *J Virol.* (2010) 84:2421–31. doi: 10.1128/JVI.02174-09

56. Perry ST, Prestwood TR, Lada SM, Benedict CA, Shresta S. Cardif-mediated signaling controls the initial innate response to dengue virus *in vivo*. *J Virol.* (2009) 83:8276–81. doi: 10.1128/JVI.00365-09
57. Schoggins JW, Rice CM. Interferon-stimulated genes and their antiviral effector functions. *Curr Opin Virol.* (2011) 1:519–25. doi: 10.1016/j.coviro.2011.10.008
58. Gack MU, Shin YC, Joo CH, Urano T, Liang C, Sun L, et al. TRIM25 RING-finger E3 ubiquitin ligase is essential for RIG-I-mediated antiviral activity. *Nature* (2007) 446:916–20. doi: 10.1038/nature05732
59. Gack MU, Kirchhofer A, Shin YC, Inn KS, Liang C, Cui S, et al. Roles of RIG-I N-terminal tandem CARD and splice variant in TRIM25-mediated antiviral signal transduction. *Proc Nat Acad Sci USA.* (2008) 105:16743–8. doi: 10.1073/pnas.0804947105
60. Peisley A, Wu B, Xu H, Chen ZJ, Hur S. Structural basis for ubiquitin-mediated antiviral signal activation by RIG-I. *Nature* (2014) 509:110–4. doi: 10.1038/nature13140
61. Liu HM, Loo YM, Horner SM, Zornetzer GA, Katze MG, Gale M, Jr. The mitochondrial targeting chaperone 14-3-3epsilon regulates a RIG-I translocon that mediates membrane association and innate antiviral immunity. *Cell Host Microbe* (2012) 11:528–37. doi: 10.1016/j.chom.2012.04.006
62. Pijlman GP, Funk A, Kondratieva N, Leung J, Torres S, van der Aa L, et al. A highly structured, nuclease-resistant, noncoding RNA produced by flaviviruses is required for pathogenicity. *Cell Host Microbe* (2008) 4:579–91. doi: 10.1016/j.chom.2008.10.007
63. Heil F, Hemmi H, Hochrein H, Ampenberger F, Kirschning C, Akira S, et al. Species-specific recognition of single-stranded RNA via toll-like receptor 7 and 8. *Science* (2004) 303:1526–9. doi: 10.1126/science.1093620
64. Tsai YT, Chang SY, Lee CN, Kao CL. Human TLR3 recognizes dengue virus and modulates viral replication *in vitro*. *Cel Microbiol.* (2009) 11:604–15. doi: 10.1111/j.1462-5822.2008.01277.x
65. Sariol CA, Martinez MI, Rivera F, Rodriguez IV, Pantoja P, Abel K, et al. Decreased dengue replication and an increased anti-viral humoral response with the use of combined Toll-like receptor 3 and 7/8 agonists in macaques. *PLoS ONE* (2011) 6:e19323. doi: 10.1371/journal.pone.0019323
66. Sparrer KM, Gack MU. Intracellular detection of viral nucleic acids. *Curr Opin Microbiol.* (2015) 26:1–9. doi: 10.1016/j.mib.2015.03.001
67. Sun L, Wu J, Du F, Chen X, Chen ZJ. Cyclic GMP-AMP synthase is a cytosolic DNA sensor that activates the type I interferon pathway. *Science* (2013) 339:786–91. doi: 10.1126/science.1232458
68. Chen Q, Sun L, Chen ZJ. Regulation and function of the cGAS-STING pathway of cytosolic DNA sensing. *Nat Immunol.* (2016) 17:1142–9. doi: 10.1038/ni.3558
69. Ishikawa H, Barber GN. STING is an endoplasmic reticulum adaptor that facilitates innate immune signalling. *Nature* (2008) 455:674–8. doi: 10.1038/nature07317
70. Zhong B, Yang Y, Li S, Wang YY, Li Y, Diao F, et al. The adaptor protein MITA links virus-sensing receptors to IRF3 transcription factor activation. *Immunity* (2008) 29:538–50. doi: 10.1016/j.immuni.2008.09.003
71. Sun W, Li Y, Chen L, Chen H, You F, Zhou X, et al. ERIS, an endoplasmic reticulum IFN stimulator, activates innate immune signaling through dimerization. *Proc Nat Acad Sci USA.* (2009) 106:8653–8. doi: 10.1073/pnas.0900850106
72. Jin L, Waterman PM, Jonscher KR, Short CM, Reisdorph NA, Cambier JC. MPYS, a novel membrane tetraspanner, is associated with major histocompatibility complex class II and mediates transduction of apoptotic signals. *Mol Cell Biol.* (2008) 28:5014–26. doi: 10.1128/MCB.00640-08
73. Abe T, Barber GN. Cytosolic-DNA-mediated, STING-dependent proinflammatory gene induction necessitates canonical NF-kappaB activation through TBK1. *J Virol.* (2014) 88:5328–41. doi: 10.1128/JVI.00037-14
74. Li Y, Wilson HL, Kiss-Toth E. Regulating STING in health and disease. *J Inflammation* (2017) 14:11. doi: 10.1186/s12950-017-0159-2
75. Zevini A, Olagnier D, Hiscott J. Crosstalk between Cytoplasmic RIG-I and STING Sensing Pathways. *Trends Immunol.* (2017) 38:194–205. doi: 10.1016/j.it.2016.12.004
76. Rodriguez-Madoz JR, Belicha-Villanueva A, Bernal-Rubio D, Ashour J, Ayllon J, Fernandez-Sesma A. Inhibition of the type I interferon response in human dendritic cells by dengue virus infection requires a catalytically active NS2B3 complex. *J Virol.* (2010) 84:9760–74. doi: 10.1128/JVI.01051-10
77. Platanias LC. Mechanisms of type-I- and type-II-interferon-mediated signalling. *Nat Rev Immunol.* (2005) 5:375–86. doi: 10.1038/nri1604
78. Ivashkiv LB, Donlin LT. Regulation of type I interferon responses. *Nat Rev Immunol.* (2014) 14:36–49. doi: 10.1038/nri3581
79. Kim TK, Maniatis T. Regulation of interferon-gamma-activated STAT1 by the ubiquitin-proteasome pathway. *Science* (1996) 273:1717–9.
80. Yeh HM, Yu CY, Yang HC, Ko SH, Liao CL, Lin YL. Ubiquitin-specific protease 13 regulates IFN signaling by stabilizing STAT1. *J Immunol.* (2013) 191:3328–36. doi: 10.4049/jimmunol.1300225
81. Su CI, Tseng CH, Yu CY, Lai MMC. SUMO modification stabilizes dengue virus nonstructural protein 5 to support virus replication. *J. Virol.* (2016) 90:4308–19. doi: 10.1128/JVI.00223-16
82. Palmer CS, Osellame LD, Stojanovski D, Ryan MT. The regulation of mitochondrial morphology: intricate mechanisms and dynamic machinery. *Cell Signal.* (2011) 23:1534–45. doi: 10.1016/j.cellsig.2011.05.021
83. Youle RJ, van der Bliek AM. Mitochondrial fission, fusion, and stress. *Science* (2012) 337:1062–5. doi: 10.1126/science.1219855
84. Hou F, Sun L, Zheng H, Skaug B, Jiang QX, Chen ZJ. MAVS forms functional prion-like aggregates to activate and propagate antiviral innate immune response. *Cell* (2011) 146:448–61. doi: 10.1016/j.cell.2011.06.041
85. Onoguchi K, Onomoto K, Takamatsu S, Jogi M, Takemura A, Morimoto S, et al. Virus-infection or 5'ppp-RNA activates antiviral signal through redistribution of IPS-1 mediated by MFN1. *PLoS Pathog.* (2010) 6:e1001012. doi: 10.1371/journal.ppat.1001012
86. Koshiba T, Yasukawa K, Yanagi Y, Kawabata S. Mitochondrial membrane potential is required for MAVS-mediated antiviral signaling. *Sci. Signal.* (2011) 4:ra7. doi: 10.1126/scisignal.2001147
87. Ishihara N, Jofuku A, Eura Y, Mihara K. Regulation of mitochondrial morphology by membrane potential, and DRP1-dependent division and FZO1-dependent fusion reaction in mammalian cells. *Biochem Biophys Res Commun.* (2003) 301:891–8. doi: 10.1016/S0006-291X(03)00050-0
88. Chatel-Chaix L, Cortese M, Romero-Brey I, Bender S, Neufeldt CJ, Fischl W, et al. Dengue virus perturbs mitochondrial morphodynamics to dampen innate immune responses. *Cell Host Microbe* (2016) 20:342–56. doi: 10.1016/j.chom.2016.07.008

10

Regulating IRFs in IFN Driven Disease

*Caroline A. Jefferies**

Department of Medicine, Division of Rheumatology and Department of Biomedical Sciences, Cedars Sinai Medical Center, Los Angeles, CA, United States

***Correspondence:**
Caroline A. Jefferies
caroline.jefferies@cshs.org

The Interferon regulatory factors (IRFs) are a family of transcription factors that play pivotal roles in many aspects of the immune response, including immune cell development and differentiation and regulating responses to pathogens. Three family members, IRF3, IRF5, and IRF7, are critical to production of type I interferons downstream of pathogen recognition receptors that detect viral RNA and DNA. A fourth family member, IRF9, regulates interferon-driven gene expression. In addition, IRF4, IRF8, and IRF5 regulate myeloid cell development and phenotype, thus playing important roles in regulating inflammatory responses. Thus, understanding how their levels and activity is regulated is of critical importance given that perturbations in either can result in dysregulated immune responses and potential autoimmune disease. This review will focus the role of IRF family members in regulating type I IFN production and responses and myeloid cell development or differentiation, with particular emphasis on how regulation of their levels and activity by ubiquitination and microRNAs may impact autoimmune disease.

Keywords: interferon, ubiquitin, E3 ligase, microRNA, monocyte

Interferon regulatory factors (IRFs) are a family of transcription factors that regulate many aspects of innate and adaptive immune responses—including driving anti-viral responses, responding to pathogens to drive pro-inflammatory responses and regulating immune cell differentiation (1). Comprised of 9 family members, the IRFs share significant homology within their N-terminal DNA-binding domain (DBD) of ~120 amino acids which forms a helix-loop-helix motif that recognizes specific DNA sequences similar to the interferon stimulated response element (ISRE). The C terminal domain is more diverse amongst family members and confers their unique function via regulating their ability to interact with each other and proteins outside of the IRF family. In general, the C terminal domain of each IRF member contains a nuclear export sequence, an autoinhibitory sequence, and an IRF-association domain which for most family members contains serine residues that are phosphorylated to regulate activity. IRF family members can both homodimerize and heterodimerize, forming both transcriptionally active or repressive complexes as discussed below [reviewed extensively elsewhere (1–3)]. Given their central role as transcriptional regulators of type I Interferon (IFN-α and -β) biology, they have been implicated in in the pathology of several autoimmune and autoinflammatory conditions, including systemic lupus erythematosus (SLE) in which overexpression of type I IFNs is thought to be a major contributor to pathology (4, 5).

This review will address the role of IRF family members in regulating type I IFN production and responses and myeloid cell development or differentiation. Specifically, it will focus on providing an update on how regulation of their levels and activity by microRNAs or ubiquitination may impact IFN-driven autoimmune disease.

IRF FAMILY—ROLE IN TYPE I IFN BIOLOGY

The type I IFN system comprises 13 subtypes of IFN-α, in addition to IFN-β, IFN-ε, IFN-λ, and IFN-θ (6, 7). The main function of these cytokines is to direct anti-viral immunity: promoting differentiation of B cells into antibody producing plasma cells, inducing differentiation of naïve T cells to effector CD4 or CD8 T cells, reducing proliferation of Treg cells and driving the expression of MHC class I and II and costimulatory molecules on dendritic cells and monocytes (8). Under normal homeostatic conditions, IFN-α and IFN-β are produced in response to detection of viral RNA and DNA by pattern recognition receptors (PRRs). Toll like receptors 3, 7, and 9 are the canonical and best described of the PRRs that recognize viral RNA and DNA, but in more recent years cytosolic PRRs that detect intracellular RNA and DNA, such as RIG-I, c-GAS, and DDX41 have been recognized as key drivers of the antiviral response and type I IFN production [reviewed in (9)]. Both TLRs and cytosolic RNA and DNA can also recognize self RNA/DNA and drive the production of type I IFNs also. Self RNA and DNA released from dead or dying cells is detected by the endosomal TLRs, TLR3, 7, and 9, whilst damaged DNA or oxidized DNA released from damaged mitochondria is detected by cytosolic DNA sensors (10). These pathways are the primary drivers of IFN overproduction and IFN-driven pathology in SLE (11).

IRFs as Regulators of IFN Expression

IRF3, IRF5, IRF7, and IRF8 have been shown to be positive regulators of type I interferon gene induction downstream of pattern recognition receptors [**Figure 1**, reviewed in (12)]. Whilst IRF1 was the first IRF to be identified as an inducer of type I IFNs (13, 14), subsequent analyses in *Irf*$^{-/-}$ MEFs suggested IRF1 was non-essential for induction of IFNs in response to cytosolic viruses (15). IRF3 and IRF7, the two family-members with greatest structural homology, are now known to be the principal mediators of IFN induction, acting downstream of cytosolic RNA and DNA receptors and the TLRs (TLR3, TLR4, TLR7, and TLR9) (9). IRF3 is ubiquitously expressed, whereas IRF7 is expressed only at very low levels, except in plasmacytoid DCs (pDCs) where it is relatively abundant (16). However, IRF7 expression is induced by type I IFNs, resulting in a feedforward loop that maximally drives type IFN expression (17). IRF3 is activated by phosphorylation (by kinases TBK1 and IKKε), promoting dimerization, nuclear translocation, association with the co-activator CREB-binding protein (CBP) and binding to canonical interferon response element sequence (IRES) in the promoter of IFN-β and IFN-α (18–21). Interestingly, a two-step phosphorylation of IRF3 has been proposed which involves TBK1 phosphorylation at site II (threonine 405 or serine 406) to relieve an autoinhibitory loop and promoting interaction with its co-factor Creb binding protein (CBP) and facilitating phosphorylation and full activation at site I (serine 385/386) (22–25). Activation of IRF3 occurs at intracellular vesicles via assembly of adaptor complexes, which then recruit in TBK1 and IKKε. TLR3 and TLR4 both use the adaptor protein TRIF to recruit in TBK1 to endosomes and phagosomes respectively, whereas RIG-I/MDA5 recruit the adaptor protein IPS-1 to recruit and activate TBK1 at the mitochondrial membrane. The growing number of cytosolic DNA-detecting PRRs (c-GAS, DDX41, IFI16) utilize the adaptor protein STING, found in the ER membrane, which once activated, translocates to the Golgi membrane to recruit and activate TBK1 (26). IRF3 can also directly induce the expression of cytokines in addition to type I IFNs, including CXCL10, RANTES, ISG56, IL-12p35, IL-23, and IL-15, whilst inhibiting IL-12β and TGF-β (27–33). However, it is currently unknown whether IRF3 activation can modulate the expression of these additional cytokines in all cells and downstream of all PRRs.

In a similar manner IRF7 is activated by TBK1/IKKε downstream of cytosolic RNA/DNA sensors and TRIF dependent pathways. Here IRF7 can either homodimerize or heterodimerize with IRF3 to induce IFN-α/β expression (34). Previously it was thought that, IRF7 was not required for IFN-β expression in the early phase of a response due to its low basal level in resting cells, and that IRF3 in complex with CBP alone was required. However, consistent with a role for IRF7 as the master regulator of IFN responses (34), we now know from work in *Irf7*$^{-/-}$ MEFs that IRF7 in complex with IRF3 and CBP is essential for both the early and late phase induction of IFNs in response to single stranded RNA viruses. In pDCs in which the TLR7/TLR9 pathway is predominantly active, phosphorylation and activation of IRF7 is independent of TBK1/IKKε and instead involves recruitment of MyD88, recruitment and activation of IRAK1/2/4 signaling complex, resulting in IKKα activation and phosphorylation of IRF7, thus driving IFN-α/β expression in response to ssRNA or DNA viruses (35).

Together with IRF3 and IRF7, IRF5 is another important member of the family involved in driving IFN production. Indeed, a risk haplotype of IRF5 is associated with SLE and results in enhanced production of type I IFN. IRF5 is expressed predominantly in B cell, monocytes, macrophages and pDCs. Activation of IRF5 involves phosphorylation by IKKβ (36, 37) at conserved residues in the IAD domain. Similar to IRF3 and IRF7, this releases an autoinhibitory loop, promoting nuclear translocation and interaction with CBP. For example, mice lacking *Irf5* showed increased levels of type I IFN in their serum following infection with the RNA viruses vesicular stomatitis virus (VSV) or Newcastle disease virus (NDV) (38). This implicated the RIG-I like receptor signaling pathway in activating IRF5, which was confirmed by over-expression of MAVs inducing IRF5 activation and IFN-induction (36). In addition, bacterial sensing via nucleotide-binding oligomerization domain containing (NOD)2 has been shown to drive IRF5 phosphorylation (both via TBK1 and RIP2), leading to enhanced type I IFN expression (39, 40). In pDCs IRF5 is key to the induction of pro-inflammatory genes (IL-12, IL-6, TNF-α, and IL-23) downstream of TLR7/9-MyD88, featuring ubiquitination of IRF5 by TRAF6. Whereas, IRF7 is activated from late endosomes in response to TLR7/9 ligation to drive IFN expression, IRF5 is activated from early endosomes to drive inflammatory gene expression by binding MD88 directly, which in turn facilitates its ubiquitination and activation. Interestingly, IRF4 binds same region of MyD88 as IRF5 and negatively regulates MyD88 dependent signaling (41).

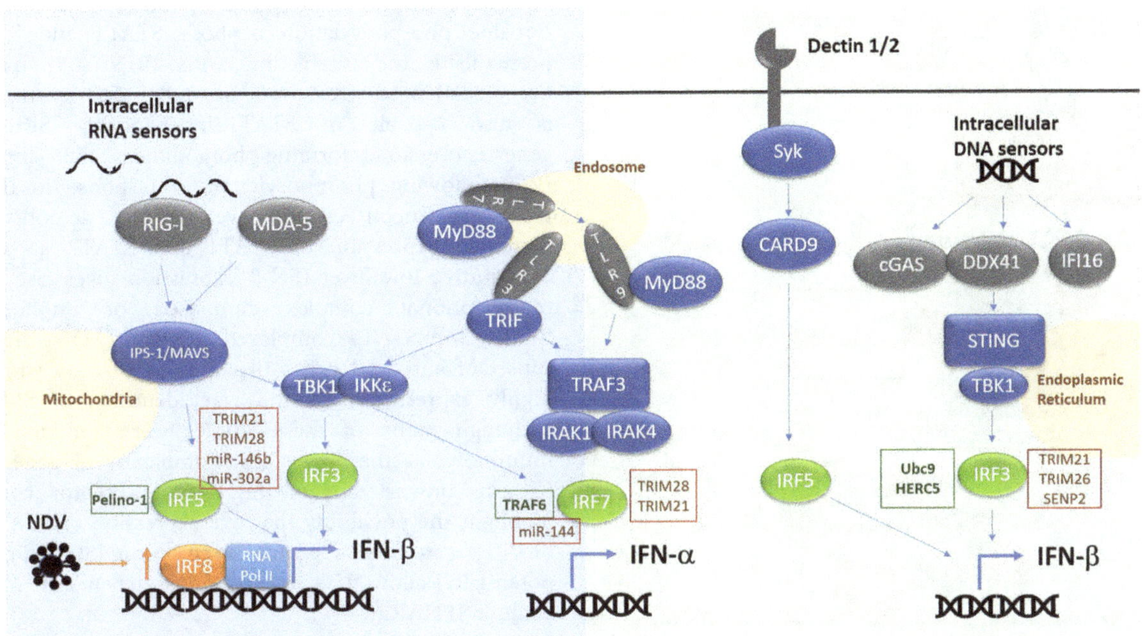

FIGURE 1 | Overview of RNA/DNA sensing pathways. E3 ligases and microRNAs regulating IRF family members are highlighted in text boxes. Green text box for positive regulators and red for negative regulators.

IRF5 is also involved in driving IFN-β expression downstream of C type lectin receptors (CLRs) such as Dectin-1 and Dectin-2 which recognize the β glucan cell wall of *C. albicans* (42). Such production requires Syk and Card9 in addition to IRF5 but is independent of other IRFs.

Thus, the co-ordinate activity of IRF3, 5, and 7 downstream of the various PRRs determines the extent of type I IFN induction and the pattern of cytokines induced. As to which IRF is activated in any given situation depends on both the initiating signal and the cell type involved. For example, in NDV-infected cells the IRF5/IRF7 heterodimer has an inhibitory effect on the *IFNA1* promoter, while IRF3 and IRF5 cooperatively activate this promoter (43, 44). In addition, overexpression of IRF5 or IRF7 results in expression of a different set of IFN-α subtypes, with IRF5-overexpressing cells driving mainly IFN-α8 expression, while IRF7-overexpressing cells produce mainly IFN-α1 (45). Thus, the potential exists that different levels of expression of IRF family members in different infection and disease settings will determine the level and subtype of type I IFN being produced. Indeed, given the central role for IRF3, 5, and 7 in regulating IFN expression, it is not surprising that they have been implicated in diseases such as systemic lupus erythematosus (SLE), which are driven in part by overexpression of type I IFNs. IRF5, for example, has a strong genetic association with disease (46), and a risk haplotype which results in enhanced IRF5 expression in SLE was found to correlate with enhanced levels of proinflammatory cytokines released from monocyte-derived cells from healthy individuals stimulated with NOD2 and TLRs ligands, thus indicating the presence of a correlation between *IRF5* genetic variants and IRF5-mediated transcriptional regulation of cytokine genes (47). Similarly, increased association of IRF3 with the promoter of IL-23 results in increased expression of this cytokine in SLE monocytes (33). A non-synonymous SNP in *IRF7* is associated with enhanced IRF7 activity and is associated with SLE (48).

A role for IRF8 in stabilizing the basal transcription machinery at type I IFN promoters to enhance IFN expression in dendritic cells (DC) and monocytes has also been reported. Whilst principally known for its role in proinflammatory gene induction, IRF8 also reportedly takes part in a second phase of interferon induction in dendritic cells in response to Newcastle Disease virus (NDV) which triggers IFN induction via activation of RIG-I dependent pathways (49). The role of IRF8 in DC-induced IFN-β requires upregulation of IRF8 expression in a feed forward loop which then works via prolonging the recruitment of the basal transcription machinery to the promoters of IFN genes in dendritic cells. This mechanism is also at play in monocytes (50). Indeed, original investigations into a possible role for IRF8 in DC function supports a role for IRF8 in mediating the development of IFN-inducing DC subsets (51–53). However, it should be noted that the role of RIG-I in IRF8-mediated IFN induction in DCs may be indirect, driving the expression of IRF8 for example rather than directly activating this transcription factor.

Signaling Downstream of IFN Alpha Receptor (IFNAR)

Canonical type I IFN signaling occurs following binding of IFN to the ubiquitously expressed type I IFN receptor (IFNAR), comprising two transmembrane proteins, IFNAR1 and

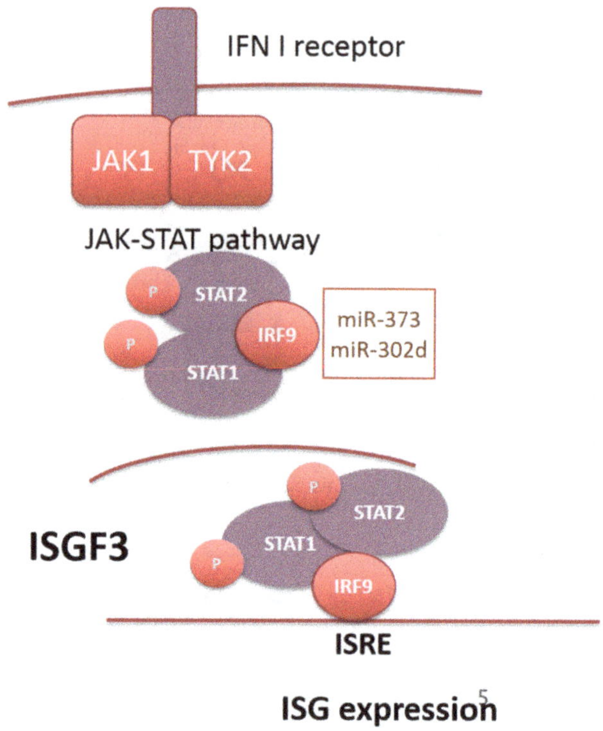

FIGURE 2 | Overview of signaling downstream of the IFN-alpha receptor. microRNAs targeting IRF9 are highlighted in the text box.

IFNAR2 (54). This results in activation of two cytoplasmic kinases JAK1 and TYK2, which subsequently phosphorylate the associated transcription factors STAT1 and STAT2 (55). Once phosphorylated STAT1 and STAT2 dimerize and interact with IRF9 to form the transcriptionally active complex, ISGF3, which binds to IFN-stimulated response elements (ISRE) in the promoter region of IFN-inducible genes (56, 57). In the ISGF3 complex, DNA binding activity is facilitated by IRF9, with STAT1 providing additional DNA contacts, thus stabilizing the complex (58). STAT2 provides a transactivation domain to enhance RNA pol II dependent gene expression but is unable to bind directly to DNA (**Figure 2**). In addition to ISGF3-dependent gene expression, STAT1 homodimers facilitate transcriptional responses to IFN-γ (and type I IFNs to a lesser extent) by binding to the IFN-γ activated site (GAS) DNA element. A type I IFN gene signature in the peripheral blood of SLE patients has been described which correlates with increased disease activity (59–61). This may result from enhanced levels of IFN-α or -β, or from constitutive activity of the JAK-STAT pathway, downstream of the IFNAR complex. For example, the JAK-STAT pathway has been shown to be activated in SLE patients (skin and kidney, specifically) (62–64) and in murine models (65, 66), with elevated levels of STAT1 protein detected both in monocytes and skin lesions from SLE patients. With respect to ISGF3, in a mouse model of pristane-inducible IFN-driven lupus, both IRF9 and STAT1 were shown to be required for autoantibody production and development of kidney disease (67).

Interestingly, the long-held paradigm that IFNα-driven tyrosine phosphorylation of both STAT1 and STAT2 is a prerequisite for interaction with IRF9 (68) has recently been challenged [reviewed in (69)]. For example, STAT2 is also capable of STAT1-independent ISRE-dependent gene expression, forming homodimers that interact with IRF9 following phosphorylation in response to IFN-α (70). However, Cheon et al. have recently demonstrated that increased expression of STAT1 and STAT2 as a result of constitutive low level IFN-β expression gives rise to a novel transcriptional complex composed of unphosphorylated STAT1 and STAT2 complexed to IRF9 (71), which drives a subset of anti-viral genes that overlap directly with the most highly expressed ISGs thus far identified in SLE patients. Although many of these studies were conducted in non-immune cells, they reveal the complexity of gene expression patterns downstream of the IFNAR receptor complex and highlight the possibility that overexpression of STAT1, STAT2, or IRF9 can have a profound effect on ISG expression and potentially allow ISG expression independent of signaling through IFNAR.

Role for IRFs in IFN-Driven Autoimmune Disease

The role of IRFs in infection, protective immunity and primary immunodeficiencies has been reviewed extensively elsewhere in this focused issue (72). Given the role of IRF proteins in regulating both the production and downstream signaling of type I (and type II) interferons, it is hardly surprising that they have been both genetically and biochemically shown to be important mediators of IFN driven autoimmunity (4, 73, 74). Systemic lupus erythematosus (SLE) is amongst the best characterized for the involvement of IFNs in disease pathology. For example, in SLE, elevated IFN-α is observed in over 50% of patients and correlates with disease severity, flare and tissue involvement (specifically skin, kidney, and central nervous system). In recent years a type I IFN gene signature in the peripheral blood of SLE patients has been described which correlates with increased disease activity (59–61). More recently, Rheumatoid Arthritis (RA) patients have been found to have a type I IFN signature which correlates with autoantibody production (75), indicating that type I IFNs play an important role in driving a subset of RA (75). The various effects of type I IFNs on both the innate and the adaptive immune system contribute to the breaking of immune tolerance to self, overactivation of myeloid cells, B and T lymphocytes and differentiation or polarization of myeloid cells (monocytes and neutrophils) and T cells to more pathogenic sub-types. With respect for a role for IRFs in mediating these effects, genetic association studies have identified IRF5 and IRF7 as being risk factors for developing SLE (76–80). IRF5, like IRF7, is an IFN-inducible gene and is found to be significantly upregulated in PBMCs from SLE patients compared to healthy controls. IRF5 was found to be constitutively activated in monocytes from SLE patients resulting in enhanced levels of IL-6, TNF-α, and IFN-α (81, 82). IRF5 has been shown to be critical for the development of SLE in MRL-LPR mice (80), with alteration in function or expression of IRF5 affecting both myeloid cells and B cells in SLE-like models (79, 83). The role for IRF7 has been suggested not only for is critical role in regulating IFN-a production by pDCs, but also genetic association studies showing certain SNPs in IRF7 to confer enhanced risk for developing SLE. Functionally these genetic variants were found to be associated with increased serum IFN-α in SLE patients with autoantibodies against DNA and the Smith autoantigen (84). Interestingly, IRF3 has also been shown to be associated with enhanced IFN-α levels in SLE patients, the study also identifying a novel genetic association in a Mexican cohort of SLE patients, suggesting that IRF3 may play an important but as yet underappreciated role in driving IFN expression in SLE (85). IRF3 is also strongly associated with RA—elevated levels of phosphorylated IRF3 have been identified in the synovial tissue of RA patients and IRF3 has also been strongly associated with ISG expression in RA (86, 87). Regarding a role for other IRFs in IFN-driven disease, we recently demonstrated that IRF9 expression is enhanced in SLE monocytes and positively correlates with ISG expression (88), indicating that perturbations of IRF9 levels may alter functional activity of the ISGF3 complex and potentially contribute to disease activity. The ability of IRFs to regulate IFN production and downstream signaling thus makes them important potential targets for therapeutic intervention—highlighting the importance of understanding how their activity is controlled in molecular detail. One aspect that is rarely considered in IRF biology is the effect that conventional treatments for autoimmune diseases via their ability to alter IFN expression may also affect the expression of IRFs in patients, given the fact that IRF3, 5 7, and 9 are all IFN-regulated genes. For example, glucocorticoids, the mainstay treatment for autoimmune and inflammatory disorders, inhibit the expression of IFN stimulated genes. They therefore not only alter the expression of IFN-regulated IRFs but can directly impact their activity by targeting an interaction between the glucocorticoid-sensitive coactivator GRIP1/NCOA2 and IRF family members—IRF9 and IRF3 specifically (89, 90). Thus, in IFN driven diseases glucocorticoid treatment would be expected to reduce the expression and activity of the IFN signature as has been shown for SLE (91) and RA (92). Another mainstay for treating IFN-driven diseases (particularly SLE) also has a direct effect on the expression of IFNs and can therefore affect IRF levels. These are the anti-malarial 4-aminoquinoline drugs chloroquine and hydroxychloroquine which accumulate in the endolysosomal compartment of cells and inhibit signaling of endosomal TLRs such as TLR3, 7, and 9 and hence IFN-induction. In SLE, patients on chloroquine/Plaquenil show a reduction in IFN levels and would therefore be expected to show corresponding changes in IFN-regulated IRF expression (93). Interestingly, chloroquine is implicated in directly regulating IRF3 activity via increased expression of the deubiquitinating enzyme USP25, which enhances IRF3 nuclear translocation and results in increased LPS-induced IFN-β expression (94). This raises the possibility that chloroquine can directly or indirectly affect the activity and expression of IRF proteins in SLE or other IFN-driven diseases.

Several anti-IFN therapies have been clinically evaluated in SLE in recent years with varying degrees of success. Sifalimumab improved disease in patients with moderate to severe active disease, reducing the level of IFN stimulated genes (ISGs) in patients with initially high ISG scores, whereas the effects of Rontalizumab were greatest in patients with low to moderate levels of ISGs (95, 96). Anifrolumab, a blocking antibody against the IFN receptor (as opposed to targeting IFN-α isoforms), has reportedly better efficacy, although responses are far from complete (97). Another contribution IFN-driven disease that cannot be discounted in the potential role of intracellular RNA/DNA receptors in regulating type I IFN production. The recent identification that mutations in *STING* or *TREX1* (which both work to regulate IFN-β production) drive monogenic forms of IFN-driven disease (interferonopathies) have suggested that dysregulation of these pathways may contribute to interferon driven diseases such as SLE or Sjogren's syndrome (98). Indeed, DNA released from stressed mitochondria in SLE neutrophils has been shown to drive IFN responses via the cGAS-STING pathway (99–101). More recently the cGAS-STING pathway has been shown to contribute to ISG regulation, independent of type I signaling through the IFNAR complex, indicating that other mechanisms may be at play in driving ISG expression in cells (102). Whether cGAS-STING activation of IRF3/IRF5 drives ISG expression directly in this scenario, or whether it drives expression of type III IFNs (IL-28A, IL-28B, and IL-29) which can also drive expression of ISGs (103), remains to be fully explored. These studies highlight the need to understand these pathways in molecular detail and underscore the complexity of targeting the IFN system therapeutically.

IMMUNE CELL DEVELOPMENT AND DIFFERENTIATION

In addition to regulating IFN production IRFs have important roles in regulating immune cell development and differentiation (**Figure 3**). Whilst IRFs have been shown to regulate both lymphoid and myeloid cell development and differentiation, possibly their most influential role is observed in regulating dendritic cell (DC) subset development and macrophage differentiation/polarization, with obvious consequences for inflammatory outcomes.

Myeloid Cell Development

Hematopoietic stem cells give rise to both the myeloid and lymphoid arms of hematopoietic lineage. Myeloid cells derive primarily from the Common Myeloid Progenitor (CMP) whereas the lymphoid arm derive from the Common Lymphoid Progenitor (CLP). The CMP can give rise to all types of myeloid cells, including monocytes, neutrophils and most types of dendritic cells (DCs). A unique subset of DCs, termed plasmacytoid DCs derive from CLP. IRFs play an integral role in both DC and monocyte development. DCs are essential for antigen presentation and act as the bridge between innate and adaptive immune responses. They comprise four main subsets of DCs—conventional DCs (cDCs), plasmacytoid DCs (pDCs),

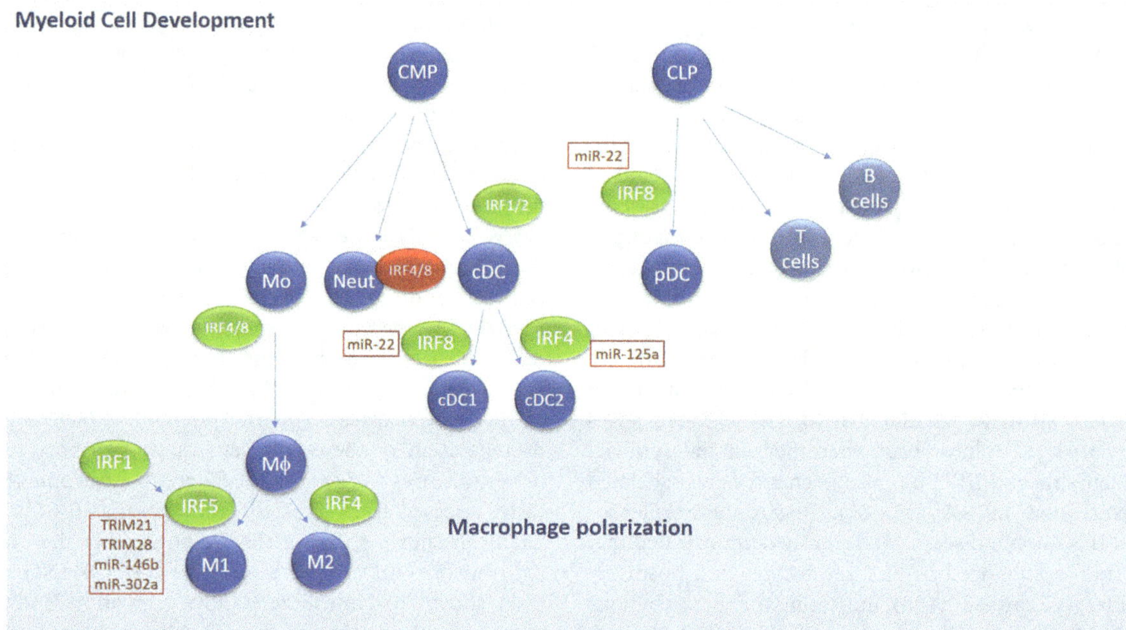

FIGURE 3 | Overview of IRF involvement in myeloid cell development and macrophage differentiation. E3 ligases and microRNAs regulating IRF family members are highlighted in text boxes. Green text box for positive regulators and red for negative regulators. CMP, common myeloid progenitor; CLP, common lymphoid progenitor; Mo, Monocyte; Neut, Neutrophil; DC, Dendritic cell; MΦ, macrophage.

monocyte-derived DCs, and Langerhans cells. Conventional DCs in mice are further sub-grouped into cDC1 and cDC2 subsets with different markers for human and murine counterparts (104).

Each DC subset develops under the control of differential expression of IRF4 and IRF8 in collaboration with transcription factors such as PU.1, ID2, and KLF4 (105–108). For conventional DCs, IRF8 regulates cDC1 subset development in mouse and humans, characterized by expression of CD8 or CD103 in mice or CD141 in humans and by the expression of IL-12 following TLR engagement. IRF4 on the other hand regulates cDC2 subsets, which express high levels of CD11b and CD172 in both mouse and humans and are highly efficient at inducing $CD4^+$ T cell effector function and expansion. High expression of IRF8 in combination with E2-2 and Bcl11A are required for development of pDCs, which secrete high amounts of type I IFN in response to stimulation. IRF1 and IRF2 also appear to be important in regulating DC subset development—*Irf*$^{-/-}$ mice show a loss of splenic and epidermal DCs (due to augmented type I IFN signaling) (109, 110) whereas *Irf1*$^{-/-}$ exhibit an increase in pDCs and a decrease in $CD8^+$ DCs in mice, along with an increase of IL-10 and TGF-β (111). In addition to regulating DC differentiation, IRF8 also promotes the commitment of myeloid progenitors to the monocyte/macrophage lineage, whilst inhibiting development of neutrophils (112). *Irf8*$^{-/-}$ mice lack bone marrow resident macrophages, in addition to $CD8^+$ DCs and pDCs in lymphoid organs (53, 113, 114). IRF4 has also been shown to promote macrophage differentiation and impair granulocyte formation, but its role in these events is secondary to IRF8 (115). A recent role for IRF4 in negatively regulating myeloid-derived suppressor cell (MDSC) development and immunosuppressive function in tumors has recently been described (116), indicating the importance of understanding IRF-dependent regulation of myeloid cell development and function for disease.

M1/M2 Macrophage Polarization

Like DCs, macrophages play an important role in sensing pathogens, initiating innate immunity, and cross-talking with the adaptive immune system to generate an appropriate immune response. Like DCs and T cells, subsets of macrophages with differing functions have been identified [reviewed extensively in (117, 118)]. Broadly speaking they can be divided into inflammatory M1 macrophages and anti-inflammatory or resolving M2 macrophages. M2 macrophages can be further subdivided into M2a-M2d subsets. Stimuli such as GM-CSF, LPS, and IFN-γ are potent drivers of M1 polarization for example, whereas fungal products, immune complexes, M-CSF and IL-4, IL-13, IL-10, and TGF-β all promote M2 macrophages. M1 macrophages are characterized as secreting high levels of TNF-α, IFN-γ, IL-12, and IL-23, promoting strong microbiocidal functions and production of reactive nitrogen and oxygen species and promotion of Th1/Th17 responses. In contrast M2 macrophages regulate parasitic infections, promote tissue remodeling and repair and secrete immunosuppressive cytokines IL-10 and TGF-β. Regarding the different M2 subsets, M2a subtype is driven by IL-4, IL-13, and fungal and helminth infections. M2b is driven by immune complexes, IL-1/IL-18 and LPS, whilst M2c is elicited by IL-10, TGF-β and glucocorticoids.

Functionally, M2a and c secrete IL-10 and TGF-β and are generally immunosuppressive, whereas M2b secrete IL-1, IL-12, and IL-10 and are implicated in inflammatory diseases such as SLE. M2d macrophages have only been identified in mice thus far and are induced from M1 macrophages following exposure to ATP (119, 120). Phenotypically they play a role in tissue remodeling and repair and have been shown to be associated with angiogenesis through secretion of VEGF (121).

Regarding IRF involvement in M1/M2 differentiation, IRF4 is strongly associated with M2 polarization, interacting with other transcription factors and chromatin remodelers to drive M2a or M2c subsets (122). The histone demethylase Jumonji domain containing-3 (Jmjd3) is involved in depressing M2-associated genes by reversing epigenetic modifications and has been shown by Satoh *et al* to work in concert with IRF4 to induce M2 polarization (123). Both IRF4 and Jmjd3 induce expression of M2-specific genes, arginase 1, FIZZ1, Ym1, and mannose receptor (MR) in response to IL-4 stimulation. Both Jmjd3 and IRF4 expression is driven by IL-4 in macrophages, and they in turn reciprocally regulate expression of each other (123, 124). Thus, IRF4 and Jmjd3 regulate M2a polarization downstream of IL-4 and IL-13. IRF4 also antagonizes IRF5 binding to MyD88 and in this way promotes M2 over M1 differentiation (125). Whether IRF4 is required for M2b, M2c, or M2d polarization is currently unknown.

IRF5 is the key transcription factor regulating M1 polarization (126, 127). Various inflammatory stimuli such as GM-CSF, LPS, and IFN-γ can upregulate the expression of IRF5. Enhanced expression of IRF5 in M1 macrophages is required to drive transcription of M1 markers such as IL-12, TNF-α, and IFN-γ and repress IL-10 (128). IRF5 has also been shown to regulate IL-23 secretion from macrophages, thus triggering the differentiation of Th17 cells (126). Thus, by influencing macrophage polarization toward an M1 phenotype, IRF5 plays an important role in regulating downstream adaptive immune responses and T helper cell differentiation toward a Th1 or Th17 phenotype. IRF1 seems to facilitate M1 polarization in general—priming expression of inflammatory genes associated with an M1 phenotype, such as IL-12p35 and IL-12p40 and synergizing with IRF8 to drive IL-12 production. IRF1 can also directly co-operate with IRF5 in order to drive M1 polarization in response to IFN-γ (125) and IRF1 and IFN-β work together to enhance IRF5 expression and as a consequence, M1 polarization in U937 cells. Thus, IRF1 promotes M1 polarization through its ability to enhance IRF5 levels and activity. The ability of IRF4 to compete with IRF5 for MyD88 binding and hence activation of downstream signals, suggests that relative levels of IRF4 and IRF5 in macrophages are important determinants of whether cells will polarize toward M1 or M2 phenotype.

POST-TRANSLATIONAL REGULATION OF IRFS—UBIQUITINATION AND NON-CODING microRNA

Given the critical function of IRF family members in regulating IFN production and downstream signaling, and their role in regulating immune cell differentiation, means to regulate their activity are critical to preventing overstimulation of pathways and cells and consequent autoimmune disease. We will discuss two mechanisms to negatively regulate IRF family members—the post-translational modification of IRFs by ubiquitin and ubiquitin-like proteins and the epigenetic mechanism of microRNA (miR) targeting.

Ubiquitination

Ubiquitination, like phosphorylation, is a reversible process regulated by E3 ligases that add ubiquitin chains to targets and de-ubiquitinases that remove these chains [reviewed in (129, 130)]. Ubiquitin itself is a small, ubiquitously expressed, 76 amino acid (8.6 kDa) protein that is conjugated to an internal lysine of a target via the formation of an isopeptide bond between its C terminal glycine reside and the ε-amino residue of the lysine on the target protein. Ubiquitin chains are then formed on this initiating ubiquitin and the internal lysine targeted for polyubiquitination determines function—for example Lysine 48 (K48) linked chains target the protein for degradation, whereas K27 and K63 linked chains alter the activity of the protein target. Again, like phosphorylation, ubiquitination is a rapid method for activating or deactivating pathways. Indeed, signaling downstream of the PRRs is widely regulated by ubiquitination, both in order to activate signaling and to turn it off pathways once the response is deemed sufficient (131, 132). For example, the adaptor protein STING is regulated by multiple E3 ligases such as TRIM56, TRIM32 and AMFR, each activated by specific pathways in order to confer a specific outcome—i.e., STING activation, inactivation or relocalization. TRIM56 and TRIM32 catalyze K63-linked polyubiquitination of STING, driving dimerization and promoting its ability to interact with TBK1 and drive IFN-β expression (133, 134). K48-linked ubiquitination of STING by RNF5 and TRIM30a has also been reported, resulting in proteasomal degradation of STING and subsequent downregulation of cytosolic DNA-mediated signaling and IFN production (135, 136). AMFR on the other hand, in complex with INSIG1, catalyzes K27-linked polyubiquitination of STING, which acts as a platform to recruit in TBK1 and facilitating translocation to perinucleosomes and antiviral gene expression (137). Recently, ubiquitination of STING on K224 by the E3 ligase MUL1 has recently been shown to regulate its trafficking from the endoplasmic reticulum (ER) to the Golgi (138). In addition to ubiquitin, SUMO (small ubiquitin-like modifier) can also be covalently linked to lysine residues in target proteins, acting to regulate localization, protein-protein interactions, and activity of target proteins, a process known as SUMOylation. Indeed, TRIM38 has also been shown to regulate SUMOylation of STING during early responses to DNA virus, to promote its stability and enhance its activity (139). Thus, ubiquitination of proteins or addition of ubiquitin-like modifiers such SUMO is a highly dynamic, versatile, and effective means of regulating protein function and levels in cells.

The activity of IRF proteins is tightly controlled through both ubiquitination and SUMOylation. In general, ubiquitination and phosphorylation of IRFs are integrally linked, with one modification often being a pre-requisite for the other to take place (140). For example, ubiquitination of IRF7 by TRAF6 at lysine 444, 446, and 452 is required prior to TBK1/IKKε driven phosphorylation at serine 477 and 479 (141). The juxtaposition of both the ubiquitination site and phospho-acceptor site on IRF7 and other IRFs suggests that such these post-translational modifications work sequentially to recruit in all the players necessary for activation. And similar to STING, it appears that competing ubiquitin or ubiquitin-like modifications work to fine-tune and regulate IRF protein stability and function. For example, both IRF3 and IRF7 are negatively regulated by SUMOylation following viral infection in order to turn off and limit responses (142). TRIM28 is the E3 ligase that regulates IRF7 SUMOylation at K444 and K446 (143).

Regulation of IRF3 activity by ubiquitination or other ubiquitin like modifiers such as SUMO or ISG15, is highly complex, and most likely is highly dependent on context and cell type. IRF3 stability is regulated by K48-linked ubiquitination by TRIM21 promoting proteasomal degradation post TLR-stimulation in order to turn off and limit responses (144). Indeed, TRIM21 deficient mice develop SLE-like symptoms, accompanied by enhanced IFN levels, accompanied by sustained IRF3 levels post TLR-activation (145). TRIM21 also plays a role in autophagy and has been shown to interact with the p62 sequestersome protein, thus facilitating removal of IRF3 by targeted autophagy (146–148). In contrast, TRIM21 ubiquitination of IRF3 has also been shown to stabilize IRF3 activity via disrupting an interaction between IRF3 and Pin1, a protein that promotes IRF3 degradation (148–150). Both published and unpublished results from our group indicate that TRIM21-mediated regulation of IRF3 is complex and that it may in fact act to stabilize IRF3 in resting cells (as evidenced by decreased basal levels of IRF3 in TRIM21-deficient BMDMs) but then become activated, potentially by phosphorylation (151), to promote ubiquitination and proteolysis of IRF3 in order to limit and turn off anti-viral responses. TRIM21 also regulates IRF7 stability downstream of viral TLRs in order to limit antiviral responses (152). Like TRIM21, the E3 ligase RAUL adds K48-linked ubiquitin chains to both IRF3 and IRF7 and ultimately acts as a brake on the system in response to viral infection (153).

Similar to IRF7, IRF3 is also regulated by other ubiquitin-like modifiers: addition of SUMO and another modifier interferon stimulated gene 15 (ISG15) to on the N terminal DBD works to sustain IRF3 levels by protecting these sites from ubiquitination. Ubc9 for example SUMOylates IRF3 (142) whilst SENP2 is a deSUMOylating enzyme that removes SUMO for IRF3, presumably then allowing TRIM26 to ubiquitinate these residues with K48-linked chains, promoting IRF3 degradation (154, 155). ISGylation of IRF3 by HERC5 inhibits the interaction between IRF3 and PIN1, thus preventing Pin1-dependent IRF3 degradation (156). Thus, competing ubiquitin-like modifications on IRF3 work to either stabilize or degrade IRF3.

IRF5 stability is also regulated by ubiquitination. K63-linked ubiquitination of IRF5 by Pelino-1 for example positively regulates M1 polarization downstream of TLR4/IFN-γ. This study also linked the Pellino-1-IRF5 axis to regulation of glucose intolerance in obesity, with BMDMs from mice lacking Pellino-1 showing improved glucose intolerance when fed a high-fat diet (157). Work from our own lab has shown that TRIM21 differentially ubiquitinates different isoforms of IRF5, with IRF5-V1 and V-5 targeted or degradation by TRIM21 whereas IRF5-V2 and IRF5-V3 (IRF5-V2 linked to susceptibility to SLE) are resistant to TRIM21-mediated degradation, with obvious implications for downstream activity (158). TRIM28, a SUMO E3 ligase, is an additional negative regulator of IRF5 activity, promoting epigenetic modifications of IRF5-dependent genes (159).

Interestingly, ubiquitination of IRF1 is linked with stability and seems to be required for IL-1-induced expression of the chemokines CXCL10 and CCL5, thus promoting inflammatory cell recruitment (160). The E3 ligase responsible is the apoptosis inhibitor cIAP2, whose activity is enhanced by the sphigosphine-1-phosphate, catalyzing the addition of K63-linked chains onto IRF1. Recently Src family kinases have been shown to positively regulate K63-linked ubiquitination and accumulation of IRF1 in response to TLR7/8 signaling in monocytes and B cells (161).

As to whether other IRF proteins that are involved in regulating IFN production or downstream signaling pathways are regulated by ubiquitin-like post-translational modification remains to be determined. Given the fact that type I IFNs themselves rapidly induce expression of both E3 ligases [particularly the TRIM family (162)] that target IRFs, it is hardly surprising that many of these mechanisms are being considered as targets for therapeutic intervention in diseases driven by interferons such as SLE.

microRNAs Targeting IRF proteins

microRNAs (miRs) are important regulators of gene expression in a whole host of cellular processes and immune responses (163, 164). They are an evolutionarily conserved family of small (~22 nucleotides long) non-coding RNAs that function to bind the 3′ UTR of mRNA targets and thus regulate gene expression. Like coding RNA, non-coding RNAs such as microRNA can be either constitutively expressed or inducible—and the inducibility of these small epigenetic modifiers allows cells to exquisitely regulate and control various pathways—including those regulated by IRF proteins. Binding can trigger degradation of the target mRNA (as occurs in the majority of cases), prevent translation, or in rarer cases, stabilize the mRNA leading to positive regulation. The biogenesis and functions of microRNA have been reviewed extensively elsewhere (165–168). The focus here will be to review the role microRNAs play in regulating the levels of IRF protein members and how this contributes to both homeostasis and to disease.

There is a body of evidence to support a role for miRs in the regulation of pathways producing type I interferons and those downstream of the IFN receptor complex. For example, miRs have been implicated at all levels of TLR signaling, including manipulation of TLR levels themselves (169, 170). Downstream of the TLRs, miR-146 has been shown to target a number of signaling molecules, including IRAK1 and TRAF6 (171–173). The ability of a single miR to target multiple players on a particular pathway is a unique feature of these epigenetic regulators and suggests that they have evolved to regulate pathways and processes in the cell rather than individual players.

Regarding the IRFs that regulate IFN-α and -β production, both IRF5 and IRF7 have been shown to be targeted by specific miRs. miR-302a for example is induced by influenza A and targets IRF5 directly, in order to control and limit IFN production (174). Regarding regulating IRF5 to influence M1/M2 transition, IL-10 induces miR-146b, which in turn directly targets IRF5 to promote M2 differentiation (175). microRNAs that target IRF7 on the other hand have been linked to its role in regulating oncogenesis and apoptosis rather than IFN induction *per se*—for example in breast cancer cells, miR-762 targets IRF7, inhibiting proliferation and invasion in a matrigel assay (176). In a separate study, miR-541 was shown to promote vascular smooth muscle cell proliferation by targeting IRF7 and thus inhibiting apoptosis (177). Regarding how microRNAs might target IRF7 in order to regulate IFN production, miR-144 was shown to target the TRAF6-IRF7 axis, targeting TRAF6 in order to attenuate attenuating the host response to influenza virus, indicating that mechanisms to regulate IRF7 activity by microRNAs exist whether direct or indirect (178).

To date however, no miR has been uncovered that specifically targets IRF3—instead many have been identified that regulate upstream adaptor proteins and hence the activity of IRF3. For example, miR-3570 targets the adaptor protein IPS-1/MAVs in order to shut-off RIG-I dependent signaling. miR-576-3p was shown to be induced in response to RNA and DNA viruses via IRF3-depependent IFN-β production, in order to shut off and limit anti-viral responses. It achieves this by targeting STING, MAVS, and TRAF3, all 3 critical players in regulating IRF3 activity or facilitating type I IFN expression. Therefore, IRF3 drives a negative regulatory loop involving miR-576-3p (179, 180).

Regarding signaling downstream of the type I IFN receptor (IFNAR), IRF9 levels and activity are critical in mediating STAT1/STAT2 driven responses. A number of microRNAs have been published that target IRF9 directly. miR-373 for example is upregulated by Hepatitis C virus (HCV) and targets IRF9 and JAK1 in order to turn off and limit anti-viral defense mechanisms (181). Our own work has shown the IRF9 is also targeted directly by miR-302d. In this study we observed that miR-302d, an estrogen regulated microRNA, is decreased in SLE monocytes, resulting in enhanced expression of IRF9 (88). The level of expression of IRF9 positively correlated with levels of interferon stimulated gene (ISG) expression and also disease activity, indicating that disruption of the microRNA balance in cells may have important consequences for immune cell function, particularly in the context of autoimmune disease.

Regarding a role for microRNAs in targeting IRFs to influence myeloid cell development or differentiation, one would expect that targeting IRF4, IRF8, or IRF5 would directly influence these events. Indeed, as mentioned above, miR-302a targets IRF5 to influence M1/M2 levels in response to viral infection (174). miR-125a has recently been shown to regulate M1/M2 differentiation and inflammation, targeting negative regulators of inflammation such as A20 and promoting an M1 or pro-inflammatory phenotype (182, 183). A recent study showed that Notch-dependent upregulation of miR-125a in tumors inhibited tumor associated macrophage function and promoted M1 macrophages via its ability to regulate HIF1-a and IRF4 (184). Regarding regulating DC development or differentiation, IRF8 is the natural target as it positively regulates pDC over cDC. In this context, miR-22 directly targets IRF8 and was shown to be highly expressed in cDCs compared with pDCs and directly influence DC differentiation (185). Thus, understanding the role of microRNAs that target IRFs involved in myeloid cell function and development may have important relevance to disease pathology.

Given the numerous roles microRNAs play in fine tuning TLR and IFN responses, it is not surprising that the dysregulation of these molecules has been implicated in SLE. To date numerous examples of dysregulated SLE associated microRNAs have been identified (186–189). Best characterized in SLE are miR-146 and miR-125, which in addition to targeting IRF5 and IRF4, also upregulate IFN-α and RANTES, respectively, thus contributing to disease activity (190, 191). miR-125a, is downregulated in SLE, has been found to negatively correlate with levels of the chemokine RANTES, a major player in organ inflammation (192) and lupus nephritis (193). Investigations into the mechanism behind this revealed a role for miR-125a in negatively regulating Kruppel-like factor 13 (KLF13) expression, a transcription factor that binds and activates the RANTES promoter, thereby inducing its expression in T cells (194). Our own work has also confirmed *miR-125a* expression decreased in SLE monocytes and identified a novel target, IL-16, which regulates *CXCL10* expression in lung epithelial cells and helps drive lung inflammation in an autoimmune context (195). Given that monocyte and neutrophil subsets in SLE patients are key drivers of inflammation, understanding how microRNA changes in patients regulate IRF protein levels and hence contribute to myeloid cell development may be key in uncovering novel therapeutic targets.

FUTURE PERSPECTIVES

Numerous mechanisms exist to control the innate immune response and myeloid cell differentiation in order to prevent inflammatory and autoimmune disease. As IRF family members are critical in this respect, tight regulation of their levels and activity is one mechanism of maintaining tolerance to self-antigens such as self-nucleic acids. But in different diseases it appears individual IRFs have greater or lesser involvement [reviewed in (4)]. For example—IRF3 seems to be more important in synovial inflammation in RA and responsible for ISG induction, whereas its involvement in SLE does not seem to be as important. IRF5 may perhaps be more important in SLE. So rather than targeting a single IRF for all IFN-mediated diseases, we must first understand the complex interplay between the individual IRFs in specific diseases 9 and potentially sub-types of disease in order to understand how targeting individual family members will impact the immune response as a whole.

Regarding potential targeting strategies: Ubiquitination of IRFs is a rapid and versatile way to regulate both levels and activity of IRFs, whereas epigenetic targeting of IRFs by microRNAs can fine tune IRF expression levels. Both work in concert to tailor immune responses appropriately. However, many questions remain regarding the IRFs and how they are regulated as it pertains to IFN biology: for example—what role do IRFs play in IFNAR-independent induction of ISGs? Is it possible that different combinations of STATs and IRFs can replace the canonical ISGF3 transcriptional complex? What role does regulation of availability of IRFs by microRNA targeting play in this process? And finally, can we target E3 ligases to fine tune IRF function and levels? Answering these questions will undoubtedly contribute to our understanding regarding how IRFs contribute to the pathology of autoimmune diseases such as SLE, but its biggest impact will be in explaining the following: firstly how we can improve on current IFN-targeting strategies—i.e., will JAK inhibition provide enhanced efficacy compared with IFNAR targeting strategies? And secondly, potentially uncover additional new therapeutic targets—be they modulators of E3 ligase activity or RNA-targeting strategies. As central regulators of monocytes function and IFN biology, addressing these questions promises to have a big impact in IFN-driven autoimmune disease.

AUTHOR CONTRIBUTIONS

The author confirms being the sole contributor of this work and has approved it for publication.

REFERENCES

1. Tamura T, Yanai H, Savitsky D, Taniguchi T. The IRF family transcription factors in immunity and oncogenesis. *Annu Rev Immunol.* (2008) 26:535–84. doi: 10.1146/annurev.immunol.26.021607.090400
2. Taniguchi T, Ogasawara K, Takaoka A, Tanaka N. IRF family of transcription factors as regulators of host defense. *Annu Rev Immunol.* (2001) 19:623–55. doi: 10.1146/annurev.immunol.19.1.623
3. Yanai H, Negishi H, Taniguchi T. The IRF family of transcription factors: inception, impact and implications in oncogenesis. *Oncoimmunology.* (2012) 1:1376–86. doi: 10.4161/onci.22475
4. Matta B, Song S, Li D, Barnes BJ. Interferon regulatory factor signaling in autoimmune disease. *Cytokine.* (2017) 98:15–26. doi: 10.1016/j.cyto.2017.02.006
5. Santana-de Anda K, Gomez-Martin D, Diaz-Zamudio M, Alcocer-Varela J. Interferon regulatory factors: beyond the antiviral response and their link to the development of autoimmune pathology. *Autoimmun Rev.* (2011) 11:98–103. doi: 10.1016/j.autrev.2011.08.006
6. Ivashkiv LB, Donlin LT. Regulation of type I interferon responses. *Nat Rev Immunol.* (2014) 14:36–49. doi: 10.1038/nri3581
7. Platanias LC. Mechanisms of type-I- and type-II-interferon-mediated signalling. *Nat Rev Immunol.* (2005) 5:375–86. doi: 10.1038/nri1604
8. Stetson DB, Medzhitov R. Type I interferons in host defense. *Immunity.* (2006) 25:373–81. doi: 10.1016/j.immuni.2006.08.007
9. Wu J, Chen ZJ. Innate immune sensing and signaling of cytosolic nucleic acids. *Annu Rev Immunol.* (2014) 32:461–88. doi: 10.1146/annurev-immunol-032713-120156
10. Roers A, Hiller B, Hornung V. Recognition of endogenous nucleic acids by the innate immune system. *Immunity.* (2016) 44:739–54. doi: 10.1016/j.immuni.2016.04.002
11. Kanneganti TD, Kundu M, Green DR. Innate immune recognition of mtDNA-an undercover signal? *Cell Metab.* (2015) 21:793–4. doi: 10.1016/j.cmet.2015.05.019
12. Honda K, Takaoka A, Taniguchi T. Type I interferon [corrected] gene induction by the interferon regulatory factor family of transcription factors. *Immunity.* (2006) 25:349–60. doi: 10.1016/j.immuni.2006.08.009
13. Fujita T, Sakakibara J, Sudo Y, Miyamoto M, Kimura Y, Taniguchi T. Evidence for a nuclear factor(s), IRF-1, mediating induction and silencing properties to human IFN-beta gene regulatory elements. *EMBO J.* (1988) 7:3397–405. doi: 10.1002/j.1460-2075.1988.tb03213.x
14. Miyamoto M, Fujita T, Kimura Y, Maruyama M, Harada H, Sudo Y, et al. Regulated expression of a gene encoding a nuclear factor, IRF-1, that specifically binds to IFN-beta gene regulatory elements. *Cell.* (1988) 54:903–13. doi: 10.1016/S0092-8674(88)91307-4
15. Matsuyama T, Kimura T, Kitagawa M, Pfeffer K, Kawakami T, Watanabe N, et al. Targeted disruption of IRF-1 or IRF-2 results in abnormal type I IFN gene induction and aberrant lymphocyte development. *Cell.* (1993) 75:83–97. doi: 10.1016/S0092-8674(05)80086-8
16. Au WC, Moore PA, LaFleur DW, Tombal B, Pitha PM. Characterization of the interferon regulatory factor-7 and its potential role in the transcription activation of interferon A genes. *J Biol Chem.* (1998) 273:29210–7. doi: 10.1074/jbc.273.44.29210
17. Marie I, Durbin JE, Levy DE. Differential viral induction of distinct interferon-alpha genes by positive feedback through interferon regulatory factor-7. *EMBO J.* (1998) 17:6660–9. doi: 10.1093/emboj/17.22.6660
18. Sharma S, tenOever BR, Grandvaux N, Zhou GP, Lin R, Hiscott J. Triggering the interferon antiviral response through an IKK-related pathway. *Science.* (2003) 300:1148–51. doi: 10.1126/science.1081315
19. Fitzgerald KA, McWhirter SM, Faia KL, Rowe DC, Latz E, Golenbock DT, et al. IKKepsilon and TBK1 are essential components of the IRF3 signaling pathway. *Nat Immunol.* (2003) 4:491–6. doi: 10.1038/ni921
20. McWhirter SM, Fitzgerald KA, Rosains J, Rowe DC, Golenbock DT, Maniatis T. IFN-regulatory factor 3-dependent gene expression is defective in Tbk1-deficient mouse embryonic fibroblasts. *Proc Natl Acad Sci USA.* (2004) 101:233–8. doi: 10.1073/pnas.2237236100
21. Yanai H, Chiba S, Hangai S, Kometani K, Inoue A, Kimura Y, et al. Revisiting the role of IRF3 in inflammation and immunity by conditional and specifically targeted gene ablation in mice. *Proc Natl Acad Sci USA.* (2018) 115:5253–8. doi: 10.1073/pnas.1803936115
22. Qin BY, Liu C, Lam SS, Srinath H, Delston R, Correia JJ, et al. Crystal structure of IRF-3 reveals mechanism of autoinhibition and virus-induced phosphoactivation. *Nat Struct Biol.* (2003) 10:913–21. doi: 10.1038/nsb1002
23. Takahasi K, Suzuki NN, Horiuchi M, Mori M, Suhara W, Okabe Y, et al. X-ray crystal structure of IRF-3 and its functional implications. *Nat Struct Biol.* (2003) 10:922–7. doi: 10.1038/nsb1001
24. Mori M, Yoneyama M, Ito T, Takahashi K, Inagaki F, Fujita T. Identification of Ser-386 of interferon regulatory factor 3 as critical target for inducible phosphorylation that determines activation. *J Biol Chem.* (2004) 279:9698–702. doi: 10.1074/jbc.M310616200
25. Panne D, McWhirter SM, Maniatis T, Harrison SC. Interferon regulatory factor 3 is regulated by a dual phosphorylation-dependent switch. *J Biol Chem.* (2007) 282:22816–22. doi: 10.1074/jbc.M703019200
26. Chen Q, Sun L, Chen ZJ. Regulation and function of the cGAS-STING pathway of cytosolic DNA sensing. *Nat Immunol.* (2016) 17:1142–9. doi: 10.1038/ni.3558
27. Sakaguchi S, Negishi H, Asagiri M, Nakajima C, Mizutani T, Takaoka A, et al. Essential role of IRF-3 in lipopolysaccharide-induced interferon-beta gene expression and endotoxin shock. *Biochem Biophys Res Commun.* (2003) 306:860–6. doi: 10.1016/S0006-291X(03)01049-0
28. Goriely S, Molle C, Nguyen M, Albarani V, Haddou NO, Lin R, et al. Interferon regulatory factor 3 is involved in Toll-like receptor 4 (TLR4)- and TLR3-induced IL-12p35 gene activation. *Blood.* (2006) 107:1078–84. doi: 10.1182/blood-2005-06-2416

29. Lin R, Mamane Y, Hiscott J. Structural and functional analysis of interferon regulatory factor 3: Localization of the transactivation and autoinhibitory domains. *Mol Cell Biol.* (1999) 19:2465–74. doi: 10.1128/MCB.19.4.2465
30. Brownell J, Bruckner J, Wagoner J, Thomas E, Loo YM, Gale M Jr., et al. Direct, interferon-independent activation of the CXCL10 promoter by NF-kappaB and interferon regulatory factor 3 during hepatitis C virus infection. *J Virol.* (2014) 88:1582–90. doi: 10.1128/JVI.02007-13
31. Koshiba R, Yanai H, Matsuda A, Goto A, Nakajima A, Negishi H, et al. Regulation of cooperative function of the Il12b enhancer and promoter by the interferon regulatory factors 3 and 5. *Biochem Biophys Res Commun.* (2013) 430:95–100. doi: 10.1016/j.bbrc.2012.11.006
32. Xu P, Bailey-Bucktrout S, Xi Y, Xu D, Du D, Zhang Q, et al. Innate antiviral host defense attenuates TGF-beta function through IRF3-mediated suppression of Smad signaling. *Mol Cell.* (2014) 56:723–37. doi: 10.1016/j.molcel.2014.11.027
33. Smith S, Gabhann JN, Higgs R, Stacey K, Wahren-Herlenius M, Espinosa A, et al. Enhanced interferon regulatory factor 3 binding to the interleukin-23p19 promoter correlates with enhanced interleukin-23 expression in systemic lupus erythematosus. *Arthritis Rheum.* (2012) 64:1601–9. doi: 10.1002/art.33494
34. Honda K, Yanai H, Negishi H, Asagiri M, Sato M, Mizutani T, et al. IRF-7 is the master regulator of type-I interferon-dependent immune responses. *Nature.* (2005) 434:772–7. doi: 10.1038/nature03464
35. Ikushima H, Negishi H, and Taniguchi T. The IRF family transcription factors at the interface of innate and adaptive immune responses. *Cold Spring Harb Symp Quant Biol.* (2013) 78:105–16. doi: 10.1101/sqb.2013.78.020321
36. Ren J, Chen X, Chen ZJ. IKKbeta is an IRF5 kinase that instigates inflammation. *Proc Natl Acad Sci USA.* (2014) 111:17438–43. doi: 10.1073/pnas.1418516111
37. Lopez-Pelaez M, Lamont DJ, Peggie M, Shpiro N, Gray NS, Cohen P. Protein kinase IKKbeta-catalyzed phosphorylation of IRF5 at Ser462 induces its dimerization and nuclear translocation in myeloid cells. *Proc Natl Acad Sci USA.* (2014) 111:17432–7. doi: 10.1073/pnas.1418399111
38. Paun A, Reinert JT, Jiang Z, Medin C, Balkhi MY, Fitzgerald KA, et al. Functional characterization of murine interferon regulatory factor 5 (IRF-5) and its role in the innate antiviral response. *J Biol Chem.* (2008) 283:14295–308. doi: 10.1074/jbc.M800501200
39. Pandey AK, Yang Y, Jiang Z, Fortune SM, Coulombe F, Behr MA, et al. NOD2, RIP2 and IRF5 play a critical role in the type I interferon response to Mycobacterium tuberculosis. *PLoS Pathog.* (2009) 5:e1000500. doi: 10.1371/journal.ppat.1000500
40. Chang Foreman HC, Van Scoy S, Cheng TF, Reich NC. Activation of interferon regulatory factor 5 by site specific phosphorylation. *PLoS ONE.* (2012) 7:e33098. doi: 10.1371/journal.pone.0033098
41. Negishi H, Ohba Y, Yanai H, Takaoka A, Honma K, Yui K, et al. Negative regulation of Toll-like-receptor signaling by IRF-4. *Proc Natl Acad Sci USA.* (2005) 102:15989–94. doi: 10.1073/pnas.0508327102
42. del Fresno C, Soulat D, Roth S, Blazek K, Udalova I, Sancho D, et al. Interferon-beta production via Dectin-1-Syk-IRF5 signaling in dendritic cells is crucial for immunity to *C. albicans*. *Immunity.* (2013) 38:1176–86. doi: 10.1016/j.immuni.2013.05.010
43. Cheng TF, Brzostek S, Ando O, Van Scoy S, Kumar KP, Reich NC. Differential activation of IFN regulatory factor (IRF)-3 and IRF-5 transcription factors during viral infection. *J Immunol.* (2006) 176:7462–70. doi: 10.4049/jimmunol.176.12.7462
44. Barnes BJ, Field AE, Pitha-Rowe PM. Virus-induced heterodimer formation between IRF-5 and IRF-7 modulates assembly of the IFNA enhanceosome *in vivo* and transcriptional activity of IFNA genes. *J Biol Chem.* (2003) 278:16630–41. doi: 10.1074/jbc.M212609200
45. Barnes BJ, Moore PA, Pitha PM. Virus-specific activation of a novel interferon regulatory factor, IRF-5, results in the induction of distinct interferon alpha genes. *J Biol Chem.* (2001) 276:23382–90. doi: 10.1074/jbc.M101216200
46. Lazzari E, Jefferies CA. IRF5-mediated signaling and implications for SLE. *Clin Immunol.* (2014) 153:343–52. doi: 10.1016/j.clim.2014.06.001
47. Hedl M, Abraham C. IRF5 risk polymorphisms contribute to interindividual variance in pattern recognition receptor-mediated cytokine secretion in human monocyte-derived cells. *J Immunol.* (2012) 188:5348–56. doi: 10.4049/jimmunol.1103319
48. Fu Q, Zhao J, Qian X, Wong JL, Kaufman KM, Yu CY, et al. Association of a functional IRF7 variant with systemic lupus erythematosus. *Arthritis Rheum.* (2011) 63:749–54. doi: 10.1002/art.30193
49. Tailor P, Tamura T, Kong HJ, Kubota T, Kubota M, Borghi P, et al. The feedback phase of type I interferon induction in dendritic cells requires interferon regulatory factor 8. *Immunity.* (2007) 27:228–39. doi: 10.1016/j.immuni.2007.06.009
50. Li P, Wong JJ, Sum C, Sin WX, Ng KQ, Koh MB, et al. IRF8 and IRF3 cooperatively regulate rapid interferon-beta induction in human blood monocytes. *Blood.* (2011) 117:2847–54. doi: 10.1182/blood-2010-07-294272
51. Schiavoni G, Mattei F, Sestili P, Borghi P, Venditti M, Morse HC, III, et al. ICSBP is essential for the development of mouse type I interferon-producing cells and for the generation and activation of CD8alpha(+) dendritic cells. *J Exp Med.* (2002) 196:1415–25. doi: 10.1084/jem.20021263
52. Tamura T, Tailor P, Yamaoka K, Kong HJ, Tsujimura H, O'Shea JJ, et al. IFN regulatory factor-4 and−8 govern dendritic cell subset development and their functional diversity. *J Immunol.* (2005) 174:2573–81. doi: 10.4049/jimmunol.174.5.2573
53. Tsujimura H, Nagamura-Inoue T, Tamura T, Ozato K. IFN consensus sequence binding protein/IFN regulatory factor-8 guides bone marrow progenitor cells toward the macrophage lineage. *J Immunol.* (2002) 169:1261–9. doi: 10.4049/jimmunol.169.3.1261
54. Ng CT, Mendoza JL, Garcia KC, Oldstone MB. Alpha and beta type 1 interferon signaling: passage for diverse biologic outcomes. *Cell.* (2016) 164:349–52. doi: 10.1016/j.cell.2015.12.027
55. Darnell JE Jr., Kerr IM, Stark GR. Jak-STAT pathways and transcriptional activation in response to IFNs and other extracellular signaling proteins. *Science.* (1994) 264:1415–21. doi: 10.1126/science.8197455
56. Levy DE, Kessler DS, Pine R, Darnell JE Jr. Cytoplasmic activation of ISGF3, the positive regulator of interferon-alpha-stimulated transcription, reconstituted *in vitro*. *Genes Dev.* (1989) 3:1362–71. doi: 10.1101/gad.3.9.1362
57. Qureshi SA, Salditt-Georgieff M, Darnell JE Jr. Tyrosine-phosphorylated Stat1 and Stat2 plus a 48-kDa protein all contact DNA in forming interferon-stimulated-gene factor 3. *Proc Natl Acad Sci USA.* (1995) 92:3829–33. doi: 10.1073/pnas.92.9.3829
58. Bluyssen HA, Levy DE. Stat2 is a transcriptional activator that requires sequence-specific contacts provided by stat1 and p48 for stable interaction with DNA. *J Biol Chem.* (1997) 272:4600–5. doi: 10.1074/jbc.272.7.4600
59. Kennedy WP, Maciuca R, Wolslegel K, Tew W, Abbas AR, Chaivorapol C, et al. Association of the interferon signature metric with serological disease manifestations but not global activity scores in multiple cohorts of patients with SLE. *Lupus Sci Med.* (2015) 2:e000080. doi: 10.1136/lupus-2014-000080
60. Petri M, Singh S, Tesfasyone H, Dedrick R, Fry K, Lal P, et al. Longitudinal expression of type I interferon responsive genes in systemic lupus erythematosus. *Lupus.* (2009) 18:980–9. doi: 10.1177/0961203309105529
61. Bauer JW, Petri M, Batliwalla FM, Koeuth T, Wilson J, Slattery C, et al. Interferon-regulated chemokines as biomarkers of systemic lupus erythematosus disease activity: a validation study. *Arthritis Rheum.* (2009) 60:3098–107. doi: 10.1002/art.24803
62. Kawasaki M, Fujishiro M, Yamaguchi A, Nozawa K, Kaneko H, Takasaki Y, et al. Possible role of the JAK/STAT pathways in the regulation of T cell-interferon related genes in systemic lupus erythematosus. *Lupus.* (2011) 20:1231–9. doi: 10.1177/0961203311409963
63. Li J, Zhao S, Yi M, Hu X, Li J, Xie H, et al. Activation of JAK-STAT1 signal transduction pathway in lesional skin and monocytes from patients with systemic lupus erythematosus. *J Central South Univ Med Sci.* (2011) 36:109–15. doi: 10.3969/j.issn.1672-7347.2011.02.003
64. Liang Y, Xu WD, Yang XK, Fang XY, Liu YY, Ni J, et al. Association of signaling transducers and activators of transcription 1 and systemic lupus erythematosus. *Autoimmunity.* (2014) 47:141–5. doi: 10.3109/08916934.2013.873415

65. Wang S, Yang N, Zhang L, Huang B, Tan H, Liang Y, et al. Jak/STAT signaling is involved in the inflammatory infiltration of the kidneys in MRL/lpr mice. *Lupus.* (2010) 19:1171–80. doi: 10.1177/0961203310367660
66. Dong J, Wang QX, Zhou CY, Ma XF, Zhang YC. Activation of the STAT1 signalling pathway in lupus nephritis in MRL/lpr mice. *Lupus.* (2007) 16:101–9. doi: 10.1177/0961203306075383
67. Thibault DL, Chu AD, Graham KL, Balboni I, Lee LY, Kohlmoos C, et al. IRF9 and STAT1 are required for IgG autoantibody production and B cell expression of TLR7 in mice. *J Clin Invest.* (2008) 118:1417–26. doi: 10.1172/JCI30065
68. Pilz A, Ramsauer K, Heidari H, Leitges M, Kovarik P, Decker T. Phosphorylation of the Stat1 transactivating domain is required for the response to type I interferons. *EMBO Rep.* (2003) 4:368–73. doi: 10.1038/sj.embor.embor802
69. Au-Yeung N, Mandhana R, Horvath CM. Transcriptional regulation by STAT1 and STAT2 in the interferon JAK-STAT pathway. *Jak Stat.* (2013) 2:e23931. doi: 10.4161/jkst.23931
70. Blaszczyk K, Olejnik A, Nowicka H, Ozgyin L, Chen YL, Chmielewski S, et al. STAT2/IRF9 directs a prolonged ISGF3-like transcriptional response and antiviral activity in the absence of STAT1. *Biochem J.* (2015) 466:511–24. doi: 10.1042/BJ20140644
71. Majoros A, Platanitis E, Szappanos D, Cheon H, Vogl C, Shukla P, et al. Response to interferons and antibacterial innate immunity in the absence of tyrosine-phosphorylated STAT1. *EMBO Rep.* (2016) 17:367–82. doi: 10.15252/embr.201540726
72. Mogensen TH. IRF and STAT Transcription factors - from basic biology to roles in infection, protective immunity, and primary immunodeficiencies. *Front Immunol.* (2018) 9:3047. doi: 10.3389/fimmu.2018.03047
73. Crow MK. Type I interferon in systemic lupus erythematosus. *Curr Top Microbiol Immunol.* (2007) 316:359–86. doi: 10.1007/978-3-540-71329-6_17
74. Ronnblom L. The importance of the type I interferon system in autoimmunity. *Clin Exp Rheumatol.* (2016) 34(4 Suppl. 98):21–4.
75. Castaneda-Delgado JE, Bastian-Hernandez Y, Macias-Segura N, Santiago-Algarra D, Castillo-Ortiz JD, Aleman-Navarro AL, et al. Type I interferon gene response is increased in early and established rheumatoid arthritis and correlates with autoantibody production. *Front Immunol.* (2017) 8:285. doi: 10.3389/fimmu.2017.00285
76. Bronson PG, Chaivorapol C, Ortmann W, Behrens TW, Graham RR. The genetics of type I interferon in systemic lupus erythematosus. *Curr Opin Immunol.* (2012) 24:530–7. doi: 10.1016/j.coi.2012.07.008
77. Byrne JC, Ni Gabhann J, Lazzari E, Mahony R, Smith S, Stacey K, et al. Genetics of SLE: functional relevance for monocytes/macrophages in disease. *Clin Dev Immunol.* (2012) 2012:582352. doi: 10.1155/2012/582352
78. Watkins AA, Yasuda K, Wilson GE, Aprahamian T, Xie Y, Maganto-Garcia E, et al. IRF5 deficiency ameliorates lupus but promotes atherosclerosis and metabolic dysfunction in a mouse model of lupus-associated atherosclerosis. *J Immunol.* (2015) 194:1467–79. doi: 10.4049/jimmunol.1402807
79. Yasuda K, Watkins AA, Kochar GS, Wilson GE, Laskow B, Richez C, et al. Interferon regulatory factor-5 deficiency ameliorates disease severity in the MRL/lpr mouse model of lupus in the absence of a mutation in DOCK2. *PLoS ONE.* (2014) 9:e103478. doi: 10.1371/journal.pone.0103478
80. Tada Y, Kondo S, Aoki S, Koarada S, Inoue H, Suematsu R, et al. Interferon regulatory factor 5 is critical for the development of lupus in MRL/lpr mice. *Arthritis Rheum.* (2011) 63:738–48. doi: 10.1002/art.30183
81. Stone RC, Feng D, Deng J, Singh S, Yang L, Fitzgerald-Bocarsly P, et al. Interferon regulatory factor 5 activation in monocytes of systemic lupus erythematosus patients is triggered by circulating autoantigens independent of type I interferons. *Arthritis Rheum.* (2012) 64:788–98. doi: 10.1002/art.33395
82. Feng D, Stone RC, Eloranta ML, Sangster-Guity N, Nordmark G, Sigurdsson S, et al. Genetic variants and disease-associated factors contribute to enhanced interferon regulatory factor 5 expression in blood cells of patients with systemic lupus erythematosus. *Arthritis Rheum.* (2010) 62:562–73. doi: 10.1002/art.27223
83. Yasuda K, Nundel K, Watkins AA, Dhawan T, Bonegio RG, Ubellacker JM, et al. Phenotype and function of B cells and dendritic cells from interferon regulatory factor 5-deficient mice with and without a mutation in DOCK2. *Int Immunol.* (2013) 25:295–306. doi: 10.1093/intimm/dxs114
84. Salloum R, Franek BS, Kariuki SN, Rhee L, Mikolaitis RA, Jolly M, et al. Genetic variation at the IRF7/PHRF1 locus is associated with autoantibody profile and serum interferon-alpha activity in lupus patients. *Arthritis Rheum.* (2010) 62:553–61. doi: 10.1002/art.27182
85. Santana-de Anda K, Gomez-Martin D, Monsivais-Urenda AE, Salgado-Bustamante M, Gonzalez-Amaro R, Alcocer-Varela J. Interferon regulatory factor 3 as key element of the interferon signature in plasmacytoid dendritic cells from systemic lupus erythematosus patients: novel genetic associations in the Mexican mestizo population. *Clin Exp Immunol.* (2014) 178:428–37. doi: 10.1111/cei.12429
86. Sweeney SE, Kimbler TB, Firestein GS. Synoviocyte innate immune responses: II. Pivotal role of IFN regulatory factor 3. *J Immunol.* (2010) 184:7162–8. doi: 10.4049/jimmunol.0903944
87. Sweeney SE, Mo L, Firestein GS. Antiviral gene expression in rheumatoid arthritis: role of IKKepsilon and interferon regulatory factor 3. *Arthritis Rheum.* (2007) 56:743–52. doi: 10.1002/art.22421
88. Smith S. MicroRNA-302d targets IRF9 to regulate the IFN-induced gene expression in SLE. (2017) 79:105–11. doi: 10.1016/j.jaut.2017.03.003
89. Flammer JR, Dobrovolna J, Kennedy MA, Chinenov Y, Glass CK, Ivashkiv LB, et al. The type I interferon signaling pathway is a target for glucocorticoid inhibition. *Mol Cell Biol.* (2010) 30:4564–74. doi: 10.1128/MCB.00146-10
90. Reily MM, Pantoja C, Hu X, Chinenov Y, and Rogatsky I. The GRIP1:IRF3 interaction as a target for glucocorticoid receptor-mediated immunosuppression. *EMBO J.* (2006) 25:108–17. doi: 10.1038/sj.emboj.7600919
91. Bennett L, Palucka AK, Arce E, Cantrell V, Borvak J, Banchereau J, et al. Interferon and granulopoiesis signatures in systemic lupus erythematosus blood. *J Exp Med.* (2003) 197:711–23. doi: 10.1084/jem.20021553
92. de Jong TD, Vosslamber S, Blits M, Wolbink G, Nurmohamed MT, van der Laken CJ, et al. Effect of prednisone on type I interferon signature in rheumatoid arthritis: consequences for response prediction to rituximab. *Arthritis Res Ther.* (2015) 17:78. doi: 10.1186/s13075-015-0564-y
93. Willis R, Seif AM, McGwin G Jr, Martinez-Martinez LA, Gonzalez EB, Dang N, et al. Effect of hydroxychloroquine treatment on pro-inflammatory cytokines and disease activity in SLE patients: data from LUMINA (LXXV), a multiethnic US cohort. *Lupus.* (2012) 21:830–5. doi: 10.1177/0961203312437270
94. Ding C, Li F, Long Y, Zheng J. Chloroquine attenuates lipopolysaccharide-induced inflammatory responses through upregulation of USP25. *Can J Physiol Pharmacol.* (2017) 95:481–91. doi: 10.1139/cjpp-2016-0303
95. Kennedy JW, Khan W. Total hip arthroplasty in systemic lupus erythematosus: a systematic review. *Int J Rheumatol.* (2015) 2015:475489. doi: 10.1155/2015/475489
96. Petri M, Wallace DJ, Spindler A, Chindalore V, Kalunian K, Mysler E, et al. Sifalimumab, a human anti-interferon-alpha monoclonal antibody, in systemic lupus erythematosus: a phase I randomized, controlled, dose-escalation study. *Arthritis Rheum.* (2013) 65:1011–21. doi: 10.1002/art.37824
97. Furie R, Khamashta M, Merrill JT, Werth VP, Kalunian K, Brohawn P, et al. Anifrolumab, an anti-interferon-alpha receptor monoclonal antibody, in moderate-to-severe systemic lupus erythematosus. *Arthritis Rheumatol.* (2017) 69:376–86. doi: 10.1002/art.39962
98. Lee-Kirsch MA. The Type I interferonopathies. *Annu Rev Med.* (2017) 68:297–315. doi: 10.1146/annurev-med-050715-104506
99. An J, Durcan L, Karr RM, Briggs TA, Rice GI, Teal TH, et al. Expression of cyclic GMP-AMP synthase in patients with systemic lupus erythematosus. *Arthritis Rheumatol.* (2017) 69:800–7. doi: 10.1002/art.40002
100. Carlucci PM, Purmalek MM, Dey AK, Temesgen-Oyelakin Y, Sakhardande S, Joshi AA, et al. Neutrophil subsets and their gene signature associate with vascular inflammation and coronary atherosclerosis in lupus. *JCI Insight.* (2018) 3:e99276. doi: 10.1172/jci.insight.99276
101. Lood C, Blanco LP, Purmalek MM, Carmona-Rivera C, De Ravin SS, Smith CK, et al. Neutrophil extracellular traps enriched in oxidized mitochondrial DNA are interferogenic and contribute to lupus-like disease. *Nat Med.* (2016) 22:146–53. doi: 10.1038/nm.4027
102. Kato Y, Park J, Takamatsu H, Konaka H, Aoki W, Aburaya S, et al. Apoptosis-derived membrane vesicles drive the cGAS-STING pathway and enhance type I IFN production in systemic lupus erythematosus. *Ann. Rheum Dis.* (2018) 77:1507–15. doi: 10.1136/annrheumdis-2018-212988

103. Wack A, Terczynska-Dyla E, Hartmann R. Guarding the frontiers: the biology of type III interferons. *Nat Immunol.* (2015) 16:802–9. doi: 10.1038/ni.3212
104. Guilliams M, Ginhoux F, Jakubzick C, Naik SH, Onai N, Schraml BU, et al. Dendritic cells, monocytes and macrophages: a unified nomenclature based on ontogeny. *Nat Rev Immunol.* (2014) 14:571–8. doi: 10.1038/nri3712
105. Chopin M, Allan RS, Belz GT. Transcriptional regulation of dendritic cell diversity. *Front Immunol.* (2012) 3:26. doi: 10.3389/fimmu.2012.00026
106. Belz GT, Nutt SL. Transcriptional programming of the dendritic cell network. *Nat Rev Immunol.* (2012) 12:101–13. doi: 10.1038/nri3149
107. Villani AC, Satija R, Reynolds G, Sarkizova S, Shekhar K, Fletcher J, et al. Single-cell RNA-seq reveals new types of human blood dendritic cells, monocytes, and progenitors. *Science.* (2017) 356:eaah4573. doi: 10.1126/science.aah4573
108. See P, Dutertre CA, Chen J, Gunther P, McGovern N, Irac SE, et al. Mapping the human DC lineage through the integration of high-dimensional techniques. *Science.* (2017) 356:eaag3009. doi: 10.1126/science.aag3009
109. Honda K, Mizutani T, Taniguchi T. Negative regulation of IFN-alpha/beta signaling by IFN regulatory factor 2 for homeostatic development of dendritic cells. *Proc Natl Acad Sci USA.* (2004) 101:2416–21. doi: 10.1073/pnas.0307336101
110. Ichikawa E, Hida S, Omatsu Y, Shimoyama S, Takahara K, Miyagawa S, et al. Defective development of splenic and epidermal CD4+ dendritic cells in mice deficient for IFN regulatory factor-2. *Proc Natl Acad Sci USA.* (2004) 101:3909–14. doi: 10.1073/pnas.0400610101
111. Gabriele L, Fragale A, Borghi P, Sestili P, Stellacci E, Venditti M, et al. IRF-1 deficiency skews the differentiation of dendritic cells toward plasmacytoid and tolerogenic features. *J Leukoc Biol.* (2006) 80:1500–11. doi: 10.1189/jlb.0406246
112. Tamura T, Nagamura-Inoue T, Shmeltzer Z, Kuwata T, Ozato K. ICSBP directs bipotential myeloid progenitor cells to differentiate into mature macrophages. *Immunity.* (2000) 13:155–65. doi: 10.1016/S1074-7613(00)00016-9
113. Scheller M, Foerster J, Heyworth CM, Waring JF, Lohler J, Gilmore GL, et al. Altered development and cytokine responses of myeloid progenitors in the absence of transcription factor, interferon consensus sequence binding protein. *Blood.* (1999) 94:3764–71.
114. Tamura T, Ozato K. ICSBP/IRF-8: its regulatory roles in the development of myeloid cells. *J Interferon Cytokine Res.* (2002) 22:145–52. doi: 10.1089/107999002753452755
115. Yamamoto M, Kato T, Hotta C, Nishiyama A, Kurotaki D, Yoshinari M, et al. Shared and distinct functions of the transcription factors IRF4 and IRF8 in myeloid cell development. *PLoS ONE.* (2011) 6:e25812. doi: 10.1371/journal.pone.0025812
116. Nam S, Kang K, Cha JS, Kim JW, Lee HG, Kim Y, et al. Interferon regulatory factor 4 (IRF4) controls myeloid-derived suppressor cell (MDSC) differentiation and function. *J Leukoc Biol.* (2016) 100:1273–84. doi: 10.1189/jlb.1A0215-068RR
117. Italiani P, Boraschi D. From monocytes to M1/M2 macrophages: phenotypical vs. functional differentiation. *Front Immunol.* (2014) 5:514. doi: 10.3389/fimmu.2014.00514
118. Roszer T. Understanding the mysterious M2 macrophage through activation markers and effector mechanisms. *Mediators Inflamm.* (2015) 2015:816460. doi: 10.1155/2015/816460
119. Ferrante CJ, Pinhal-Enfield G, Elson G, Cronstein BN, Hasko G, Outram S, et al. The adenosine-dependent angiogenic switch of macrophages to an M2-like phenotype is independent of interleukin-4 receptor alpha (IL-4Ralpha) signaling. *Inflammation.* (2013) 36:921–31. doi: 10.1007/s10753-013-9621-3
120. Pinhal-Enfield G, Ramanathan M, Hasko G, Vogel SN, Salzman AL, Boons GJ, et al. An angiogenic switch in macrophages involving synergy between Toll-like receptors 2, 4, 7, and 9 and adenosine A(2A) receptors. *Am J Pathol.* (2003) 163:711–21. doi: 10.1016/S0002-9440(10)63698-X
121. Corliss BA, Azimi MS, Munson JM, Peirce SM, Murfee WL. Macrophages: an inflammatory link between angiogenesis and lymphangiogenesis. *Microcirculation.* (2016) 23:95–121. doi: 10.1111/micc.12259
122. Gunthner R, Anders HJ. Interferon-regulatory factors determine macrophage phenotype polarization. *Mediators Inflamm.* (2013) 2013:731023. doi: 10.1155/2013/731023
123. Satoh T, Takeuchi O, Vandenbon A, Yasuda K, Tanaka Y, Kumagai Y, et al. The Jmjd3-Irf4 axis regulates M2 macrophage polarization and host responses against helminth infection. *Nat Immunol.* (2010) 11:936–44. doi: 10.1038/ni.1920
124. Ishii M, Wen H, Corsa CA, Liu T, Coelho AL, Allen RM, et al. Epigenetic regulation of the alternatively activated macrophage phenotype. *Blood.* (2009) 114:3244–54. doi: 10.1182/blood-2009-04-217620
125. Negishi H, Fujita Y, Yanai H, Sakaguchi S, Ouyang X, Shinohara M, et al. Evidence for licensing of IFN-gamma-induced IFN regulatory factor 1 transcription factor by MyD88 in Toll-like receptor-dependent gene induction program. *Proc Natl Acad Sci USA.* (2006) 103:15136–41. doi: 10.1073/pnas.0607181103
126. Krausgruber T, Blazek K, Smallie T, Alzabin S, Lockstone H, Sahgal N, et al. IRF5 promotes inflammatory macrophage polarization and TH1-TH17 responses. *Nat Immunol.* (2011) 12:231–8. doi: 10.1038/ni.1990
127. Weiss M, Blazek K, Byrne AJ, Perocheau DP, Udalova IA. IRF5 is a specific marker of inflammatory macrophages *in vivo*. *Mediators Inflamm.* (2013) 2013:245804. doi: 10.1155/2013/245804
128. Lawrence T, Natoli G. Transcriptional regulation of macrophage polarization: enabling diversity with identity. *Nat Rev Immunol.* (2011) 11:750–61. doi: 10.1038/nri3088
129. Komander D, Rape M. The ubiquitin code. *Annu Rev Biochem.* (2012) 81:203–29. doi: 10.1146/annurev-biochem-060310-170328
130. Zheng N, Shabek N. Ubiquitin ligases: structure, function, and regulation. *Annu Rev Biochem.* (2017) 86:129–57. doi: 10.1146/annurev-biochem-060815-014922
131. Heaton SM, Borg NA, Dixit VM. Ubiquitin in the activation and attenuation of innate antiviral immunity. *J Exp Med.* (2016) 213:1–13. doi: 10.1084/jem.20151531
132. Jefferies C, Wynne C, Higgs R. Antiviral TRIMs: friend or foe in autoimmune and autoinflammatory disease? *Nat Rev Immunol.* (2011) 11:617–25. doi: 10.1038/nri3043
133. Zhang J, Hu MM, Wang YY, Shu HB. TRIM32 protein modulates type I interferon induction and cellular antiviral response by targeting MITA/STING protein for K63-linked ubiquitination. *J Biol Chem.* (2012) 287:28646–55. doi: 10.1074/jbc.M112.362608
134. Tsuchida T, Zou J, Saitoh T, Kumar H, Abe T, Matsuura Y, et al. The ubiquitin ligase TRIM56 regulates innate immune responses to intracellular double-stranded DNA. *Immunity.* (2010) 33:765–76. doi: 10.1016/j.immuni.2010.10.013
135. Zhong B, Zhang L, Lei C, Li Y, Mao AP, Yang Y, et al. The ubiquitin ligase RNF5 regulates antiviral responses by mediating degradation of the adaptor protein MITA. *Immunity.* (2009) 30:397–407. doi: 10.1016/j.immuni.2009.01.008
136. Wang Y, Lian Q, Yang B, Yan S, Zhou H, He L, et al. TRIM30alpha Is a negative-feedback regulator of the intracellular DNA and DNA virus-triggered response by targeting STING. *PLoS Pathog.* (2015) 11:e1005012. doi: 10.1371/journal.ppat.1005012
137. Wang Q, Liu X, Cui Y, Tang Y, Chen W, Li S, et al. The E3 ubiquitin ligase AMFR and INSIG1 bridge the activation of TBK1 kinase by modifying the adaptor STING. *Immunity.* (2014) 41:919–33. doi: 10.1016/j.immuni.2014.11.011
138. Ni G, Konno H, Barber GN. Ubiquitination of STING at lysine 224 controls IRF3 activation. *Sci Immunol.* (2017) 2:eaah7119. doi: 10.1126/sciimmunol.aah7119
139. Hu MM, Yang Q, Xie XQ, Liao CY, Lin H, Liu TT, et al. Sumoylation promotes the stability of the DNA sensor cGAS and the adaptor STING to regulate the kinetics of response to DNA virus. *Immunity.* (2016) 45:555–69. doi: 10.1016/j.immuni.2016.08.014
140. Higgs R, Jefferies CA. Targeting IRFs by ubiquitination: regulating antiviral responses. *Biochem Soc Trans.* (2008) 36(Pt 3):453–8. doi: 10.1042/BST0360453
141. Ning S, Campos AD, Darnay BG, Bentz GL, Pagano JS. TRAF6 and the three C-terminal lysine sites on IRF7 are required for its ubiquitination-mediated activation by the tumor necrosis factor receptor family member latent membrane protein 1. *Mol Cell Biol.* (2008) 28:6536–46. doi: 10.1128/MCB.00785-08

142. Kubota T, Matsuoka M, Chang TH, Tailor P, Sasaki T, Tashiro M, et al. Virus infection triggers SUMOylation of IRF3 and IRF7, leading to the negative regulation of type I interferon gene expression. *J Biol Chem.* (2008) 283:25660–70. doi: 10.1074/jbc.M804479200
143. Liang Q, Deng H, Li X, Wu X, Tang Q, Chang TH, et al. Tripartite motif-containing protein 28 is a small ubiquitin-related modifier E3 ligase and negative regulator of IFN regulatory factor 7. *J Immunol.* (2011) 187:4754–63. doi: 10.4049/jimmunol.1101704
144. Higgs R, Ni Gabhann J, Ben Larbi N, Breen EP, Fitzgerald KA, Jefferies CA. The E3 ubiquitin ligase Ro52 negatively regulates IFN-beta production post-pathogen recognition by polyubiquitin-mediated degradation of IRF3. *J Immunol.* (2008) 181:1780–6. doi: 10.4049/jimmunol.181.3.1780
145. Espinosa A, Dardalhon V, Brauner S, Ambrosi A, Higgs R, Quintana FJ, et al. Loss of the lupus autoantigen Ro52/Trim21 induces tissue inflammation and systemic autoimmunity by disregulating the IL-23-Th17 pathway. *J Exp Med.* (2009) 206:1661–71. doi: 10.1084/jem.20090585
146. Pan JA, Sun Y, Jiang YP, Bott AJ, Jaber N, Dou Z, et al. TRIM21 Ubiquitylates SQSTM1/p62 and suppresses protein sequestration to regulate redox homeostasis. *Mol Cell.* (2016) 61:720–33. doi: 10.1016/j.molcel.2016.02.007
147. Kim JY, Ozato K. The sequestosome 1/p62 attenuates cytokine gene expression in activated macrophages by inhibiting IFN regulatory factor 8 and TNF receptor-associated factor 6/NF-kappaB activity. *J Immunol.* (2009) 182:2131–40. doi: 10.4049/jimmunol.0802755
148. Kimura T, Jain A, Choi SW, Mandell MA, Schroder K, Johansen T, et al. TRIM-mediated precision autophagy targets cytoplasmic regulators of innate immunity. *J Cell Biol.* (2015) 210:973–89. doi: 10.1083/jcb.201503023
149. Saitoh T, Tun-Kyi A, Ryo A, Yamamoto M, Finn G, Fujita T, et al. Negative regulation of interferon-regulatory factor 3-dependent innate antiviral response by the prolyl isomerase Pin1. *Nat Immunol.* (2006) 7:598–605. doi: 10.1038/ni1347
150. Yang K, Shi HX, Liu XY, Shan YF, Wei B, Chen S, et al. TRIM21 is essential to sustain IFN regulatory factor 3 activation during antiviral response. *J Immunol.* (2009) 182:3782–92. doi: 10.4049/jimmunol.0803126
151. Stacey KB, Breen E, Jefferies CA. Tyrosine phosphorylation of the E3 ubiquitin ligase TRIM21 positively regulates interaction with IRF3 and hence TRIM21 activity. *PLoS ONE.* (2012) 7:e34041. doi: 10.1371/journal.pone.0034041
152. Higgs R, Lazzari E, Wynne C, Ni Gabhann J, Espinosa A, Wahren-Herlenius M, et al. Self protection from anti-viral responses–Ro52 promotes degradation of the transcription factor IRF7 downstream of the viral Toll-Like receptors. *PLoS ONE.* (2010) 5:e11776. doi: 10.1371/journal.pone.0011776
153. Yu Y, Hayward GS. The ubiquitin E3 ligase RAUL negatively regulates type i interferon through ubiquitination of the transcription factors IRF7 and IRF3. *Immunity.* (2010) 33:863–77. doi: 10.1016/j.immuni.2010.11.027
154. Ran Y, Liu TT, Zhou Q, Li S, Mao AP, Li Y, et al. SENP2 negatively regulates cellular antiviral response by deSUMOylating IRF3 and conditioning it for ubiquitination and degradation. *J Mol Cell Biol.* (2011) 3:283–92. doi: 10.1093/jmcb/mjr020
155. Wang P, Zhao W, Zhao K, Zhang L, Gao C. TRIM26 negatively regulates interferon-beta production and antiviral response through polyubiquitination and degradation of nuclear IRF3. *PLoS Pathog.* (2015) 11:e1004726. doi: 10.1371/journal.ppat.1004726
156. Shi HX, Yang K, Liu X, Liu XY, Wei B, Shan YF, et al. Positive regulation of interferon regulatory factor 3 activation by Herc5 via ISG15 modification. *Mol Cell Biol.* (2010) 30:2424–36. doi: 10.1128/MCB.01466-09
157. Kim D, Lee H, Koh J, Ko JS, Yoon BR, Jeon YK, et al. Cytosolic pellino-1-mediated K63-linked ubiquitination of IRF5 in M1 macrophages regulates glucose intolerance in obesity. *Cell Rep.* (2017) 20:832–45. doi: 10.1016/j.celrep.2017.06.088
158. Lazzari E, Korczeniewska J, Ni Gabhann J, Smith S, Barnes BJ, Jefferies CA. TRIpartite motif 21 (TRIM21) differentially regulates the stability of interferon regulatory factor 5 (IRF5) isoforms. *PLoS ONE.* (2014) 9:e103609. doi: 10.1371/journal.pone.0103609
159. Eames HL, Saliba DG, Krausgruber T, Lanfrancotti A, Ryzhakov G, Udalova IA. KAP1/TRIM28: an inhibitor of IRF5 function in inflammatory macrophages. *Immunobiology.* (2012) 217:1315–24. doi: 10.1016/j.imbio.2012.07.026
160. Harikumar KB, Yester JW, Surace MJ, Oyeniran C, Price MM, Huang WC, et al. K63-linked polyubiquitination of transcription factor IRF1 is essential for IL-1-induced production of chemokines CXCL10 and CCL5. *Nat Immunol.* (2014) 15:231–8. doi: 10.1038/ni.2810
161. Tulli L, Cattaneo F, Vinot J, Baldari CT, D'Oro U. Src family kinases regulate interferon regulatory factor 1 K63 ubiquitination following activation by TLR7/8 vaccine adjuvant in human monocytes and B cells. *Front Immunol.* (2018) 9:330. doi: 10.3389/fimmu.2018.00330
162. Carthagena L, Bergamaschi A, Luna JM, David A, Uchil PD, Margottin-Goguet F, et al. Human TRIM gene expression in response to interferons. *PLoS ONE.* (2009) 4:e4894. doi: 10.1371/journal.pone.0004894
163. Mehta A, Baltimore D. microRNAs as regulatory elements in immune system logic. *Nat Rev Immunol.* (2016) 16:279–94. doi: 10.1038/nri.2016.40
164. Davidson-Moncada J, Papavasiliou FN, Tam W. microRNAs of the immune system: roles in inflammation and cancer. *Ann N Y Acad Sci.* (2010) 1183:183–94. doi: 10.1111/j.1749-6632.2009.05121.x
165. Ha M, Kim VN. Regulation of microRNA biogenesis. *Nat Rev Mol Cell Biol.* (2014) 15:509–24. doi: 10.1038/nrm3838
166. Bartel DP. microRNAs: target recognition and regulatory functions. *Cell.* (2009) 136:215–33. doi: 10.1016/j.cell.2009.01.002
167. He L, Hannon GJ. microRNAs: small RNAs with a big role in gene regulation. *Nat Rev Genet.* (2004) 5:522–31. doi: 10.1038/nrg1379
168. O'Brien J, Hayder H, Zayed Y, Peng C. Overview of MicroRNA biogenesis, mechanisms of actions, and circulation. *Front Endocrinol.* (2018) 9:402. doi: 10.3389/fendo.2018.00402
169. He X, Jing Z, Cheng G. microRNAs: new regulators of Toll-like receptor signalling pathways. *Biomed Res Int.* (2014) 2014:945169. doi: 10.1155/2014/945169
170. Nahid MA, Satoh M, Chan EK. MicroRNA in TLR signaling and endotoxin tolerance. *Cell Mol Immunol.* (2011) 8:388–403. doi: 10.1038/cmi.2011.26
171. Hou J, Wang P, Lin L, Liu X, Ma F, An H, et al. MicroRNA-146a feedback inhibits RIG-I-dependent Type I IFN production in macrophages by targeting TRAF6, IRAK1, and IRAK2. *J Immunol.* (2009) 183:2150–8. doi: 10.4049/jimmunol.0900707
172. Taganov KD, Boldin MP, Chang KJ, Baltimore D. NF-kappaB-dependent induction of microRNA miR-146, an inhibitor targeted to signaling proteins of innate immune responses. *Proc Natl Acad Sci USA.* (2006) 103:12481–6. doi: 10.1073/pnas.0605298103
173. Jurkin J, Schichl YM, Koeffel R, Bauer T, Richter S, Konradi S, et al. miR-146a is differentially expressed by myeloid dendritic cell subsets and desensitizes cells to TLR2-dependent activation. *J Immunol.* (2010) 184:4955–65. doi: 10.4049/jimmunol.0903021
174. Chen X, Zhou L, Peng N, Yu H, Li M, Cao Z, et al. MicroRNA-302a suppresses influenza A virus-stimulated interferon regulatory factor-5 expression and cytokine storm induction. *J Biol Chem.* (2017) 292:21291–303. doi: 10.1074/jbc.M117.805937
175. Peng L, Zhang H, Hao Y, Xu F, Yang J, Zhang R, et al. Reprogramming macrophage orientation by microRNA 146b targeting transcription factor IRF5. *EBiomedicine.* (2016) 14:83–96. doi: 10.1016/j.ebiom.2016.10.041
176. Li Y, Huang R, Wang L, Hao J, Zhang Q, Ling R, et al. microRNA-762 promotes breast cancer cell proliferation and invasion by targeting IRF7 expression. *Cell Prolif.* (2015) 48:643–9. doi: 10.1111/cpr.12223
177. Yang F, Xu Z, Duan S, Luo M. MicroRNA-541 promotes the proliferation of vascular smooth muscle cells by targeting IRF7. *Am J Transl Res.* (2016) 8:506–15.
178. Rosenberger CM, Podyminogin RL, Diercks AH, Treuting PM, Peschon JJ, Rodriguez D, et al. miR-144 attenuates the host response to influenza virus by targeting the TRAF6-IRF7 signaling axis. *PLoS Pathog.* (2017) 13:e1006305. doi: 10.1371/journal.ppat.1006305
179. Xu T, Chu Q, Cui J, Bi D. Inducible MicroRNA-3570 feedback inhibits the RIG-I-dependent innate immune response to rhabdovirus in teleost fish by targeting MAVS/IPS-1. *J Virol.* (2018) 92:e01594-17. doi: 10.1128/JVI.01594-17
180. Yarbrough ML, Zhang K, Sakthivel R, Forst CV, Posner BA, Barber GN, et al. Primate-specific miR-576-3p sets host defense signalling threshold. *Nat Commun.* (2014) 5:4963. doi: 10.1038/ncomms5963

181. Mukherjee A, Di Bisceglie AM, Ray RB. Hepatitis C virus-mediated enhancement of microRNA miR-373 impairs the JAK/STAT signaling pathway. *J Virol.* (2015) 89:3356–65. doi: 10.1128/JVI.03085-14
182. Banerjee S, Cui H, Xie N, Tan Z, Yang S, Icyuz M, et al. miR-125a-5p regulates differential activation of macrophages and inflammation. *J Biol Chem.* (2013) 288:35428–36. doi: 10.1074/jbc.M112.426866
183. Kim SW, Ramasamy K, Bouamar H, Lin AP, Jiang D, Aguiar RC. microRNAs miR-125a and miR-125b constitutively activate the NF-kappaB pathway by targeting the tumor necrosis factor alpha-induced protein 3 (TNFAIP3, A20). *Proc Natl Acad Sci USA.* (2012) 109:7865–70. doi: 10.1073/pnas.1200081109
184. Zhao JL, Huang F, He F, Gao CC, Liang SQ, Ma PF, et al. Forced activation of notch in macrophages represses tumor growth by upregulating miR-125a and disabling tumor-associated macrophages. *Cancer Res.* (2016) 76:1403–15. doi: 10.1158/0008-5472.CAN-15-2019
185. Li HS, Greeley N, Sugimoto N, Liu YJ, Watowich SS. miR-22 controls Irf8 mRNA abundance and murine dendritic cell development. *PLoS ONE.* (2012) 7:e52341. doi: 10.1371/journal.pone.0052341
186. Dai Y, Sui W, Lan H, Yan Q, Huang H, Huang Y. Comprehensive analysis of microRNA expression patterns in renal biopsies of lupus nephritis patients. *Rheumatol Int.* (2009) 29:749–54. doi: 10.1007/s00296-008-0758-6
187. Stagakis E, Bertsias G, Verginis P, Nakou M, Hatziapostolou M, Kritikos H, et al. Identification of novel microRNA signatures linked to human lupus disease activity and pathogenesis: miR-21 regulates aberrant T cell responses through regulation of PDCD4 expression. *Ann Rheum Dis.* (2011) 70:1496–506. doi: 10.1136/ard.2010.139857
188. Dai Y, Huang YS, Tang M, Lv TY, Hu CX, Tan YH, et al. Microarray analysis of microRNA expression in peripheral blood cells of systemic lupus erythematosus patients. *Lupus.* (2007) 16:939–46. doi: 10.1177/0961203307084158
189. Tang Y, Luo X, Cui H, Ni X, Yuan M, Guo Y, et al. MicroRNA-146A contributes to abnormal activation of the type I interferon pathway in human lupus by targeting the key signaling proteins. *Arthritis Rheum.* (2009) 60:1065–75. doi: 10.1002/art.24436
190. Pan W, Zhu S, Yuan M, Cui H, Wang L, Luo X, et al. MicroRNA-21 and microRNA-148a contribute to DNA hypomethylation in lupus CD4+ T cells by directly and indirectly targeting DNA methyltransferase 1. *J Immunol.* (2010) 184:6773–81. doi: 10.4049/jimmunol.0904060
191. Zhao S, Wang Y, Liang Y, Zhao M, Long H, Ding S, et al. MicroRNA-126 regulates DNA methylation in CD4+ T cells and contributes to systemic lupus erythematosus by targeting DNA methyltransferase 1. *Arthritis Rheum.* (2011) 63:1376–86. doi: 10.1002/art.30196
192. Conti P, DiGioacchino M. MCP-1 and RANTES are mediators of acute and chronic inflammation. *Allergy Asthma Proc.* (2001) 22:133–7. doi: 10.2500/108854101778148737
193. Moore KJ, Wada T, Barbee SD, Kelley VR. Gene transfer of RANTES elicits autoimmune renal injury in MRL-Faslpr mice. *Kidney Int.* (1998) 53:1631–41. doi: 10.1046/j.1523-1755.1998.00911.x
194. Zhao X, Tang Y, Qu B, Cui H, Wang S, Wang L, et al. MicroRNA-125a contributes to elevated inflammatory chemokine RANTES levels via targeting KLF13 in systemic lupus erythematosus. *Arthritis Rheum.* (2010) 62:3425–35. doi: 10.1002/art.27632
195. Smith S, Wu PW, Seo JJ, Fernando T, Jin M, Contreras J, et al. IL-16/miR-125a axis controls neutrophil recruitment in pristane-induced lung inflammation. *JCI Insight.* (2018) 3:120798. doi: 10.1172/jci.insight.120798

11

Fine-Tuning of Type I Interferon Response by STAT3

Ming-Hsun Tsai[1], *Li-Mei Pai*[2,3,4] *and Chien-Kuo Lee*[1*]

[1] Graduate Institute of Immunology, National Taiwan University College of Medicine, Taipei, Taiwan, [2] Department of Biochemistry and Molecular Biology, Chang Gung University, Taoyuan, Taiwan, [3] Molecular Medicine Research Center, Chang Gung University, Taoyuan, Taiwan, [4] Liver Research Center, Chang Gung Memorial Hospital, Taoyuan, Taiwan

***Correspondence:**
Chien-Kuo Lee
leeck@ntu.edu.tw*

Type I interferon (IFN-I) is induced during innate immune response and is required for initiating antiviral activity, growth inhibition, and immunomodulation. STAT1, STAT2, and STAT3 are activated in response to IFN-I stimulation. STAT1, STAT2, and IRF9 form ISGF3 complex which transactivates downstream IFN-stimulated genes and mediates antiviral response. However, the role of STAT3 remains to be characterized. Here, we review the multiple actions of STAT3 on suppressing IFN-I responses, including blocking IFN-I signaling, downregulating the expression of ISGF3 components, and antagonizing the transcriptional activity of ISGF3. Finally, we discuss the evolution of the suppressive activity of STAT3 and the therapeutic potential of STAT3 inhibitors in host defense against viral infections and IFN-I-associated diseases.

Keywords: type I interferon (IFN-I), STAT3, phospholipid scramblase 2, antiviral immunity, SOCS3

STAT3, AN OVERLOOKED SIGNAL MEDIATOR OF IFN-I

STAT3 was originally identified as acute-phase response factor (APRF) that is activated by IL-6 and binds to the promoters of acute-phase protein genes in hepatocytes to regulate inflammatory responses (1–4). It is now known that STAT3 is widely expressed in different cells and is activated by an array of cytokines and growth factors to mediate various activities (5–8). Total body ablation of STAT3 results in embryonic lethality (9, 10), whereas tissue-specific knockout of STAT3 reveals multiple functions in immune system, including regulation of homeostasis of immune cells, such as B-cells (11) and granulocytes (12), survival and/or proliferation of thymocytes (13), and differentiation of plasma cells (14), Th2 (15), Treg (16), and follicular helper T (Tfh) cells (17). Although STAT3 controls RORγt expression and Th17 development (18, 19), it, however, is not required for generation of type 3 innate lymphoid cells (ILC3) whose master regulator is also RORγt (20).

Like other STAT proteins, the activity of STAT3 is also regulated by acetylation, methylation and other post-translational modification such as SUMOylation in addition to phosphorylation (21, 22). STAT3 is activated primarily by tyrosine phosphorylation at Y705. In addition, serine phosphorylation at S727 is required for full transactivation ability of STAT3. However, unphosphorylated STAT3 can still form dimers through its N-terminal domain (NTD) and induce transcription (23). Moreover, acetylation of STAT3 plays a positive role in STAT3 transcription ability. Mutation of STAT3 at lysine residue K685, a p300-acetylation site, inhibits dimerization of STAT3 (24, 25). In addition to K685, K49, and K87 at NTD of STAT3 can be acetylated by p300 in response to IL-6, which affects STAT3 downstream gene expression (26). Other than acetylation, K140 and K49 of STAT3 can be methylated and negatively and positively modulate STAT3-mediated transcription, respectively (27, 28). Furthermore, removal of sumoylation of STAT3 at

K451 enhances its transcriptional activity by enhancing phosphorylation states (29). Together, these results suggest that multiple post-translational modifications of STAT3 modulate its activation and gene transcription.

Engagement of IFN-I to IFN receptor complex leads to activation of STAT1, STAT2, and STAT3 by tyrosine phosphorylation. STAT1 and STAT2 are considered to be the primordial signal mediators of IFN-I, as genetic ablation (30–33), hypomorphic mutation (33–35) or functional inactivation (35–38) of either molecule severely impairs the induction of IFN-stimulated genes (ISG) and IFN-I-mediated antiviral response in mice and humans. Nevertheless, STAT2 has also been reported to negatively regulate IFN-I response, either by constitutive phosphorylation at T387 to block ISGF3 formation and its DNA binding (39) or by IFN-I-induced phosphorylation at S287 (40) or S734 (41) with mechanisms yet to be defined. Moreover, STAT2 can serve as an adaptor to bridge the interaction between USP18 and IFNAR2, which inhibits ligand binding to the receptor, resulting in decreased receptor dimerization and signaling (42). These results suggest an emerging role of IFN-I signaling mediators in negative feedback regulation of IFN-I response.

While STAT3 is activated by IFN-I stimulation in various cell types in addition to STAT1 and STAT2 (43–47), the actual functions and biological significance of STAT3 in IFN-I response are less appreciated, probably due to relatively transient activation compared to STAT1 (3, 48, 49), impaired IFN-I-mediated, STAT3-dependent transcriptional activity (50, 51) or a dispensable role in some IFN-I mediated activities (52–54). For example, IFN-I-induced growth stimulatory activity in the absence of either STAT1 or STAT2 is independent of STAT3 (52). STAT3 is non-essential and cannot compensate the loss of STAT1 for IFN-I- or IFN-II-induced antiviral response in U3A, a human epithelial cell line (53). Moreover, during Tfh differentiation, STAT3 is not involved in IFN-I-induced, STAT1-mediated upregulation of the key transcription factor Bcl6 in CD4 T cells (54). In fact, it has also been shown that low or no IFN-I-activated STAT3 is found in CD4 T cells of patients with relapsing remitting multiple sclerosis (55) and in normal melanocytes or melanoma cells from patients (56). However, it is still unclear why STAT3 is selectively activated by IFN-I in different cell types.

However, it becomes clear that STAT3 is not just activated by IFN-I, it also regulates IFN activity. In fact, emerging evidence suggests that STAT3 may function to fine-tune IFN-I response (57–60). Gain- and loss-of-function analyses suggest that STAT3 negatively regulates IFN-α-induced ISG expression and antiviral activity (60). STAT3KO Tfh cells displays a markedly elevated levels of a number of ISGs in addition to T-bet expression, resembling a Th1-like effector phenotype, which leads to impaired germinal center (GC) formation and antibody production during LCMV infection (61). Blockade of IFN-I signaling rescues the defect in LCMV-infected mice, suggesting a requirement of STAT3 for Tfh cell and a fine balance in signaling pathways following acute viral infection. Similarly, knockdown of STAT3 in highly STAT3 activated diffuse large B cell lymphoma (DLBCL) cells results in increased expression of several ISGs (58). Inhibition of STAT3 synergizes with lenalidomide, an IFN-I inducing agent, in suppressing the growth of DLBCL by augmenting IFN-I-induced cytotoxicity. In addition to ISGs, STAT3 deficiency also upregulates IFN-I production, which may contribute to enhanced antiviral response (60) and improved chemotherapeutic activity in tumors (62). Interestingly, STAT1 deficiency in murine macrophage results in a sustained activation of STAT3 in response to combined stimulation of TLR and IFN, leading to repressed production of cytokines like TNF and IL-12 (63). STAT3 depletion restores TLR-dependent inflammatory response in the absence of STAT1, suggesting a functional cross-regulation of STAT1 and STAT3 and an anti-inflammatory role of STAT3 in IFN and TLR response. Together, these studies suggest that STAT3 may function as one of the key regulatory molecules for IFN response.

Several potential mechanisms have been described to illustrate the direct and indirect actions of STAT3 to suppress IFN-I response. For example, STAT3 may sequester STAT1 and prevent it from forming functional homodimers, STAT3 can cooperate with repressors to inhibit ISGF3 binding to DNA, and STAT3 can directly reduce the expression of ISGF3 components. STAT3 can also induce a suppressor to attenuate IFN-I signaling or a miRNA to reduce the expression of ISGF3 components to indirectly block IFN-I response. These mechanisms will be elaborated further in the following section.

MECHANISMS OF NEGATIVE REGULATION OF IFN-I BY STAT3

Sequestration of STAT1

Engagement of IFN-I to IFN receptor triggers the activation of STAT1, STAT2, and STAT3 and the formation of ISGF3 heterotrimer, consisting of STAT1, STAT2, and IRF9, and homodimers of STAT1:STAT1 or STAT3:STAT3 and heterodimer of STAT1:STAT3. It is conceivable that increased amounts of activated STAT3 can compete for binding with STAT1 to prevent the formation of STAT1:STAT1 homodimer. Indeed, overexpression of IFN-α-activated STAT3 inhibits STAT1-dependent gene expression, thereby downregulating the induction of proinflammatory cytokines, including CXCL9 and CXCL10 and a transcription factor IRF1, probably by sequestering activated STAT1 into STAT1:STAT3 heterodimers and reducing DNA binding of STAT1:STAT1 homodimers (57). Interestingly, increased amounts of activated STAT3 does not reduce ISGF3-driven expression of OAS and Mx2 genes. Instead, STAT3 seems to positively regulate their expression. Conversely, in mouse embryonic fibroblast cells lacking STAT3, IL-6 mediates IFNγ-like response with increased expression of MHC class II and antiviral state by inducing prolonged STAT1 activation and shifting homodimers of STAT1 or STAST3 and heterodimer of STAT1:STAT3 toward STAT1 homodimer only (64). Under physiological conditions, prolonged IFN-α treatment also affects STAT3-dependent IL-6 signaling by promoting formation of STAT1:STAT3 and STAT1:STAT1 complex, resulting in downregulation of STAT3 targets such as Bcl-X_L, Mcl-1, and survivin and increased apoptosis (65). Likewise, IFN-α priming results in acquisition of pro-inflammatory function of IL-10, leading to expression of IFN-γ-inducible, STAT1-depedent genes (66). Therefore, IFN-I signaling can be antagonized by STAT3, at least, in two ways: to compete for STAT1 association and for DNA binding (**Figure 1A**).

Cooperation With Repressors

STAT3 is reported to interact with many nuclear proteins to either activate or suppress the functions of STAT3 in transactivation ability and signaling pathways (67). For example, PDZ and LIM domain 2 (PDLIM2), a nuclear E3 ligase, which can interact with STAT3 and terminate its transcription by promoting degradation of STAT3 (68). HDAC1/2 forms a complex with SIN3 transcription regulator homolog A (Sin3a) to suppress the transcriptional activity of STAT3:STAT3 dimers through deacetylation (69, 70). In addition, DAXX directly interacts with STAT3 in the nucleus, leading to suppressing STAT3-mediated transactivation, probably through recruitment of a DNA methyltransferase (71, 72). STAT3 activation is therefore tightly regulated at multiple levels to prevent hyperactivation of STAT3-mediated pathologies, including cancers, autoimmune and inflammatory disorders (73).

However, these proteins are mainly limited to the control of the functions of STAT3 *per se*. Recently, we found that STAT3 interacts and cooperates with phospholipid scramblase 2 (PLSCR2) to negatively regulate IFN-I response (59). PLSCR2 is also an ISG and is predominantly located to the nucleus. PLSCR2 does not affect IFN-I-dependent phosphorylation of STAT1 and STAT2, nuclear translocation of activated STATs, or assembly of ISGF3 complex. Instead, PLSCR2 suppresses the recruitment of ISGF3 to ISRE of ISGs, in a STAT3-dependent manner, to fine-tune IFN-I response (**Figure 1B**). PLSCR2 deficiency results in increased ISG expression and antiviral activity. Mutations in palmitoylation motif of PLSCR2 impairs the interactions between PLSCR2 and STAT3, leading to blockade of the suppressive activity. Interestingly, expression profile analysis reveals that in addition to ISGs, genes involved in inflammatory response are also highly enriched in PLSCR2KO cells in response to IFN-I stimulation (59). This is consistent with enhanced inflammatory response upon TLR stimulation (74, 75) and in bowl diseases in the absence of STAT3 due to incapability of inducing SOCS3, a negative regulator of cytokine signaling (76–78) and the lack of signaling through the receptor of an anti-inflammatory cytokine such as IL-10 (79).

Reduction of ISGF3 Components

Constitutive STAT3 activation by autocrine production of IL-6 and IL-10 is found in activated B cell-like (ABC) diffused large B cell lymphoma cell lines (DLBCL) (80, 81). Genome-wide analysis has identified ~2,200 STAT3 direct target genes which control different aspects of B cells, including activation, survival, proliferation, differentiation, and migration (58). STAT3 also regulates multiple oncogenic signaling pathways, including NF-κB, a cell-cycle checkpoint, PI3K/AKT/mTORC1, and STAT3 itself. Interestingly, constitutive STAT3 activation also suppresses the expression of ISGF3 components, such as IRF9, STAT1 and STAT2, and IRF7, a transcription factor for IFN-I production, through direct binding to the promoters of the genes (58). Therefore, STAT3 is able to directly reduce the levels of critical components in signaling pathway to weaken IFN-I response (**Figure 1C**).

MicroRNAs (miRs) are known to regulate IFN signaling pathways (82, 83). IFN-γ-activated STAT1 binds directly to the promoter of miR155 and induces its expression (84). Moreover, virus infection-induced miR155 also targets SOCS1 to feedback promote IFN-I-mediated antiviral activity (85). Therefore, STAT1 activation positively regulates its function by up-regulating miR-155 and down-regulating a STAT inhibitory factor SOCS1. STAT3, on other hand, stimulates miR-221/222 expression, which in turn targets PDLIM2 to stabilize and increase STAT3 levels (86). Knockdown of miR-221/222 results in upregulation of members of the IFN-α signaling pathway, including STAT1, STAT2, IRF9, and several ISGs in a human glioma cell line (87). Virus infection-induced upregulation of miR221 in peritoneal macrophages negatively regulates innate antiviral response against VSV (88). Therefore, STAT3-dependent transcription of miR-221/222 may function to downregulate STAT1 and STAT2 expression indirectly to antagonize IFN-I response (**Figure 2A**).

Induction of Negative Regulators

Suppressors of cytokine signaling (SOCS) family proteins are ISGs that feedback regulate cytokine signaling through various ways, including blocking receptor docking by activated STATs, inhibiting JAK kinase activity, and promoting degradation of activated JAKs and receptors (89, 90). IFN-I induces SOCS1 and SOCS3 expression in a STAT1- and STAT3-dependent manner, respectively (91). In addition to feedback regulation, the signaling pathways of STAT1 and STAT3 can cross-regulate by the induced SOCS1 and SOCS3 reciprocally (92, 93). Constitutive expression of SOCS3 inhibits IFN-α-induced STAT1 phosphorylation, ISG expression and anti-proliferative activity (94). HSV-1 (95) or IAV (96) infection-induced SOCS3 is responsible for the suppression of signaling and production of IFN-I and impaired antiviral response. Moreover, hepatic SOCS3 expression is also strongly associated with non-responsiveness to IFN-I therapy in HCV patients (97). Therefore, STAT3 can indirectly cross-regulate STAT1-mediated signaling and ISG expression at multiple layers of feedback control through induced SOCS3 (**Figure 2B**).

VIRAL STRATEGIES TO EXPLOIT STAT3

Given that STAT3 can exert negative effects on IFN-I response, it is conceivable that viruses may exploit STAT3 to evade IFN-I-mediated antiviral immunity to facilitate their replication. Indeed, porcine epidemic diarrhea virus is shown to trigger STAT3 activation via stimulated EGFR signaling to enhance virus replication in an intestinal epithelial cell line (98). Inhibitors or siRNA to EGFR result in augmented expression of IFN-I and ISG genes and decreased viral yield. Similar results are also observed using the same approaches to block STAT3 activation, suggesting that attenuation of antiviral activity by EGFR activation requires STAT3 signaling pathway. EGFR- and IFN-signaling crosstalk is also known to play a role in regulating HCV replication

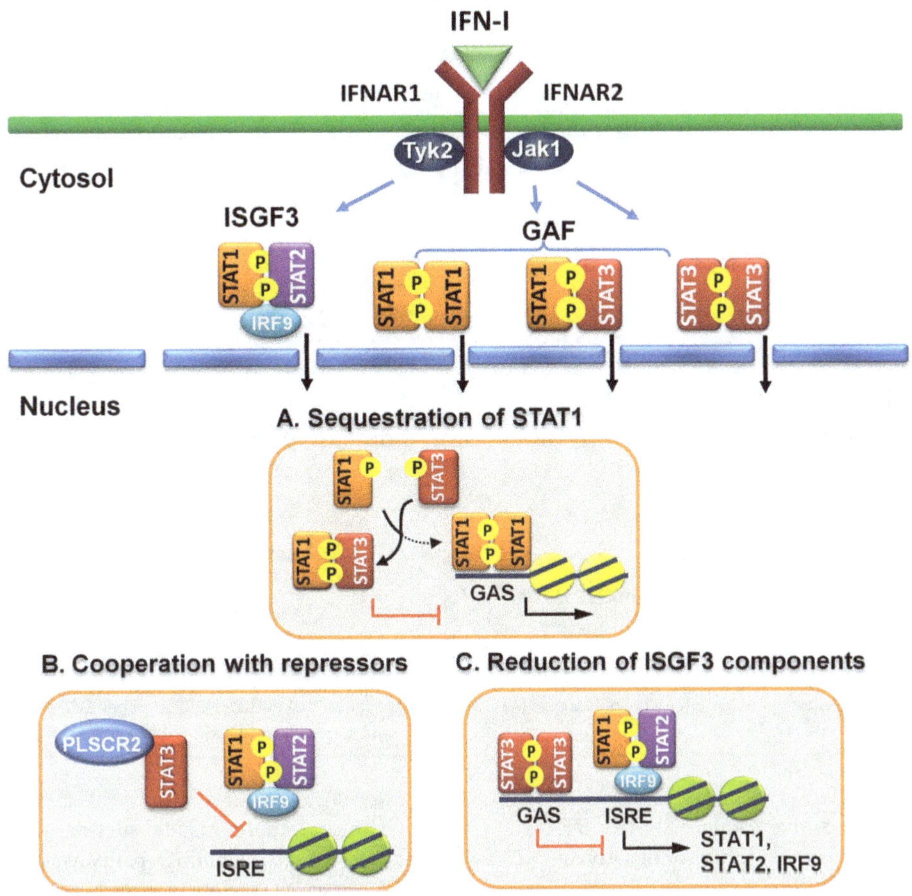

FIGURE 1 | Direct regulatory mechanisms of STAT3 for IFN-I response. **(A)** Activated STAT3 sequesters activated STAT1 to form heterodimers and prevents STAT1 from forming functional homodimers to transactivate downstream genes. **(B)** STAT3 cooperates with other repressors, such as PLSCR2 to prevent ISGF3 from binding to DNA. **(C)** STAT3 binds directly to the promoters of ISGF3 components, including STAT1, STAT2, and IRF9 and suppress their expression.

(99). Erlotinib, an EGFR inhibitor, and IFN-α synergize to inhibit HCV infection in a hepatoma cell line (100). While STAT3 silencing or inhibition suppresses HCV infection, SOCS silencing impairs the synergistic antiviral activity of IFN-α and erlotinib. Therefore, EGFR may impair IFN antiviral response by suppressing SOCS3 expression, which relieves SOCS3-mediated antagonism of STAT3, thereby promoting virus replication (100).

Although virus targeting and inhibiting STAT3 seems to be counterintuitive because of its negative role in IFN-I response (57–60), several viruses are reported to degrade STAT3 protein or suppress its functions. For example, the V protein of Mumps virus (MuV) catalyzes proteasomal degradation of STAT1 and STAT3, resulting in blockade of IFN-I, IFN-II, and prevention of the responses to interleukin-6 and v-Src signals and induction of apoptosis in STAT3-dependent multiple myeloma cells and transformed murine fibroblasts (101). Hepatitis E virus (HEV) viral ORF3 protein (pORF3) blocks the nuclear translocation of p-STAT3, probably by impeding endocytosis of EGFR, resulting in downregulation of STAT3-stimulated acute-phase gene-driven reporter activity (102). While, the absence of STAT3 during MuV infection may reduce pro-inflammatory activity of IL-6 and IFN-γ, functional blockade of STAT3 by HEV may result in downregulation of the acute-phase response, a major determinant of inflammation in the host.

In fact, several viruses also boost or attenuate STAT3 functions to perturb immune response, alter cell architecture and tissue organization, prevent apoptosis or trigger cellular transformation to facilitate their replication, which have been thoroughly reviewed elsewhere (103, 104) and will not be discussed further.

EVOLUTIONARILY CONSERVED FEEDBACK REGULATION BY STAT

The cytokine receptor (CytoR)-JAK-STAT is a highly conserved signaling pathway, which expands extensively in bilateria during early vertebrate evolution and is concurrent with the development of adaptive immune system (105, 106). In early jawed vertebrates, the regulation of IFN has been established through two rounds of whole-genome duplication that occurs between invertebrates and vertebrates to provide expanded

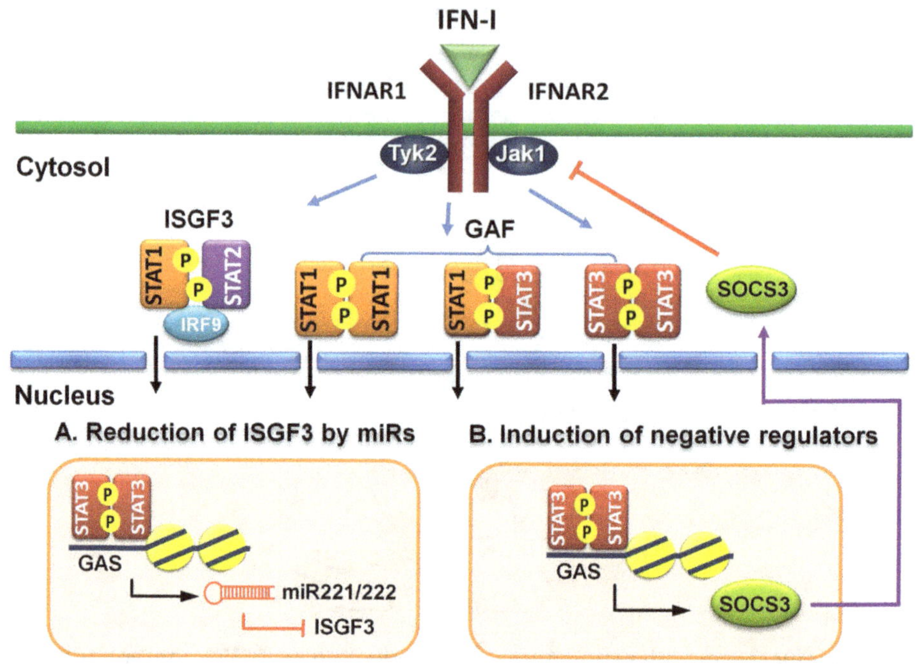

FIGURE 2 | Indirect regulatory mechanisms of STAT3 for IFN-I responses. **(A)** STAT3 induces microRNA miR-221/222 to target ISGF3 components, including STAT1, STAT2, and IRF9 to reduce their *de novo* protein synthesis. **(B)** STAT3 induces a negative regulator, such as SOCS3 to block IFN-I signaling.

signaling molecules, such as positive regulators, JAKs, STATs and IRFs, and negative regulators, protein inhibitor of activated STAT (PIAS) and SOCS (107).

There is only one STAT protein in *Drosophila* that is stat92E which is required for normal development of several tissues, including embryonic segmentation, imaginal discs, blood cells, and germ cells (108). A crustacean Pm-STAT is also identified from giant tiger prawn (*Penaeus monodon*) and the phosphorylated form of Pm-STAT is increased in lymphoid organ of the shrimp following white spot syndrome virus (WSSV) infection (109). RNA silencing of Lv-STAT in whiteleg shrimp (*Litopenaeus vannamei*) significantly reduces the copy number of WSSV and the mortality caused by WSSV infection (110). Moreover, treatment of a specific inhibitor of STAT3 (S3I-201) in hematopoietic tissue of crayfish (*Cherax quadricarinatus*) also decreases WSSV titers, suggesting a proviral role of the invertebrate STAT protein (110).

In addition to shrimp, an Ec-STAT3 identified from orange-spotted grouper (*Epinephelus coioides*) is activated and induced to translocate into nucleus following Singapore grouper iridovirus (SGIV) infection. Inhibition of Ec-STAT3 by RNA silencing or a small molecule inhibitor decreases SGIV replication and induces cell cycle arrest and downregulates the expression of prosurvival genes, such as Bcl-2, Bcl-x_L, and Bax. Ec-STAT3 is also activated in fish by red-spotted grouper nervous necrosis virus (RGNNV). While inhibition of Ec-STAT3 does not affect RGNNV replication, virus infection-induced vacuolation and autophagy are significantly increased (111). Moreover, the expression of several proinflammatory factors, including TNFα, IL-1β, and IL-8, is also mediated by Ec-STAT3 during infection.

Therefore, these results suggest that microbial infection-triggered STAT signaling pathway is well conserved from invertebrates to vertebrates and that proviral and prosurvial role of STAT3 are probably also preserved from shrimp, fish to mammals, although the feedback regulation of IFN-I response by STAT3 in shrimp and fish remains unclear.

IS STAT3 DRUGGABLE OR UNDRUGGABLE?

As an oncogene and is activated in a wide range of malignant cells, STAT3 is considered to be one of the most important therapeutic targets, particularly, for cancers (112). However, there are still lack of clinically available STAT3 inhibitors due to insufficient potency and/or selectivity (113, 114). Currently, the STAT3 inhibitors under development include three categories: small molecule compounds, peptide-based molecules, and double-stranded oligodeoxynucleotide decoy (ODN-decoy) (115). Usually, small molecule compounds and peptide-based inhibitors are designed in a way to effectively reduce tyrosine phosphorylation and/or dimerization of STAT3 and block STAT3-mediated transcriptional activity. For example, SH2 domain of STAT3 is the main target of STAT3 inhibitors which are known to occupy or dock to pY-Tyr705-binding pocket. However, it is also highly homologous to SH2 domain of STAT1. Likewise, the DBD of STAT3 is also highly similar to that of STAT1. Therefore, the chances of cross-reacting and simultaneous suppression of the activity of STAT1 and STAT3 by an inhibitor are high. Indeed, inhibitors like Stattic and S3I-201 that target STAT3 SH2 domain are also reported to inhibit STAT1 phosphorylation and nuclear translocation (116, 117).

Since both STAT3 and STAT1 can recognize the same GAS element of some genes, it comes as no surprise that STAT3 DBD-targeting decoy ODN also binds STAT1 and reduces STAT1-dependent IFNγ-induced cell death (118). Therefore, the inhibitors targeting to either SH2 or DBD domain of STAT3 are likely to suppress STAT1-mediated signaling. In addition, targeting upstream of STAT3, such as JAKs, is also likely to exert a board spectrum of inhibitory effect on different STAT proteins. For example, AG490, AZD1480, and Sorafenib are also able to potently suppress STAT1 phosphorylation in addition to STAT3 phosphorylation (119–121).

When STAT3 inhibitors are used to boost antiviral responses, it is anticipated that STAT1-mediated antiviral responses will also be attenuated due to cross-reactivity. Nevertheless, several STAT3 inhibitors have been shown to enhance antiviral response *in vitro* or *in vivo* and display some therapeutic potential. For example, pretreatment of S3I-201 can reduce viral replication in human cytomegalovirus (HCMV), varicella-zoster virus, SGIV, or vesicular stomatitis virus (122–126). Moreover, Stattic can also reduce HCMV replication (126). Although these studies usually attribute the reduced viral replication to the proviral role of STAT3, it is also likely that reduced SOCS3 expression derepresses STAT1 to contribute to antiviral responses.

Despite the concerns raised in many literatures about the potential problems in developing STAT3 inhibitors, some of them are already in clinical trials, including 3 inhibitors targeting to SH2 of STAT3 and 1 inhibitor as an antisense ODN (127). Therefore, there is no definitely answer yet as STAT3 is druggable or not. Nevertheless, different approaches may need to be implanted to provide viable solutions for developing drugs that can selectively block the activity of STAT3.

CONCLUSIONS AND PERSPECTIVES

While accumulating evidence suggests that STAT3 is a negative regulator of the IFN-I response, it only represents one of many other regulatory mechanisms for IFN-I signaling (128), suggesting the importance of balancing the pluripotent activities of IFN-I. In fact, this notion becomes evident with the emerging type I interferonopathies of autoinflammatory diseases, which are Mendelian disorders associated with an up-regulation of IFN-I signaling as a novel type of human inborn errors of immunity, including Aicardi-Goutières syndromes (AGS), familial chilblain lupus (FCL), bilateral striatal necrosis (BSN), STING-associated vasculopathy with onset in infancy (SAVI)…etc. (129). Mutations in STAT3 is known to cause many diseases in humans, including loss-of-function-induced autosomal dominant hyper IgE syndrome (AD-HIES), gain-of-function-induced malignancies and autoimmunity (73). However, it remains to be determined if functional deficiency of STAT3 will lead to type I interferonopathies.

Targeting STAT3 as a therapeutic approach for cancers and other diseases must take the multifaceted functions of STAT3 into consideration. As shown in this review that STAT3 not just possesses proviral and prosurvival activities, it also exhibits seemingly paradoxical roles in inflammation (130) and immune modulation (5, 131, 132). Moreover, due to sequence conservation between STAT1 and STAT3, developing highly selective drugs for STAT3 without affecting STAT1 is desirable, which is also the challenge for precision medicine to deal with these diseases.

AUTHOR CONTRIBUTIONS

All authors listed have made a substantial, direct and intellectual contribution to the work, and approved it for publication.

ACKNOWLEDGMENTS

This study was supported by research grants from the Ministry of Science and Technology Taiwan (MOST 102-2320-B-002-030-MY3) and (MOST 105-2911-I-002-509), National Health Research Institutes, Taiwan (NHRI-EX107-10632SI) and the Excellent Translational Medicine Research Projects of National Taiwan University College of Medicine and National Taiwan University Hospital to C-KL and Chang Gung Memorial Hospital (CMRPD1H0191) to L-MP.

REFERENCES

1. Akira S, Nishio Y, Inoue M, Wang XJ, Wei S, Matsusaka T, et al. Molecular cloning of APRF, a novel IFN-stimulated gene factor 3 p91-related transcription factor involved in the gp130-mediated signaling pathway. *Cell.* (1994) 77:63–71. doi: 10.1016/0092-8674(94)90235-6
2. Lutticken C, Wegenka UM, Yuan J, Buschmann J, Schindler C, Ziemiecki A, et al. Association of transcription factor APRF and protein kinase Jak1 with the interleukin-6 signal transducer gp130. *Science.* (1994) 263:89–92. doi: 10.1126/science.8272872
3. Raz R, Durbin JE, Levy DE. Acute phase response factor and additional members of the interferon-stimulated gene factor 3 family integrate diverse signals from cytokines, interferons, and growth factors. *J Biol Chem.* (1994) 269:24391–5.
4. Zhong Z, Wen Z, Darnell JE Jr. Stat3: a STAT family member activated by tyrosine phosphorylation in response to epidermal growth factor and interleukin-6. *Science.* (1994) 264:95–8. doi: 10.1126/science.8140422
5. Hillmer EJ, Zhang H, Li HS, Watowich SS. STAT3 signaling in immunity. *Cytokine Growth Factor Rev.* (2016) 31:1–15. doi: 10.1016/j.cytogfr.2016.05.001
6. Huynh J, Chand A, Gough D, Ernst M. Therapeutically exploiting STAT3 activity in cancer - using tissue repair as a road map. *Nat Rev Cancer.* (2019) 19:82–96. doi: 10.1038/s41568-018-0090-8
7. Levy DE, Lee CK. What does Stat3 do? *J Clin Invest.* (2002) 109:1143–8. doi: 10.1172/JCI200215650
8. Yu H, Lee H, Herrmann A, Buettner R, Jove R. Revisiting STAT3 signalling in cancer: new and unexpected biological functions. *Nat Rev Cancer.* (2014) 14:736–46. doi: 10.1038/nrc3818
9. Takeda K, Noguchi K, Shi W, Tanaka T, Matsumoto M, Yoshida N, et al. Targeted disruption of the mouse Stat3 gene leads to early embryonic lethality. *Proc Natl Acad Sci USA.* (1997) 94:3801–4. doi: 10.1073/pnas.94.8.3801
10. Raz R, Lee CK, Cannizzaro LA, d'Eustachio P, Levy DE. Essential role of STAT3 for embryonic stem cell pluripotency. *Proc Natl Acad Sci USA.* (1999) 96:2846–51. doi: 10.1073/pnas.96.6.2846

11. Chou WC, Levy DE, Lee CK. STAT3 positively regulates an early step in B-cell development. *Blood.* (2006) 108:3005–11. doi: 10.1182/blood-2006-05-024430
12. Lee C, Raz R, Gimeno R, Gertner R, Wistinghausen B, Takeshita K, et al. STAT3 is a negative regulator of granulopoiesis but is not required for G-CSF-dependent differentiation. *Immunity.* (2002) 17:63. doi: 10.1016/S1074-7613(02)00336-9
13. Sano S, Takahama Y, Sugawara T, Kosaka H, Itami S, Yoshikawa K, et al. Stat3 in thymic epithelial cells is essential for postnatal maintenance of thymic architecture and thymocyte survival. *Immunity.* (2001) 15:261–73. doi: 10.1016/S1074-7613(01)00180-7
14. Diehl SA, Schmidlin H, Nagasawa M, van Haren SD, Kwakkenbos MJ, Yasuda E, et al. STAT3-mediated up-regulation of BLIMP1 Is coordinated with BCL6 down-regulation to control human plasma cell differentiation. *J Immunol.* (2008) 180:4805–15. doi: 10.4049/jimmunol.180.7.4805
15. Stritesky GL, Muthukrishnan R, Sehra S, Goswami R, Pham D, Travers J, et al. The transcription factor STAT3 is required for T helper 2 cell development. *Immunity.* (2011) 34:39–49. doi: 10.1016/j.immuni.2010.12.013
16. Bettelli E, Carrier Y, Gao W, Korn T, Strom TB, Oukka M, et al. Reciprocal developmental pathways for the generation of pathogenic effector TH17 and regulatory T cells. *Nature.* (2006) 441:235–8. doi: 10.1038/nature04753
17. Eddahri F, Denanglaire S, Bureau F, Spolski R, Leonard WJ, Leo O, et al. Interleukin-6/STAT3 signaling regulates the ability of naive T cells to acquire B-cell help capacities. *Blood.* (2009) 113:2426–33. doi: 10.1182/blood-2008-04-154682
18. Harris TJ, Grosso JF, Yen HR, Xin H, Kortylewski M, Albesiano E, et al. Cutting edge: an *in vivo* requirement for STAT3 signaling in TH17 development and TH17-dependent autoimmunity. *J Immunol.* (2007) 179:4313–7. doi: 10.4049/jimmunol.179.7.4313
19. Mathur AN, Chang HC, Zisoulis DG, Stritesky GL, Yu Q, O'Malley JT, et al. Stat3 and Stat4 direct development of IL-17-secreting Th cells. *J Immunol.* (2007) 178:4901–7. doi: 10.4049/jimmunol.178.8.4901
20. Guo X, Qiu J, Tu T, Yang X, Deng L, Anders RA, et al. Induction of innate lymphoid cell-derived interleukin-22 by the transcription factor STAT3 mediates protection against intestinal infection. *Immunity.* (2014) 40:25–39. doi: 10.1016/j.immuni.2013.10.021
21. Zhuang S. Regulation of STAT signaling by acetylation. *Cell Signal.* (2013) 25:1924–31. doi: 10.1016/j.cellsig.2013.05.007
22. Qi QR, Yang ZM. Regulation and function of signal transducer and activator of transcription 3. *World J Biol Chem.* (2014) 5:231–9. doi: 10.4331/wjbc.v5.i2.231
23. Yang J, Stark GR. Roles of unphosphorylated STATs in signaling. *Cell Res.* (2008) 18:443–51. doi: 10.1038/cr.2008.41
24. Wang R, Cherukuri P, Luo J. Activation of Stat3 sequence-specific DNA binding and transcription by p300/CREB-binding protein-mediated acetylation. *J Biol Chem.* (2005) 280:11528–34. doi: 10.1074/jbc.M413930200
25. Yuan ZL, Guan YJ, Chatterjee D, Chin YE. Stat3 dimerization regulated by reversible acetylation of a single lysine residue. *Science.* (2005) 307:269–73. doi: 10.1126/science.1105166
26. Ray S, Boldogh I, Brasier AR. STAT3 NH2-terminal acetylation is activated by the hepatic acute-phase response and required for IL-6 induction of angiotensinogen. *Gastroenterology.* (2005) 129:1616–32. doi: 10.1053/j.gastro.2005.07.055
27. Yang J, Huang J, Dasgupta M, Sears N, Miyagi M, Wang B, et al. Reversible methylation of promoter-bound STAT3 by histone-modifying enzymes. *Proc Natl Acad Sci USA.* (2010) 107:21499–504. doi: 10.1073/pnas.1016147107
28. Dasgupta M, Dermawan JK, Willard B, Stark GR. STAT3-driven transcription depends upon the dimethylation of K49 by EZH2. *Proc Natl Acad Sci USA.* (2015) 112:3985–90. doi: 10.1073/pnas.1503152112
29. Zhou Z, Wang M, Li J, Xiao M, Chin YE, Cheng J, et al. SUMOylation and SENP3 regulate STAT3 activation in head and neck cancer. *Oncogene.* (2016) 35:5826–38. doi: 10.1038/onc.2016.124
30. Durbin JE, Hackenmiller R, Simon MC, Levy DE. Targeted disruption of the mouse Stat1 gene results in compromised innate immunity to viral disease. *Cell.* (1996) 84:443–50. doi: 10.1016/S0092-8674(00)81289-1
31. Meraz MA, White JM, Sheehan KC, Bach EA, Rodig SJ, Dighe AS, et al. Targeted disruption of the Stat1 gene in mice reveals unexpected physiologic specificity in the JAK-STAT signaling pathway. *Cell.* (1996) 84:431–42. doi: 10.1016/S0092-8674(00)81288-X
32. Park C, Li S, Cha E, Schindler C. Immune response in Stat2 knockout mice. *Immunity.* (2000) 13:795–804. doi: 10.1016/S1074-7613(00)00077-7
33. Hambleton S, Goodbourn S, Young DF, Dickinson P, Mohamad SM, Valappil M, et al. STAT2 deficiency and susceptibility to viral illness in humans. *Proc Natl Acad Sci USA.* (2013) 110:3053–8. doi: 10.1073/pnas.1220098110
34. Chen LS, Wei PC, Liu T, Kao CH, Pai LM, Lee CK. STAT2 hypomorphic mutant mice display impaired dendritic cell development and antiviral response. *J Biomed Sci.* (2009) 16:22. doi: 10.1186/1423-0127-16-22
35. Dupuis S, Jouanguy E, Al-Hajjar S, Fieschi C, Al-Mohsen IZ, Al-Jumaah S, et al. Impaired response to interferon-alpha/beta and lethal viral disease in human STAT1 deficiency. *Nat Genet.* (2003) 33:388–91. doi: 10.1038/ng1097
36. Dupuis S, Dargemont C, Fieschi C, Thomassin N, Rosenzweig S, Harris J, et al. Impairment of mycobacterial but not viral immunity by a germline human STAT1 mutation. *Science.* (2001) 293:300–3. doi: 10.1126/science.1061154
37. Sampaio EP, Bax HI, Hsu AP, Kristosturyan E, Pechacek J, Chandrasekaran P, et al. A novel STAT1 mutation associated with disseminated mycobacterial disease. *J Clin Immunol.* (2012) 32:681–9. doi: 10.1007/s10875-012-9659-2
38. Tsumura M, Okada S, Sakai H, Yasunaga S, Ohtsubo M, Murata T, et al. Dominant-negative STAT1 SH2 domain mutations in unrelated patients with Mendelian susceptibility to mycobacterial disease. *Hum Mutat.* (2012) 33:1377–87. doi: 10.1002/humu.22113
39. Wang Y, Nan J, Willard B, Wang X, Yang J, Stark GR. Negative regulation of type I IFN signaling by phosphorylation of STAT2 on T387. *EMBO J.* (2017) 36:202–12. doi: 10.15252/embj.201694834
40. Steen HC, Nogusa S, Thapa RJ, Basagoudanavar SH, Gill AL, Merali S, et al. Identification of STAT2 serine 287 as a novel regulatory phosphorylation site in type I interferon-induced cellular responses. *J Biol Chem.* (2013) 288:747–58. doi: 10.1074/jbc.M112.402529
41. Steen HC, Kotredes KP, Nogusa S, Harris MY, Balachandran S, Gamero AM. Phosphorylation of STAT2 on serine-734 negatively regulates the IFN-alpha-induced antiviral response. *J Cell Sci.* (2016) 129:4190–9. doi: 10.1242/jcs.185421
42. Arimoto KI, Lochte S, Stoner SA, Burkart C, Zhang Y, Miyauchi S, et al. STAT2 is an essential adaptor in USP18-mediated suppression of type I interferon signaling. *Nat Struct Mol Biol.* (2017) 24:279–89. doi: 10.1038/nsmb.3378
43. Gonzalez-Navajas JM, Lee J, David M, Raz E. Immunomodulatory functions of type I interferons. *Nat Rev Immunol.* (2012) 12:125–35. doi: 10.1038/nri3133
44. Ivashkiv LB, Donlin LT. Regulation of type I interferon responses. *Nat Rev Immunol.* (2014) 14:36–49. doi: 10.1038/nri3581
45. Katze MG, He Y, Gale M Jr. Viruses and interferon: a fight for supremacy. *Nat Rev Immunol.* (2002) 2:675–87. doi: 10.1038/nri888
46. Platanias LC. Mechanisms of type-I- and type-II-interferon-mediated signalling. *Nat Rev Immunol.* (2005) 5:375–86. doi: 10.1038/nri1604
47. van Boxel-Dezaire AH, Rani MR, Stark GR. Complex modulation of cell type-specific signaling in response to type I interferons. *Immunity.* (2006) 25:361–72. doi: 10.1016/j.immuni.2006.08.014
48. Tomic J, Lichty B, Spaner DE. Aberrant interferon-signaling is associated with aggressive chronic lymphocytic leukemia. *Blood.* (2011) 117:2668–80. doi: 10.1182/blood-2010-05-285999
49. van Boxel-Dezaire AH, Zula JA, Xu Y, Ransohoff RM, Jacobberger JW, Stark GR. Major differences in the responses of primary human leukocyte subsets to IFN-beta. *J Immunol.* (2010) 185:5888–99. doi: 10.4049/jimmunol.0902314
50. Icardi L, Lievens S, Mori R, Piessevaux J, De Cauwer L, De Bosscher K, et al. Opposed regulation of type I IFN-induced STAT3 and ISGF3 transcriptional activities by histone deacetylases (HDACS) 1 and 2. *FASEB J.* (2012) 26:240–9. doi: 10.1096/fj.11-191122
51. Icardi L, Mori R, Gesellchen V, Eyckerman S, De Cauwer L, Verhelst J, et al. The Sin3a repressor complex is a master regulator of STAT

transcriptional activity. *Proc Natl Acad Sci USA.* (2012) 109:12058–63. doi: 10.1073/pnas.1206458109

52. Gimeno R, Lee CK, Schindler C, Levy DE. Stat1 and Stat2 but not Stat3 arbitrate contradictory growth signals elicited by alpha/beta interferon in T lymphocytes. *Mol Cell Biol.* (2005) 25:5456–65. doi: 10.1128/MCB.25.13.5456-5465.2005
53. Horvath CM, Darnell JE, Jr. The antiviral state induced by alpha interferon and gamma interferon requires transcriptionally active Stat1 protein. *J Virol.* (1996) 70:647–50.
54. Nakayamada S, Poholek AC, Lu KT, Takahashi H, Kato M, Iwata S, et al. Type I IFN induces binding of STAT1 to Bcl6: divergent roles of STAT family transcription factors in the T follicular helper cell genetic program. *J Immunol.* (2014) 192:2156–66. doi: 10.4049/jimmunol.1300675
55. Zula JA, Green HC, Ransohoff RM, Rudick RA, Stark GR, van Boxel-Dezaire AH. The role of cell type-specific responses in IFN-beta therapy of multiple sclerosis. *Proc Natl Acad Sci USA.* (2011) 108:19689–94. doi: 10.1073/pnas.1117347108
56. Humpolikova-Adamkova L, Kovarik J, Dusek L, Lauerova L, Boudny V, Fait V, et al. Interferon-alpha treatment may negatively influence disease progression in melanoma patients by hyperactivation of STAT3 protein. *Eur J Cancer.* (2009) 45:1315–23. doi: 10.1016/j.ejca.2009.01.009
57. Ho HH, Ivashkiv LB. Role of STAT3 in type I interferon responses. Negative regulation of STAT1-dependent inflammatory gene activation. *J Biol Chem.* (2006) 281:14111–8. doi: 10.1074/jbc.M511797200
58. Lu L, Zhu F, Zhang M, Li Y, Drennan AC, Kimpara S, et al. Gene regulation and suppression of type I interferon signaling by STAT3 in diffuse large B cell lymphoma. *Proc Natl Acad Sci USA.* (2018) 115:E498-e505. doi: 10.1073/pnas.1715118115
59. Tsai MH, Lee CK. STAT3 cooperates with phospholipid scramblase 2 to suppress type I interferon response. *Front Immunol.* (2018) 9:1886. doi: 10.3389/fimmu.2018.01886
60. Wang WB, Levy DE, Lee CK. STAT3 negatively regulates type I IFN-mediated antiviral response. *J Immunol.* (2011) 187:2578–85. doi: 10.4049/jimmunol.1004128
61. Ray JP, Marshall HD, Laidlaw BJ, Staron MM, Kaech SM, Craft J. Transcription factor STAT3 and type I interferons are corepressive insulators for differentiation of follicular helper and T helper 1 cells. *Immunity.* (2014) 40:367–77. doi: 10.1016/j.immuni.2014.02.005
62. Yang H, Yamazaki T, Pietrocola F, Zhou H, Zitvogel L, Ma Y, et al. STAT3 Inhibition enhances the therapeutic efficacy of immunogenic chemotherapy by stimulating type 1 interferon production by cancer cells. *Cancer Res.* (2015) 75:3812–22. doi: 10.1158/0008-5472.CAN-15-1122
63. Kim HS, Kim DC, Kim HM, Kwon HJ, Kwon SJ, Kang SJ, et al. STAT1 deficiency redirects IFN signalling toward suppression of TLR response through a feedback activation of STAT3. *Sci Rep.* (2015) 5:13414. doi: 10.1038/srep13414
64. Costa-Pereira AP, Tininini S, Strobl B, Alonzi T, Schlaak JF, Is'harc H, et al. Mutational switch of an IL-6 response to an interferon-gamma-like response. *Proc Natl Acad Sci USA.* (2002) 99:8043–7. doi: 10.1073/pnas.122236099
65. Thyrell L, Arulampalam V, Hjortsberg L, Farnebo M, Grander D, Pokrovskaja Tamm K. Interferon alpha induces cell death through interference with interleukin 6 signaling and inhibition of STAT3 activity. *Exp Cell Res.* (2007) 313:4015–24. doi: 10.1016/j.yexcr.2007.08.007
66. Sharif MN, Tassiulas I, Hu Y, Mecklenbrauker I, Tarakhovsky A, Ivashkiv LB. IFN-alpha priming results in a gain of proinflammatory function by IL-10: implications for systemic lupus erythematosus pathogenesis. *J Immunol.* (2004) 172:6476–81. doi: 10.4049/jimmunol.172.10.6476
67. Matsuda T, Muromoto R, Sekine Y, Togi S, Kitai Y, Kon S, et al. Signal transducer and activator of transcription 3 regulation by novel binding partners. *World J Biol Chem.* (2015) 6:324–32. doi: 10.4331/wjbc.v6.i4.324
68. Tanaka T, Yamamoto Y, Muromoto R, Ikeda O, Sekine Y, Grusby MJ, et al. PDLIM2 inhibits T helper 17 cell development and granulomatous inflammation through degradation of STAT3. *Sci Signal.* (2011) 4:ra85. doi: 10.1126/scisignal.2001637
69. Yang XJ, Seto E. The Rpd3/Hda1 family of lysine deacetylases: from bacteria and yeast to mice and men. *Nat Rev Mol Cell Biol.* (2008) 9:206–18. doi: 10.1038/nrm2346
70. Marie IJ, Chang HM, Levy DE. HDAC stimulates gene expression through BRD4 availability in response to IFN and in interferonopathies. *J Exp Med.* (2018) 2018:520. doi: 10.1084/jem.20180520
71. Muromoto R, Nakao K, Watanabe T, Sato N, Sekine Y, Sugiyama K, et al. Physical and functional interactions between Daxx and STAT3. *Oncogene.* (2006) 25:2131–6. doi: 10.1038/sj.onc.1209235
72. Puto LA, Reed JC. Daxx represses RelB target promoters via DNA methyltransferase recruitment and DNA hypermethylation. *Genes Dev.* (2008) 22:998–1010. doi: 10.1101/gad.1632208
73. Vogel TP, Milner JD, Cooper MA. The ying and yang of STAT3 in human disease. *J Clin Immunol.* (2015) 35:615–23. doi: 10.1007/s10875-015-0187-8
74. Murray PJ. Understanding and exploiting the endogenous interleukin-10/STAT3-mediated anti-inflammatory response. *Curr Opin Pharmacol.* (2006) 6:379–86. doi: 10.1016/j.coph.2006.01.010
75. Hu X, Chakravarty SD, Ivashkiv LB. Regulation of interferon and Toll-like receptor signaling during macrophage activation by opposing feedforward and feedback inhibition mechanisms. *Immunol Rev.* (2008) 226:41–56. doi: 10.1111/j.1600-065X.2008.00707.x
76. Suzuki A, Hanada T, Mitsuyama K, Yoshida T, Kamizono S, Hoshino T, et al. CIS3/SOCS3/SSI3 plays a negative regulatory role in STAT3 activation and intestinal inflammation. *J Exp Med.* (2001) 193:471–81. doi: 10.1084/jem.193.4.471
77. Takeda K, Clausen BE, Kaisho T, Tsujimura T, Terada N, Forster I, et al. Enhanced Th1 activity and development of chronic enterocolitis in mice devoid of Stat3 in macrophages and neutrophils. *Immunity.* (1999) 10:39–49. doi: 10.1016/S1074-7613(00)80005-9
78. Melillo JA, Song L, Bhagat G, Blazquez AB, Plumlee CR, Lee C, et al. Dendritic cell (DC)-specific targeting reveals Stat3 as a negative regulator of DC function. *J Immunol.* (2010) 184:2638–45. doi: 10.4049/jimmunol.0902960
79. Murray PJ. The primary mechanism of the IL-10-regulated antiinflammatory response is to selectively inhibit transcription. *Proc Natl Acad Sci USA.* (2005) 102:8686–91. doi: 10.1073/pnas.0500419102
80. Ding BB, Yu JJ, Yu RY, Mendez LM, Shaknovich R, Zhang Y, et al. Constitutively activated STAT3 promotes cell proliferation and survival in the activated B-cell subtype of diffuse large B-cell lymphomas. *Blood.* (2008) 111:1515–23. doi: 10.1182/blood-2007-04-087734
81. Lam LT, Wright G, Davis RE, Lenz G, Farinha P, Dang L, et al. Cooperative signaling through the signal transducer and activator of transcription 3 and nuclear factor-{kappa}B pathways in subtypes of diffuse large B-cell lymphoma. *Blood.* (2008) 111:3701–13. doi: 10.1182/blood-2007-09-111948
82. Forster SC, Tate MD, Hertzog PJ. MicroRNA as type I interferon-regulated transcripts and modulators of the innate immune response. *Front Immunol.* (2015) 6:334. doi: 10.3389/fimmu.2015.00334
83. Kohanbash G, Okada H. MicroRNAs and STAT interplay. *Semin Cancer Biol.* (2012) 22:70–5. doi: 10.1016/j.semcancer.2011.12.010
84. Kutty RK, Nagineni CN, Samuel W, Vijayasarathy C, Hooks JJ, Redmond TM. Inflammatory cytokines regulate microRNA-155 expression in human retinal pigment epithelial cells by activating JAK/STAT pathway. *Biochem Biophys Res Commun.* (2010) 402:390–5. doi: 10.1016/j.bbrc.2010.10.042
85. Wang P, Hou J, Lin L, Wang C, Liu X, Li D, et al. Inducible microRNA-155 feedback promotes type I IFN signaling in antiviral innate immunity by targeting suppressor of cytokine signaling 1. *J Immunol.* (2010) 185:6226–33. doi: 10.4049/jimmunol.1000491
86. Liu S, Sun X, Wang M, Hou Y, Zhan Y, Jiang Y, et al. A microRNA 221- and 222-mediated feedback loop maintains constitutive activation of NFkappaB and STAT3 in colorectal cancer cells. *Gastroenterology.* (2014) 147:847–59 e11. doi: 10.1053/j.gastro.2014.06.006
87. Zhang C, Han L, Zhang A, Yang W, Zhou X, Pu P, et al. Global changes of mRNA expression reveals an increased activity of the interferon-induced signal transducer and activator of transcription (STAT) pathway by repression of miR-221/222 in glioblastoma U251 cells. *Int J Oncol.* (2010) 36:1503–12. doi: 10.3892/ijo_00000637

88. Du H, Cui S, Li Y, Yang G, Wang P, Fikrig E, et al. MiR-221 negatively regulates innate anti-viral response. *PLoS ONE.* (2018) 13:e0200385. doi: 10.1371/journal.pone.0200385
89. Alexander WS, Hilton DJ. The role of suppressors of cytokine signaling (SOCS) proteins in regulation of the immune response. *Annu Rev Immunol.* (2004) 22:503–29. doi: 10.1146/annurev.immunol.22.091003.090312
90. Yasukawa H, Sasaki A, Yoshimura A. Negative regulation of cytokine signaling pathways. *Ann Rev Immunol.* (2000) 18:143–64. doi: 10.1146/annurev.immunol.18.1.143
91. Qin H, Niyongere SA, Lee SJ, Baker BJ, Benveniste EN. Expression and functional significance of SOCS-1 and SOCS-3 in astrocytes. *J Immunol.* (2008) 181:3167–76. doi: 10.4049/jimmunol.181.5.3167
92. Croker BA, Krebs DL, Zhang JG, Wormald S, Willson TA, Stanley EG, et al. SOCS3 negatively regulates IL-6 signaling *in vivo*. *Nat Immunol.* (2003) 4:540–5. doi: 10.1038/ni931
93. Hong F, Jaruga B, Kim WH, Radaeva S, El-Assal ON, Tian Z, et al. Opposing roles of STAT1 and STAT3 in T cell-mediated hepatitis: regulation by SOCS. *J Clin Invest.* (2002) 110:1503–13. doi: 10.1172/JCI0215841
94. Sakai I, Takeuchi K, Yamauchi H, Narumi H, Fujita S. Constitutive expression of SOCS3 confers resistance to IFN-alpha in chronic myelogenous leukemia cells. *Blood.* (2002) 100:2926–31. doi: 10.1182/blood-2002-01-0073
95. Yokota S, Yokosawa N, Okabayashi T, Suzutani T, Miura S, Jimbow K, et al. Induction of suppressor of cytokine signaling-3 by herpes simplex virus type 1 contributes to inhibition of the interferon signaling pathway. *J Virol.* (2004) 78:6282–6. doi: 10.1128/JVI.78.12.6282-6286.2004
96. Pauli EK, Schmolke M, Wolff T, Viemann D, Roth J, Bode JG, et al. Influenza A virus inhibits type I IFN signaling via NF-kappaB-dependent induction of SOCS-3 expression. *PLoS Pathog.* (2008) 4:e1000196. doi: 10.1371/journal.ppat.1000196
97. Kim KA, Lin W, Tai AW, Shao RX, Weinberg E, De Sa Borges CB, et al. Hepatic SOCS3 expression is strongly associated with non-response to therapy and race in HCV and HCV/HIV infection. *J Hepatol.* (2009) 50:705–11. doi: 10.1016/j.jhep.2008.12.021
98. Yang L, Xu J, Guo L, Guo T, Zhang L, Feng L, et al. Porcine epidemic diarrhea virus-induced epidermal growth factor receptor activation impairs the antiviral activity of type I interferon. *J Virol.* (2018) 92:17. doi: 10.1128/JVI.02095-17
99. Schoggins JW. Regulating interferon antiviral activity: a role for epidermal growth factor receptor. *Hepatology.* (2013) 58:1200–2. doi: 10.1002/hep.26486
100. Lupberger J, Duong FH, Fofana I, Zona L, Xiao F, Thumann C, et al. Epidermal growth factor receptor signaling impairs the antiviral activity of interferon-alpha. *Hepatology.* (2013) 58:1225–35. doi: 10.1002/hep.26404
101. Ulane CM, Rodriguez JJ, Parisien JP, Horvath CM. STAT3 ubiquitylation and degradation by mumps virus suppress cytokine and oncogene signaling. *J Virol.* (2003) 77:6385–93. doi: 10.1128/JVI.77.11.6385-6393.2003
102. Chandra V, Kar-Roy A, Kumari S, Mayor S, Jameel S. The hepatitis E virus ORF3 protein modulates epidermal growth factor receptor trafficking, STAT3 translocation, and the acute-phase response. *J Virol.* (2008) 82:7100–10. doi: 10.1128/JVI.00403-08
103. Roca Suarez AA, Van Renne N, Baumert TF, Lupberger J. Viral manipulation of STAT3: Evade, exploit, and injure. *PLoS Pathog.* (2018) 14:e1006839. doi: 10.1371/journal.ppat.1006839
104. Kuchipudi SV. The complex role of STAT3 in viral infections. *J Immunol Res.* (2015) 2015:272359. doi: 10.1155/2015/272359
105. Liongue C, Taznin T, Ward AC. Signaling via the CytoR/JAK/STAT/SOCS pathway: emergence during evolution. *Mol Immunol.* (2016) 71:166–75. doi: 10.1016/j.molimm.2016.02.002
106. Liongue C, Sertori R, Ward AC. Evolution of cytokine receptor signaling. *J Immunol.* (2016) 197:11–8. doi: 10.4049/jimmunol.1600372
107. Secombes CJ, Zou J. Evolution of interferons and interferon receptors. *Front Immunol.* (2017) 8:209. doi: 10.3389/fimmu.2017.00209
108. Arbouzova NI, Zeidler MP. JAK/STAT signalling in Drosophila: insights into conserved regulatory and cellular functions. *Development.* (2006) 133:2605–16. doi: 10.1242/dev.02411
109. Chen WY, Ho KC, Leu JH, Liu KF, Wang HC, Kou GH, et al. WSSV infection activates STAT in shrimp. *Dev Compar Immunol.* (2008) 32:1142–50. doi: 10.1016/j.dci.2008.03.003
110. Wen R, Li F, Li S, Xiang J. Function of shrimp STAT during WSSV infection. *Fish Shellfish Immunol.* (2014) 38:354–60. doi: 10.1016/j.fsi.2014.04.002
111. Huang Y, Huang X, Yang Y, Wang W, Yu Y, Qin Q. Involvement of fish signal transducer and activator of transcription 3 (STAT3) in nodavirus infection induced cell death. *Fish Shellfish Immunol.* (2015) 43:241–8. doi: 10.1016/j.fsi.2014.12.031
112. Huynh J, Etemadi N, Hollande F, Ernst M, Buchert M. The JAK/STAT3 axis: a comprehensive drug target for solid malignancies. *Semin Cancer Biol.* (2017) 45:13–22. doi: 10.1016/j.semcancer.2017.06.001
113. Xiong A, Yang Z, Shen Y, Zhou J, Shen Q. Transcription factor STAT3 as a novel molecular target for cancer prevention. *Cancers.* (2014) 6:926–57. doi: 10.3390/cancers6020926
114. Wong ALA, Hirpara JL, Pervaiz S, Eu JQ, Sethi G, Goh BC. Do STAT3 inhibitors have potential in the future for cancer therapy? *Expert Opin Investig Drugs.* (2017) 26:883–7. doi: 10.1080/13543784.2017.1351941
115. Wake MS, Watson CJ. STAT3 the oncogene - still eluding therapy? *FEBS J.* (2015) 282:2600–11. doi: 10.1111/febs.13285
116. Schust J, Sperl B, Hollis A, Mayer TU, Berg T. Stattic: a small-molecule inhibitor of STAT3 activation and dimerization. *Chem Biol.* (2006) 13:1235–42. doi: 10.1016/j.chembiol.2006.09.018
117. Lin L, Benson DM, Jr., DeAngelis S, Bakan CE, Li PK, Li C, et al. A small molecule, LLL12 inhibits constitutive STAT3 and IL-6-induced STAT3 signaling and exhibits potent growth suppressive activity in human multiple myeloma cells. *Int J Cancer.* (2012) 130:1459–69. doi: 10.1002/ijc.26152
118. Tadlaoui Hbibi A, Laguillier C, Souissi I, Lesage D, Le Coquil S, Cao A, et al. Efficient killing of SW480 colon carcinoma cells by a signal transducer and activator of transcription (STAT) 3 hairpin decoy oligodeoxynucleotide–interference with interferon-gamma-STAT1-mediated killing. *FEBS J.* (2009) 276:2505–15. doi: 10.1111/j.1742-4658.2009.06975.x
119. Derenzini E, Lemoine M, Buglio D, Katayama H, Ji Y, Davis RE, et al. The JAK inhibitor AZD1480 regulates proliferation and immunity in Hodgkin lymphoma. *Blood Cancer J.* (2011) 1:e46. doi: 10.1038/bcj.2011.46
120. Kobayashi A, Tanizaki Y, Kimura A, Ishida Y, Nosaka M, Toujima S, et al. AG490, a Jak2 inhibitor, suppressed the progression of murine ovarian cancer. *Eur J Pharmacol.* (2015) 766:63–75. doi: 10.1016/j.ejphar.2015.09.039
121. Martin del Campo SE, Levine KM, Mundy-Bosse BL, Grignol VP, Fairchild ET, Campbell AR, et al. The Raf kinase inhibitor sorafenib inhibits JAK-STAT signal transduction in human immune cells. *J Immunol.* (2015) 195:1995–2005. doi: 10.4049/jimmunol.1400084
122. Marozin S, Altomonte J, Munoz-Alvarez KA, Rizzani A, De Toni EN, Thasler WE, et al. STAT3 inhibition reduces toxicity of oncolytic VSV and provides a potentially synergistic combination therapy for hepatocellular carcinoma. *Cancer Gene Ther.* (2015) 22:317–25. doi: 10.1038/cgt.2015.23
123. Sen N, Che X, Rajamani J, Zerboni L, Sung P, Ptacek J, et al. Signal transducer and activator of transcription 3 (STAT3) and survivin induction by varicella-zoster virus promote replication and skin pathogenesis. *Proc Natl Acad Sci USA.* (2012) 109:600–5. doi: 10.1073/pnas.1114232109
124. Huang X, Huang Y, Yang Y, Wei S, Qin Q. Involvement of fish signal transducer and activator of transcription 3 (STAT3) in SGIV replication and virus induced paraptosis. *Fish Shellfish Immunol.* (2014) 41:308–16. doi: 10.1016/j.fsi.2014.09.011
125. Reitsma JM, Terhune SS. Inhibition of cellular STAT3 synergizes with the cytomegalovirus kinase inhibitor maribavir to disrupt infection. *Antiviral Res.* (2013) 100:321–7. doi: 10.1016/j.antiviral.2013.09.011
126. Reitsma JM, Sato H, Nevels M, Terhune SS, Paulus C. Human cytomegalovirus IE1 protein disrupts interleukin-6 signaling by sequestering STAT3 in the nucleus. *J Virol.* (2013) 87:10763–76. doi: 10.1128/JVI.01197-13

127. Johnson DE, O'Keefe RA, Grandis JR. Targeting the IL-6/JAK/STAT3 signalling axis in cancer. *Nat Rev Clin Oncol.* (2018) 15:234–48. doi: 10.1038/nrclinonc.2018.8
128. Arimoto KI, Miyauchi S, Stoner SA, Fan JB, Zhang DE. Negative regulation of type I IFN signaling. *J Leukocyte Biol.* (2018) 103:1099–116. doi: 10.1002/JLB.2MIR0817-342R
129. Rodero MP, Crow YJ. Type I interferon-mediated monogenic autoinflammation: the type I interferonopathies, a conceptual overview. *J Exp Med.* (2016) 213:2527–38. doi: 10.1084/jem.20161596
130. Scheller J, Chalaris A, Schmidt-Arras D, Rose-John S. The pro- and anti-inflammatory properties of the cytokine interleukin-6. *Biochim Biophys Acta.* (2011) 1813:878–88. doi: 10.1016/j.bbamcr.2011.01.034
131. Yu H, Kortylewski M, Pardoll D. Crosstalk between cancer and immune cells: role of STAT3 in the tumour microenvironment. *Nat Rev Immunol.* (2007) 7:41–51. doi: 10.1038/nri1995
132. Yu H, Pardoll D, Jove R. STATs in cancer inflammation and immunity: a leading role for STAT3. *Nat Rev Cancer.* (2009) 9:798–809. doi: 10.1038/nrc2734

12

IRF and STAT Transcription Factors - From Basic Biology to Roles in Infection, Protective Immunity and Primary Immunodeficiencies

Trine H. Mogensen [1,2,3*]

[1] Department of Infectious diseases, Aarhus University Hospital, Aarhus, Denmark, [2] Department of Biomedicine, Aarhus University, Aarhus, Denmark, [3] Department of Clinical Medicine, Aarhus University, Aarhus, Denmark

***Correspondence:**
Trine H. Mogensen
trine.mogensen@biomed.au.dk

The induction and action of type I interferon (IFN) is of fundamental importance in human immune defenses toward microbial pathogens, particularly viruses. Basic discoveries within the molecular and cellular signaling pathways regulating type I IFN induction and downstream actions have shown the essential role of the IFN regulatory factor (IRF) and the signal transducer and activator of transcription (STAT) families, respectively. However, the exact biological and immunological functions of these factors have been most clearly revealed through the study of inborn errors of immunity and the resultant infectious phenotypes in humans. The spectrum of human inborn errors of immunity caused by mutations in IRFs and STATs has proven very diverse. These diseases encompass herpes simplex encephalitis (HSE) and severe influenza in IRF3- and IRF7/IRF9 deficiency, respectively. They also include Mendelian susceptibility to mycobacterial infection (MSMD) in STAT1 deficiency, through disseminated measles infection associated with STAT2 deficiency, and finally staphylococcal abscesses and chronic mucocutaneous candidiasis (CMC) classically described with Hyper-IgE syndrome (HIES) in the case of STAT3 deficiency. More recently, increasing focus has been on aspects of autoimmunity and autoinflammation playing an important part in many primary immunodeficiency diseases (PID)s, as exemplified by STAT1 gain-of-function causing CMC and autoimmune thyroiditis, as well as a recently described autoinflammatory syndrome with hypogammaglobulinemia and lymphoproliferation as a result of STAT3 gain-of-function. Here I review the infectious, inflammatory, and autoimmune disorders arising from mutations in IRF and STAT transcription factors in humans, highlightning the underlying molecular mechanisms and immunopathogenesis as well as the clinical/therapeutic perspectives of these new insights.

Keywords: IRF, STAT, interferon, antiviral, proinflammatory, primary immunodeficiency, genetics

INTRODUCTION

Several decades of research uncovering the basic biology, regulation; and functions of the machinery for induction and responses to type I interferon (IFN) have paved the way for an understanding of a number of very diverse human diseases arising when one or more molecules in these pathways are defective. In this manner, the study of humans with primary immunodeficiencies (PID)s provides important understanding of specific protective immunity in humans, an insight that cannot always be gained by studying experimental animal models. Moreover, the study of individuals with defects in these pathways may teach us valuable lessons about principles of basic cell biology and infection immunology. Finally, detailed knowledge on the fundamental immunopathogenesis allows for rapid and specific diagnosis and not least for targeted treatments for individuals with these rare inborn errors of immunity.

Several PIDs have been associated to the defective expression or function of molecules belonging to innate immune signaling receptors or pathways (1, 2). These discoveries have been accelerated by the introduction of whole exome sequencing (WES) techniques. Moreover, with the advent of such sequencing methologies, an increasing number of monogenic diseases caused by gain-of-function (GOF) mutations have emerged (3). This expands the spectrum of PIDs to also include conditions characterized by autoimmunity and autoinflammation.

BASIC STRUCTURE, SIGNALING, AND BIOLOGY OF IRF AND STAT TRANSCRIPTION FACTORS

Recognition of Microbial Pathogens and Induction of IFNs by IRFs

The innate immune system utilizes pattern recognition receptors (PRR)s to detect pathogen-associated molecular patterns (PAMP)s to mount protective immune responses, including production of cytokines and IFN (4). Production of type I IFN is induced following recognition of nucleic acids, mainly of foreign origin, but under certain pathological conditions deriving from the host. Different classes of PRRs are involved in induction of IFN, including membrane-associated Toll-like receptors (TLR)s, cytosolic RNA sensing retinoic acid inducible gene (RIG)-like receptors (RLR)s, and DNA sensors (4, 5). Each of these classes of PRRs activate IFN regulatory factor (IRF)s through unique adaptor molecules, known as TIR-domain-containing adapter inducing IFNβ (TRIF), mitochondrial antiviral signaling protein (MAVS) and stimulator of IFN genes (STING), respectively, to which IRF binds in order to become phosphorylated (6) (**Figure 1**).

IRFs

In mammals nine different IRF family members have been described. All IRF proteins have a conserved amino-terminal DNA binding domain (DBD) with a helix-loop-helix structure and a motif containing five tryptophan residues. IRF-association domains (IAD)1 and 2 at the carboxyterminal region of IRFs mediate homodimeric and heterodimeric interactions with other IRF family members, transcription factors, and co-factors. Whereas IRF3 has restricted DNA binding properties, IRF7 exhibits broader DNA binding specificity, accounting for its capacity to induce several IFNα subtypes. The C-terminal signal response domain of IRF proteins contains several possible phosphorylation sites, of which phosphorylation at serine 386 for IRF3 or serine 477 and 479 at IRF7 are believed to represent the main activation sites (7). In addition, poly-ubiquitination of IRF7 at K63 by TRAF6 and the E2 enzyme complex Ubc13/Uev1A is required for IRF7 activation (8).

Transcriptional activation of the IFNβ promoter by IRF3/7 has been extensively studied (9, 10), and proceeds with phosphorylation of IRF3/7 by the kinase TKB1, leading to dimerization and translocation of IRF3/7 homo-or hetero-dimers to the nucleus together with other transcription factors, such as nuclear factor (NF)-κB and activator protein (AP)-1 (11). Assembly of the enhanceosome on the IFNβ promoter leads to histone acetylation and displacement of the nucleosome, hereby allowing initiation of IFNβ gene transcription. Importantly, NF-κB can cooperate in the induction of IFNs, at least at the IFNβ promoter, whereas IRFs, on the other hand, do not take part in induction of proinflammatory cytokines, although they may indirectly stimulate their synthesis (12, 13). IRF3 appears to be constitutively expressed in many cell types, residing in the cytoplasm in an inactive form, which upon upstream activating signals induces transcription of a set of early transcribed type I and type III IFN genes (mostly IFNβ, IFNα4, and IFNα1) (13, 14). IRF7 on the other hand, is a lymphoid transcription factor constitutively expressed only in B cells, monocytes and plasmacytoid dendritic cells (pDC)s (15). pDCs in particular express high levels of IRF7, while in most other cell types IRF7 is inducible from low levels of expression (16). Thus, early during infection IRF7 only has a minor contribution to the production of type I and type III IFNs. However, at later stages of infection, as more IRF7 is induced by type I IFNs, IRF7 induces the production of a delayed set of IFNα genes, including IFNα2, α5, α6, and α8, as well as IFNβ2 and IFNβ3 (14, 17, 18) (**Figure 1**). This generates a positive feedback loop, as type I and III IFNs induce more IRF7, thus leading to production of even more type I and type III IFNs, and this amplification loop is believed to play an important role in the generation of an immediate and potent response to virus infection (16).

The Interferons

Type I IFNs were initially discovered as soluble factors mediating viral interference (19), and subsequent work allowed the cloning, sequencing, and functional characterization of this group of cytokines (11, 20–24). Whereas type I IFNs (IFNα and IFNβ) are predominantly expressed by innate immune cells, the functionally similar type III IFNs, (IFNλ1-4), discovered in 2003, are more restricted and primarily act on epithelial surfaces (17, 25). Finally, type II IFN (IFNγ), discovered in 1965, is being synthesized by Natural killer (NK) cells and T cells and exerts antiviral functions mainly by activating macrophages (25). Type I IFNs exert a broad range of antiviral activities, including induction of the classically described molecules dsRNA-activated protein kinase R (PKR) which inhibits the cellular translational machinery, 2′-5′-oligoadenylate synthetase (OAS)/RNAseL with the capacity to degrade foreign RNA, and Mx proteins that mainly restrict influenza virus through an itranuclear GTPase activity (11). Moreover, a wide range of IFN-inducible genes (ISG)s with diverse effects on antiviral defenses and cell proliferation and differentiation are induced and mediate the pleiotropic effects of type I (and III) IFNs (11).

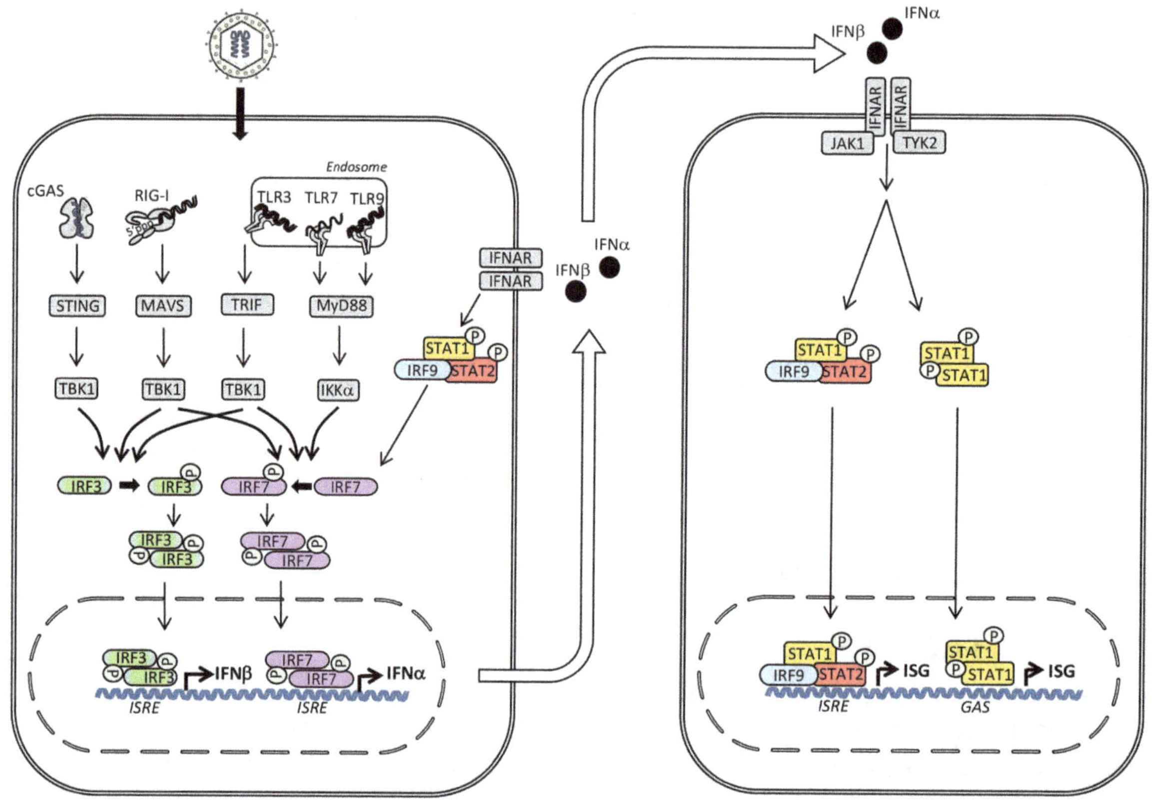

FIGURE 1 | Induction of type I interferon (IFN) and signaling by the type I IFN receptor. The presence of microbial or self-nucleic acid in the cytosol or within the endosomal compartment activates pattern recognition receptors (PRR)s. RNA activates retinoic acid-inducible receptor (RIG)-I in the cytosol and Toll-like receptor (TLR)3 and TLR7 in the endosomal compartment, whereas DNA is sensed by cyclic GMP-AMP synthase (cGAS) in the cytosol and by TLR9 within endosomes. These events trigger signaling pathways through the adaptor molecules stimulator of IFN genes (STING), mitochondrial antiviral signaling protein (MAVS), TIR-domain-containing adapter-inducing interferon-β (TRIF), and Myeloid differentiation primary response (MyD)88 leading to phosphorylation and activation of the TANK binding kinase (TBK)1, which in turn phosphorylates the transcription factors IFN regulatory factor (IRF)3 and IRF7. Whereas IRF3 is constitutively present, IRF7 is expressed at low levels but may be secondarily induced by type I IFN. Phosphorylation of IRF3 and IRF7 leads to homodimerization, nuclear translocation, and expression of type I IFNs (IFNα and IFNβ) acting on neighboring cells with type I IFN receptors. Type I IFN binds to IFNα/β receptor (IFNAR)2 leading to recruitment of IFNAR1 and formation of a complex that activates the receptor-associated Janus-associated kinase (JAK)1 and tyrosine kinase (TYK)2 and subsequent tyrosine phosphorylation of STAT1 and STAT2. These activated transcription factors together with IRF9 form the heterotrimeric transcription factor IFN-stimulated gene factor (ISGF)3 complex which binds to IFN-stimulated regulatory elements (ISRE) in DNA. In addition, STAT1 homodimers form the IFN-γ-activated factor (GAF) complex which binds to IFNg-activated sequences (GAS). Altogether, these transcription factors induce a broad spectrum of IFN-stimulated genes (ISG)s that mediate the complex "antiviral state" of IFNs.

JAK-STAT Molecules

The evolutionarily conserved Janus kinase-signal transducers and activators of transcription (JAK-STAT) signaling pathway mediates responses to a number of important cytokines and growth factors (26) (**Figures 1, 2**). The specific responses to JAK-STAT signaling are therefore highly dependent on the cellular context and include proliferation, differentiation, migration, apoptosis, and cell survival (27). As a consequence, JAK-STAT pathways are involved in various physiological processes, including innate and adaptive immune responses, hematopoiesis, growth, and development (28). The identification of the JAK-STAT pathway was the result of seminal work performed by several scientists, including Darnell, Stark, and Kerr in the search for molecules mediating IFN-induced signaling (29). Four members of the JAK family (JAK1, 2, 3, and tyrosine kinase (TYK)2 and seven members of the STAT family (STAT1, 2, 3, 4, 5A, 5B, and 6) have been identified (28). JAKs belong to a class of tyrosine kinases characterized by containing both a catalytic domain and a kinase-like domain with autoregulatory function (29). By functional screening, these kinases were subsequently functionally linked to the transcription factors STATs (26). The overall structure of STAT proteins consists of coiled coil (CC) domain, a DNA binding domain (DBD), and an SH2 domain (29).

JAK-STAT Signaling Downstream of the IFN Receptor

Type I IFNs act via the IFNα/β receptor (IFNAR)1 and IFNAR2, type III IFN signals through IFNLR1 and IL10R2, whereas IFNγ acts via IFNGR1 and IFNGR2 (11) (**Figure 1**). The binding of type I IFN induces formation of a receptor complex between

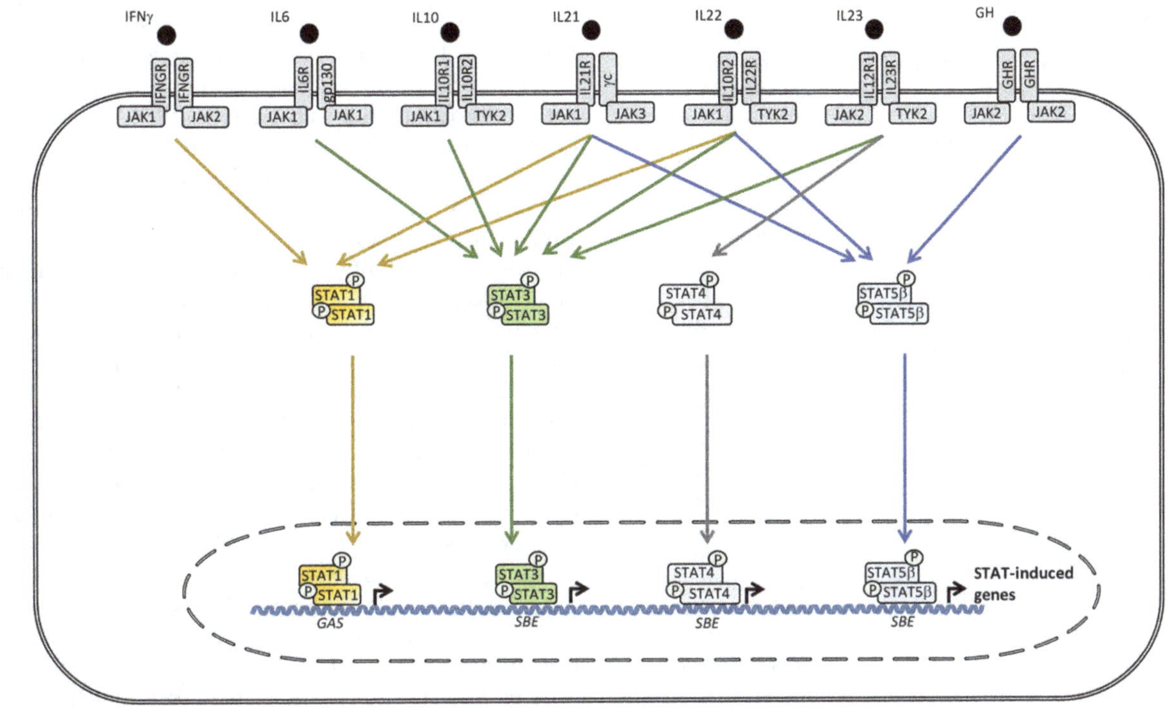

FIGURE 2 | A wide range of cytokines, including interleukin (IL)6, IL10, IL21, IL22, IL23, IFNγ, and growth factors activate receptors utilizing different combinations of the tyrosine kinases janus activated kinase (JAK)1, JAK2, and tyrosine kinase (TYK)2 which trigger signaling pathways involving signal transducer and activator of transcription (STAT)1, STAT3, STAT4, and STAT5A/B. Phosphorylated STAT3 can homo- or heterodimerize with other STAT3 molecules or STAT1 or STAT5, respectively. STAT complexes modulate transcription of various genes, including increased IL6, IL10, IL17A/17F, IL22, transforming growth factor (TGF)β, and monocytic chemotactic protein (MCP)1 production, as well as decreased tumor necrosis factor (TNF)α, IL12, and IFNγ synthesis. SBE, STAT binding element. GAS, γ-IFN-activated sequence.

IFNAR1 and IFNAR2, leading to activation of the receptor-associated JAK1 and TYK2 kinases (11, 22, 25). This is followed by recruitment and tyrosine phosphorylation of STAT1 and STAT2, which together with the transcription factor IRF9 form the heterotrimeric IFN-stimulated gene factor (ISGF)3 complex that binds to IFN-stimulated regulatory elements (ISRE) (26, 28, 29). In addition, phosphorylated STAT1 homodimers, termed IFN-γ-activated factor (GAF), are activated and in a similar manner induce transcription from γ-IFN activation sequence (GAS) (30) (**Figure 1**). Signaling from the type III IFN receptor is similar. In the case of type II IFN, binding of IFNγ induces homodimerization of IFNGR1 subunits and recruitment of IFNGR2 subunits, and this association induces phosphorylation and activation of JAK1 and JAK2 kinases, ultimately leading to phosphorylation of STAT1 to form the GAF complex as well as weak activation of the ISGF3 complex (11).

STAT3 Signaling Downstream of Multiple Cytokine and Growth Factor Receptors

The STAT3 molecule was discovered by Akira et al. by purification and cloning and was found to bind to the interleukin (IL)6 responsive element of the acute phase response promoter (31). Simultaneously STAT3 was described by another group as a DNA binding protein downstream of the epidermal growth factor receptor (32). Pathways involving STAT3 activation are triggered by a number of cytokines and growth factors (27) (**Figure 2**). Receptor binding of the ligand leads to recruitment of intracellular JAK2 and TYK2, resulting in specific phosphorylation on STAT3 at tyrosine 705, allowing dimerization, nuclear translocation, and transcriptional activation of target genes (27). Phosphorylated STAT3 primarily homodimerize but also has the capacity to heterodimerize with STAT1 and STAT5, thereby inducing differentiated transcriptional programs (**Figure 2**). The 770 amino acid STAT3 molecule may be further post-translationally modified by phosphorylation, methylation, and acetylation, contributing to functional regulation (27, 28). The set of genes induced by actvated STAT3 is extraordinarily high and diverse, including IL10, IL17A/F, IL22, IL26, transforming growth factor (TGF)β, IL6, and monocytic chemotactic protein (MCP) 1. In contrast, pro-inflammatory mediators, such as tumor necrosis factor (TNF)α, IFNγ, and IL12, are downregulated through STAT3-mediated signaling pathways (27) (**Figure 2**).

DISEASES ASSOCIATED WITH DEFECTIVE IRF SIGNALING

In the second part of this review, presently known PIDs associated with defects in IRF and STAT transcription factors

TABLE 1 | Mutations in IRFs and STATs, functional impact, and associated PID/infectious phenotype.

Gene	Inheritance	Allele	PID and infectious phenotype
IRF3	AD/IP	LOF	Herpes simplex encephalitis (HSE)
IRF7	AR	LOF	Severe influenza
IRF8	AR	LOF	Mendelian susceptibility to mycobacterial infection (MSMD)
IRF9	AR	LOF	Severe influenza
STAT1	AD/AR	LOF	MSMD, HSE, fungi
STAT1	AD	GOF	Chronic mucocutaneous candidiasis (CMC), progressive multifocal leukoencephalopathy (PML)/JC virus
STAT3	AD	LOF	Hyper-IgE syndrome (HIES), *Staphylococcus aureus*, *Candida albicans*, aspergillus, EBV
STAT3	AD	GOF	Autoinflammation, hypogammaglobulinemia
STAT5B	AD	LOF	Growth hormone insensitivity syndrome (GHIS) with a broad infectious phenotype

IRF, interferon (IFN) regulatory factor; STAT, signal transducer and activator of transcription; AD, autosomal dominant, AR, autosomal recessive; LOF, loss-of-function; GOF, gain-of-function.

are described, including the clinical presentation, infectious phenotype and the genetic and immunological basis of disease. An overview of individual genetic defects and associated PIDs is given in **Table 1**, and the signaling pathways and transcription factors affected by either defective or excessive function of IRFs and STATs are illustrated in **Figures 3, 4**.

IRF3 Deficiency and Herpes Simplex Encephalitis

A number of seminal discoveries by Casanova and colleagues described an essential non-redundant role of TLR3 signaling, including TLR3, UNC93B, TRIF, TRAF3, and TBK1, and the generation of type I IFN responses in the central nervous system (CNS) in protection against herpes simplex encephalitis (HSE) (33–37). Based on this work, our group additionally described a patient with defective IRF3 signaling and HSE (38) (**Figure 3**). The patient, who was a 16-year-old adolescent, suffered from a severe episode of HSE with convulsions and neurological deficits and was found to have impaired type I IFN production in response to HSV-1 and a number of viral PAMPs. More specifically, the R285Q *IRF3* mutation resulted in change from the positively charged arginine to the neutral glutamine, causing functionally defective phosphorylation, dimerization, and transcriptional activation of IRF3 (38). Since no dominant negative effect of the IRF3 variant could be demonstrated, it was concluded that the mechanism was haploinsufficiency and that the inheritance was autosomal dominant (AD) with incomplete penetrance. The causal relationship between heterozygous IRF3 deficiency and HSE was supported by the reconstitution of patient fibroblasts with wild-type (wt) IRF3, resulting in normal production of type I and III IFN in response to HSV and the TLR3 ligand Poly(IC). The infectious history of the patient, like the vast majority of previously described HSE patients with defects in TLR3 signaling pathways, was notable for no previously reported increased susceptibility to other infections, suggesting specificity in the susceptibility to HSV-1 infection and development of CNS infection (38). This very narrow infectious phenotype caused by a defect of a transcription factor, which represents a point of convergence downstream of several IFN-inducing PRRs appears surprising. However, this observation may be, at least partly, explained by the more pronounced impact of the specific R285Q *IRF3* mutation on the functional interaction with the TLR3 pathway adaptor molecule TRIF, than between IRF3 and the adaptor molecules MAVS and STING of the RIG-I and DNA sensor signaling pathways, respectively, (6, 38). Importantly, a second patient with a different IRF3 variant was subsequently described in a cohort of adult patients with HSE, providing further support for IRF3 as a genetic etiology for HSE (39). Also of relevance is a case report describing the presence of a TLR3 variant in a patient with recurrent HSV-2 meningitis (Mollaret's meningitis), thus adding another piece of data to the notion of an important role of the TLR3 signaling pathway for mounting protective IFN responses during HSV-1 and HSV2 neuroinfections (40). Importantly, this is paralleled by an earlier study showing increased susceptibility to HSV-1 infection in the brain in IRF3-deficient mice (41).

IRF7 and IRF9 Deficiency and Severe Influenza

Despite a number of single nucleotide polymorphisms (SNP)s identified by genome wide association studies (GWAS) in patients with severe disseminated influenza infection, as well as evidence from mouse studies of an essential role of IFN in antiviral defenses against Influenza virus, the first monogenic defect associated with severe influenza was only described in 2015 (42, 43). The authors described homozygous IRF7 deficiency in a 2.5-year-old girl with severe influenza and acute respiratory distress syndrome (**Figure 3**). Functional studies demonstrated abolished type I IFN production in pDCs in response to Influenza A virus (IAV) and consequently elevated IAV replication in fibroblasts. The results were were further supported by including airway epithelial cells derived from induced pluripotent stem cells from the patient revealing impaired IAV replication and reduced IFN production (42).

Again the common theme is a relatively narrow infectious phenotype of the patient in contrast to *Irf7* knock-out mice which exhibit elevated susceptibility to a number of RNA- and DNA viruses (44, 45). Finally, there are some remaining pieces to the puzzle, since the infectious phenotype of patients with mutations in IRF3 and STAT1 that impair induction and responsiveness to type I IFN, respectively, have not revealed a similar increased risk

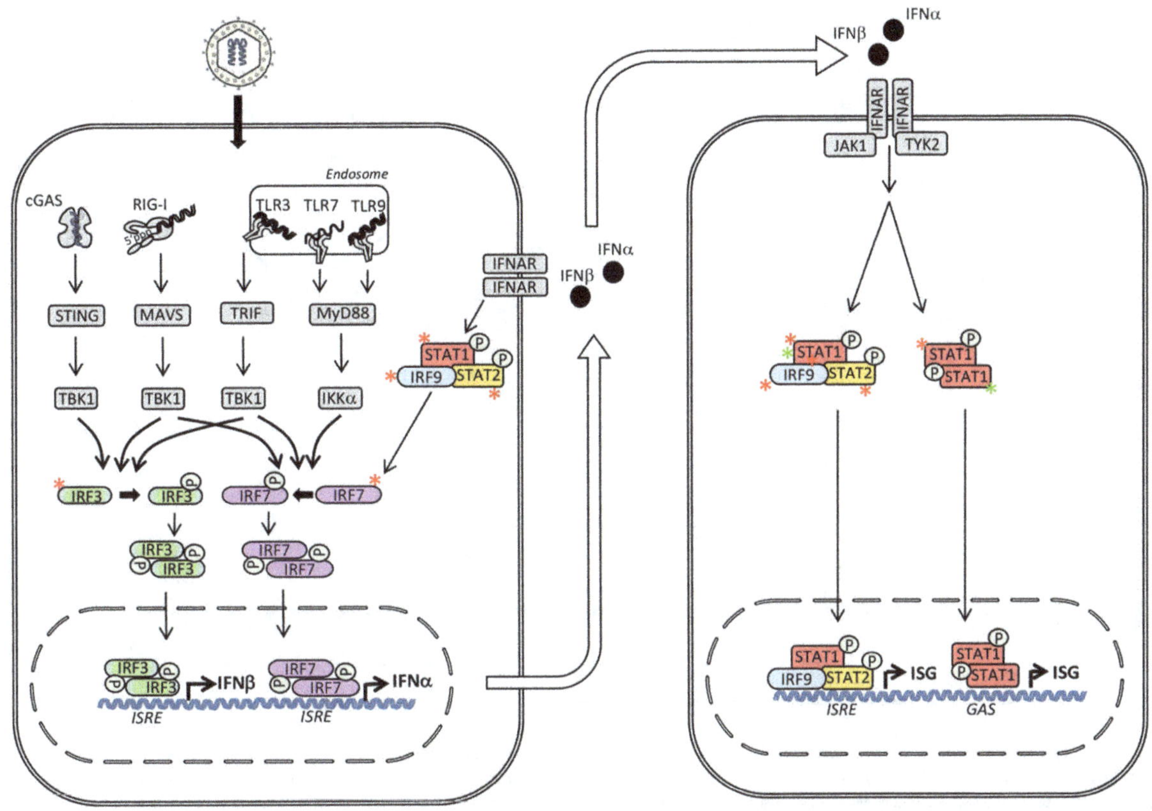

FIGURE 3 | Inborn errors of immunity in interferon (IFN) regulatory factors (IRF)s and signal transducers and activators of transcription (STAT)s may lead to either loss-of-function (LOF) (red asterisk) or gain of-function (GOF) (green asterisk) of the molecule and result in different primary immunodeficiencies (PID)s and infectious phenotypes. Within the IFN inducing signaling pathways defects in IRF3, IRF7, IRF9, and IRF8 result in herpes simplex encephalitis (HSE), severe influenza, and Mendelian susceptibility to mycobacterial disease (MSMD), respectively. Defects downstream of the type I IFN receptor in STAT1, STAT2 or IRF9 cause MSMD, susceptibility to measles, and severe influenza, respectively. In contrast, STAT1 GOF causes chronic mucocutaneous candidiasis (CMC). ISRE, IFN stimulated response element; GAS, γ-IFN-activated sequence.

of severe influenza infection (38, 46). This intriguing observation may suggest a particularly important role of the IRF3-IRF7 amplification loop for rapid production of large amounts of IFNβ as well as multiple IFNα subtypes in antiviral defense against IAV in lung tissue and/or alveolar macrophages (43).

Recently, life-threatening influenza was also reported in a child with autosomal recessive (AR) homozygous IRF9 deficiency (47) (**Figure 3**). Since IRF9 acts downstream of type IFN as part of the ISGF3 complex, IRF9 deficiency represents a defect in the response to IFN rather than in the induction of IFN responses. Prior to admission with severe influenza at the age of 5 years, the patient had an infectious history with several hospital admissions with RSV bronchiolitis, severe disease with biliary perforation presumably secondary to vaccination with the measles-mumps-rubella (MMR) vaccine, and frequent fevers. Based on serological evidence of infections with HSV, cytomegalovirus (CMV), rhinoviruses, and enteroviruses without particularly severe clinical infections, the report suggested a relatively narrow phenotype of IRF9 deficiency (47). The authors demonstrated normal responses to STAT1 homodimers and STAT1/2 heterodimers from a GAS promoter in contrast to impaired responses from an ISRE promoter downstream of the heterotrimer STAT1/STAT2/IRF9 (47) (**Figure 3**). The causal relationship between homozygous IRF9 deficiency and increased susceptibility to influenza was convincingly demonstrated by the rescue of IFN responses and control of viral replication after expression of wt IRF9 in patient cells (47). In addition to IRF7 and IRF9 deficiency predisposing to severe influenza, a *RIG-I* variant has also been described in an adult patient with severe influenza (48). Altogether, these reports demonstrate an important role of type I (and possibly type III) IFN in antiviral immunity to influenza virus in humans.

DISEASES ASSOCIATED WITH DEFECTIVE STAT SIGNALING

STAT1- and IRF8 Deficiency and Mendelian Susceptibility to Mycobacterial Disease

AD STAT1 deficiency was among the first genetic etiologies of mycobacterial disease to be described (49) (**Figure 3**). This condition, which was termed Mendelian susceptibility to mycobacterial disease (MSMD), primarily leads to severe infection with atypical mycobacteria and the weakly virulent

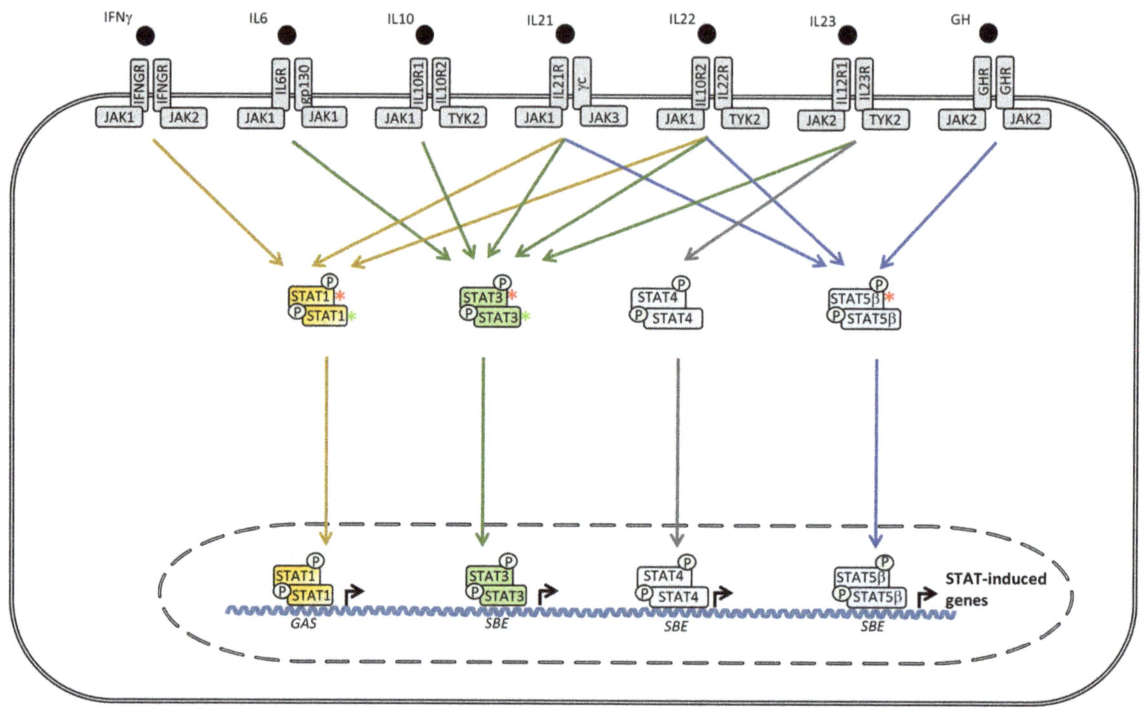

FIGURE 4 | Defects downstream of various receptors utilizing signal transcducer and activator of transcription (STAT)1, STAT3, or STAT5B cause Mendelian susceptibility to mycobacterial disease (MSMD), hyper-IgE syndrome (HIES) and growth hormone insensitivity syndrome (GHIS), respectively. In contrast, STAT1 GOF causes chronic mucocutaneous candidiasis (CMC), whereas, STAT3 GOF leads to an autoinflammatory condition with hypogammaglobulinemia, lymphoproliferation, and a broad infectious phenotype. SBE, STAT bindinf element; GAS, γ-IFN-activated sequence.

Bacille-Calmette-Guerin (BCG) vaccine strain. However, severe viral infections, particularly HSE, and increased susceptibility to certain intracellular bacteria, including *Listeria monocytogenes* and salmonella species, as well as fungi have also been described (50–52). The fundamental and non-redundant role of the IL12-IFNγ circuit in the intercellular communication between macrophages/dendritic myeloid cells and T/NK cells in immunity to mycobacteria has been reinforced by the reports of several defective molecules within these pathways giving rise to MSMD with a very similar phenotype. Thus, MSMD can also originate from defects in IL12 p40, IL12RB1, IFNGR1, IFNGR2, NEMO, ISG15, TYK2, CYBB, IRF8, and most recently in SPPL2a (50–63). In addition, mycobacterial infection is a prominent feature of the MonoMAC syndrome caused by *GATA2* mutations (64, 65). While various heterozygous *STAT1* mutations were described to be associated with impaired IFNγ responses (49, 66), an intriguing aspect of AD STAT1 heterozygous dominant MSMD is the apparent partial preservation of IFNα/IFNβ responses and lack of broad susceptibility to viruses, as might have been expected, given the central position of STAT1 downstream of the type I IFN receptor (29, 67, 68) (**Figure 3**). However, when the first patient with AR STAT1 defect, with complete loss of STAT1 function, was identified, it turned out that this phenotype indeed does show increased susceptibility to a broad range of viral infections in addition to MSMD (2, 58). In addition, patient cells are unresponsive to both IFNγ as well as to IFNα and IFNβ, and even also to IFNλ and IL27 (69). Finally, hypomorphic STAT1 alleles have been described to underlie AR STAT1 deficiency and display a milder, partial phenotype (46, 70–72).

Altogether, MSMD is a clear example of a PID with a relatively narrow infectious phenotype that may originate from a number of molecules belonging to the same functionally connected immunological pathway.

STAT2 Deficiency and Fulminating Vaccine Strain Measles Virus Infection

Whereas STAT1 deficiency, together with other genetic abnormalities in the macrophage - T cell circuit governing IL12-IFNγ immunity, gives rise to MSMD, STAT2 deficiency was reported in 2013 to cause a narrow infectious phenotype with a fulminating disease course in a 5-year old child following MMR vaccination (73) (**Figure 3**). Moreover, an infant brother died from a febrile illness following a presumed viral infection of unknown etiology. Detailed studies revealed a homozygous mutation in intron 4 of *STAT2* preventing correct RNA splicing in patient cells. In addition, the authors demonstrated absence of STAT2 protein expression, significantly impaired type I IFN signaling, as well as abnormal permissiveness to viral replication in patient cells *in vitro* (73). Intriguingly however, patients with STAT2 deficiency have not been described to suffer from neither mycobacterial infection, nor a broad spectrum of viral infections, which might have been anticipated based on profoundly defective IFN responses found *in vitro*. This may suggest partial redundancy between STAT1 and STAT2 with a dominating role of STAT1 in terms of immunity to mycobacteria, i.e., in individuals with STAT1 deficiency STAT2 can partially compensate with regards to mycobacterial infection, whereas STAT1 cannot compensate for the lack of STAT2 when it comes to measles virus infection.

STAT3 Defect and Hyper-IgE Syndrome With Prominent Infectious- and Somatic Phenotypes

Already in the initial description Hyper-IgE syndrome (HIES), originally termed Job's syndrome, "cold" abscesses caused by *Staphylococcus aureus* was described as a prominent feature (74). Other characteristics include eczematoid rashes presenting already during the neonatal period, recurrent sinopulmonary infections, skin abscesses, chronic mucocutaneous candidiasis (CMC), and eosinophilia, in combination with significantly elevated serum IgE>2,000IU/mL, and frequently even higher (75, 76). Fungal infections with *Pneumocystic jirovecii*, histoplasma, coccidioides and cryptococcus have been described to cause mucocutaneous- and gastrointestinal infections as well as meningitis. Moreover, AD HIES patients have been reported to exhibit increased susceptibility to VZV reactivation and Epstein-Barr virus (EBV) viremia (77, 78). The complexity of AD HIES pathogenesis is evidenced by the extensive list of non-immunological manifestations reported (76, 78). Abnormal craniofacial features include characteristic facies, craniosynostosis, high-arched palate, and sometimes retained childhood dentition (79, 80). Within the musculoskeletal system hyperextensibility, scoliosis, osteoporosis, and minimal trauma fractures are observed (76). Increasing awareness has also been on vascular abnormalities, including coronary artery aneurisms and hypertension (81). Similarly to many other PIDs, AD-HIES patients are at an increased risk of developing malignancies, particularly non-Hodgkin lymphoma (82).

The identification of STAT3 as the genetic origin of HIES in 2007 paved the way for a much more detailed understanding of the pathogenesis underlying the immunological abnormalities and infectious disease spectrum as well as the somatic features observed in this disease (83, 84) (**Figure 4**). The first study, revealed increased innate immune responses and impaired IL6 signaling, and further identified both inherited familial and sporadic mutations within the *STAT3* locus in patients with HIES (83). These *STAT3* mutations were either missense mutations or in-frame deletions and appeared to be localized primarily within the SH2-domain or the DBD of the molecule and act by a dominatint negative mechanism (83, 84). However, when mutations were present within the DBD of *STAT3*, expression, phosphorylation, and nuclear translocation of STAT3 were found to be normal compared to the situation in healthy controls (84). In contrast, in patients harboring *STAT3* mutations affecting the SH2 domain or the trans-activating domain, cellular STAT3 phosphorylation at tyrosine 705 was reduced (85). The specific mechanism, by which STAT3 mutations abolish the function of the molecule, therefore remains to be fully clarified.

The central role played by STAT3 in signaling downstream of IL6 is believed to explain a substantial part of the immunodeficiency observed in AD HIES patients (83). This notion is supported by a report describing severe staphylococcal infection in a child with anti-IL6-antibodies, providing further evidence that IL6 is critical in response to human infection with staphylococci (86). Moreover, STAT3 has been shown to negatively regulate type I IFN responses and inflammatory TLR signaling (87). A hallmark of AD HIES is the presence of impaired Th17 responses, and accordingly STAT3 mutations have been demonstrated to result in a failure of Th17 T cell differentiation (88, 89). IL17 signaling also plays a role in neutrophil proliferation and chemotaxis, possibly explaining abnormal neutrophil responses and - recruitment to lung and skin causing recurrent staphylococcal infection in these organs and tissues in HIES (90, 91). Concerning the origin of the highly elevated IgE levels characteristic of the disorder, this feature has been suggested to reflect a role for STAT3 downstream of IL21 receptor signaling, based on the observation of elevated IgE levels in mice deficient in IL21R (83, 92) (**Figure 4**). Notably, HIES also exists in an AR form that may be caused by defects in either TYK2, dedicator of cytokinesis (DOCK)8, or phosphoglucomutase (PGN)3, although these present with a somewhat different phenotype, including a more pronounced tendency toward cutaneous viral infections and without the somatic phenotype characteristic of AD HIES resulting from *STAT3* mutations (78, 93–95). However, TYK2 deficiency as a genetic cause of HIES remains controversial, since TYK2 deficient patients presenting with mycobacterial and viral infections in the absence of HIES have been reported (56).

STAT5B Deficiency in Patients With Short Stature and Immunodeficiency

STAT5B plays a key role downstream of the IL2 receptor and the growth hormone receptor (GHR), explaining why STAT5B defect causes Growth hormone insensitivity syndrome (GHIS) with a complex infectious and somatic phenotype (**Figure 4**). This medical condition was first described by Kofoed et al. in 2003 and constitutes a syndrome with short stature, facial dysmorphism, autoimmune manifestations, and severe infections (9, 10). The spectrum of autoimmune manifestations include autoimmune thyroiditis, idiopathic thrombocytopenic purpura, lymphocytic interstitial pneumonitis, and eczema (9, 10, 96). Although STAT5A and STAT5B molecules are very similar and share a high degree of identity, they differ in both DNA binding- and transactivation domains, providing and explanation for the non-redundant roles of STAT5B in human growth and immunity. The immunological phenotype includes a reduced number of $CD4^{+}CD25high$ $Foxp3^{+}$ cells in STAT5B patients, which is thought to contribute to the immune dysregulation of the disease (67). Indeed, studies in *Stat5a/Stat5b* double-deficient mice have demonstrated reduced numbers of Treg cells, functionally connected to the development of autoimmunity and lymphocytic infiltrations (97). Moreover, based on the immune phenotype in mice, an increased rate of T cell apoptosis has been suggested to contribute to T cell lymphopenia and the broad susceptibility to infections observed in STAT5B deficient patients (67). Finally the insensitivity to GH originates from the role of STAT5B in inducing expression of insulin growth factor (IGF)-1 following GHR activation and STAT5B phosphorylation by JAK2 (67) (**Figure 4**).

DISEASES ASSOCIATED WITH EXCESSIVE STAT SIGNALING

STAT1 Gain-of-Function in Th17 Deficiency and Chronic Mucocutaneous Candidiasis

A common theme in several PIDs is that different mutations in a given molecule may have rather different functional consequences and impact and hence may result in entirely different clinical pictures (3). A good example of this is the major difference between STAT1 deficiency (described above) as opposed to the disease caused by STAT1 gain-of-function (GOF) (**Figures 3, 4**). Two groups of investigators independently established heterozygous STAT1 GOF as a cause of Th17 deficiency and AD CMC. Van de Veerdonk et al. analyzed 5 different families constituting 14 cases of AD CMC, leading to the finding of defective production of IFNβ, IL17, and IL22 in response to candida, and the identification of heterozygous mutations within conserved residues in exon 10 encoding the CC domain of *STAT1* (98). Simultaneously, Liu et al. identified heterozygous variations in the *STAT1* gene within the CC domain by WES (16). Functional analyses of the mutant alleles revealed GOF mutations by a mechanism involving impaired nuclear dephosphorylation of Stat1, and indeed, nuclear dephosporylation rather than cytosolic hyperphosphorylation may be the dominant molecular mechanism underlying the immunological abnormalities in STAT1 GOF (99). Altogether, several different amino acid changes have been reported to cause either STAT1 LOF or GOF, most prominently in the CC domain and the DB domain of the molecule, although the precise functional impact of individual mutations may be difficult to estimate by bioinformatics alone, but requires mutagenesis studies (89, 98–104). Moreover, autoimmunity is a common feature of this patient population. Thyroid disease, enteropathy, alopecia, autoimmune cytopenias, type I diabetes and systemic lupus erythematosus-like disease have been reported (105). More recently, progressive multifocal leukoencephalopathy (PML) caused by reactivation of JC virus was described in a small number of patients with STAT1 GOF, indicating a profound T cell deficiency in this condition (98).

Several hypotheses have been presented to explain the molecular mechanism, whereby *STAT1* GOF impairs the development of Th17 cells and IL17 responses (89). One of these states that STAT1 counteracts the gene expression induced by STAT3 downstream of Th17 cell differentiating- and generating signals, such as IL6, IL21, and IL23 signaling (106) (**Figure 4**). Another idea is that exaggerated IFNα/β- and IL27 responses inhibit the development of the Th17 subset of T cells (67, 107). However, the precise molecular mechanisms behind impaired STAT3 signaling in these patients remains unknown. As to the pathogenesis of the autoimmune phenomena sometimes associated with STAT1 GOF, this is not readily explained by decreased numbers of Treg cells, which appear to be normal (108). However, based on the observation that some of the features in STAT1 GOF patients overlap with the group of monogenic diseases termed interferonopathies, including an elevated IFN signature, i.e., upregulation of ISGs in the blood, this may account for some aspects of the autoimmunity present (109–111).

STAT3 GOF in an Autoinflammatory Phenotype With Hypogammaglobulinemia and Lymphoproliferation

Defective STAT3 has been described above as the genetic origin of AD HIES. However, more recently it has been appreciated that the opposite, namely *STAT3* GOF mutations, can cause early-onset lymphoproliferation and autoimmunity (3, 112–114) (**Figure 4**). This severe pleiotrophic phenotype with multiorgan involvement encompasses hypogammaglobulinemia without fulfilling the criteria for common variable immunodeficiency (CVID), together with autoimmune cytopenias, lymphocytic interstitial pneumonia, enteropathy, hepatitis, and arthritis. Examination of the immunological phenotype revealed hypogammaglobulinemia, T cell lymphopenia (with increased fraction of double-negative T cells), impairment in switched memory B cells, decreased pDCs, as well as reduced regulatory T cells, in accordance with autoimmunity as a dominating feature (77, 112–114).

PROPHYLAXIS AND TREATMENT OF DISEASES AFFECTING IRFs AND STATs

A number of prophylactic and therapeutic strategies are currently available to prevent and treat PIDs in general, including those involving IRFs and STATs. Overall, since these conditions are generally severe and life threatening and often diagnosed early in life, they need correction by bone marrow transplantation (BMT) or hematopoietic stem cell transplantation (HSCT), where results are generally excellent, particularly in the case of early treatment, although depending on the underlying condition and genetic etiology. Thus, survival and cure is currently reached in up to 90% of patients undergoing HSCT for severe PIDs (115, 116). A prerequisite for these positive results, however, is early diagnosis and HSCT before secondary complications develop. This goal may be achieved in the future by introducing advanced programs for newborn screening for some of the major PIDs, which has proven possible in the case of SCID, even in developing countries (117, 118). Among the PIDs related to IRF and STAT deficiencies covered in the present review, HSCT are used for MSMD, HIES, GHIS as well as for STAT1 GOF and STAT3 GOF (119).

I addition, general vaccination strategies are relevant in the case of severe influenza in IRF7 and IRF9 deficiency. Prophylaxis with antibiotics (for example co-trimoxazole) and antifungals (such as intraconazole) are broadly employed with good results in conditions, such as HIES, CMC, GHIS, and MSMD (119). Prophylactic aciclovir treatment may be recommended in some cases of HSE caused by IRF3 deficiency, at least in recurrent cases. In many conditions dominated by abnormalities in B cell development and -responses with resulting hypogammaglobulinemia, immunoglobulin substitution therapy is a cornerstone of maintenance prophylaxis against infection with many years of experience and good evidence of beneficial effects in various PIDs (115, 119).

Novel medications include use of selective JAK inhibitors for the treatment of excessive production of type I IFN in the group of interferonopathies caused by mutations in STING or other molecules within the DNA sensing pathways (111, 120). Such approaches may also be relevant in a number of the described PIDs, such as STAT1 GOF and HIES, in which type I IFN is believed to play a role in generating the autoimmune state. On the other hand, HSE associated with impaired antiviral type I IFN responses might be treated with type I IFN as an adjunctive to the current standard therapy with antiviral aciclovir, although large clinical trials are ongoing but need to prove efficacy of this treatment approach.

Finally, looking into the future, new powerful technologies, such as CRISPR/Cas editing of genetic defects in PIDs is a promising avenue, which has already demonstrated potential success for medical conditions such as β-globin expression in thalassemia, and more recently in the case of certain PIDs, most notably chronic granulomatous disease (CGD) and adenosine deaminase (ADA)-severe combined immunodeficiency (SCID) (121–124). It seems highly likely that the CRISPR/Cas technique will be more widely applicable, also to some of the PIDs described here involving IRFs and STATs. Among these STAT1 and STAT3 deficiency in MSMD and AD HIES might be good candidates for gene correction.

CONCLUSION AND FUTURE PERSPECTIVES

Lessons learned from the fascinating decade long unraveling of PIDs are numerous and have provided fundamental new insight into basic infection immunology and the correlates of protective immunity against bacterial, viral, and fungal pathogens in humans. More recently, it has also brought new knowledge about the pathogenesis of a number of conditions with underlying autoimmunity and autoinflammation. Importantly, these discoveries have been taken directly into clinical medicine and are thus the basis, upon which the invention and development of specific prophylactic and therapeutic strategies for patients are based.

Notably, this journey has repeatedly demonstrated significant differences between mouse and human immunity, which underscores the importance and strength of studying human patients to understand basic innate and adaptive immunology in humans. Moreover, with the increasing awareness of the major contribution of autoimmunity and autoinflammation as part of many PIDs, there is now a need for the development of approaches to treating these complex pathologies (114). Again, this reinforces the essential need for understanding basic molecular and cellular mechanisms underlying these states of dysregulated immunity.

In conclusion, improved understanding of the genetic defects and immunopathogenesis of various currently known PIDs is of fundamental importance to identify new targets and immunomodulatory agents in future management of conditions of immune dysregulation, infection, and inflammation. Given that this field of research is in a rapidly expanding phase, it is to be anticipated that many additional human inborn errors of immunity will be uncovered within the next few years. Finally, despite the extensive list of PIDs caused by mutations in IRFs and STATs as described in the present review, we are likely to learn even more in the future, thus providing new insights into both basic biology, signaling, and regulation of these transcription factors and the human pathologies their dysregulation may cause.

AUTHOR CONTRIBUTIONS

The author confirms being the sole contributor of this work and has approved it for publication.

REFERENCES

1. Bucciol G, Moens L, Bosch B, Bossuyt X, Casanova JL, Puel A, et al. Lessons learned from the study of human inborn errors of innate immunity. *J Allergy Clin Immunol.* (2018). doi: 10.1016/j.jaci.2018.07.013. [Epub ahead of print].
2. Sancho-Shimizu V, Perez de Diego R, Jouanguy E, Zhang SY, Casanova JL. Inborn errors of anti-viral interferon immunity in humans. *Curr Opin Virol.* (2011) 1:487–96. doi: 10.1016/j.coviro.2011.10.016
3. Jhamnani RD, Rosenzweig SD. An update on gain-of-function mutations in primary immunodeficiency diseases. *Curr Opin Allergy Clin Immunol.* (2017) 17:391–7. doi: 10.1097/ACI.0000000000000401
4. Mogensen TH. Pathogen recognition and inflammatory signaling in innate immune defenses. *Clin Microbiol Rev.* (2009) 22:240–73. doi: 10.1128/CMR.00046-08
5. Paludan SR, Bowie AG. Immune sensing of DNA. *Immunity* (2013) 38:870–80. doi: 10.1016/j.immuni.2013.05.004
6. Liu S, Cai X, Wu J, Cong Q, Chen X, Li T, et al. Phosphorylation of innate immune adaptor proteins MAVS, STING, and TRIF induces IRF3 activation. *Science* (2015) 347:aaa2630. doi: 10.1126/science.aaa2630
7. Ning S, Pagano JS, Barber GN. IRF7: activation, regulation, modification and function. *Genes Immun.* (2011) 12:399–414. doi: 10.1038/gene.2011.21
8. Bao M, Liu YJ. Regulation of TLR7/9 signaling in plasmacytoid dendritic cells. *Protein Cell* (2013) 4:40–52. doi: 10.1007/s13238-012-2104-8
9. Kofoed EM, Hwa V, Little B, Woods KA, Buckway CK, Tsubaki J, et al. Growth hormone insensitivity associated with a STAT5b mutation. *N Engl J Med.* (2003) 349:1139–47. doi: 10.1056/NEJMoa022926
10. Nadeau K, Hwa V, Rosenfeld RG. STAT5b deficiency: an unsuspected cause of growth failure, immunodeficiency, and severe pulmonary disease. *J Pediatr.* (2011) 158:701–8. doi: 10.1016/j.jpeds.2010.12.042
11. Stark GR, Kerr IM, Williams BR, Silverman RH, Schreiber RD. How cells respond to interferons. *Annu Rev Biochem.* (1998) 67:227–64. doi: 10.1146/annurev.biochem.67.1.227

12. Kim TK, Maniatis T. The mechanism of transcriptional synergy of an *in vitro* assembled interferon-beta enhanceosome. *Mol Cell* (1997) 1:119–29. doi: 10.1016/S1097-2765(00)80013-1
13. Honda K, Taniguchi T. IRFs: master regulators of signalling by Toll-like receptors and cytosolic pattern-recognition receptors. *Nat Rev Immunol.* (2006) 6:644–58. doi: 10.1038/nri1900
14. Osterlund PI, Pietila TE, Veckman V, Kotenko SV, Julkunen I. IFN regulatory factor family members differentially regulate the expression of type III IFN (IFN-lambda) genes. *J Immunol.* (2007) 179:3434–42. doi: 10.4049/jimmunol.179.6.3434
15. Au WC, Moore PA, LaFleur DW, Tombal B, Pitha PM. Characterization of the interferon regulatory factor-7 and its potential role in the transcription activation of interferon A genes. *J Biol Chem.* (1998) 273:29210–7. doi: 10.1074/jbc.273.44.29210
16. Marie I, Durbin JE, Levy DE. Differential viral induction of distinct interferon-alpha genes by positive feedback through interferon regulatory factor-7. *EMBO J.* (1998) 17:6660–9. doi: 10.1093/emboj/17.22.6660
17. Iversen MB, Paludan SR. Mechanisms of type III interferon expression. *J Interferon Cytokine Res.* (2010) 30:573–8. doi: 10.1089/jir.2010.0063
18. Civas A, Island ML, Genin P, Morin P, Navarro S. Regulation of virus-induced interferon-A genes. *Biochimie* (2002) 84:643–54. doi: 10.1016/S0300-9084(02)01431-1
19. Isaacs A, Lindenmann J. Virus interference. I. The interferon. *Proc R Soc Lond B Biol Sci.* (1957) 147:258–67. doi: 10.1098/rspb.1957.0048
20. Taniguchi T, Fujii-Kuriyama Y, Muramatsu M. Molecular cloning of human interferon cDNA. *Proc Natl Acad Sci USA.* (1980) 77:4003–6. doi: 10.1073/pnas.77.7.4003
21. Maeda S, McCandliss R, Gross M, Sloma A, Familletti PC, Tabor JM, et al. Construction and identification of bacterial plasmids containing nucleotide sequence for human leukocyte interferon. *Proc Natl Acad Sci USA.* (1980) 77:7010–3. doi: 10.1073/pnas.77.12.7010
22. Levy DE, Garcia-Sastre A. The virus battles: IFN induction of the antiviral state and mechanisms of viral evasion. *Cytokine Growth Factor Rev.* (2001) 12:143–56. doi: 10.1016/S1359-6101(00)00027-7
23. Katze MG, He Y, Gale M Jr. Viruses and interferon: a fight for supremacy. *Nat Rev Immunol.* (2002) 2:675–87. doi: 10.1038/nri888
24. Pestka S, Krause CD, Walter MR. Interferons, interferon-like cytokines, and their receptors. *Immunol Rev.* (2004) 202:8–32. doi: 10.1111/j.0105-2896.2004.00204.x
25. Negishi H, Taniguchi T, Yanai H. The Interferon (IFN) class of cytokines and the IFN Regulatory Factor (IRF) Transcription factor family. *Cold Spring Harb Perspect Biol.* (2017) 10. doi: 10.1101/cshperspect.a028423
26. Darnell JE Jr. Studies of IFN-induced transcriptional activation uncover the Jak-Stat pathway. *J Interferon Cytokine Res.* (1998) 18:549–54.
27. Stark GR, Darnell JE Jr. The JAK-STAT pathway at twenty. *Immunity* (2012) 36:503–14. doi: 10.1016/j.immuni.2012.03.013
28. Briscoe J, Guschin D, Rogers NC, Watling D, Muller M, Horn F, et al. JAKs, STATs and signal transduction in response to the interferons and other cytokines. *Philos Trans R Soc Lond B Biol Sci.* (1996) 351:167–71. doi: 10.1098/rstb.1996.0013
29. Darnell JE Jr, Kerr IM, Stark GR. Jak-STAT pathways and transcriptional activation in response to IFNs and other extracellular signaling proteins. *Science* (1994) 264:1415–21. doi: 10.1126/science.8197455
30. Decker T, Kovarik P, Meinke A. GAS elements: a few nucleotides with a major impact on cytokine-induced gene expression. *J Interferon Cytokine Res.* (1997) 17:121–34. doi: 10.1089/jir.1997.17.121
31. Akira S, Nishio Y, Inoue M, Wang XJ, Wei S, Matsusaka T, et al. Molecular cloning of APRF, a novel IFN-stimulated gene factor 3 p91-related transcription factor involved in the gp130-mediated signaling pathway. *Cell* (1994) 77:63–71. doi: 10.1016/0092-8674(94)90235-6
32. Zhong Z, Wen Z, Darnell JE Jr. Stat3: a STAT family member activated by tyrosine phosphorylation in response to epidermal growth factor and interleukin-6. *Science* (1994) 264:95–8. doi: 10.1126/science.8140422
33. Casrouge A, Zhang SY, Eidenschenk C, Jouanguy E, Puel A, Yang K, et al. Herpes simplex virus encephalitis in human UNC-93B deficiency. *Science* (2006) 314:308–12. doi: 10.1126/science.1128346
34. Zhang SY, Jouanguy E, Ugolini S, Smahi A, Elain G, Romero P, et al. TLR3 deficiency in patients with herpes simplex encephalitis. *Science* (2007) 317:1522–7. doi: 10.1126/science.1139522
35. Sancho-Shimizu V, Perez de Diego R, Lorenzo L, Halwani R, Alangari A, Israelsson E, et al. Herpes simplex encephalitis in children with autosomal recessive and dominant TRIF deficiency. *J Clin Invest.* (2011) 121:4889–902. doi: 10.1172/JCI59259
36. Perez de Diego R, Sancho-Shimizu V, Lorenzo L, Puel A, Plancoulaine S, Picard C, et al. Human TRAF3 adaptor molecule deficiency leads to impaired Toll-like receptor 3 response and susceptibility to herpes simplex encephalitis. *Immunity* (2010) 33:400–11. doi: 10.1016/j.immuni.2010.08.014
37. Herman M, Ciancanelli M, Ou YH, Lorenzo L, Klaudel-Dreszler M, Pauwels E, et al. Heterozygous TBK1 mutations impair TLR3 immunity and underlie herpes simplex encephalitis of childhood. *J Exp Med.* (2012) 209:1567–82. doi: 10.1084/jem.20111316
38. Andersen LL, Mork N, Reinert LS, Kofod-Olsen E, Narita R, Jorgensen SE, et al. Functional IRF3 deficiency in a patient with herpes simplex encephalitis. *J Exp Med.* (2015) 212:1371–9. doi: 10.1084/jem.20142274
39. Mork N, Kofod-Olsen E, Sorensen KB, Bach E, Orntoft TF, Ostergaard L, et al. Mutations in the TLR3 signaling pathway and beyond in adult patients with herpes simplex encephalitis. *Genes Immun.* (2015) 16:552–66. doi: 10.1038/gene.2015.46
40. Willmann O, Ahmad-Nejad P, Neumaier M, Hennerici MG, Fatar M. Toll-like receptor 3 immune deficiency may be causative for HSV-2-associated mollaret meningitis. *Eur Neurol.* (2010) 63:249–51. doi: 10.1159/000287585
41. Menachery VD, Pasieka TJ, Leib DA. Interferon regulatory factor 3-dependent pathways are critical for control of herpes simplex virus type 1 central nervous system infection. *J Virol.* (2010) 84:9685–94. doi: 10.1128/JVI.00706-10
42. Ciancanelli MJ, Huang SX, Luthra P, Garner H, Itan Y, Volpi S, et al. Infectious disease. Life-threatening influenza and impaired interferon amplification in human IRF7 deficiency. *Science* (2015) 348:448–53. doi: 10.1126/science.aaa1578
43. Ciancanelli MJ, Abel L, Zhang SY, Casanova JL. Host genetics of severe influenza: from mouse Mx1 to human IRF7. *Curr Opin Immunol.* (2016) 38:109–20. doi: 10.1016/j.coi.2015.12.002
44. Chen HW, King K, Tu J, Sanchez M, Luster AD, Shresta S. The roles of IRF-3 and IRF-7 in innate antiviral immunity against dengue virus. *J Immunol.* (2013) 191:4194–201. doi: 10.4049/jimmunol.1300799
45. Li W, Hofer MJ, Nocon AL, Manders P, Campbell IL. Interferon regulatory factor 7 (IRF7) is required for the optimal initial control but not subsequent clearance of lymphocytic choriomeningitis virus infection in mice. *Virology* (2013) 439:152–62. doi: 10.1016/j.virol.2013.02.015
46. Boisson-Dupuis S, Kong XF, Okada S, Cypowyj S, Puel A, Abel L, et al. Inborn errors of human STAT1: allelic heterogeneity governs the diversity of immunological and infectious phenotypes. *Curr Opin Immunol.* (2012) 24:364–78. doi: 10.1016/j.coi.2012.04.011
47. Hernandez N, Melki I, Jing H, Habib T, Huang SSY, Danielson J, et al. Life-threatening influenza pneumonitis in a child with inherited IRF9 deficiency. *J Exp Med.* (2018) 215:2567–85. doi: 10.1084/jem.20180628
48. Jorgensen SE, Christiansen M, Ryo LB, Gad HH, Gjedsted J, Staeheli P, et al. Defective RNA sensing by RIG-I in severe influenza virus infection. *Clin Exp Immunol.* (2018) 192:366–76. doi: 10.1111/cei.13120
49. Dupuis S, Dargemont C, Fieschi C, Thomassin N, Rosenzweig S, Harris J, et al. Impairment of mycobacterial but not viral immunity by a germline human STAT1 mutation. *Science* (2001) 293:300–3. doi: 10.1126/science.1061154
50. Abel L, El-Baghdadi J, Bousfiha AA, Casanova JL, Schurr E. Human genetics of tuberculosis: a long and winding road. *Philos Trans R Soc Lond B Biol Sci.* (2014) 369:20130428. doi: 10.1098/rstb.2013.0428
51. Boisson-Dupuis S, Bustamante J, El-Baghdadi J, Camcioglu Y, Parvaneh N, El Azbaoui S, et al. Inherited and acquired immunodeficiencies underlying tuberculosis in childhood. *Immunol Rev.* (2015) 264:103–20. doi: 10.1111/imr.12272
52. Bustamante J, Picard C, Boisson-Dupuis S, Abel L, Casanova JL. Genetic lessons learned from X-linked Mendelian susceptibility to

mycobacterial diseases. *Ann N Y Acad Sci.* (2011) 1246:92–101. doi: 10.1111/j.1749-6632.2011.06273.x
53. Bogunovic D, Byun M, Durfee LA, Abhyankar A, Sanal O, Mansouri D, et al. Mycobacterial disease and impaired IFN-gamma immunity in humans with inherited ISG15 deficiency. *Science* (2012) 337:1684–8. doi: 10.1126/science.1224026
54. Bustamante J, Arias AA, Vogt G, Picard C, Galicia LB, Prando C, et al. Germline CYBB mutations that selectively affect macrophages in kindreds with X-linked predisposition to tuberculous mycobacterial disease. *Nat Immunol.* (2011) 12:213–21. doi: 10.1038/ni.1992
55. Filipe-Santos O, Bustamante J, Haverkamp MH, Vinolo E, Ku CL, Puel A, et al. X-linked susceptibility to mycobacteria is caused by mutations in NEMO impairing CD40-dependent IL-12 production. *J Exp Med.* (2006) 203:1745–59. doi: 10.1084/jem.20060085
56. Kreins AY, Ciancanelli MJ, Okada S, Kong XF, Ramirez-Alejo N, Kilic SS, et al. Human TYK2 deficiency: mycobacterial and viral infections without hyper-IgE syndrome. *J Exp Med.* (2015) 212:1641–62. doi: 10.1084/jem.20140280
57. Altare F, Lammas D, Revy P, Jouanguy E, Doffinger R, Lamhamedi S, et al. Inherited interleukin 12 deficiency in a child with bacille Calmette-Guerin and Salmonella enteritidis disseminated infection. *J Clin Invest.* (1998) 102:2035–40. doi: 10.1172/JCI4950
58. Dupuis S, Jouanguy E, Al-Hajjar S, Fieschi C, Al-Mohsen IZ, Al-Jumaah S, et al. Impaired response to interferon-alpha/beta and lethal viral disease in human STAT1 deficiency. *Nat Genet.* (2003) 33:388–91. doi: 10.1038/ng1097
59. Dorman SE, Picard C, Lammas D, Heyne K, van Dissel JT, Baretto R, et al. Clinical features of dominant and recessive interferon gamma receptor 1 deficiencies. *Lancet* (2004) 364:2113–21. doi: 10.1016/S0140-6736(04)17552-1
60. Kong XF, Martinez-Barricarte R, Kennedy J, Mele F, Lazarov T, Deenick EK, et al. Disruption of an antimycobacterial circuit between dendritic and helper T cells in human SPPL2a deficiency. *Nat Immunol.* (2018) 19:973–85. doi: 10.1038/s41590-018-0178-z
61. Jouanguy E, Altare F, Lamhamedi S, Revy P, Emile JF, Newport M, et al. Interferon-gamma-receptor deficiency in an infant with fatal bacille Calmette-Guerin infection. *N Engl J Med.* (1996) 335:1956–61. doi: 10.1056/NEJM199612263352604
62. Doffinger R, Jouanguy E, Dupuis S, Fondaneche MC, Stephan JL, Emile JF, et al. Partial interferon-gamma receptor signaling chain deficiency in a patient with bacille Calmette-Guerin and Mycobacterium abscessus infection. *J Infect Dis.* (2000) 181:379–84. doi: 10.1086/315197
63. Koscielniak E, de Boer T, Dupuis S, Naumann L, Casanova JL, Ottenhoff TH. Disseminated Mycobacterium peregrinum infection in a child with complete interferon-gamma receptor-1 deficiency. *Pediatr Infect Dis J.* (2003) 22:378–80. doi: 10.1097/01.inf.0000060181.71042.b5
64. Hsu AP, Sampaio EP, Khan J, Calvo KR, Lemieux JE, Patel SY, et al. Mutations in GATA2 are associated with the autosomal dominant and sporadic monocytopenia and mycobacterial infection (MonoMAC) syndrome. *Blood* (2011) 118:2653–5. doi: 10.1182/blood-2011-05-356352
65. Camargo JF, Lobo SA, Hsu AP, Zerbe CS, Wormser GP, Holland SM. MonoMAC syndrome in a patient with a GATA2 mutation: case report and review of the literature. *Clin Infect Dis.* (2013) 57:697–9. doi: 10.1093/cid/cit368
66. Sampaio EP, Bax HI, Hsu AP, Kristosturyan E, Pechacek J, Chandrasekaran P, et al. A novel STAT1 mutation associated with disseminated mycobacterial disease. *J Clin Immunol.* (2012) 32:681–9. doi: 10.1007/s10875-012-9659-2
67. Casanova JL, Holland SM, Notarangelo LD. Inborn errors of human JAKs and STATs. *Immunity* (2012) 36:515–28. doi: 10.1016/j.immuni.2012.03.016
68. Schindler C, Darnell JE Jr. Transcriptional responses to polypeptide ligands: the JAK-STAT pathway. *Annu Rev Biochem.* (1995) 64:621–51.
69. Vairo D, Tassone L, Tabellini G, Tamassia N, Gasperini S, Bazzoni F, et al. Severe impairment of IFN-gamma and IFN-alpha responses in cells of a patient with a novel STAT1 splicing mutation. *Blood* (2011) 118:1806–17. doi: 10.1182/blood-2011-01-330571
70. Averbuch D, Chapgier A, Boisson-Dupuis S, Casanova JL, Engelhard D. The clinical spectrum of patients with deficiency of Signal Transducer and Activator of Transcription-1. *Pediatr Infect Dis J.* (2011) 30:352–5. doi: 10.1097/INF.0b013e3181fdff4a
71. Chapgier A, Boisson-Dupuis S, Jouanguy E, Vogt G, Feinberg J, Prochnicka-Chalufour A, et al. Novel STAT1 alleles in otherwise healthy patients with mycobacterial disease. *PLoS Genet.* (2006) 2:e131. doi: 10.1371/journal.pgen.0020131
72. Kristensen IA, Veirum JE, Moller BK, Christiansen M. Novel STAT1 alleles in a patient with impaired resistance to mycobacteria. *J Clin Immunol.* (2011) 31:265–71. doi: 10.1007/s10875-010-9480-8
73. Hambleton S, Goodbourn S, Young DF, Dickinson P, Mohamad SM, Valappil M, et al. STAT2 deficiency and susceptibility to viral illness in humans. *Proc Natl Acad Sci USA.* (2013) 110:3053–8. doi: 10.1073/pnas.1220098110
74. Davis SD, Schaller J, Wedgwood RJ. Job's Syndrome. Recurrent, "cold", staphylococcal abscesses. *Lancet* (1966) 1:1013–5. doi: 10.1016/S0140-6736(66)90119-X
75. Buckley RH, Wray BB, Belmaker EZ. Extreme hyperimmunoglobulinemia E and undue susceptibility to infection. *Pediatrics* (1972) 49:59–70.
76. Grimbacher B, Holland SM, Gallin JI, Greenberg F, Hill SC, Malech HL, et al. Hyper-IgE syndrome with recurrent infections–an autosomal dominant multisystem disorder. *N Engl J Med.* (1999) 340:692–702. doi: 10.1056/NEJM199903043400904
77. Siegel AM, Heimall J, Freeman AF, Hsu AP, Brittain E, Brenchley JM, et al. A critical role for STAT3 transcription factor signaling in the development and maintenance of human T cell memory. *Immunity* (2011) 35:806–18. doi: 10.1016/j.immuni.2011.09.016
78. Sowerwine KJ, Holland SM, Freeman AF. Hyper-IgE syndrome update. *Ann N Y Acad Sci.* (2012) 1250:25–32. doi: 10.1111/j.1749-6632.2011.06387.x
79. Smithwick EM, Finelt M, Pahwa S, Good RA, Naspitz CK, Mendes NF, et al. Cranial synostosis in Job's syndrome. *Lancet* (1978) 1:826. doi: 10.1016/S0140-6736(78)93028-3
80. O'Connell AC, Puck JM, Grimbacher B, Facchetti F, Majorana A, Gallin JI, et al. Delayed eruption of permanent teeth in hyperimmunoglobulinemia E recurrent infection syndrome. *Oral Surg Oral Med Oral Pathol Oral Radiol Endod.* (2000) 89:177–85. doi: 10.1067/moe.2000.103129
81. Freeman AF, Avila EM, Shaw PA, Davis J, Hsu AP, Welch P, et al. Coronary artery abnormalities in Hyper-IgE syndrome. *J Clin Immunol.* (2011) 31:338–45. doi: 10.1007/s10875-011-9515-9
82. Leonard GD, Posadas E, Herrmann PC, Anderson VL, Jaffe ES, Holland SM, et al. Non-Hodgkin's lymphoma in Job's syndrome: a case report and literature review. *Leuk Lymphoma* (2004) 45:2521–5. doi: 10.1080/10428190400004463
83. Holland SM, DeLeo FR, Elloumi HZ, Hsu AP, Uzel G, Brodsky N, et al. STAT3 mutations in the hyper-IgE syndrome. *N Engl J Med.* (2007) 357:1608–19. doi: 10.1056/NEJMoa073687
84. Minegishi Y, Saito M, Tsuchiya S, Tsuge I, Takada H, Hara T, et al. Dominant-negative mutations in the DNA-binding domain of STAT3 cause hyper-IgE syndrome. *Nature* (2007) 448:1058–62. doi: 10.1038/nature06096
85. Renner ED, Rylaarsdam S, Anover-Sombke S, Rack AL, Reichenbach J, Carey JC, et al. Novel signal transducer and activator of transcription 3 (STAT3) mutations, reduced T(H)17 cell numbers, and variably defective STAT3 phosphorylation in hyper-IgE syndrome. *J Allergy Clin Immunol.* (2008) 122:181–7. doi: 10.1016/j.jaci.2008.04.037
86. Puel A, Picard C, Lorrot M, Pons C, Chrabieh M, Lorenzo L, et al. Recurrent staphylococcal cellulitis and subcutaneous abscesses in a child with autoantibodies against IL-6. *J Immunol.* (2008) 180:647–54. doi: 10.4049/jimmunol.180.1.647
87. Wang WB, Levy DE, Lee CK. STAT3 negatively regulates type I IFN-mediated antiviral response. *J Immunol.* (2011) 187:2578–85. doi: 10.4049/jimmunol.1004128
88. Milner JD, Brenchley JM, Laurence A, Freeman AF, Hill BJ, Elias KM, et al. Impaired T(H)17 cell differentiation in subjects with autosomal dominant hyper-IgE syndrome. *Nature* (2008) 452:773–6. doi: 10.1038/nature06764
89. Puel A, Cypowyj S, Bustamante J, Wright JF, Liu L, Lim HK, et al. Chronic mucocutaneous candidiasis in humans with inborn errors of interleukin-17 immunity. *Science* (2011) 332:65–8. doi: 10.1126/science.1200439
90. Laan M, Cui ZH, Hoshino H, Lotvall J, Sjostrand M, Gruenert DC, et al. Neutrophil recruitment by human IL-17 via C-X-C chemokine release in the airways. *J Immunol.* (1999) 162:2347–52.
91. Hill HR, Ochs HD, Quie PG, Clark RA, Pabst HF, Klebanoff SJ, et al. Defect in neutrophil granulocyte chemotaxis in Job's syndrome

of recurrent "cold" staphylococcal abscesses. *Lancet* (1974) 2:617–9. doi: 10.1016/S0140-6736(74)91942-4
92. Ozaki K, Spolski R, Feng CG, Qi CF, Cheng J, Sher A, et al. A critical role for IL-21 in regulating immunoglobulin production. *Science* (2002) 298:1630–4. doi: 10.1126/science.1077002
93. Engelhardt KR, McGhee S, Winkler S, Sassi A, Woellner C, Lopez-Herrera G, et al. Large deletions and point mutations involving the dedicator of cytokinesis 8 (DOCK8) in the autosomal-recessive form of hyper-IgE syndrome. *J Allergy Clin Immunol.* (2009) 124:1289–302.e4. doi: 10.1016/j.jaci.2009.10.038
94. Woellner C, Schaffer AA, Puck JM, Renner ED, Knebel C, Holland SM, et al. The hyper IgE syndrome and mutations in TYK2. *Immunity* (2007) 26:535. doi: 10.1016/j.immuni.2007.05.007
95. Yang L, Fliegauf M, Grimbacher B. Hyper-IgE syndromes: reviewing PGM3 deficiency. *Curr Opin Pediatr.* (2014) 26:697–703. doi: 10.1097/MOP.0000000000000158
96. Pugliese-Pires PN, Tonelli CA, Dora JM, Silva PC, Czepielewski M, Simoni G, et al. A novel STAT5B mutation causing GH insensitivity syndrome associated with hyperprolactinemia and immune dysfunction in two male siblings. *Eur J Endocrinol.* (2010) 163:349–55. doi: 10.1530/EJE-10-0272
97. Snow JW, Abraham N, Ma MC, Herndier BG, Pastuszak AW, Goldsmith MA. Loss of tolerance and autoimmunity affecting multiple organs in STAT5A/5B-deficient mice. *J Immunol.* (2003) 171:5042–50. doi: 10.4049/jimmunol.171.10.5042
98. van de Veerdonk FL, Plantinga TS, Hoischen A, Smeekens SP, Joosten LA, Gilissen C, et al. STAT1 mutations in autosomal dominant chronic mucocutaneous candidiasis. *N Engl J Med.* (2011) 365:54–61. doi: 10.1056/NEJMoa1100102
99. Liu L, Okada S, Kong XF, Kreins AY, Cypowyj S, Abhyankar A, et al. Gain-of-function human STAT1 mutations impair IL-17 immunity and underlie chronic mucocutaneous candidiasis. *J Exp Med.* (2011) 208:1635–48. doi: 10.1084/jem.20110958
100. Takezaki S, Yamada M, Kato M, Park MJ, Maruyama K, Yamazaki Y, et al. Chronic mucocutaneous candidiasis caused by a gain-of-function mutation in the STAT1 DNA-binding domain. *J Immunol.* (2012) 189:1521–6. doi: 10.4049/jimmunol.1200926
101. Yamazaki Y, Yamada M, Kawai T, Morio T, Onodera M, Ueki M, et al. Two novel gain-of-function mutations of STAT1 responsible for chronic mucocutaneous candidiasis disease: impaired production of IL-17A and IL-22, and the presence of anti-IL-17F autoantibody. *J Immunol.* (2014) 193:4880–7. doi: 10.4049/jimmunol.1401467
102. Smeekens SP, Plantinga TS, van de Veerdonk FL, Heinhuis B, Hoischen A, Joosten LA, et al. STAT1 hyperphosphorylation and defective IL12R/IL23R signaling underlie defective immunity in autosomal dominant chronic mucocutaneous candidiasis. *PLoS ONE* (2011) 6:e29248. doi: 10.1371/journal.pone.0029248
103. Nielsen J, Kofod-Olsen E, Spaun E, Larsen CS, Christiansen M, Mogensen TH. A STAT1-gain-of-function mutation causing Th17 deficiency with chronic mucocutaneous candidiasis, psoriasiform hyperkeratosis and dermatophytosis. *BMJ Case Rep.* (2015) 2015. doi: 10.1136/bcr-2015-211372
104. Kagawa R, Fujiki R, Tsumura M, Sakata S, Nishimura S, Itan Y, et al. Alanine-scanning mutagenesis of human signal transducer and activator of transcription 1 to estimate loss- or gain-of-function variants. *J Allergy Clin Immunol.* (2017) 140:232–41. doi: 10.1016/j.jaci.2016.09.035
105. Toubiana J, Okada S, Hiller J, Oleastro M, Lagos Gomez M, Aldave Becerra JC, et al. Heterozygous STAT1 gain-of-function mutations underlie an unexpectedly broad clinical phenotype. *Blood* (2016) 127:3154–64. doi: 10.1182/blood-2015-11-679902
106. Zhou L, Ivanov II, Spolski R, Min R, Shenderov K, Egawa T, et al. IL-6 programs T(H)-17 cell differentiation by promoting sequential engagement of the IL-21 and IL-23 pathways. *Nat Immunol.* (2007) 8:967–74. doi: 10.1038/ni1488
107. Chen M, Chen G, Nie H, Zhang X, Niu X, Zang YC, et al. Regulatory effects of IFN-beta on production of osteopontin and IL-17 by CD4+ T Cells in MS. *Eur J Immunol.* (2009) 39:2525–36. doi: 10.1002/eji.2008 38879
108. Uzel G, Sampaio EP, Lawrence MG, Hsu AP, Hackett M, Dorsey MJ, et al. Dominant gain-of-function STAT1 mutations in FOXP3 wild-type immune dysregulation-polyendocrinopathy-enteropathy-X-linked-like syndrome. *J Allergy Clin Immunol.* (2013) 131:1611–23. doi: 10.1016/j.jaci.2012.11.054
109. Crow YJ. Type I interferonopathies: a novel set of inborn errors of immunity. *Ann N Y Acad Sci.* (2011) 1238:91–8. doi: 10.1111/j.1749-6632.2011.06220.x
110. Liu BC, Sarhan J, Poltorak A. Host-intrinsic interferon status in infection and immunity. *Trends Mol Med.* (2018) 24:658–68. doi: 10.1016/j.molmed.2018.06.004
111. Rodero MP, Crow YJ. Type I interferon-mediated monogenic autoinflammation: the type I interferonopathies, a conceptual overview. *J Exp Med.* (2016) 213:2527–38. doi: 10.1084/jem.20161596
112. Flanagan SE, Haapaniemi E, Russell MA, Caswell R, Allen HL, De Franco E, et al. Activating germline mutations in STAT3 cause early-onset multi-organ autoimmune disease. *Nat Genet.* (2014) 46:812–4. doi: 10.1038/ng.3040
113. Milner JD, Vogel TP, Forbes L, Ma CA, Stray-Pedersen A, Niemela JE, et al. Early-onset lymphoproliferation and autoimmunity caused by germline STAT3 gain-of-function mutations. *Blood* (2015) 125:591–9. doi: 10.1182/blood-2014-09-602763
114. Haapaniemi EM, Kaustio M, Rajala HL, van Adrichem AJ, Kainulainen L, Glumoff V, et al. Autoimmunity, hypogammaglobulinemia, lymphoproliferation, and mycobacterial disease in patients with activating mutations in STAT3. *Blood* (2015) 125:639–48. doi: 10.1182/blood-2014-04-570101
115. Mahlaoui N, Warnatz K, Jones A, Workman S, Cant A. Advances in the care of Primary Immunodeficiencies (PIDs): from birth to adulthood. *J Clin Immunol.* (2017) 37:452–60. doi: 10.1007/s10875-017-0401-y
116. Marsh R, Hebert KM, Keesler D, Boelens JJ, Dvorak C, Eckrich MJ, et al. Practice pattern changes and improvements in hematopoietic cell transplantation for primary immunodeficiencies. *J Allergy Clin Immunol.* (2018) 142:2004–7. doi: 10.1016/j.jaci.2018.08.010
117. King JR, Hammarstrom L. Newborn screening for primary immunodeficiency diseases: history, current and future practice. *J Clin Immunol.* (2018) 38:56–66. doi: 10.1007/s10875-017-0455-x
118. Al-Mousa H, Al-Dakheel G, Jabr A, Elbadaoui F, Abouelhoda M, Baig M, et al. High incidence of severe combined immunodeficiency disease in Saudi Arabia detected through combined T cell receptor excision circle and next generation sequencing of newborn dried blood spots. *Front Immunol.* (2018) 9:782. doi: 10.3389/fimmu.2018.00782
119. Bonilla FA, Khan DA, Ballas ZK, Chinen J, Frank MM, Hsu JT, et al. Practice parameter for the diagnosis and management of primary immunodeficiency. *J Allergy Clin Immunol.* (2015) 136:1186–205.e1-78. doi: 10.1016/j.jaci.2015.04.049
120. Rodero MP, Fremond ML, Rice GI, Neven B, Crow YJ. JAK inhibition in STING-associated interferonopathy. *Ann Rheum Dis.* (2016) 75:e75. doi: 10.1136/annrheumdis-2016-210504
121. Dever DP, Bak RO, Reinisch A, Camarena J, Washington G, Nicolas CE, et al. CRISPR/Cas9 beta-globin gene targeting in human haematopoietic stem cells. *Nature* (2016) 539:384–9. doi: 10.1038/nature20134
122. De Ravin SS, Li L, Wu X, Choi U, Allen C, Koontz S, et al. CRISPR-Cas9 gene repair of hematopoietic stem cells from patients with X-linked chronic granulomatous disease. *Sci Transl Med.* (2017) 9:eaah3480. doi: 10.1126/scitranslmed.aah3480
123. Schiroli G, Ferrari S, Conway A, Jacob A, Capo V, Albano L, et al. Preclinical modeling highlights the therapeutic potential of hematopoietic stem cell gene editing for correction of SCID-X1. *Sci Transl Med.* (2017) 9:eaan0820. doi: 10.1126/scitranslmed.aan0820
124. Chinen J, Cowan MJ. Advances series, advances and highlights in primary immunodeficiencies 2017. *J Allergy Clin Immunol.* (2018) 142:1041–51. doi: 10.1016/j.jaci.2018.08.016

13

Genome-Wide Inhibition of Pro-Atherogenic Gene Expression by Multi-STAT Targeting Compounds as a Novel Treatment Strategy of CVDs

Martyna Plens-Galaska [1†], Malgorzata Szelag [1†], Aida Collado [2,3], Patrice Marques [2,3], Susana Vallejo [4,5], Mariella Ramos-González [4,5], Joanna Wesoly [6], María Jesus Sanz [2,3], Concepción Peiró [4,5] and Hans A. R. Bluyssen [1]*

[1] Department of Human Molecular Genetics, Institute of Molecular Biology and Biotechnology, Adam Mickiewicz University, Poznan, Poland, [2] Department of Pharmacology, Faculty of Medicine, University of Valencia, Valencia, Spain, [3] Institute of Health Research INCLIVA, University Clinic Hospital of Valencia, Valencia, Spain, [4] Department of Pharmacology, School of Medicine, Universidad Autónoma de Madrid, Madrid, Spain, [5] Instituto de Investigación Sanitaria Hospital Universitario La Paz (IdiPAZ), Madrid, Spain, [6] Laboratory of High Throughput Technologies, Institute of Molecular Biology and Biotechnology, Faculty of Biology, Adam Mickiewicz University, Poznan, Poland

***Correspondence:**
Hans A. R. Bluyssen
h.bluyss@amu.edu.pl

† These authors have contributed equally to this work

Cardiovascular diseases (CVDs), including atherosclerosis, are globally the leading cause of death. Key factors contributing to onset and progression of atherosclerosis include the pro-inflammatory cytokines Interferon (IFN)α and IFNγ and the Pattern Recognition Receptor (PRR) Toll-like receptor 4 (TLR4). Together, they trigger activation of Signal Transducer and Activator of Transcription (STAT)s. Searches for compounds targeting the pTyr-SH2 interaction area of STAT3, yielded many small molecules, including STATTIC and STX-0119. However, many of these inhibitors do not seem STAT3-specific. We hypothesized that multi-STAT-inhibitors that simultaneously block STAT1, STAT2, and STAT3 activity and pro-inflammatory target gene expression may be a promising strategy to treat CVDs. Using comparative *in silico* docking of multiple STAT-SH2 models on multi-million compound libraries, we identified the novel multi-STAT inhibitor, C01L_F03. This compound targets the SH2 domain of STAT1, STAT2, and STAT3 with the same affinity and simultaneously blocks their activity and expression of multiple STAT-target genes in HMECs in response to IFNα. The same *in silico* and *in vitro* multi-STAT inhibiting capacity was shown for STATTIC and STX-0119. Moreover, C01L_F03, STATTIC and STX-0119 were also able to affect genome-wide interactions between IFNγ and TLR4 by commonly inhibiting pro-inflammatory and pro-atherogenic gene expression directed by cooperative involvement of STATs with IRFs and/or NF-κB. Moreover, we observed that multi-STAT inhibitors could be used to inhibit IFNγ+LPS-induced HMECs migration, leukocyte adhesion to ECs as well as impairment of mesenteric artery contractility. Together, this implicates that application of a multi-STAT inhibitory strategy could provide great promise for the treatment of CVDs.

Keywords: vascular inflammation, STAT, *in silico* docking, multi-STAT inhibitors, CVDs treatment strategy

INTRODUCTION

Cardiovascular diseases (CVDs) are globally the leading cause of death in Western Countries. Atherosclerosis is preceded by endothelial dysfunction, a prothrombotic and pro-inflammatory state of the endothelium which involves the increased expression of cell surface adhesion molecules, the production of inflammatory cytokines and chemokines and altered contractility of vascular smooth muscle cells (VSMCs) (1). Blood leukocytes are recruited to the injured vascular endothelium. This process is a hallmark of the initiation and progression of atherosclerosis. Recruitment of blood leukocytes involves many inflammatory mediators, modulated by cells of both innate and adaptive immunity (1). Pro-inflammatory cytokines Interferon (IFN)α, IFNγ and Toll-like receptor 4 (TLR4) activators are key factors contributing to early stages of atherosclerosis (2). IFNα and IFNγ induce phosphorylation of STATs through Janus-kinases (JAK)s. Thus, IFNα stimulates formation of STAT1 and STAT2 heterodimers, that complexed with IRF9 form ISGF3 and regulate expression of ISRE-containing genes. On the other hand, IFNα and IFNγ activate STAT1 or STAT3 homo-/heterodimer formation, which regulate expression of a distinct set of GAS-driven genes. IFNs also activate members of the IRF family including IRF1 and IRF8, that modulate a second wave of ISRE-dependent gene expression (3, 4).

Rapid activation of nuclear factor-κB (NF-κB) and IRFs is a result of TLR4 ligation (4–7). This leads to amplification of the initial inflammatory response, exertion of antimicrobial activities and initiation of acquired immunity. Several of the cytokines that are upregulated in the initial wave of immediate early gene expression e.g., IFNβ and TNFα, induce a secondary wave of STAT1 and STAT2 dependent gene expression and NF-κB signaling, respectively (4, 8, 9). On the other hand, IL-6 leads to the activation of STAT3.

IFNγ and TLR4 participate in signaling cross-talk through combinatorial actions of distinct and overlapping transcription factors on ISRE, GAS, ISRE/GAS, ISRE/NF-κB or GAS/NF-κB binding sites. As such, inflammation-induced activation of STAT1, STAT2, and STAT3, NF-κB and different IRFs coordinates robust expression of multiple chemokines, adhesion molecules, antiviral and antimicrobial proteins. Thus, signal integration between IFNγ and LPS in vascular cells and atheroma interacting immune cells modulates important aspects of inflammation, with STATs being important mediators (7, 10).

JAK-STAT pathway inhibitory strategies are numerous and one of the most promising is development of JAK inhibitors (Jakinibs), which exhibit the pan-JAK effect, defined as cross-binding to few JAKs e.g., FDA approved tofacitinib inhibits both Jak1 and Jak2. The concept of STAT inhibition is the more targeted approach, since STAT inhibitory strategies focus on affecting STAT dimerization. By exploring the pTyr-SH2 interaction area of STAT3, searches for STAT3-targeting compounds are numerous and yielded many small molecules, which can be called Statinibs (11, 12). Compared to Jakinibs these compounds affect expression of pro-inflammatory cytokines directly. Statinibs do not affect JAK-STAT signaling cascade upstream of the STAT phosphorylation and do not abrogate JAK action. Jakinibs might also influence, as a side effect, other JAK targets like SOCS or other kinases (e.g., Src and Abl). Of these STAT3-interacting compounds, STATTIC was shown to inhibit activation, dimerization, nuclear translocation of STAT3, and to increase apoptosis in STAT3-dependent cancer cell lines [reviewed in (7, 13)]. Similarly, the small-molecule STX-0119 was able to inhibit STAT3 dimerization and suppress human lymphoma SCC3 cell growth, through apoptosis and downregulation of known STAT3 targets. STX-0119 also exhibited potent antitumor effects *in vivo* of SCC3 tumor-bearing nude mice (14). Recently, we proposed a STAT cross-binding mechanism for STATTIC and STX-0119, in which both compounds target the SH2 domain of STAT1, STAT2, and STAT3 with similar affinity. We hypothesized that non-specific STAT-inhibitors, by simultaneous blocking STAT1, STAT2, and STAT3 activity (pan-STAT action) and expression of pro-inflammatory target genes, may be a promising avenue for the treatment of CVDs.

To prove this, we developed a pipeline approach which combines comparative *in silico* docking of multi-million CL and CDL libraries to multiple STAT-SH2 models with *in vitro* STAT inhibition validation, as a novel selection strategy for STAT-targeting inhibitors. This approach allowed us to identify a new type of multi-STAT inhibitor, C01L_F03 targeting the SH2 domain of STAT1, 2, and 3 with equal affinity. Moreover, we observed a similar STAT cross-binding mechanism for STATTIC and STX-0119, leading to genome-wide inhibition of pro-atherogenic gene expression directed by cooperative involvement of STATs with IRFs and/or NF-κB. Consequently, a

Abbreviations: ACTB, Actin Beta; APOL1, Apolipoprotein L1; BCA, Bicinchoninic acid; BID, BH3 Interacting Domain Death Agonist; BS, Binding Score value; CAVS, Comparative Approach for Virtual Screening; CBAV, Comparative Binding Affinity Value; CCL3L3, C-C Motif Chemokine Ligand 3 Like 3; CCL5, C-C Motif Chemokine Ligand 5; CCL7, C-C Motif Chemokine Ligand 7; CCL8, C-C Motif Chemokine Ligand 8; CCND1, Cyclin D1; CD74, Cluster of Differentiation 74; CDL, Clean Drug-Like; CL, Clean Leads; CVDs, Cardiovascular Diseases; CXCL10, C-X-C motif chemokine 10; CXCL9, C-X-C motif chemokine 9; ECs, Endothelial Cells; EGF, Endothelial Growth Factor; FAS, Fas Cell Surface Death Receptor; FBS, Fetal Bovine Serum; FC, Fold Change; GAS, Interferon-Gamma Activated Sequence; GBP4, Guanylate Binding Protein 4; GBP5, Guanylate Binding Protein 5; GO, Gene Ontology; HMECs, Human Microvascular Endothelial Cells; HRP, Horseradish Peroxidase; HUVECs, Human Umbilical Vein Endothelial Cells; ICAM1, Intercellular Adhesion Molecule 1; IFI44L, Interferon Induced Protein 44 Like; IFIT1, Interferon Induced Protein with Tetratricopeptide Repeats 1; IFIT2, Interferon Induced Protein with Tetratricopeptide Repeats 2; IFIT3, Interferon Induced Protein with Tetratricopeptide Repeats 3; IFN, Interferon; INDO, Indoleamine 2,3-Dioxygenase 1; IRF, Interferon Regulatory Factor; IRF1, Interferon Regulatory Factor 1; IRF8, Interferon Regulatory Factor 8; ISG15, Interferon-Stimulated Gene 15; ISRE, Interferon-Stimulated Response Element; LBPV, Ligand Binding Pose Variation; LPS, Lipopolysaccharide; MMP12, Matrix Metalloproteinase-12; MMP3, Matrix Metalloproteinase-3; NF-κB, Nuclear Factor κB; OAS1, 2′-5′-Oligoadenylate Synthetase 1; OAS2, 2′-5′-Oligoadenylate Synthetase 2; PBS, Phosphate Buffered Saline; PIM1, Pim-1 Proto-Oncogene; S1PR1, Sphingosine-1-Phosphate Receptor 1; SCC3, Sister-Chromatid Cohesion protein 3; SH2, Src Homology 2 Domain; SOCS3, Suppressor of Cytokine Signaling 3; STAT, Signal Transducer and Activator of Transcription; TLR4, Toll-like Receptor 4; TNF, Tumor Necrosis Factor; UBD, Ubiquitin D; VCAM1, Vascular Cell Adhesion Molecule 1; VEGF, Vascular Endothelial Growth Factor; VSMCs, Vascular Smooth Muscle Cells.

multi-STAT inhibitory strategy was applied to inhibit endothelial cell (EC) migration, leukocyte adhesion to ECs and impairment of mesenteric artery contractility under inflammatory conditions.

MATERIALS AND METHODS

Protein Model Preparation

Three-dimensional models of STAT1, STAT2, and STAT3 were prepared based on the existing crystal structures for STATs deposited in RCSB Protein Data Bank: 1YVL, unphosphorylated STAT1 monomer; 1BF5, phosphorylated STAT1 dimer and 1BG1, phosphorylated STAT3 dimer [detailed description see Czerwoniec et al. (15) and Szelag et al. (16)]. Based on Chimera Dock Prep protocol AMBER ff99SB charges were applied to human STAT1, 2, and 3 models (17). Highly conserved pTyr-binding pocket (pY+0) and hydrophobic side-pocket (pY-X) in SH2 domain were selected for docking and virtual screening procedures. At the level of protein structures these SH2 domain superficial cavities are essential for STAT activation and binding of inhibitors (16, 18). To generate a "protomol," "a pre-computed molecular representation of an idealized ligand" we used a ligand-based approach implemented in Surflex-Dock 2.6 (19). By definition protomol acts as the molecular probe of the active site to which ligands are matched (20). Ligand used to generate the protomol for STATs included a four amino acids from STAT-SH2 specific pTyr-linker matching the selected sub-pockets [STAT1, G**pY^{701}**IK; STAT2, K**pY^{690}**LK; STAT3, P**pY^{705}**LK (15)].

Compound Library Selection and Small Inhibitors Preparation

Two small compound libraries of Clean Leads (CL) and Clean Drug-Like (CDL) were selected and downloaded from ZINC Database, with ready-to-dock parameters of protonation state and partial atomic charges (21). CL with molecular weight between 250 and 350 g/mol are smaller than most drugs. CDL chemical parameters fulfill criteria of the Lipinski's rule of five (22, 23). CL are in general more soluble than their bigger CDL cousins, and thus more likely to actually be assayed *in vitro*. In 2011 for the purpose of primary virtual screening (pre-screen) a CL subset has been downloaded, containing at that time 712,426 compounds. During the next step, similarity screening in 2013, CL subset in number of 4,591,276 and CDL subset in number of 13,195,609 compounds were selected.

Geometries of STAT3 inhibitors used for docking, STATTIC (24) and STX-0119 (25) were obtained from ZINC Database (code names ZINC00162014 and ZINC04107278 respectively). The structures were provided in ready-to-dock, 3D formats with molecules represented in biologically relevant forms (21).

Virtual Screening of Small Compound Libraries

To select the top STAT1 inhibitors novel six-step virtual screening procedure was employed. The applied strategy is an antecedent to our more advanced protocol for big-scale virtual screening, named CAVS [see Czerwoniec et al. (15)]. The procedure used here is characterized by the following steps:

1. ***Pre-screen:*** For the CL library (712,426 compounds) docking simulations to STAT1 were carried out using Surflex-Dock 2.6 (19). Pscreen algorithm with fast screening parameter settings was employed (15, 20). For each compound we obtained 10 binding poses in the predefined area of the STAT1-SH2 domain. Additionally, each binding pose was supplied with a Binding Score value (BS) representing the total predicted binding affinity of the compound to the STAT1-SH2 domain. Moreover, input of polar interactions to the BS (represented by Polar Score) and the error rate of binding (represented by Crash) were also calculated.
2. ***Primary filtering of inhibitors:*** For each compound the best of ten binding poses was filtered out for further analysis. Then, we compared the binding quality between different compounds by using the STAT1-BS. Compounds with the highest STAT1-BS values were selected, checked for availability and 12 compounds (A01-L01) have been purchased for initial experimental validation.
3. ***Similarity screen:*** Based on the experimental results the best three compounds for STAT1 inhibition (C01, E01, and F01 from CL library) were used to perform a structural similarity screening. The CL list containing now 4,591,276 structures was screened with the criteria of at least 50% similarity to C01, E01, and F01. 1129 CL compounds fulfilled these criteria. Similarly, the CDL list with 13,195,609 structures was screened for compounds with >50% similarity and a molecular weight of ≥300 g/mol, to include bigger structures which could target a larger area of the SH2 domain. These criteria were fulfilled by 832 CDL compounds. Then for a total of 1,961 compounds, similarity scores (SIM and RMSD) were calculated using Surflex-Sim 2.6 (19) to assess the level of similarity to C01, E01, and F01.
4. ***Re-screen:*** Repeated docking simulations of a total of 1,961 compounds from the similarity screen to STAT1, 2 and 3-SH2 were carried employing the Surflex-Dock 2.6 pgeom algorithm which is recommended for detailed studies of relative alignments. More exhaustive parameter settings were used for optimal pose prediction of the compounds (15, 20). As a result, in the predefined area of STAT-SH2 domain we obtained 20 binding poses of each compound.
5. ***Secondary filtering of inhibitors:*** For each compound the best of 20 binding poses was filtered out for further analysis. Then by using the "Comparative Binding Affinity Value" for STAT1 [STAT1-CBAV, more details see Czerwoniec et al. (15)] the binding between STAT1, 2 and 3 was compared for each compound. Compounds with STAT1-CBAV≥0 were selected for graphical validation.
6. ***Binding diversity of conformers:*** Finally, graphical validation of the selected compounds was represented by the "ligand binding pose variation" (LBPV). This parameter reflects the docking accuracy. For detailed description of this procedure, see Czerwoniec et al. (15). The LBPV range of [0.8–1.0] represents low conformer diversity with very good binding specificity of the compound to STAT-SH2, whereas the range of [0.0–0.2] denotes high conformer diversity with poor binding specificity. Finally, compounds with the highest STAT1-CBAV and STAT1-LBPV values were selected, checked

for availability and six compounds (C01L_A03 to C01L_F03) have been purchased for further experimental validation.

Comparative Docking of STATTIC, STX-0119, and C01L_F03

In order to compare STATTIC and STX-0119 with compounds obtained from CL and CDL virtual screening, docking simulations of STATTIC and STX-0119 to STAT1, 2 and 3 SH2 domain were performed with the pgeom algorithm (15, 20) implemented in Surflex-Dock 2.6 (19). For each structure in the predefined area of STAT-SH2 domain we obtained 20 binding poses. Then, for each compound the best of twenty binding poses was filtered out for further analysis. Finally, STAT1-CBAV was determined to compare the binding between STAT1, STAT2, and STAT3 for both compounds. Also, LBPV was used to validate the docking accuracy.

Moreover, we performed more exact docking simulations of STATTIC; two STATTIC analogs STB and STC; STX-0119; C01 and C01L_F03 for STAT1, 2 and 3 [see Szelag et al. (16)]. Geometries of two STATTIC analogs, which displayed lesser inhibition of STAT3 binding *in vitro* (13), were obtained from ZINC Database (code names ZINC00162015 and ZINC00162011 respectively). The structures were provided in ready-to-dock, 3D formats with molecules represented in biologically relevant forms (21). For all studied complexes of STAT1, 2 and 3 with STATTIC, STB, STC, STX-0119, C01, and C01L_F03 HADDOCK ligand docking protocol (26, 27) was used with addition of Surflex-Dock protocol (pgeomx algorithm) (16) to estimate the ΔG^0 (free enthalpy change), which corresponds to the stability of the complex in a protein-ligand interaction in the equilibrium. More negative ΔG^0 (higher free enthalpy change) corresponds to stronger interaction between ligand and the protein, which reflects better complex stability.

In silico STAT-SH2 Mutagenesis

We have performed docking studies of STATTIC, STX-0119 and C01L_F03 to wt and mutated STAT1, 2, 3 [with our STAT 3D models described in (16)]. For this purpose, HADDOCK ligand docking protocol (26, 27) was used with addition of Surflex-Dock protocol (16) to estimate the ΔG^0 (free enthalpy change), which corresponds to the stability of the complex in a protein-ligand interaction in the equilibrium. We assumed that mutation of selected a.a. to alanine would impair binding of studied inhibitors to STAT1, 2, and 3-SH2 domain.

Cell Culture Experiments

Recombinant IFNα and IFNγ were purchased from Merck, while LPS was provided by Sigma-Aldrich. C01 and C01L_A03-C01L_F03 were purchased from Enamine; E01 from Asinex; F01 from ChemDiv; STX-0119 from Merck and STATTIC from Sigma-Aldrich. Rabbit polyclonal antibodies against STAT1-pTyr^{701}, tSTAT1, tSTAT2, tSTAT3 were obtained from Santa Cruz, STAT2-pTyr^{689} and STAT3-pTyr^{705} form Merck. Tubulin antibody was purchased from Merck and anti-rabbit HRP-conjugated antibody from Sigma-Aldrich. Human Microvascular Endothelial Cells (HMECs) (28) were provided by the Center for Disease Control and Prevention (Atlanta, GA) and cultured in MCDB-131 medium (IITD PAN, Wroclaw, Poland) containing 10% of fetal bovine serum (FBS) (Gibco, Thermo Fisher Scientific), 100 U/ml penicillin, 100 μg/ml streptomycin, 0.01 μg/ml EGF, 0.05 μM hydrocortisone and 2 mM L-glutamine. At least 12 h before the experiment, full medium was exchanged for serum starved-medium (containing 1% of FBS instead of 10%). After minimum 12 h-starvation HMECs were pre-treated with various concentrations of inhibitors: C01, E01, F01 (40 h) or C01L_F03 (48 h) or STATTIC (8 h) or STX-0119 (24 h). Additionally, HMECs were treated with 200 U/ml of IFNα (1 h for protein isolation or 4 h for RNA isolation), 10 ng/ml IFNγ (24 h or 8 h) and/or 1 μg/ml LPS (8 h or 4 h) or IL-6 (1 h) 100 ng/ml.

Western Blot Analysis

HMECs were washed with phosphate buffered saline (PBS) and lysed using radio-immune precipitation assay (RIPA) lysis buffer (50 mM Tris-HCl, pH = 8.0, 150 mM NaCl, 1% Nonidet-40, 0.5% sodium deoxycholate, 0.1% SDS, 1% protein inhibitor cocktail, 1% EDTA, 0.1% PMSF) and stored at −80°C, as described in Sikorski et al. (4). Lysates were quantified using bicinchoninic acid (BCA) kit (Perce). Thirty micrograms of protein were loaded on Blot 4–12% Bis-Tris Plus Gels, electrophoresed and transferred to PVDF membranes (Santa Cruz). All western blot analyses were performed with Snap ID system (Merck). Membranes were blocked in 0.125% non-fat dry milk or 1% BSA in TBS-Tween (TBS-T) and incubated with primary antibodies (1:1000 pSTAT1, 1:500 tSTAT1, 1:500 pSTAT2, 1:500 tSTAT2, 1:3500 pSTAT3, 1:500 tSTAT3, 1:2000 tubulin) and then with secondary anti-rabbit HRP-conjugated antibody (1:2,0000). Immunoreactive bands were visualized by enhanced chemiluminescence (ECL) using Luminata Forte HRP Substrate (Merck) and detected with G:Box System (Syngene). After detection membranes were stripped with buffer containing 25 mM glycine, 1% SDS, pH = 2.0 and re-probed. The software Image Studio Lite from LI-COR Biosciences was used for western blot quantification with α-tubulin as reference protein.

ChIP qPCR

ChIP experiments were performed as described by Daniel et al. in (29) with minor modifications (29). Briefly, 15 mln cells were seeded and pre-treated with 50 μM of C01L_F03 48 h and for 1 h with 200 U/ml of IFNα. Cross-linking with DSG (Sigma) was performed for 45 min and then with formaldehyde (Sigma) for 10 min. After fixation chromatin was sonicated with a Diagenode Bioruptor Plus to generate fragments with length of 200–1,000 bp. Chromatin was immunoprecipitated with antibodies against pSTAT1, pSTAT2, pSTAT3, and NF-κB p65 (Cell Signaling Technology®). Chromatin-antibody complexes were precipitated with anti-IgA and anti-IgG paramagnetic beads (Life Technologies). After four washing steps, complexes were eluted and the cross-links reversed. DNA fragments were column purified (Qiagen, MinElute). DNA was quantified with a Qubit fluorometer (Invitrogen). After immunoprecipitation DNA was quantified using quantitative PCR (qPCR) and normalized to values obtained after amplification of unprecipitated (input) DNA. Oligonucleotides sequences (Genomed) are in **Table 1**.

TABLE 1 | List of primer sequences used in experimental procedures.

Gene Name	Primer Sequence (5′ → 3′order)	
	Forward	**Reverse**
ACTB	ACAGAGCCTCGCCTTTGCCGAT	ATCATCCATGGTGAGCTGGCGG
CXCL10	GCAGAGGAACCTCCAGTCTCAGCA	AGAGAGAGGTACTCCTTGAATGCCAC
CXCL9	GTGGTGTTCTTTTCCTCTTGGG	CTCACTACTGGGGTTCCTTGC
IFIT2	TCTTCCGTGTCTGTTCCATTC	AGCTGAAAGTTGCCATACCG
IRF1	GTCCAGCCGAGATGCTAAGAGC	TCTTCCGTGTCTGTTCCATTC
OAS2	CAATCAGCGAGGCCAGTAAT	TCCAGGTTGGGAGAAGTCAA
CCL5	CCATATTCCTCGGACACCAC	GGGTGACAAAGACGACTGCT
ICAM	CAGCGGCTGACGTGTGCAGTAA	TTGGGCGCCGGAAAGCTGTA
VCAM	TCCAGGTGGAGCTCTACTCATTCCC	TCCCATTCACGAGGCCACCACT
OAS2_ChIP	CGCTGCAGTGGGTGGAGAGA	GCCGGCAAGACAGTGAATGG
SOCS3_ChIP	CCATTCGGGAGTTCCTGGAC	TTGGCTTCTTGTGCTTGTGC
IRF1_ChIP STAT1	CCAAACACTTAGCGGGATTC	GAAATGACGGCACGCAG
IER3_ChIP	CCACCACCAGACTTCATCCC	GGAACTGCGGCAAAGTAGGA
IRF1_ChIP NF-κB	CTCAACAGCCAAGTGTGACC	GGCCAGCTTTACACCACAAG

RNA Isolation and Quantitative Reverse Transcription-PCR (qRT-PCR) Analysis

Total RNA was isolated using GeneMATRIX Universal RNA Purification Kit (EURx, Gdansk, Poland). 500 ng of total RNA was subjected to reverse transcription and PCR amplification was performed in Maxima SYBR Green/ROX qRT-PCR Master Mix (Thermo Fisher Scientific) on the Eco qRT-PCR System (Illumina). The amount of target gene in each sample was normalized to β-actin (ACTB) endogenous control (ΔCT). Data were transformed as described previously (30). Forward and reverse primers used in experiments are depicted in **Table 1.**

Microarray Analysis

Firstly, before treatment HMECs were starved for 12 h in 1% MCDB medium (IITD PAN, Wroclaw, Poland). Then cells were incubated with C01L_F03 (50 μM, 48 h) or STX-0119 (25 μM, 24 h) or STATTIC (10 μM, 8 h), IFNγ (10 ng/ml, 8 h) and LPS (1 μg/ml, 4 h) before RNA isolation. RNA was isolated from harvested cells with GeneMATRIX Universal RNA Purification Kit (EURx, Gdansk, Poland) and then labeled with Illumina® TotalPrep™ RNA Amplification Kit (Thermo Fisher Scientific). To obtain raw data Standard Illumina Expression BeadChip HumanHT-12v4 hybridization protocol was used. To avoid false results in case of all negative signals their value was changed to one, then signals were log-transformed. For further analysis, statistically significant average gene expression signals from two independent biological repeats were taken for statistical testing (GEO accession: GSE101508). Background subtraction and quantile normalization were applied and genes significantly (p-value $\leq$ 0.05) up-regulated at least 2-fold in any sample were selected for further analysis. IFNγ+LPS responsive genes that were commonly inhibited by C01L_F03, STATTIC or STX-0119 were selected according to the following formula: Fold Change $(FC)_{IFN\gamma+LPS}/FC_{IFN\gamma+LPS+inhibitor}$ value ≥ 4. Lists of inhibited genes were compared by Venn diagram analysis in the VennDiagram package in R (31). Identification of overlapping genes was based on "Gene ID and name."

Gene Ontology Enrichment Analysis

Two datasets from microarray analysis (IFNγ+LPS induced genes; 731 in total; IFNγ+LPS responsive genes commonly inhibited by C01L_F03, STATTIC, and STX-0119) were mapped to gene ontology terms of biological process category using GOrilla webserver (32, 33). A p-value of 10^{-3} was used as a threshold and Illumina gene list from HumanHT-12v4 served as a background model. Then all statistically significant enriched GO categories were analyzed by REVIGO webserver (34) with medium similarity (0.7) and SimRel semantic similarity measure and mapped to *Homo sapiens* background to generate lists without redundant GO terms. Finally, the top 12 enriched GO terms with the highest fold enrichment for cells stimulated with IFNγ+LPS were selected and compared to those treated with tested compounds in presence of IFNγ+LPS.

Promoter Analysis

The initial list of 731 IFNγ+LPS induced genes was used for promoter analysis. The list was uploaded into pSCAN webserver (35) in search for ISRE, GAS and NF-κB binding sites. We analyzed 950 bp upstream and 50 bp downstream of the transcription start sites and obtained lists of overrepresented transcription factor binding sites, including matrix similarity score. Based on the results produced by pSCAN we chose matrices for further analysis. For checking distribution of: ISRE sequence we chose matrices: MA0652.1, MA0137.1, MA0.517.1; for GAS sequence: MA0137.2 and MA0137.3 and for NF-κB binding site: MA0105.1, MA0105.3. To prevent false positive results, we introduced threshold of matrix similarity score ≥ 0.85 for potential GAS, ISRE and ≥ 0.90 for potential NF-κB binding sites. To confirm "STAT specificity" of tested inhibitors, produced gene lists were merged for each individual binding site and compared with gene list of 159 genes inhibited commonly by C01L_F03, STATTIC and STX-0119 [by Venn diagram analysis by VennDiagram package in R (31)]. Identification of overlapping genes was based on "Gene ID and name." The next step was to check if identified sequences may appear in one gene simultaneously. For that purpose, lists of genes containing either ISRE, GAS, NF-κB binding site were compared by Venn diagram analysis according to previously used protocol.

In vitro Wound Healing Assay

HMEC cells were split on 100 mm dishes and plated to reach high confluency. Cells then were starved in MCDB medium (IITD PAN, Wroclaw, Poland) with 0.1% of FBS for 12 h. Next step was to treat 2 dishes with 25 μM of C01L_F03 and 2 dishes with 25 μM of STX-0119. After 12 h of pre-incubation with C01L_F03 or STX-0119 scratches in these dishes were made. Another set of 2 dishes was treated with 10 μM of STATTIC 12 h before pictures were taken. At the same time 10 ng/ml of IFNγ and 1 μg/ml of LPS were added to one dish from each pair treated with C01L_F03, STX-0119 or STATTIC. Additionally, scratches were also made in set of 2 dishes that remained not treated with any inhibitor, one was used as an untreated control and to the second only IFNγ and LPS were added. Pictures were taken with Axio Observer.Z1 Microscope (Zeiss) after 12 h since the moment when scratches were made. The images acquired for each sample from two independent repeats were further analyzed quantitatively by ImageJ (36). For each image, 20 distances between one side of scratch and the other were measured at certain intervals (μm). By comparing the images from or inhibitor (with or without IFNγ+LPS treatment) to control, the distances of each scratch closure were obtained. Analysis of HMECs migration according to wound healing *in vitro*, which was performed according to Liang et al. (37).

Leukocyte-Endothelial Cell Interactions Under Flow Conditions

Human umbilical vein endothelial cells (HUVECs) were isolated by collagenase treatment (38, 39) and maintained in human endothelial cell specific medium (EBM-2, Lonza, Verviers, Belgium), supplemented with endothelial growth media (EGM-2, Lonza) and 10% fetal bovine serum (FBS, Lonza). Cells up to passage 1 were grown to confluence to preserve endothelial features. Cells were incubated for 24 h in medium containing 1% FBS prior to every experiment.

Mononuclear cells were obtained from buffy coats of healthy donors by Ficoll Hypaque density gradient centrifugation (39, 40). The Glycotech flow chamber was assembled and placed on an inverted microscope stage. Freshly isolated mononuclear cells (1×10^6/ml) were then perfused across the endothelial monolayers (HUVECs) unstimulated or stimulated with IFNγ (10 ng/ml, PreproTech, London, UK) for 24 h and LPS (1 μg/ml, Sigma Aldrich, Madrid, Spain) for 4 h. In the experiments cells were incubated with STATTIC 5 μM for 4 h or 1 μM for 24 h, STX-0119 25 μM or C01L_F03 50 μM for 24 h. In all experiments, leukocyte interactions were determined after 5 min at 0.5 dyn/cm^2. Cells interacting with the surface of the endothelium were visualized and recorded (×20 objective, ×10 eyepiece) using phase-contrast microscopy (Axio Observer A1 Carl Zeiss microscope, Thornwood, NY) (41).

Ex vivo Contractility Studies

Four-month-old male C57Bl/6 mice were used for vascular reactivity experiments. Animals were maintained under standardized conditions with an artificial 12 h dark-light cycle, with free access to food and water. All animal studies were performed according to national guidelines and approved by the institutional animal care committees of Spain.

Immediately following sacrifice, the mesentery was removed, and placed in a Petri dish containing Krebs-Henseleit solution (KHS) at 4°C. The first branch mesenteric arteries (mean internal diameter ranged between 200 and 250 μm with non-significant differences observed among the different groups of mice) were dissected and mounted as ring preparations on a small-vessel myograph (DMT, Aarhus, Denmark) to measure isometric tension (42). The microvessels were exposed to 125 mM KCl to achieve a stable contraction, after which they were washed three times with KHS and a further 30 min. washout period was allowed. At this point, the vascular segments were maintained for 4 h prior to the exposure to increasing concentrations of noradrenaline (NA; 10^{-10} to 10^{-6}M) to assess vascular contraction. In some experiments, the vascular segments were exposed to STATTIC (1 nM), STX-0119 (10 nM) or C01L_F03 (1 μM), IFNγ (10 ng/ml for 3 h prior to NA stimulation), and/or LPS (1 μg/ml for 1.5 h prior to NA stimulation) based on a previous report (10). Because of incubation time limitations of the system (<8 h), we were able to test STATTIC, C01L_F03 and STX-0119 only for 4 h prior to NA stimulation.

Statistical Analysis

Results of qRT-PCR assay are presented as mean ± SEM for three independent repeats. Results of wound healing assay are presented as mean ± SEM for two independent repeats. Data for both experiments were compared by two-way ANOVA and unpaired two-tailed student *T*-test as indicated. A probability value $p < 0.0001$ was considered statistically significant. Results of mononuclear cell adhesion to HUVEC assay are presented as mean ± SEM for five to seven independent repeats. Data were compared by one-way ANOVA and unpaired two-tailed student *T*-test. A probability value $p < 0.05$ was considered statistically significant. Results of *ex vivo* contractility studies are presented as mean ± SEM for six to eighteen independent repeats. Data were compared by two-way ANOVA. A probability value $p < 0.05$ was considered statistically significant. All statistical tests were performed with GraphPad Prism version 7.0a for Mac OS X, GraphPad Software, La Jolla California USA, www.graphpad.com.

RESULTS

Identification of C01, E01 and F01 as Novel Low Potent STAT1-SH2 Inhibitory Compounds

Potential STAT1-targeting inhibitors were selected from a CL library, using the pre-screen algorithm (see Materials and Methods), according to STAT1-BS. Compounds with the highest STAT1-BS were checked for availability and 12 of them were purchased (**Table 2**). These compounds, named A01 to L01, displayed STAT1-BS from 8.51 for J01 (the highest) to 7.56 for A01 (the lowest). To test the inhibitory capacity of these compounds toward STAT1 phosphorylation *in vitro*, we first treated HMECs with LPS (1 μg/ml for 4 h) in the presence or absence of the individual compounds (200 μM for 40 h). Except for C01, E01, and F01 (**Figures 1A,B**), none of the other compounds were able to inhibit STAT1 phosphorylation (not shown). A representative experiment is shown in **Figure 1A**, in which the phosphorylation and expression of STAT1, was followed. Indeed, a dramatic reduction in phosphorylation, but not total expression, of STAT1 could be observed in LPS-stimulated cells pre-treated with C01, E01, or F01. Notably, treatment with C01 resulted in partial inhibition, whereas E01 and F01 completely inhibited STAT1 phosphorylation (**Figure 1B**). Under similar conditions, 100 μM of E01 and F01 only partially inhibited STAT1 phosphorylation, while in case of 50 or 25 μM no inhibition could be observed (data not shown). Next, we examined the *in silico* binding affinity of C01, E01, and F01 to the SH2 domain of STAT1, including the pTyr-binding pocket (pY + 0) and the hydrophobic pocket (pY-X). C01 (ZINC08344970, structure shown in **Figure S1**) exhibited binding affinity to pY+0 and pY-X of STAT1 (**Figure 1C**), in the same way as F01 (ZINC13362660, structure shown in **Figure S1**). On the other hand, E01 (ZINC09970661, structure shown in **Figure S1**) only showed affinity for pY+0, but not to pY-X and shifted toward the Ile-binding sub-site of the STAT1 pTyr-linker (**Figure 1C**). STAT1-BS was the highest for E01 (8.36) as compared to C01 (8.09) and F01 (7.78). Among these three compounds C01 displayed a higher input of polar interactions to the BS (6.9), than E01 (6.05) and F01 (6.62), but at the same time the highest error rate of binding, represented by Crash value of −1.66. E01 and F01 had significantly lower penalty score for inappropriate binding to STAT1-SH2 domain, −1.27 and −1.04 respectively (**Table 2**). Together, this suggested that C01, E01, and F01 inhibit STAT1 phosphorylation by targeting the pY+0 and pY-X of its SH2 domain, however with low potency.

TABLE 2 | Docking characteristics (pscreen algorithm, STAT1-BS, Crash, and Polar Score) of top 12 selected compounds from Clean Leads primary screen bound to STAT1-SH2 domain.

	ZINC ID	STAT1-BS	Crash	Polar score
A01	ZINC04943450	7.56	−1.12	6.96
B01	ZINC05362485	7.71	−1.66	8.67
C01	ZINC08344970	8.09	−1.66	6.9
D01	ZINC09418732	7.63	−1.11	7.57
E01	ZINC09970661	8.36	−1.27	6.05
F01	ZINC13362660	7.78	−1.04	6.62
G01	ZINC13443544	7.81	−1.77	4.94
H01	ZINC15772297	7.79	−0.99	5.98
I01	ZINC20069236	7.76	−1.72	8.99
J01	ZINC20312047	8.51	−0.85	6.87
K01	ZINC07047084	7.58	−1.4	8.94
L01	ZINC08477975	7.66	−1.32	6.92

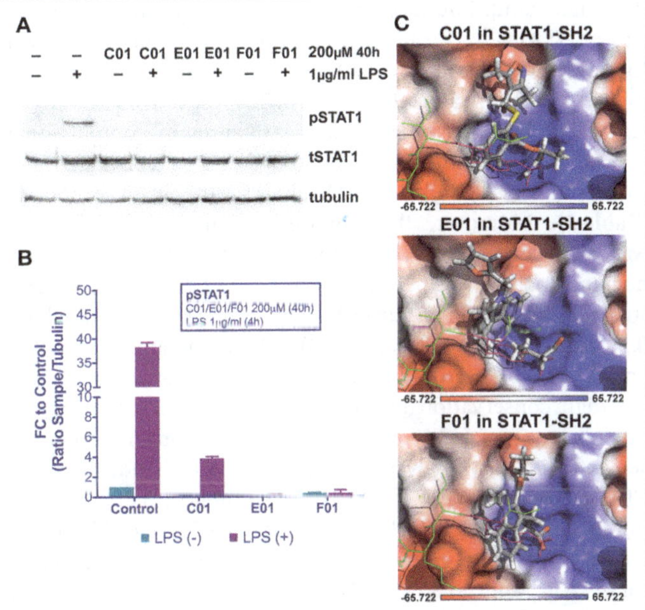

FIGURE 1 | C01, E01, and F01 inhibit LPS-induced STAT1 phosphorylation **(A)**. HMECs were treated with 200 μM of tested compounds for 40 h and with 1 μg/ml of LPS for 4 h. Protein extracts were collected and levels of pSTAT1, tSTAT1 and α-tubulin were assessed by western blotting. Western quantification **(B)**. Bars represent mean quantification form 3 individual repeats ± SEM as error bars. Top-scored binding conformations of C01, E01, and F01 in the SH2 domain of STAT1 **(C)**. C01, E01, and F01 compounds are shown in stick representation and colored according to the atomic structure. pTyr-linker is represented by green lines with pink pTyr residue. SH2 domain of STAT1 in the surface representation is colored based on the distribution of the APBS electrostatic surface potential (43). Positively charged regions are indicated in blue and negatively charged regions in red. Docking simulations were performed using Surflex-Dock 2.6 program (19, 20).

C01L_F03 Exhibits Similarity to C01 and Shows Potent STAT-SH2 Cross-Binding

To identify more potent variants of the above characterized STAT1 inhibitors, a similarity screen on the CL list and the CDL list of the ZINC database was performed for compounds with a similarity of 50% to C01, E01, or F01. Moreover, to target multiple sites of the SH2 domain only CDL compounds with a molecular weight >300 g/mol were included. Altogether 1961 compounds were analyzed for C01, E01, and F01 similarity by Surflex-Sim 2.6 and docked to the SH2 domains of STAT1, STAT2, and STAT3, using the more accurate screening method with pgeom parameter settings in Surflex-Dock 2.6 (20). The compounds were filtered by STAT1-CBAV(STAT2) >0 and STAT1-CBAV(STAT3) >0 to compare binding affinities between STAT1, 2, and 3.

Two important observations could be made from the data analysis. First, the most interesting compounds were all from the CDL list with a molecular weight exceeding 300 g/mol. Second, these compounds were mostly C01-like. Accordingly, six compounds C01L_A03 to C01L_F03 (accompanying structures are shown in **Figure S2**) were selected with STAT1-CBAV >0 (**Table 3**). Their STAT1-BS as well as their STAT1-CBAV values were higher than those for E01 and F01, calculated using the same pgeom parameter setting. In comparison to C01 all six compounds displayed significant higher STAT1-BS, but in case of STAT1-CBAV differences were not always observed. For example, C01L_A03 contained the highest STAT1-BS (9.84), as well as STAT1-CBAV (3.6 for STAT2 and 4.14 for STAT3). In the docking model of STAT1 C01L_A03 bound to pY+0, pY-X and partially the Ile sub-site (data not shown). C01L_C03, on the other hand, bound to pY+0, while pY-X and the Ile sub-site of STAT1 were only partially targeted (data not shown). In case of C01-similarity, C01L_D03 and C01L_A03 displayed highest C01-SIM values, 0.846 and 0.785, respectively. C01L_E03 and C01L_F03 had more similar structures in comparison to the other compounds (see **Figure S2**). This correlated with similar STAT1-BS and C01-SIM values for these two compounds (**Table 3**). Moreover, their binding position in STAT1-SH2 was also comparable (data not shown). A more exhaustive docking analysis was performed for C01L_F03 (ZINC05312694, structure shown in **Figure S2**). The C01L_F03's STAT1-BS of 8.23 and a STAT1-CBAV(STAT3)< 1 (0.22), suggested STAT1 and STAT3-SH2 cross-binding (**Table 3**). This coincides with the high conservation between these two STATs, sharing 50% of global amino acid sequence homology, according to pairwise sequence identity analysis (44). On the other hand, the higher STAT1-CBAV(STAT2) for C01L_F03 (**Table 3**; 3.36) predicted lower affinity for STAT2 than for STAT1 and STAT3. In contrast, the C01 compound displayed similar STAT1-CBAV for STAT2 and STAT3, 1.74 and 2.08 respectively, whereas the STAT1-BS was lower by 1.5 than for C01L_F03 (**Table 3**). The binding affinity of C01L_F03 to the individual STAT-SH2 domains, corresponded with the graphical analysis. According to **Table 3**, from the top 20 optimized binding conformations of C01L_F03 to STAT1-SH2, 19 (95%) favored pY+0 and pY-X simultaneously. LBPV analyses for other STAT-SH2 revealed that C01L_F03 also shares high affinity for pY+0 and pY-X in case of STAT3 with $LBPV_{0+X} = 0.75$ and much lower for STAT2 with $LBPV_{0+X} = 0.2$ (**Table 4**). These calculations were supported by graphical presentation of the docking results (**Figure 2A**) in which the top scored conformation of C01L_F03 for each individual STAT competed with pTyr binding to the particular STAT-SH2 domain. In the docking model of STAT1-SH2, C01L_F03 bound to pY+0 and pY-X similar to C01. The same conformation could be observed in the STAT3-SH2. In case of STAT2-SH2, C01L_F03 predominantly bound to pY+0, but not to pY-X and shifted toward the Leu-binding sub-site of the STAT2 pTyr-linker (**Figure 2A**). C01 in the STAT2-SH2 domain, on the other hand, remained in a similar position as in STAT1 and STAT3-SH2 domains. Together, the docking results of C01 and C01L_F03 suggest higher potency of the latter toward STAT1 inhibition, although with a certain degree of STAT-SH2 cross-binding.

TABLE 3 | Docking characteristics (pgeom algorithm, STAT1-BS, STAT1-CBAV) of C01L_A03-C01L_F03 bound to STAT1, STAT2, and STAT3-SH2 domain in comparison to C01, E01 and F01 from primary screening, as well as C01-like similarity analysis (C01-SIM, C01-RMSD).

Compound	ZINC ID	C01-SIM	C01-RMSD	STAT1-BS	STAT1-CBAV (STAT2)	STAT1-CBAV (STAT3)
C01	ZINC08344970	1.000	0.00	6.73	1.74	2.08
E01	ZINC09970661	0.604	2.96	6.95	−1.65	−0.73
F01	ZINC13362660	0.567	2.40	6.38	−0.09	−0.19
C01L_A03	ZINC03470000	0.785	2.28	9.84	3.60	4.14
C01L_B03	ZINC05585448	0.771	2.82	8.31	2.19	1.19
C01L_C03	ZINC08712870	0.760	2.47	7.08	0.70	1.00
C01L_D03	ZINC08712921	0.846	2.84	7.30	1.50	1.78
C01L_E03	ZINC21128441	0.777	2.13	8.01	2.94	2.68
C01L_F03	ZINC05312694	0.767	2.75	8.23	3.36	0.22

C01L_F03 Inhibits IFNα and IL-6 Induced Phosphorylation of STAT1, STAT2 and STAT3 and Binding to Target Gene Promoters and Their Expression

In addition to the docking experiments, the six compounds from the similarity screen were tested for their potential to block IFNα induced STAT phosphorylation. This led to the selection of C01L_F03 as our most potent candidate (not shown).

To address STAT cross-binding specificity of C01L_F03 we pre-treated HMECs for 48 or 24 h (data not shown) with various concentrations of the compound (50, 25, and 10 μM) in the presence or absence of IFNα (200 U/ml) or IL-6 (100 ng/ml), which were added 1 h before protein isolation. A representative experiment is shown in **Figure 2B** and **Figure S3** in which the phosphorylation of STAT1, STAT2, and STAT3 was followed. These results stand in line with our docking studies. IFNα induced phosphorylation of all three STATs was almost fully inhibited in the presence of 50 μM and 25 μM, and partially of 10 μM and 5 μM of C01L_F03 for 48 h (**Figure 2C**). A similar inhibition pattern was observed for STAT3 phosphorylation upon IL-6 treatment (**Figure S3**). Twenty-Four hour treatment with C01L_F03 resulted only in partial inhibition with the highest concentration (data not shown). Under the same conditions levels of total STAT proteins were not influenced by C01L_F03 treatment. After 48 h treatment with 50 μM C01L_F03 exhibited cytotoxic effect causing death of approximately 30% of cells (not shown). However, at a concentration of 25 μM barely any toxicity was visible. What is more 24 h treatment with 50 μM of C01L_F03 showed no toxicity (not shown). The inhibitory effect of C01L_F03 was also studied at the

TABLE 4 | Docking characteristics (pgeom algorithm, STAT1-BS, STAT1-CBAV, LBPV) of STATTIC, STX-0119, C01, E01, F01, and C01L_F03 bound to STAT1, STAT2, and STAT3-SH2 domain.

Compound	STAT1-BS	STAT1-CBAV (STAT2)	STAT1-CBAV (STAT3)	STAT1-LBPV		STAT2-LBPV		STAT3-LBPV	
STATTIC	4.70	−0.86	0.39	0.7_{0}	0.2_{X}	0.9_{0}	0.05_{X}	0.3_{0}	0.55_{X}
STX-0119	4.36	−0.32	0.25	0.45_{0+X}		0.3_{0+X}		0.25_{0+X}	
C01	6.73	1.74	2.08	0.5_{0+X}		0.45_{0+X}		0.35_{0+X}	
E01	6.95	−1.65	−0.73	0.65_{0+X}		0.3_{0+X}		0.3_{0+X}	
F01	6.38	−0.09	−0.19	0.2_{0+X}		0.2_{0+X}		0.3_{0+X}	
C01L_F03	8.23	3.36	0.22	0.95_{0+X}		0.2_{0+X}		0.75_{0+X}	

gene expression level. In agreement with the STAT cross-binding characteristics from our docking results, C01L_F03 was able to completely inhibit IFNα-induced expression of the multiple STAT- and IRF-target genes, CXCL10, IFIT2, and OAS2 at 25 μM and partially for 10 μM pre-treated for 48 h (**Figure 3A**). The same was true for the STAT1 target gene, IRF1 and the STAT3 target gene, SOCS3. To further demonstrate that the effect of C01L_F03 on STAT target gene expression was mediated by inhibiting binding of STATs to target gene promoters, we performed immunoprecipitation followed by qPCR on Chromatin extracted from untreated or IFNα treated HMECs in the absence or presence of 50 μM C01L_F03. Accordingly, using antibodies against pSTAT1, pSTAT2, or pSTAT3, treatment with IFNα caused enhanced binding of pSTAT1 and pSTAT2 to the promoter ISRE element of OAS2 (**Figure 3B**), and respectively of pSTAT1 and pSTAT3 to IRF1 and SOCS3 containing GAS sites as compared to untreated controls (**Figure 3B**). More important, the presence of CO1L_F03 dramatically reduced this DNA-binding of the different STATs (**Figure 3B**) and correlated with inhibition of target gene expression (**Figure 3A**).

Stattic and STX-0119 Exhibit STAT Cross-Binding in Analogy to C01L_F03

Recently, we proposed a similar STAT cross-binding mechanism for STATTIC and STX-0119 (16), chemical structures of STATTIC and STX-0119 are displayed in **Figure S1**. They were previously discovered as direct STAT3 inhibitors by high throughput screening (13) and virtual screening (25), respectively. In analogy to C01L_F03, we decided to examine this in more detail, by using a comparative docking strategy combined with western and Real-time PCR analysis. Using the pgeom algorithm, docking simulation of STATTIC and STX-0119 in the STAT1, 2 and 3 SH2 domain resulted in 20 optimized conformations for each compound. Moreover, corresponding BS values were calculated for each individual STAT (not shown). **Table 3** shows the top STAT1-BS of STATTIC (4.70) and of STX-0119 (4.36), as well as STAT1-CBAVs (STATTIC: −0.86 for STAT2 and 0.39 for STAT3; STX-0119: −0.32 for STAT2 and 0.25 for STAT3). As becomes clear from the calculated STAT1-CBAVs, both compounds exhibited nearly identical binding affinity to the STAT1, 2 and 3 SH2 domain. In addition, STATTIC and STX-0119 LBPV toward the STAT-SH2 pY+0 and pY-X cavities were determined. Thus, the conformational tendencies of STATTIC and STX-0119 to the STAT3-SH2 were calculated. According to **Table 4**, from the top 20 optimized binding conformations of STATTIC to STAT3-SH2, 6 (30%) favor pY+0 and 11 (55%) fit to pY-X. LBPV analyses for other STAT-SH2 revealed that STATTIC also shares partial affinity between pY+0 and pY-X in case of STAT1 and STAT2 (**Table 4**) similar to STAT3. From the top 20 optimized binding conformations of STX-0119 to STAT3-SH2, only 5 (25%) of them favor both cavities simultaneously, which is in the same range in case of STAT1 and STAT2 (**Table 4**). Graphical analysis of the docking results (**Figure 4A**) was performed as a supplement to the numerical values. For each individual STAT the top scored conformation of STATTIC and STX-0119 competes with pTyr in binding to the STAT-SH2 domain. Due to its small size and low molecular weight STATTIC lacks STAT-SH2 binding specificity, which is supported by our recent docking results. Because of targeting both cavities (pY-0 and pY-X) with low BS difference (based on CBAV) and weak affinity (based on LBPV) the same is true for STX-0119.

Stattic and STX-0119 Inhibit IFNα-Induced STAT1, STAT2 and STAT3 Phosphorylation and Target Gene Expression

These findings were further validated in HMECs *in vitro*, by testing the potential of STATTIC and STX-0119 at varying concentrations to inhibit STAT phosphorylation induced by IFNα. For STATTIC and STX-0119 (**Figures 4B,C**), we observed inhibition of phosphorylation of STAT1, STAT2 and STAT3 in a concentration dependent manner (STATTIC: between 10 and 2.5 μM for 8 h; STX-0119: between 25 and 6.25 μM for 24 h). Corresponding with the effects shown at the STAT-phosphorylation level both inhibitors also efficiently decreased IFNα-induced gene expression of the multi-STAT and IRF-targets CXCL10, OAS2 and IFIT2, the STAT1-only target IRF1 and STAT3-only target SOCS3 (**Figures 5A,B**). In comparison to C01L_F03, STATTIC was the most potent one of the three tested compounds. Moreover, all three compounds exhibited a certain degree of cytotoxicity only at the highest used concentrations (not shown).

Together our data provide a molecular basis for STAT-cross-binding specificity of C01L_F03, STATTIC, and STX-0119 and their potential to inhibit multi-STAT and IRF-target genes.

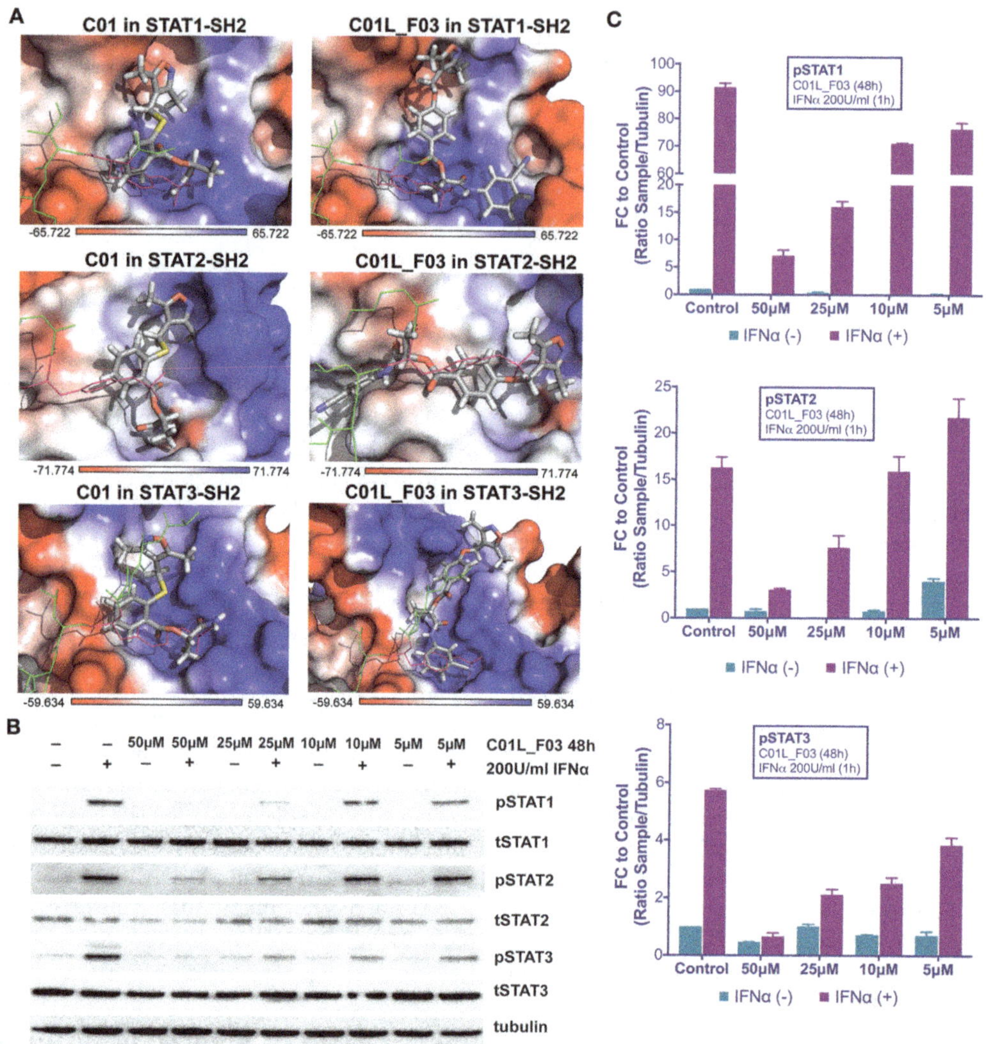

FIGURE 2 | Top-scored binding conformations of C01 and C01L_F03 in the SH2 domain of STAT1, STAT2, and STAT3 **(A)**. C01 and C01L_F03 compounds are shown in stick representation and colored according to the atomic structure. pTyr-linker is represented by green lines with pink pTyr residue. SH2 domains of STAT1, 2 and 3 in the surface representation are colored based on the distribution of the APBS electrostatic surface potential (43). Positively charged regions are indicated in blue and negatively charged regions in red. Docking simulations were performed using Surflex-Dock 2.6 program (19, 20). C01L_F03 inhibits IFNα induced phosphorylation of STAT1, STAT2 and STAT3 **(B)**. HMECs were treated with 50, 25, 10, and 5 μM C01L_F03 for 48 h and with 200 U/ml of IFNα for 1 h. Protein extracts were collected and levels of pSTAT1, pSTAT2, pSTAT3, tSTAT1, tSTAT2, tSTAT3 and α-tubulin were assessed by western blotting. Western quantification **(C)**. Bars represent mean quantification form 3 individual repeats ± SEM as error bars.

C01L_F03, STATTIC and STX-0119 Interact With the SH2 Domain of STAT1, STAT2, and STAT3

To provide evidence that STATTIC, STX-0119 and C01L_F03 concert their inhibitory actions through direct interaction with the STAT-SH2 domain we performed docking simulations in combination with STAT-SH2 *in silico* mutagenesis (see Materials and Methods). As presented in **Figure 6A,** mutating a.a. R602 in STAT1 (45), R601 in STAT2 (46) and R609 in STAT3 (47), resulted in a significant decrease in binding stability (ΔG^0) between the SH2 domains of STAT1, STAT2 and STAT3 and all three inhibitors. The same was true, after mutating a second important a.a. K584 in STAT1 (48), R583 in STAT2 and K591 in STAT3 (18), albeit to a lesser extent (**Figure 6A**). A similar approach was used to compare binding stability of STATTIC and published STATTIC analogs, STB and STC, **Figure S1** (13), and of C01L_F03 and C01 which differ in *in silico* binding affinity for STAT1, 2, and 3 (**Table 4**). As becomes clear from **Figure 6B**, STATTIC analogs exhibit lower binding stability (ΔG^0) for the SH2 domains of STAT1, 2 and 3 as compared to wt STATTIC. Likewise, interaction between C01 and STAT1, 2 and 3, corresponds with a lower binding stability (ΔG^0) in relation to C01L_F03.

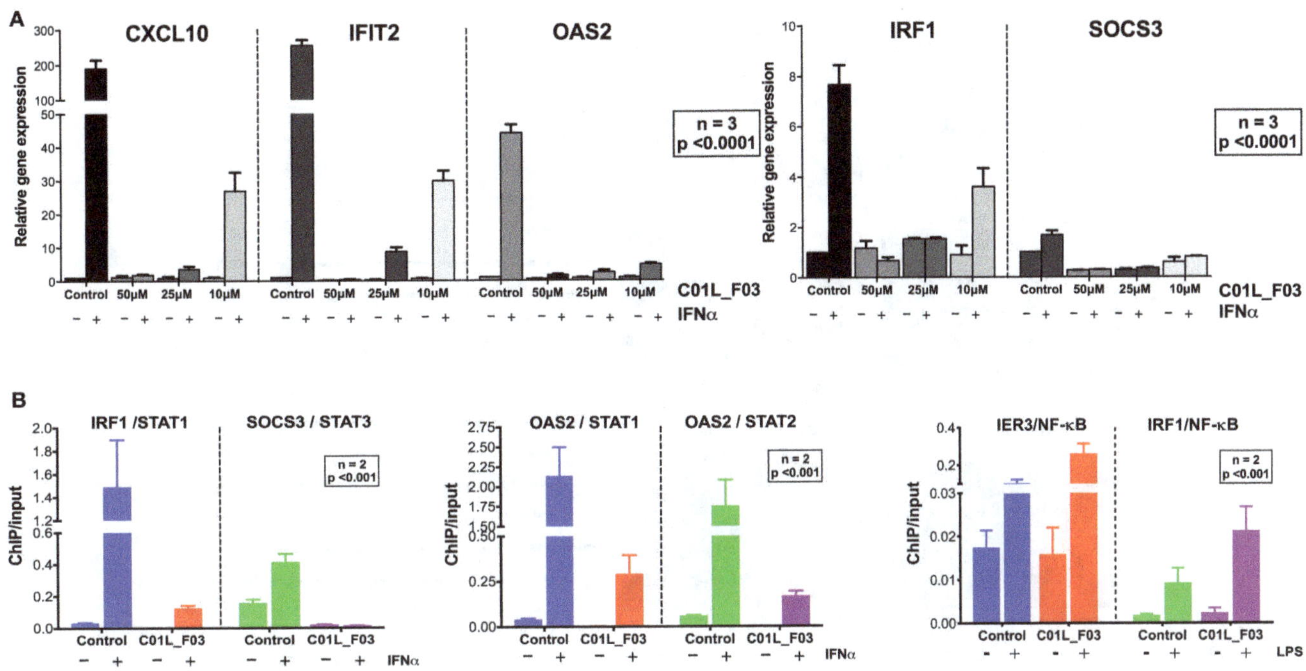

FIGURE 3 | C01L_F03 inhibits IFNα induced gene expression of CXCL10, IFIT2, OAS2, IRF1, and SOCS3 **(A)**. HMECs were treated with 50, 25, 10 of C01L_F03 for 48 h and with 200 U/ml of IFNα for 4 h. RNA was isolated and subjected to qPCR analysis. Experiments were performed in 3 individual repeats, which were compared by two-way ANOVA test and unpaired two-tailed student *T*-test. C01L_F03 inhibits IFNα stimulated binding of STAT1, STAT2 and STAT3 to the ISRE of OAS2, and GAS of IRF1 and SOCS3, and LPS stimulated binding of p65 to the NF-κB binding site of IER3 and IRF1 **(B)**. HMECs were treated with 50 μM of C01L_F03 for 48 h. Chromatin was isolated and subjected to IP with antibodies against pSTAT1, pSTAT2, pSTAT3 or NF-κB (p65), followed by qPCR analysis (primers are listed in **Table 1**). Experiments were performed in 2 individual repeats, which were compared by two-way ANOVA test and unpaired two-tailed student *T*-test.

C01L_F03, STATTIC and STX-0119 Commonly Inhibit Cross-Talk Between IFNγ and LPS in a "Multi-STAT" and "STAT-Only" Manner

In a second set of experiments HMECs were treated with IFNγ and LPS to further investigate the ability of C01L_F03, STATTIC, and STX-0119 to inhibit pro-inflammatory and pro-atherogenic signaling depending on multiple STATs, IRFs and NF-κB. As shown in **Figure 7**, pre-treatment of HMECs with C01L_F03, STATTIC or STX-0119 resulted in inhibition of IFNγ+LPS induced gene expression of IFIT2, OAS2, CCL5, CXCL10, CXCL9, ICAM1 and VCAM1, in a concentration dependent manner. Pre-treating HMECs with IFNγ+LPS, followed by STATTIC, or simultaneous treatment of IFNγ+LPS with C01L_F03 or STX-0119 (representing a more therapeutic mode), likewise resulted in potent inhibition of CXCL10, IFIT2, and OAS2 expression (**Figure S4**). In general, the different compounds displayed similar inhibition characteristics, although sometimes minor variations could be observed. These data suggested that C01L_F03, STATTIC and STX-0119 may commonly block STAT cooperative promotor activation with IRF and NF-κB mediated by IFNγ and LPS in human microvascular endothelial cells. To provide further evidence for this, we decided to study the genome-wide effect of C01L_F03, STATTIC and STX-0119 on IFNγ+LPS-mediated vascular inflammation. For this, we performed a microarray experiment on RNA isolated from HMECs treated with IFNγ+LPS in the presence or absence of: 50 μM of C01L_F03, 25 μM of STX-0119 or 10 μM of STATTIC (GEO accession: GSE101508). IFNγ+LPS increased the expression of 731 genes at least two-fold or higher as compared to untreated cells, of which the top-25 are shown in **Table 5**.

These included many known IFNγ and LPS target genes associated with: chemotaxis/migration (CXCL9, CXCL10, CCL7, CCL8, CCL3L3, MMP3, MMP12), adhesion (VCAM1, CD74), immune response to viral infection (UBD, GBP4, GBP5, OAS2, MX2, INDO, OASL, IFI44L, MX2). GO analysis of the complete list of IFNγ+LPS responsive genes revealed enrichment of biological functions mainly involved in: cytokine-mediated signaling pathway (GO:0019221); defense response and immune system process (GO:0006952 and GO:0002376); regulation of cytokine production (GO:0001817), inflammatory response (GO:0006954), regulation of cell adhesion (GO:0030155) or cell migration (GO:0030334), (see **Table 5**, **Figure 8A**).

Next, we aimed at identifying the IFNγ+LPS target genes that were commonly inhibited by C01L_F03, STX-0119 and STATTIC. For this, genes were considered of which the expression was more than 4 times inhibited by all three inhibitors as compared to IFNγ+LPS alone (see Materials and Methods). As such, out of the 731 up-regulated genes C01L_F03 inhibited

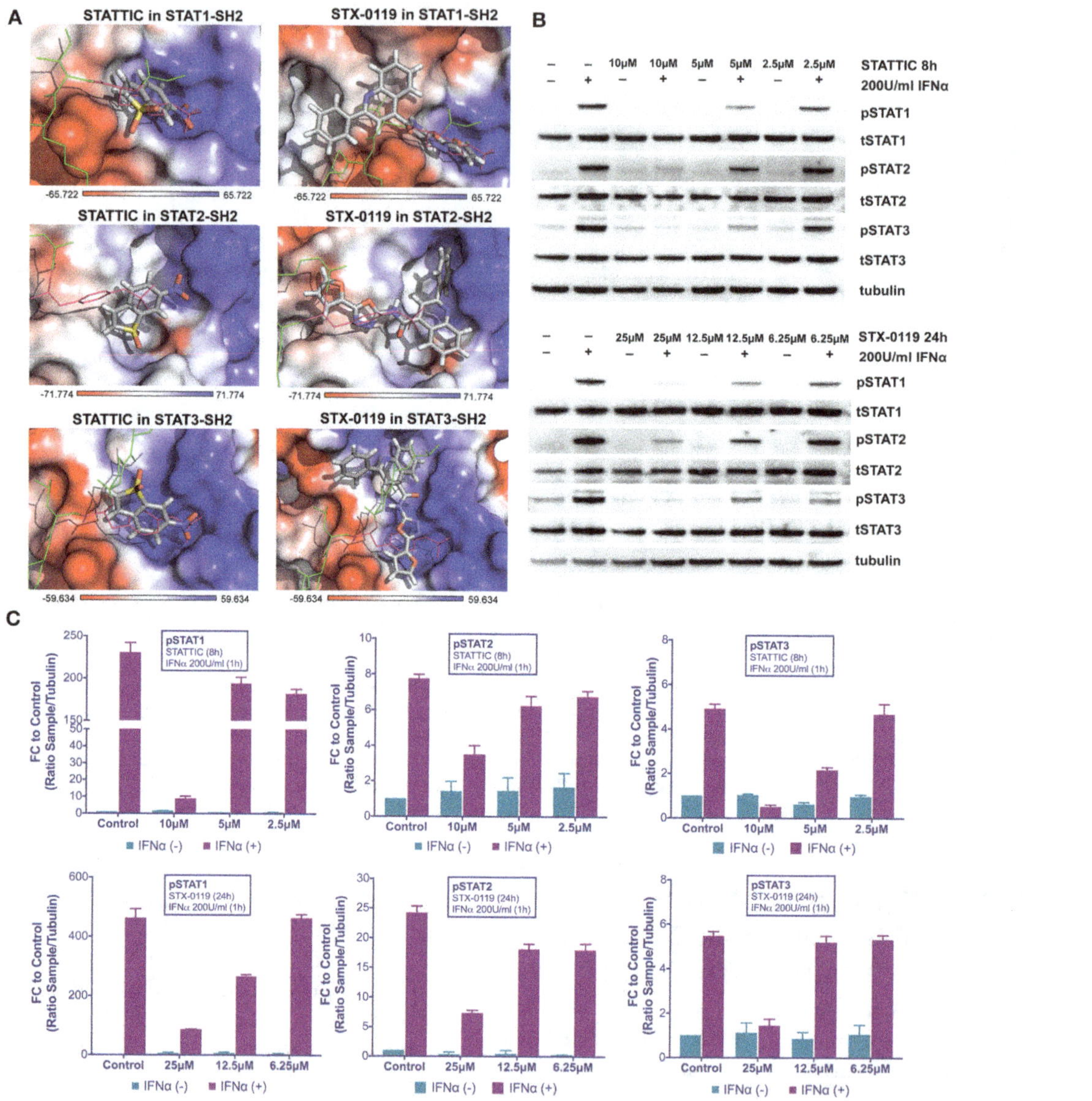

FIGURE 4 | Top-scored binding conformations of STATTIC and STX-0119 in the SH2 domain of STAT1, STAT2, and STAT3 **(A)**. STATTIC and STX-0119 compounds are in stick representation and colored according to the atomic structure. pTyr-linker is represented by green lines with pink pTyr residue. SH2 domains of STAT1, 2 and 3 in the surface representation are colored based on the distribution of the APBS electrostatic surface potential (43). Positively charged regions are indicated in blue and negatively charged regions in red. Docking simulations were performed using Surflex-Dock 2.6 program (19, 20). STATTIC and STX-0119 inhibit IFNα induced phosphorylation of STAT1, STAT2 and STAT3 **(B)**. HMECs were treated with 10, 5, 2.5 μM of STATTIC for 8 h or with 25, 12.5, 6.25 μM of STX-0119 for 24 h and with 200 U/ml of IFNα for 1 h. Protein extracts were collected and levels of pSTAT1, pSTAT2, pSTAT3, tSTAT1, tSTAT2, tSTAT3 and α-tubulin were assessed by western blotting. Western quantification **(C)**. Bars represent mean quantification form 3 individual repeats ± SEM as error bars.

expression of 259, STATTIC of 244 genes and STX-0119 of 292 genes (**Figure 8B**). What is more, expression of 159 genes was commonly inhibited by C01L_F03, STATTIC and STX-0119 (according to the requirements specified in Materials & Methods), of which the inhibition pattern of the top-25 is displayed in **Figure 8C**. Among those we could recognize the ones which were already validated by Real-time PCR (**Figures 3A, 5A,B, 7**) e.g., CXCL10, IFIT2, OAS2, or VCAM1, as well as many known STAT target genes (i.e., SOCS1, IRF1, IRF8, APOL1, BID as STAT1 targets; IFIT1, IFIT2, IFIT3, OAS1, OAS2, MX1, MX2, ISG15 as STAT1-STAT2 targets; SOCS3, CCND1, MMP3, FAS PIM1, VEGF, S1PR1 as STAT3 targets). GO analysis of the 159 commonly inhibited genes furthermore revealed enrichment of biological functions connected to pro-inflammatory and pro-atherogenic responses (**Figure 8C**). The complete list of up and down-regulated genes in response to IFNγ+LPS in the presence or absence of C01L_F03, STATTIC and STX-0119 is shown in **Table S1**.

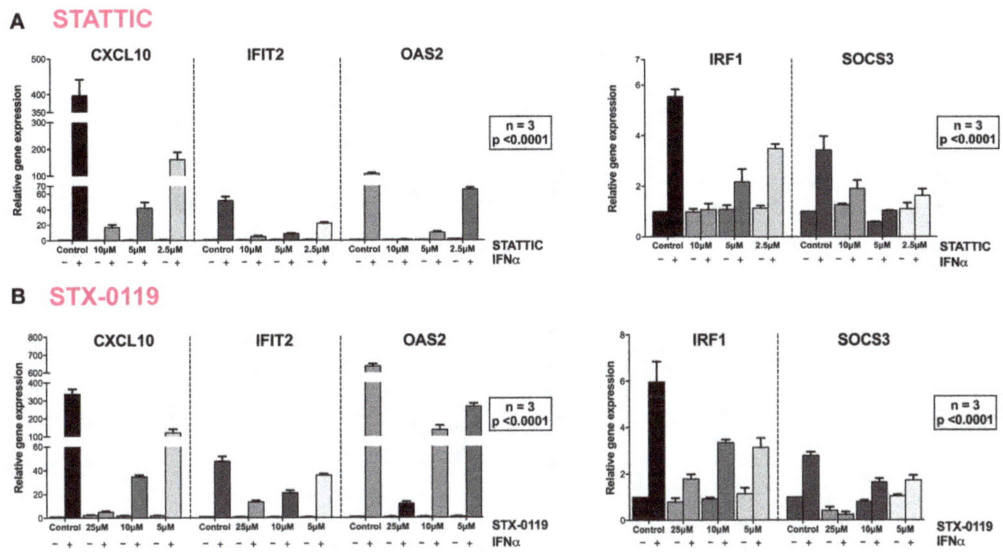

FIGURE 5 | STATTIC and STX-0119 inhibits IFNα induced gene expression of CXCL10, IFIT2, OAS2, IRF1, and SOCS3. HMECs were treated with **(A)** 10, 5, 2.5 μM of STATTIC for 8 h or **(B)** with 25, 12.5, 6.25 μM of STX-0119 for 24 h and with 200 U/ml of IFNα for 4 h. RNA was isolated and subjected to qPCR analysis. Experiments were performed in 3 individual repeats, which were compared by two-way ANOVA test and unpaired two-tailed student *T*-test.

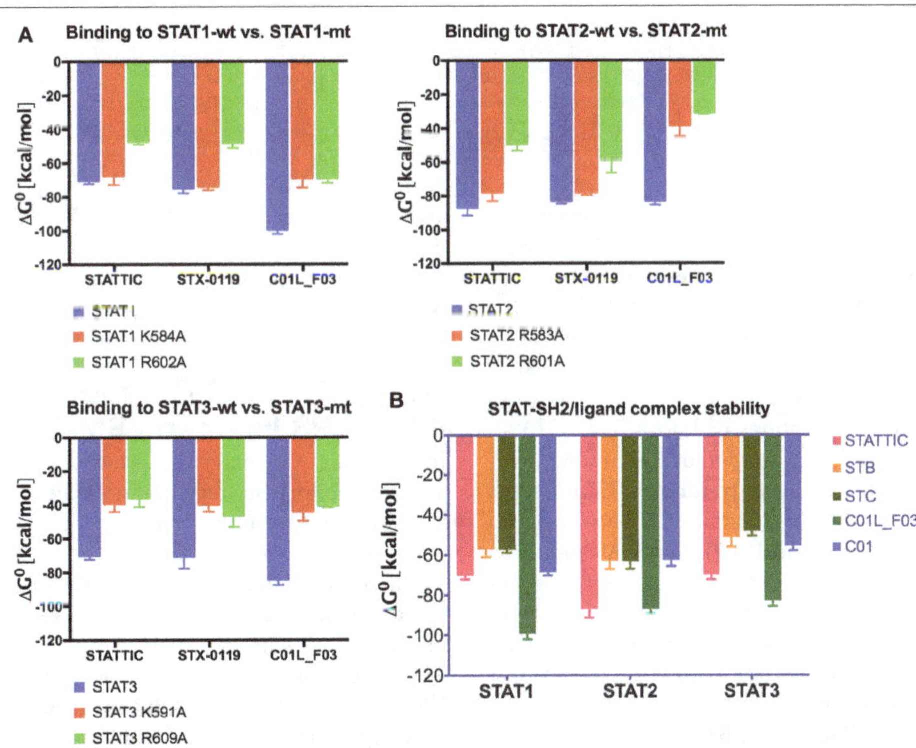

FIGURE 6 | Comparison of wt and mutated STAT-SH2/ligand complex stability **(A)**. STAT1, 2 or 3, wild type and with single point mutation to Ala, complexes with STATTIC, STX-0119 or C01L_F03 have been subjected to the *in silico* studies of binding stability in the equilibrium. ΔG^0 (free enthalpy change), which is a measure of the strength of the complex formation was estimated [based on HADDOCK ligand docking protocol (26, 27) with addition of Surflex-Dock protocol (16)]. More negative ΔG^0 (higher free enthalpy change) corresponds to stronger interaction between ligand and the protein, which reflects better complex stability. Comparison of STAT-SH2/ligand complex stability **(B)**. Complexes of STAT1, 2 and 3, with STATTIC and its analogs STB and STC, as well as C01 and C01L_F03 have been subjected to the *in silico* studies of binding stability in the equilibrium as in **(A)**.

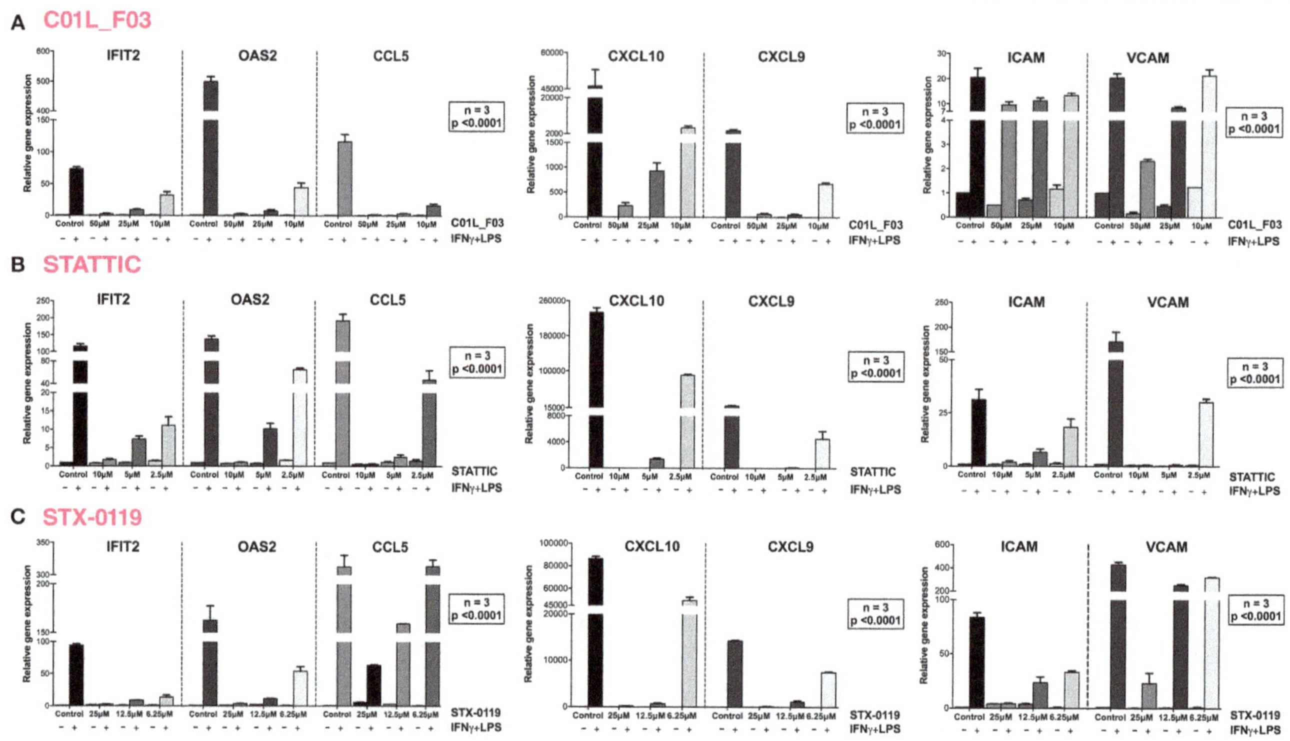

FIGURE 7 | C01L_F03, STATTIC and STX-0119 inhibit IFNγ+LPS induced gene expression of IFIT2, OAS2, CCL5, CXCL10, CXCL9, ICAM1, and VCAM1. HMECs were treated with **(A)** 50, 25, 10 μM of C01L_F03 for 48 h or **(B)** 10, 5, 2.5 μM of STATTIC for 8 h or **(C)** with 25, 12.5, 6.25 μM of STX-0119 for 24 h and for 8 h with IFNγ + 4 h with LPS. RNA was isolated and subjected to qPCR analysis. Experiments were performed in 3 individual repeats, which were compared by two-way ANOVA test and unpaired two-tailed student *T*-test.

To address the "multi-STAT" and "STAT-only" characteristics of these three inhibitors, we subsequently performed promoter analysis on the 159 commonly inhibited genes, for the presence of ISRE, STAT or NF-κB binding sites. **Figure 8D** shows the predicted representation of individual or combined ISRE, STAT or NF-κB binding sites, in their proximal promoters (−950 to +100). The majority of these genes contained single ISRE (14.9%) or GAS (17.5%) sites, or combinations of ISRE+GAS (19.3%), ISRE+NF-κB (5.3%), GAS+NF-κB (18.4%) or ISRE+GAS+NF-κB (22.8%). In general, under these conditions ISRE motifs correspond to potential binding of multiple STATs (STAT1 and STAT2) and IRFs (IRF1, IRF8, and IRF9), and GAS motifs to that of multiple STATs (STAT1 and STAT3). Surprisingly, 2 genes (1.8%), IL7R, USP18 were assigned to the group with only an NF-κB site in their proximal promoter. However, both genes contained either a GAS (IL7R) or ISRE (USP18) sequence just outside the 950 bp selected promoter area (not shown). To further proof that DNA binding of NF-κB (p65) was not affected under these conditions we performed ChIP qPCR on genes containing either both STAT1 and NF-κB binding sites (IRF1) or only an NF-κB binding element (IER3) (**Figure 3B**). Indeed, C01L_F03 did not effect the LPS-induced DNA binding of p65 to the promoter of these two genes, which correlated with the partial (IRF1) or lack of inhibition (IER3) of their expression as observed in our microarray experiment (**Table S1**). These results strongly suggest that C01L_F03, STATTIC and STX-0119 are "multi-STAT" and "STAT-only" inhibitors that commonly inhibit pro-inflammatory and pro-atherogenic gene expression directed by cooperative involvement of STATs with IRFs and/or NF-κB.

C01L_F03, STATTIC and STX-0119 Inhibit IFNγ+LPS Induced VSMC Migration

In addition, we aimed at providing evidence that a multi-STAT inhibitory strategy could be used to inhibit IFNγ+LPS induced vascular inflammation in different models. First, we performed a wound healing assay to examine the effect of all three compounds on IFNγ+LPS induced ECs migration (**Figure 9A**). Cells stimulated with IFNγ+LPS showed increased capacity of migration, resulting in almost 80% wound coverage after 12-h of treatment (**Figure 9B**). In contrast, HMECs treated additionally with C01L_F03, STATTIC or STX-0119 demonstrated drastic reduction of movement. All three inhibitors caused decrease of IFNγ+LPS induced wound healing to less than 15% (**Figure 9B**), whereas in the absence of IFNγ+LPS they were not capable of closing more than 10% of the artificial wound (**Figure 9B**). In agreement with the effect on IFNγ+LPS-induced gene expression (**Figure 8**), based on concentration and time of treatment, STATTIC was the most potent of the three compounds.

TABLE 5 | Representative top-25 genes induced by IFNγ+LPS, displaying significant inhibition by all three compounds.

Gene id	Fold change relative to control			
	IFNγ+LPS	C01L_F03	STATTIC	STX-0119
CXCL10	9298.61	615.79	15.14	223.90
CCL8	2118.86	6.83	6.31	0.79
UBD	1860.83	129.28	2.09	62.19
CXCL9	1565.00	2.26	1.00	6.31
GBP4	793.16	38.79	16.30	8.61
GBP5	435.89	20.26	5.26	11.63
OAS2	329.65	2.61	6.29	1.48
VCAM1	326.83	33.01	1.36	8.12
CCL7	289.01	1.00	3.41	1.00
INDO	209.33	1.00	1.80	1.00
MMP3	192.62	2.22	28.96	2.89
IDO1	178.80	1.62	6.03	1.42
CCL3L3	165.18	4.69	1.52	20.25
OASL	160.22	3.99	1.21	14.16
LYPD5	127.07	6.75	6.90	7.66
LTB	125.33	1.00	0.75	0.95
MMP12	111.79	0.70	0.70	0.70
IFI44L	100.04	1.14	1.14	1.21
LOC730249	91.23	0.60	0.96	0.78
CD74	88.67	1.18	0.76	0.84
LOC100129681	76.64	1.31	2.35	0.18
MX2	68.99	0.40	0.74	1.23
DLL1	68.78	3.30	10.80	8.11
C1S	64.57	4.22	5.98	2.39
TNFSF10	64.45	0.67	1.22	0.21

Gene expression levels were presented as fold change relative to control.

C01L_F03, STATTIC and STX-0119 Inhibit IFNγ and LPS Induced Mononuclear Leukocyte Adhesion to HUVECs

Our previous studies reported increased adhesion of monocytes to ECs *in vitro* under static conditions in response to IFNγ and LPS in a STAT1-dependent manner (4). We next evaluated the effect of IFNγ for 24 h followed by LPS for another 4 h challenge on mononuclear-endothelial cell interactions *in vitro* using the dynamic flow chamber assay. Thus, freshly-isolated human mononuclear cells were perfused across HUVECs monolayers stimulated or not with the IFNγ+LPS combination. Significant increases in mononuclear cell adhesion were detected in stimulated cells compared to untreated cells (**Figure 10**). Treatment with C01L_F03 (50 μM; **Figure 10A**), STATTIC (5 μM; **Figure 10B**) or STX-0119 (25 μM; **Figure 10C**) for 4 h or 24 h resulted in significant inhibition of mononuclear cell adhesion to ECs induced by the IFNγ+LPS combination. In the presence of a lower concentration of STATTIC, 1 μM (24 h), a similar drastic reduction in the number of adhered mononuclear cells induced by the IFNγ+LPS combination was observed >70% inhibition, **Figure 10B**).

C01L_F03, STATTIC and STX-0119 Protect Against IFNγ and LPS Induced Impairment of Mesenteric Artery Contractility

Recently we also observed that among the genes that were highly amplified upon treatment with IFNγ and LPS in primary mouse VSMCs, appeared inducible nitric oxide synthase (iNOS, Nos2). Dysregulation of Nos2 expression and its activity affect vessel function. Thus, we evaluated the physiological ramifications of these experimental conditions using a wire myograph/organ chamber setting. Here we examined the possible protective effect of a multi-STAT inhibitory strategy under similar conditions. As expected, stimulation of the mesenteric arteries isolated from WT animals with IFNγ+LPS resulted in drastic impairment of contractility after subjection to NA treatment as compared to matched control arteries (**Figure 11A**). Nevertheless, pre-incubation with C01L_F03 (1 μM), STATTIC (1 nM) or STX-0119 (10 nM) prevented the impaired response to NA elicited by IFNγ+LPS (**Figures 11B–D** respectively). Notably, STATTIC and STX-0119 could only be used in the nM range, without causing IFNγ+LPS-independent impairment of vessel function and integrity (not shown).

DISCUSSION

Abnormal activation of STAT pathways is present in many human diseases, including CVDs. This fact marks these proteins as highly interesting therapeutic targets (49, 50). By exploring the pTyr-SH2 interaction area of STAT3, searches for STAT3-targeting compounds yielded many small molecules including STATTIC and STX-0119. Only a few inhibitors for other STATs are described. In our pursuit for novel STAT inhibitors, we used a comparative *in silico* docking strategy on CL library from ZINC in combination with 3D structure models for human (h)STAT1, 2 and 3. We selected three novel STAT1 inhibitors C01, E01, and F01 that inhibit STAT1 phosphorylation by targeting the pY+0 and pY-X of its SH2 domain, however with low potency (**Figure 1**). To find more potent variants of these compounds, a similarity screen on the CL and the CDL libraries of the ZINC database was performed for compounds with a similarity of ≥ 50% to C01, E01 or F01 (**Tables 3, 4**). Consequently, we identified the novel multi-STAT inhibitor C01L_F03, which targets the SH2 domain of STAT1, STAT2, and STAT3 with the same affinity (**Figure 2**). In addition, it was shown to simultaneously block phosphorylation and DNA-binding of these three STATs and expression of a selection of target genes in ECs in response to IFNα (**Figures 2, 3**). These included the multiple STAT (STAT1/STAT2)-target genes, CXCL10, IFIT2 and OAS2, as well as the STAT1 target gene, IRF1 and the STAT3 target gene, SOCS3. It also predicts anti-inflammatory potential of C01L_F03 by simultaneous inhibiting STAT1, STAT2, and STAT3 activity.

According to a similar docking strategy, recently we obtained further insight into the STAT-SH2 cross-binding specificity of a pre-selection of known STAT3 inhibitors, including STATTIC and STX-0119 (16) (**Table 4**). All the studied compounds targeted the highly conserved pTyr-SH2 binding pocket of all STATs. We concluded, based on the binding affinity scores (BS) and graphic

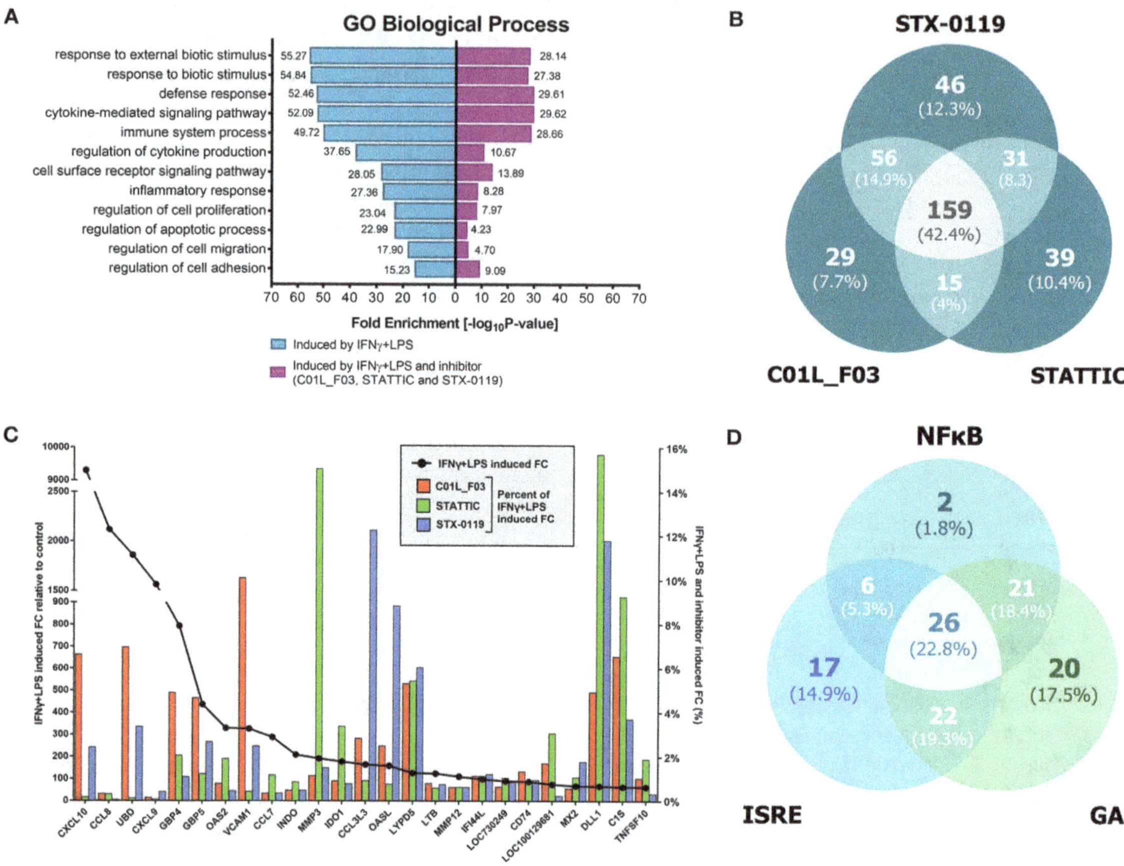

FIGURE 8 | Comparison of top GO terms **(A)**. Terms were selected based on Fold Enrichment values, between genes induced by treatment with IFNγ+LPS and group of IFNγ+LPS induced and inhibited simultaneously by three compounds. Venn diagram distribution of IFNγ+LPS induced and inhibited (C01L_F03, STATTIC, STX-0119) genes **(B)**. Data were obtained from HMECs treated with 50 μM of C01L_F03, 10 μM of STATTIC and 25 μM of STX-0119 and IFNγ+LPS. Three lists of inhibited genes were uploaded and analyzed by VennDiagram package in R (31). The diagram shows how many genes are induced by IFNγ+LPS and simultaneously inhibited by two or three inhibitors or only by one compound. Representative genes induced by IFNγ+LPS, displaying significant inhibition by all three compounds **(C)**. Expression levels of IFNγ+LPS-induced genes (displayed as •, left Y-axis) were presented as fold change (FC) relative to control. Expression of C01L_F03 or STATTIC or STX-0119 inhibited genes (displayed as colored bars, right Y-axis) was presented as percent of IFNγ+LPS-induced FC. Venn diagram distribution of ISRE, GAS, NF-κB binding sites among genes inhibited simultaneously by three compounds **(D)**. Three lists of inhibited genes were uploaded and analyzed by VennDiagram package in R (31).

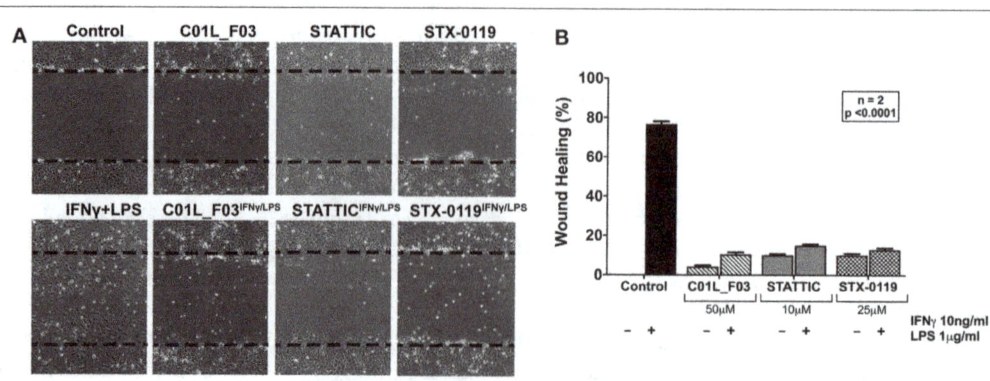

FIGURE 9 | Wound healing assay performed on HMECs treated with C01L_F03, STATTIC and STX-0119 with or without IFNγ+LPS presence **(A)**. Dashed lines determine scratch borders at the beginning of the experiment. Statistical evaluation of wound healing assay **(B)**. Graph shows percentage of healed wound in comparison to 0 h control. Experiment was performed in 2 individual repeats (40 distance measurements in total), which were compared by two-way ANOVA test.

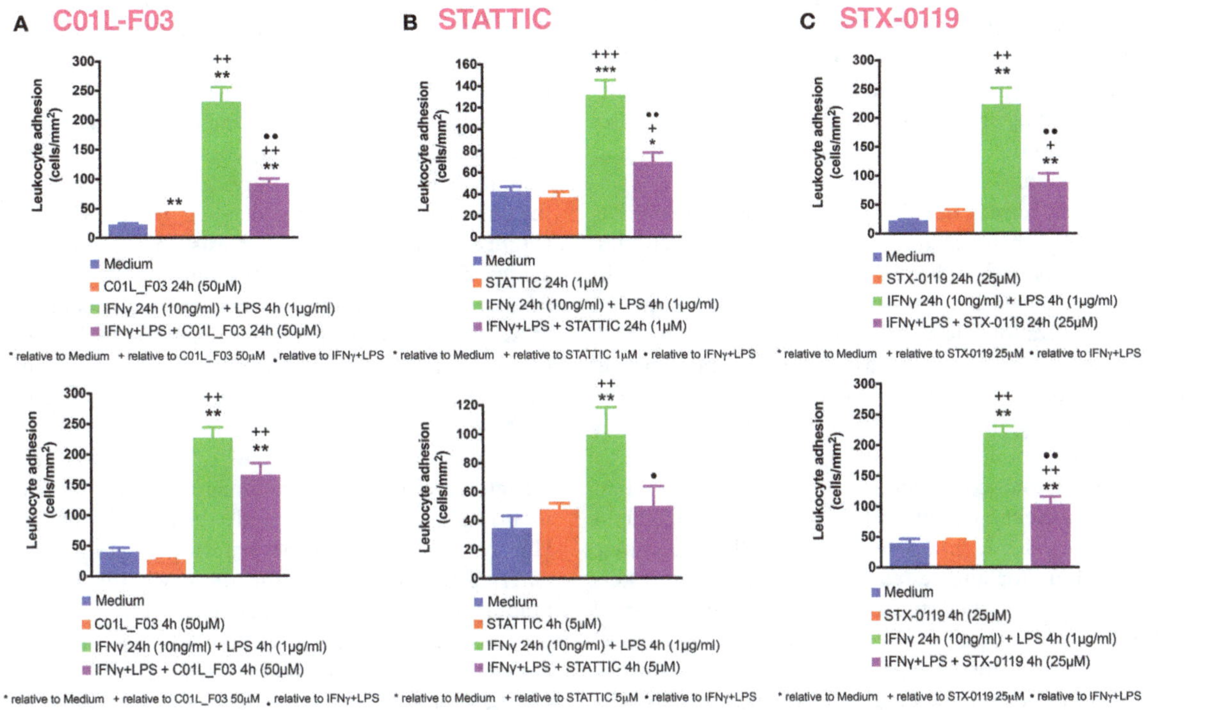

FIGURE 10 | C01L_F03, STATTIC, STX-0119 and inhibit IFNγ+LPS-induced HUVECs mononuclear cell adhesion under physiological flow. HUVECs were stimulated with IFNγ (10 ng/ml) for 24 h and LPS (1 μg/ml) for 4 h. In the experiments, cells were pretreated with **(A)** C01L_F03 50μM for 4 h or C01L_F03 50 μM for 24 h; **(B)** STATTIC 5 μM for 4 h or STATTIC 1 μM for 24 h; **(C)** STX-0119 25 μM for 4 h or STX-0119 25 μM for 24 h. Freshly isolated human mononuclear cells (106 cells/ml) were perfused across the endothelial monolayers for 5 min. at 0.5 dyn/cm^2 and leukocyte adhesion quantified. Experiments were performed in 5–7 individual repeats, which were compared by one way ANOVA test and unpaired two-tailed student *T*-test with *$p < 0.05$; **$p < 0.01$ and ***$p < 0.001$.

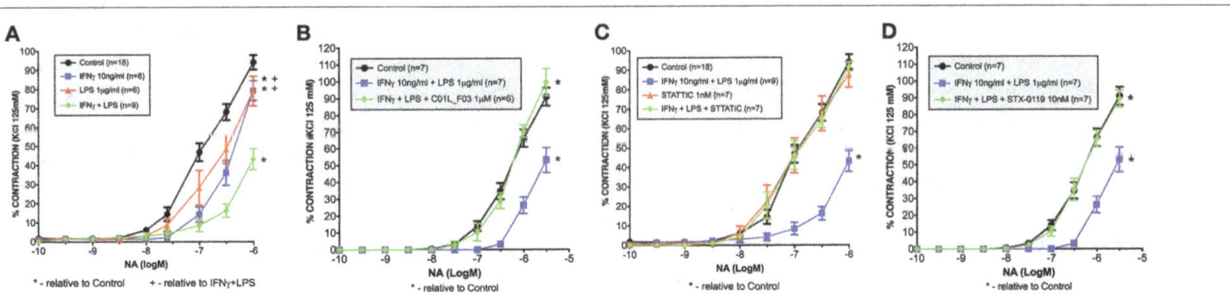

FIGURE 11 | Ameliorated response to noradrenaline in mesenteric arteries stimulated with IFNγ and LPS **(A)**. Isolated mesenteric arteries from WT mice were incubated with IFNγ (10 ng/ml for 3 h prior to NA stimulation), and/or LPS (1 μg/ml for 1.5 h prior to NA stimulation). Next, response to noradrenaline was tested on the small-vessel myograph. C01L_F03, STATTIC and STX-0119 prevent the impaired response to NA elicited by IFNγ+LPS treatment. Isolated mesenteric arteries from WT mice were pre-incubated with **(B)** C01L_F03 (1 μM for 4 h) or **(C)** STATTIC (1 nM for 4 h) or **(D)** STX-0119 (10 nM for 4 h) prior to NA stimulation and/or IFNγ (10 ng/ml for 3 h prior to NA stimulation) and LPS (1 μg/ml for 1.5 h prior to NA stimulation). Next, response to noradrenaline was tested on the small-vessel myograph. Response to noradrenaline in WT mice presented as a percentage of the maximal contraction to KCl. Two-way ANOVA test was used with *$p < 0.05$ vs. Control and +$p < 0.05$ vs. IFNγ+LPS.

representation in the SH2 domain of hSTAT1, hSTAT2 and hSTAT3, that none of these compounds are STAT3-specific. Here, we followed up on the proposed STAT cross-binding specificity of STATTIC and STX-0119. As compared to C01L_F03, a similar *in silico* and *in vitro* multi-STAT inhibiting capacity was shown for STATTIC and STX-0119 (**Figures 4**, **5**). STATTIC was the most potent of the three compounds, reflected by the time of treatment and concentration used. This could agree with the fact that STATTIC is the smallest compound of the three, and equally targeted the pTyr-binding or hydrophobic SH2 cavity. In addition, the covalent binding of STATTIC has shown to contribute to its potent inhibitory activity toward STAT3 (51). In contrast, the larger two compounds C01L_F03 and STX-0119 covered both pTyr-binding and hydrophobic SH2 cavities for binding, at the same time. Not surprisingly, the non-specific *in silico* binding of STATTIC and STX-0119 toward all STATs (STAT1-STAT6) (16), could also be observed for C01L_F03 (data not shown). Together our data provide a molecular basis for STAT-cross-binding specificity of C01L_F03, STATTIC, and STX-0119 and their potential to inhibit multi-STAT-activity and target gene expression.

In general STAT direct inhibitors are a very heterogenous group considering their chemical attributes e.g., peptides, peptidomimetics, natural and synthetic small compounds. In our work we concentrated on small compounds targeting STAT-STAT dimerization plane between pTyr linker and SH2 domain, with pTyr-binding cavity as a main interaction site. Since interaction between negatively charged pTyr residue and positively charged Arg and Lys in the cavity is very relevant for STAT-STAT dimerization, the main driving force of the binding are polar and electrostatic interactions. Thus, we postulate that the general common chemical attribute of STAT inhibitors might be negatively charged side group analogous to pTyr phosphate (which is common for the tested compounds). Our results are in agreement with other studies on the binding mode of STAT inhibitors, e.g., Arpin et al. (52) who reported a novel STAT3 small molecule inhibitor PG-S3-001 as a pancreatic cancer therapeutic. They performed detailed *in silico* characteristics of its binding to the STAT3-SH2 domain. Similar to their results, in our docking studies STATTIC, STX-0119, and C01L_F03 targeted the pTyr-binding cavity and exhibited polar and electrostatic interactions between negatively charged side groups and the same amino acids as reported by Arpin et al. (52) For example, PG-S3-001 binds with Arg609, Lys591 and Ser611 by carboxyl group, whereas STATTIC interacts with the same amino acids in STAT3 by the nitro group and the corresponding amino acids in STAT1 and STAT2. Moreover, STX-0119 and C01L_F03 possess a relatively flexible glycine core similarly to PG-S3-001.

The comparative docking simulations and *in vitro* inhibition studies related to STAT-cross-binding specificity correspond to other studies. For example, Bill et al. provided evidence for cross-binding of curcumin to STAT3 and STAT1 (53). Other natural products like cryptotanshinone (54) and resveratrol analogs (RSVA314 and RSVA405) (55) exhibited similar characteristics. Sanseverino et al. found that STATTIC inhibits not only STAT3 activation but also that of STAT1 and to a lesser extent of STAT2, in response to cell activation by IL-6 or IFNβ based on studies using human monocyte-derived dendritic cells (56). This correlates with our finding, that STATTIC is not STAT3 specific. Inhibition of STAT1 phosphorylation by STATTIC has also been described in human ovarian cancer cells (57) and melanoma cells (58). Therefore, evidence accumulates that many of the known STAT3 inhibitors do not seem STAT3 specific.

Docking simulations of C01L_F03, STATTIC, and STX-0119 in combination with *in silico* STAT-SH2 mutagenesis provided further evidence to suggest that these compounds directly interact with hSTAT1, hSTAT2, and hSTAT3 (**Figure 6**). In this respect, docking simulations highly correlated with *in vitro* mutagenesis studies of a.a. R602 in STAT1, R601 in STAT2 and R609 in STAT3, which were experimentally proven to be crucial for STAT phosphorylation and reciprocal binding of the pTyr-linker to the STAT-SH2 domain [STAT1-R602 (45); STAT2-R601 (46); STAT3-R609 (47)]. The same was true, for the second mutation a.a. K584 in STAT1 (48), R583 in STAT2 and K591 in STAT3 (18). In case of STATTIC and its selective binding to STAT3, the lower STAT3 binding affinity of published STATTIC analogs, STB and STC (13)] coincided with decreased binding stability toward STAT-SH2 models (**Figure 6**). Combined with the observed *in vitro* effects of C01L_F03 on STAT DNA-binding (**Figure 3**) this strongly suggests that all three compounds act as direct STAT-inhibitors. This is also in line with the finding that the activation state of the tyrosine kinases JAK1, JAK2, and c-Src, which are considered to be responsible for phosphorylation of STAT3 Tyr705, was not significantly inhibited by the presence of 10 or 20 mM STATTIC in breast cancer cells (13).

Of all STATs especially STAT1, STAT2, and STAT3 have been recognized as prominent modulators of inflammation, especially in immune and vascular cells during atherosclerosis (7, 59). However, STAT-inhibitory strategies targeting CVDs, still await entering the clinic. Based on the newly identified STAT cross-binding mechanism for C01L_F03, STATTIC, and STX-0119, we subsequently pursued a multi-STAT inhibitory approach as a novel strategy in the treatment of vascular inflammation and CVDs. Along these lines, we first tested the effect of C01L_F03, STATTIC, and STX-0119 on signal integration between IFNγ and LPS, which in vascular cells and atheroma interacting immune cells modulates important aspects of vascular inflammation (10) (**Table 6**). Indeed, pre-treatment of ECs with C01L_F03, STATTIC, or STX-0119 resulted in a similar inhibition pattern of IFNγ+LPS induced expression of the genes IFIT2, OAS2, CCL5, CXCL10, CXCL9, ICAM1, and VCAM1, with STATTIC being the most potent one (**Figure 7**). Likewise, STATTIC potently inhibited expression of the pro-inflammatory and pro-atherogenic genes CXCL9, CXCL10, CCL5, Nos2, IFIT1, and OAS2 in VSMCs treated with IFNγ and LPS (not shown). This suggested that C01L_F03, STATTIC, and STX-0119 may commonly block STAT cooperative promotor activation with IRF and NF-κB mediated by IFNγ and LPS in ECs and VSMCs. To provide further evidence for this, we decided to study the genome-wide effect of C01L_F03, STATTIC and STX-0119 on IFNγ+LPS-mediated vascular inflammation (**Figure 8**). Thus, IFNγ+LPS increased the expression of 731 genes, of which 159 were commonly inhibited by C01L_F03, STATTIC, and STX-0119. These 159 genes generally represented the ones with the highest IFNγ+LPS inducible levels and their biological functions reflected strong inhibitory potential of C01L_F03, STATTIC, and STX-0119 toward pro-inflammatory and proatherogenic responses. Among those genes many known STAT target genes (i.e., SOCS1, IRF1, IRF8, APOL1, BID as STAT1 targets; IFIT1, IFIT2, IFIT3, OAS1, OAS2, MX1, MX2, ISG15 as STAT1-STAT2 targets; SOCS3, CCND1, MMP3, FAS PIM1, VEGF, S1PR1 as STAT3 targets) could be recognized. More important, promoter analysis of the 159 commonly inhibited genes, for the presence of ISRE, STAT or NF-κB binding sites provided additional evidence that C01L_F03, STATTIC, and STX-0119 are "multi-STAT" as well as "STAT-only" inhibitors that commonly inhibit pro-inflammatory and pro-atherogenic gene expression directed

TABLE 6 | Comparison of top-12 GO terms, selected based on Fold enrichment values, between genes induced by treatment with IFNγ+LPS and group of IFNγ+LPS induced and inhibited simultaneously by C01L_F03, STATTIC, and STX-0119.

GO Term	Biological process	Induced by IFNγ and LPS			Inhibited by C01L_F03, STATTIC and STX-0119		
		Fold enrichment	Uniqueness	Dispensability	Fold enrichment	Uniqueness	Dispensability
GO:0043207	Response to external biotic stimulus	55.28	0.84	0.00	28.14	0.82	0.11
GO:0009607	Response to biotic stimulus	54.84	0.92	0.12	27.38	0.92	0.12
GO:0006952	Defense response	52.46	0.88	0.43	29.61	0.88	0.43
GO:0019221	Cytokine-mediated signaling pathway	52.09	0.74	0.11	29.62	0.76	0.00
GO:0002376	Immune system process	49.72	1.00	0.00	28.66	0.99	0.00
GO:0001817	Regulation of cytokine production	37.65	0.83	0.00	10.67	0.81	0.05
GO:0007166	Cell surface receptor signaling pathway	28.05	0.79	0.28	13.89	0.81	0.28
GO:0006954	Inflammatory response	27.36	0.86	0.68	8.28	0.87	0.68
GO:0042127	Regulation of cell proliferation	23.04	0.86	0.71	7.97	0.87	0.71
GO:0042981	Regulation of apoptotic process	22.99	0.82	0.83	4.23	0.86	0.83
GO:0030334	Regulation of cell migration	17.90	0.81	0.05	4.70	0.72	0.76
GO:0030155	Regulation of cell adhesion	15.23	0.88	0.05	9.09	0.86	0.05

by cooperative involvement of multiple STATs with IRFs and/or NF-κB.

Based on the previous studies, transcription of genes containing STAT-, ISRE- and NF-κB-binding sites in their promoter regions are under the cooperative regulation by extracellular stimuli activating STATs, IRFs and NF-κB, such as IFNγ, IFNα and TNFα, IL-1β or LPS (60–68). In general it is believed that in immune cells, but also in vascular cells, multiple inflammatory stimuli culminate in gene expression that requires cooperation of STATs with IRFs and/or NF-κB (69). They are responsible for promoting type I immune actions associated with host-defense mechanisms against viral and bacterial infections and excessive immune responses (70) at the basis of different diseases, including CVDs. This correlates with our recent data mining studies of atherosclerotic plaque transcriptomes. In this study we performed detailed promoter analysis of differentially expressed inflammatory genes in coronary and carotid plaques and predicted cooperative involvement of NF-κB, STATs, and IRFs (on ISRE, GAS, ISRE/GAS, ISRE/NF-κB, or GAS/NF-κB binding sites) (71). Combined with our findings here, this suggests strong inhibitory potential of C01L_F03, STATTIC, and STX-0119 toward vascular inflammation and vascular dysfunction.

The fact that among the 159 genes that were commonly inhibited by C01L_F03, STATTIC and STX-0119 were multiple chemokines and adhesion molecules, prompted us to investigate the effect of a multi-STAT inhibitory strategy on IFNγ+LPS dependent ECs migration and leukocyte adhesion to ECs. The endothelial scratch wound (migration) assay has been described as a simple and well-developed method to measure cell migration *in vitro* (37), which reflects vascular and immune cell migration during atherosclerosis. In addition, pathological angiogenesis of the vessel wall is a consistent feature of atherosclerotic plaque development and progression of the disease (72). Indeed, a significant decrease in IFNγ+LPS-induced "wound healing" of scratched ECs could be detected in the presence of C01L_F03, STATTIC, and STX-0119 (**Figure 9**). Interestingly a subset of C01L_F03, STATTIC and STX-0119 inhibited chemokines, including CXCL9, CXCL10, CCL7, CCL8, CCL3L3, CCL5, and CCRL2 (**Table 5**), has been reported to be increased in cells from the vasculature. Also, transcriptional regulation of a number of these genes in response to IFNγ and LPS in various cell types was shown to involve multiple STATs, IRFs and or NF-κB (10, 71). This coincides with our results here, but also with our recently published data, in which elevated expression of the chemokines CXCL9 and CXCL10 mirrored pSTAT1 levels in VSMCs and ECs of human atherosclerotic plaques (10). Moreover, it was proved that chemokines cooperate in leukocyte recruitment to the injured artery during vascular remodeling (73–75) and as such are involved in the pathogenesis of atherosclerosis. Our observation that C01L_F03, STATTIC, and STX-0119 were also able to significantly inhibit IFNγ-and LPS-dependent expression of VCAM1 and ICAM1 (**Figures 7**, **8**, **Table 5**, **Table S1**) as well as dramatically reduce adhesion of leukocytes to ECs under dynamic flow conditions (**Figure 10**), is in line with a prominent role for both adhesion molecules in these phenomena (59). Moreover, the transcriptional regulation of both ICAM1 and VCAM1 has shown to depend on several transcription factors, including multiple STATs, IRFs, and NF-κB (59, 62, 76). This could provide an explanation for the potent inhibitory effect of C01L_F03, STATTIC, and STX-0119 on IFNγ+LPS-induced adhesion of leukocytes to ECs, however we cannot exclude the possibility that other adhesion molecules may also be involved.

Finally, a multi-STAT inhibitory strategy was tested for the potential to inhibit IFNγ+LPS induced impairment of mesenteric artery contractility (**Figure 11**). Previously, we observed that the signal integration between IFNγ and LPS in mesenteric artery segments resulted in impaired contractility (**Figure 11A**). This finding overlapped with a dramatic increase in VSMC-specific expression of Nos2 (10), which is associated with progression of atherosclerosis by participating in vascular dysfunction (77, 78). Now we prove for the first time that C01L_F03, STATTIC, and STX-0119 are able to protect against IFNγ and LPS induced impairment of mesenteric artery contractility, likely by inhibiting Nos2 expression. The transcriptional regulation of Nos2 in response to IFNγ and LPS also has shown to depend on several transcription factors, including STATs, IRFs, and NF-κB (61, 79).

STATTIC as well as STX-0119 have shown to increase the apoptotic rate of a variety of cancer cell lines *in vitro* and in tumors *in vivo*, in a STAT3-dependent manner. In our studies, STATTIC and STX-0119, but also C01L_F03 exhibited cytotoxic effects at the highest used concentrations. It is possible that this cell death is mediated by inhibiting the anti-apoptotic effects of STAT3. However, at lower concentrations at which all three inhibitors potently inhibited STAT-dependent pro-inflammatory and pro-atherogenic gene expression, this cell death was not visible. Surprisingly, in the mesenteric artery contractility experiments STATTIC and STX-0119 could only be used in the nM range, without causing IFNγ+LPS-independent impairment of vessel function and integrity. This is a thousand fold less as in the wound healing and adhesion assay and could point to a greater sensitivity of STATTIC and STX-0119 *in vivo* as compared to *in vitro*.

In agreement with literature, targeting the STAT3 pathway is an upcoming therapeutic approach in the treatment of a rising number of inflammatory or proliferative diseases, like myelofibrosis, myeloproliferative disorders, rheumatoid arthritis and colitis ulcerosa also has a modulating effect on vascular cell function. Several FDA-approved indirect STAT3 inhibitors (Ruxolitinib: JAK1/2-inhibition; Tocilizumab: IL-6 receptor antibody; Tofacitinib: pan-JAK inhibition) as well as currently tested known drugs in clinical trials for CVDs treatment (Sirukumab: IL-6 binding antibody; Baricitinib: JAK1/JAK2 inhibitor), predict the use of STAT3-inhibiting clinical strategies in the near future (80). Recently, Johnson et al. for the first time showed that STATTIC and S3I-201 protect against AngII-induced oxidative stress, endothelial dysfunction, and hypertension in mice (81). Because AngII promotes vascular disease in the presence of multiple cardiovascular risk factors, the authors suggested that selective targeting of STAT3 might have substantial therapeutic potential. However, as S3I-201 and STATTIC are not STAT3-specific (16), an additional role of other STATs like STAT1 cannot be ruled out (82–85).

A large number of independent studies confirm the potency of STATTIC as a direct STAT3 inhibitor and support its utility in combating tumor cells. These studies demonstrate the potent anticancer activities of STATTIC, including activity against glioma cell migration on three-dimensional nanofiber scaffolds (86), colon cancer-initiating cells (87), and against outgrowth of breast cancer cells in an *ex vivo* model (88), and extend to *in vivo* activity of STATTIC in a mouse xenograft model for head and neck squamous cell carcinoma (89). Likewise, STX-0119 also demonstrated potent antitumor effects *in vivo* in SCC3-bearing nude mice in a STAT3-dependent manner (14). With their ability to function as multi-STAT inhibitors, like C01L_F03, they could additionally act as potent inhibitors of vascular inflammation in atherosclerosis.

In conclusion, our STAT-inhibitory studies of C01L_F03, STATTIC and STX-0119 and our previous revelation of STAT cross-binding of a pre-selection of known STAT3 inhibitors in combination with the literature, collectively provide evidence for a novel class of multi-STAT inhibitory compounds that target cooperative involvement of multiple STATs with NF-κB and/or IRFs (on ISRE, GAS, ISRE/GAS, ISRE/NF-κB, or GAS/NF-κB binding sites) in the regulation of crucial pro-inflammatory and pro-atherogenic target genes (7). Based on this we propose their potential as a potent clinical application in CVDs apart from their established role in cancer treatment and prevention. It should be noted that the primary aim of our study was to test our novel comparative *in silico* docking STAT-inhibitor selection strategy and offer support for the possibility of using a multi-STAT inhibitory approach in the context of vascular inflammation. However, our future studies will be dedicated to optimize our selection strategy and identify new STAT inhibitors with higher potency and bioavailability. Further testing and optimizing of already available non-specific STAT inhibitors like STATTIC, i.e., by chemical modification, may also be a promising avenue. In this respect it is also important to consider that STATs are essential factors to maintain normal homeostasis in many body organs and tissues. Consequently, for the treatment of single atherosclerotic lesions and to prevent systemic effects on other STATs, a local, "targeted" application with negligible systemic side effects might be a favorable scenario. Finally, it is important to emphasize that IL-10 and IL-6 produced by macrophages in the atherosclerotic plaque both regulate STAT3, yet generate different cellular responses. IL-6 is primarily a pro-inflammatory cytokine, whereas IL-10 generates a strong anti-inflammatory response. IL-6 and IL-10 each bind to their cognate receptor, leading to STAT3 phosphorylation, nuclear localization, and a cytokine-specific gene activation pattern. Thus, within the same cell type STAT3 can be pro- and anti-inflammatory (90, 91). When responding to certain stimuli such as inflammatory mediators or microbial products, macrophages have the ability to be polarized into M1 and M2 subtypes. M1 macrophages express low levels of IL-10, M2 macrophages express abundant IL-10 and can both be detected in atherosclerotic lesions. A macrophage phenotypic switch from M2 to M1 occurs with lesion progression and M1 macrophages dominate over M2 macrophages in the rupture-prone shoulder regions of the plaque, whereas M2 polarized cells are found in stable plaques (91). Current strategies of STAT3 inhibition do not consider IL-10 action. Thus, for the anti-atherosclerotic treatment with Statinibs to be most effective a treatment strategy should be considered during the stages were the M1 phenotype is dominant over the M2 phenotype, which correlates with low IL-10 levels and during which activation of STAT3 by IL-6 shifts to pro-inflammatory responses.

AUTHOR CONTRIBUTIONS

All the authors significantly contributed to research and to experimental process. Under the supervision of HB, MS performed *in silico* docking of STAT-SH2 models and MP-G performed *in vitro* STAT inhibition validation. Both were also involved in statistical analysis, microarray data analysis and manuscript preparation. JW assisted in microarray experiments and counseled during the process of data analysis. AC, PM, and MJS from the University of Valencia performed leukocyte adhesion experiments. SV, MR-G, and CP from Universidad Autónoma de Madrid performed *ex vivo* contractility studies. Both groups, from Valencia and Madrid were also involved in manuscript preparation/writing process.

ACKNOWLEDGMENTS

We would like to acknowledge David Schaller for testing the first set of compounds and performing Western blot experiments.

REFERENCES

1. Hansson GK, Hermansson A. The immune system in atherosclerosis. *Nat Immunol.* (2011) 12:204–12. doi: 10.1038/ni.2001
2. Stark GR, Darnell JE Jr. The JAK-STAT pathway at twenty. *Immunity* (2012) 36:503–14. doi: 10.1016/j.immuni.2012.03.013
3. Gough DJ, Levy DE, Johnstone RW, Clarke CJ. IFNgamma signaling-does it mean JAK-STAT? *Cytokine Growth Factor Rev.* (2008) 19:383–94. doi: 10.1016/j.cytogfr.2008.08.004
4. Sikorski K, Chmielewski S, Przybyl L, Heemann U, Wesoly J, Baumann M, et al. STAT1-mediated signal integration between IFNgamma and LPS leads to increased EC and SMC activation and monocyte adhesion. *Am J Physiol Cell Physiol.* (2011) 300:C1337–44. doi: 10.1152/ajpcell.00276.2010
5. Jones BW, Means TK, Heldwein KA, Keen MA, Hill PJ, Belisle JT, et al. Different toll-like receptor agonists induce distinct macrophage responses. *J Leukoc Biol.* (2001) 69:1036–44. doi: 10.1189/jlb.69.6.1036
6. Kawai T, Akira S. The role of pattern-recognition receptors in innate immunity: update on Toll-like receptors. *Nat Immunol.* (2010) 11:373–84. doi: 10.1038/ni.1863
7. Szelag M, Piaszyk-Borychowska A, Plens-Galaska M, Wesoly J, Bluyssen HA. Targeted inhibition of STATs and IRFs as a potential treatment strategy in cardiovascular disease. *Oncotarget* (2016) 7:48788–812. doi: 10.18632/oncotarget.9195
8. Decker T, Muller M, Stockinger S. The yin and yang of type I interferon activity in bacterial infection. *Nat Rev Immunol.* (2005) 5:675–87. doi: 10.1038/nri1684
9. O'Neill LA, Bowie AG. The family of five: TIR-domain-containing adaptors in toll-like receptor signalling. *Nat Rev Immunol.* (2007) 7:353–64. doi: 10.1038/nri2079
10. Chmielewski S, Olejnik A, Sikorski K, Pelisek J, Blaszczyk K, Aoqui C, et al. STAT1-dependent signal integration between IFNgamma and TLR4 in vascular cells reflect pro-atherogenic responses in human atherosclerosis. *PLoS ONE* (2014) 9:e113318. doi: 10.1371/journal.pone.0113318
11. Furqan M, Akinleye A, Mukhi N, Mittal V, Chen Y, Liu D. STAT inhibitors for cancer therapy. *J Hematol Oncol.* (2013) 6:90. doi: 10.1186/1756-8722-6-90
12. Miklossy G, Hilliard TS, Turkson J. Therapeutic modulators of STAT signalling for human diseases. *Nat Rev Drug Discov.* (2013) 12:611–29. doi: 10.1038/nrd4088
13. Schust J, Sperl B, Hollis A, Mayer TU, Berg T. Stattic: a small-molecule inhibitor of STAT3 activation and dimerization. *Chem Biol.* (2006) 13:1235–42. doi: 10.1016/j.chembiol.2006.09.018
14. Ashizawa T, Miyata H, Ishii H, Oshita C, Matsuno K, Masuda Y, et al. Antitumor activity of a novel small molecule STAT3 inhibitor against a human lymphoma cell line with high STAT3 activation. *Int J Oncol.* (2011) 38:1245–52. doi: 10.3892/ijo.2011.957
15. Czerwoniec A, Szelag M, Juszczak K, Wesoly J, Bluyssen HAR. CAVS—novel *in silico* selection strategy of specific STAT inhibitory compounds. *J Comput Sci.* (2015) 10:186–94. doi: 10.1016/j.jocs.2015.03.001
16. Szelag M, Czerwoniec A, Wesoly J, Bluyssen HA. Identification of STAT1 and STAT3 specific inhibitors using comparative virtual screening and docking validation. *PLoS ONE* (2015) 10:e0116688. doi: 10.1371/journal.pone.0116688
17. Pettersen EF, Goddard TD, Huang CC, Couch GS, Greenblatt DM, Meng EC, et al. UCSF Chimera–a visualization system for exploratory research and analysis. *J Comput Chem.* (2004) 25:1605–12. doi: 10.1002/jcc.20084
18. Park IH, Li C. Characterization of molecular recognition of STAT3 SH2 domain inhibitors through molecular simulation. *J Mol Recognit.* (2011) 24:254–65. doi: 10.1002/jmr.1047
19. Jain AN. Surflex: fully automatic flexible molecular docking using a molecular similarity-based search engine. *J Med Chem.* (2003) 46:499–511. doi: 10.1021/jm020406h
20. Jain AN. Surflex-Dock 2.1: robust performance from ligand energetic modeling, ring flexibility, and knowledge-based search. *J Comput Aided Mol Des.* (2007) 21:281–306. doi: 10.1007/s10822-007-9114-2
21. Irwin JJ, Shoichet BK. ZINC–a free database of commercially available compounds for virtual screening. *J Chem Inf Model.* (2005) 45:177–82. doi: 10.1021/ci049714+
22. Lipinski CA, Lombardo F, Dominy BW, Feeney PJ. Experimental and computational approaches to estimate solubility and permeability in drug discovery and development settings. *Adv Drug Deliv Rev.* (2001) 46:3–26. doi: 10.1016/S0169-409X(00)00129-0
23. Lipinski CA. Lead- and drug-like compounds: the rule-of-five revolution. *Drug Discov Today Technol.* (2004) 1:337–41. doi: 10.1016/j.ddtec.2004.11.007
24. McMurray JS. A new small-molecule Stat3 inhibitor. *Chem Biol.* (2006) 13:1123–4. doi: 10.1016/j.chembiol.2006.11.001
25. Matsuno K, Masuda Y, Uehara Y, Sato H, Muroya A, Takahashi O, et al. Identification of a new series of STAT3 inhibitors by virtual screening. *ACS Med Chem Lett.* (2010) 1:371–5. doi: 10.1021/ml1000273
26. Bonvin AM. (2007). *HADDOCK Small Molecule Binding Site Screening* [Online]. Available online at: http://www.bonvinlab.org/education/HADDOCK-binding-sites/ (Accessed January 10, 2018).
27. Sennhauser G, Amstutz P, Briand C, Storchenegger O, Grutter MG. Drug export pathway of multidrug exporter AcrB revealed by DARPin inhibitors. *PLoS Biol.* (2007) 5:e7. doi: 10.1371/journal.pbio.0050007
28. Ades EW, Candal FJ, Swerlick RA, George VG, Summers S, Bosse DC, et al. HMEC-1: establishment of an immortalized human microvascular endothelial cell line. *J Invest Dermatol.* (1992) 99:683–90.
29. Daniel B, Nagy G, Hah N, Horvath A, Czimmerer Z, Poliska S, et al. The active enhancer network operated by liganded RXR supports angiogenic activity in macrophages. *Genes Dev.* (2014) 28:1562–77. doi: 10.1101/gad.242685.114
30. Willems E, Leyns L, Vandesompele J. Standardization of real-time PCR gene expression data from independent biological replicates. *Anal Biochem.* (2008) 379:127–9. doi: 10.1016/j.ab.2008.04.036
31. Chen H, Boutros PC. VennDiagram: a package for the generation of highly-customizable Venn and Euler diagrams in R. *BMC Bioinformatics* (2011) 12:35. doi: 10.1186/1471-2105-12-35
32. Eden E, Lipson D, Yogev S, Yakhini Z. Discovering motifs in ranked lists of DNA sequences. *PLoS Comput Biol.* (2007) 3:e39. doi: 10.1371/journal.pcbi.0030039
33. Eden E, Navon R, Steinfeld I, Lipson D, Yakhini Z. GOrilla: a tool for discovery and visualization of enriched GO terms in ranked gene lists. *BMC Bioinformatics* (2009) 10:48. doi: 10.1186/1471-2105-10-48
34. Supek F, Bosnjak M, Skunca N, Smuc T. REVIGO summarizes and visualizes long lists of gene ontology terms. *PLoS ONE* (2011) 6:e21800. doi: 10.1371/journal.pone.0021800
35. Zambelli F, Pesole G, Pavesi G. Pscan: finding over-represented transcription factor binding site motifs in sequences from co-regulated or co-expressed genes. *Nucleic Acids Res.* (2009) 37(Web Server issue):W247–52. doi: 10.1093/nar/gkp464

36. Schneider CA, Rasband WS, Eliceiri KW. NIH Image to ImageJ: 25 years of image analysis. *Nat. Methods* (2012) 9:671–5. doi: 10.1038/nmeth.2089
37. Liang CC, Park AY, Guan JL. *In vitro* scratch assay: a convenient and inexpensive method for analysis of cell migration *in vitro*. *Nat Protoc.* (2007) 2:329–33. doi: 10.1038/nprot.2007.30
38. Rius C, Piqueras L, Gonzalez-Navarro H, Albertos F, Company C, Lopez-Gines C, et al. Arterial and venous endothelia display differential functional fractalkine (CX3CL1) expression by angiotensin-II. *Arterioscler Thromb Vasc Biol.* (2013) 33:96–104. doi: 10.1161/ATVBAHA.112.254870
39. Marques P, Collado A, Escudero P, Rius C, Gonzalez C, Servera E, et al. Cigarette smoke increases endothelial CXCL16-leukocyte CXCR6 adhesion *in vitro* and *in vivo*. Potential consequences in chronic obstructive pulmonary disease. *Front Immunol.* (2017) 8:1766. doi: 10.3389/fimmu.2017.01766
40. Mateo T, Naim Abu Nabah Y, Losada M, Estelles R, Company C, Bedrina B, et al. A critical role for TNFalpha in the selective attachment of mononuclear leukocytes to angiotensin-II-stimulated arterioles. *Blood* (2007) 110:1895–902. doi: 10.1182/blood-2007-01-070607
41. Rius C, Company C, Piqueras L, Cerda-Nicolas JM, Gonzalez C, Servera E, et al. Critical role of fractalkine (CX3CL1) in cigarette smoke-induced mononuclear cell adhesion to the arterial endothelium. *Thorax* (2013) 68:177–86. doi: 10.1136/thoraxjnl-2012-202212
42. Sobrino A, Vallejo S, Novella S, Lazaro-Franco M, Mompeon A, Bueno-Beti C, et al. Mas receptor is involved in the estrogen-receptor induced nitric oxide-dependent vasorelaxation. *Biochem Pharmacol.* (2017) 129:67–72. doi: 10.1016/j.bcp.2017.01.012
43. Unni S, Huang Y, Hanson RM, Tobias M, Krishnan S, Li WW, et al. Web servers and services for electrostatics calculations with APBS and PDB2PQR. *J Comput Chem.* (2011) 32:1488–91. doi: 10.1002/jcc.21720
44. Lin J, Buettner R, Yuan YC, Yip R, Horne D, Jove R, et al. Molecular dynamics simulations of the conformational changes in signal transducers and activators of transcription, Stat1 and Stat3. *J Mol Graph Model.* (2009) 28:347–56. doi: 10.1016/j.jmgm.2009.08.013
45. McBride KM, Banninger G, McDonald C, Reich NC. Regulated nuclear import of the STAT1 transcription factor by direct binding of importin-alpha. *EMBO J.* (2002) 21:1754–63. doi: 10.1093/emboj/21.7.1754
46. Gupta S, Yan H, Wong LH, Ralph S, Krolewski J, Schindler C. The SH2 domains of Stat1 and Stat2 mediate multiple interactions in the transduction of IFN-alpha signals. *EMBO J.* (1996) 15:1075–84.
47. Kretzschmar AK, Dinger MC, Henze C, Brocke-Heidrich K, Horn F. Analysis of Stat3 (signal transducer and activator of transcription 3) dimerization by fluorescence resonance energy transfer in living cells. *Biochem J.* (2004) 377(Pt 2):289–97. doi: 10.1042/BJ20030708
48. Devaux P, Priniski L, Cattaneo R. The measles virus phosphoprotein interacts with the linker domain of STAT1. *Virology* (2013) 444:250–6. doi: 10.1016/j.virol.2013.06.019
49. Grote K, Luchtefeld M, Schieffer B. JANUS under stress–role of JAK/STAT signaling pathway in vascular diseases. *Vascul Pharmacol.* (2005) 43:357–63. doi: 10.1016/j.vph.2005.08.021
50. Sun H, Wang Y. Interferon regulatory factors in heart: stress response beyond inflammation. *Hypertension* (2014) 63:663–4. doi: 10.1161/HYPERTENSIONAHA.113.02795
51. Furtek SL, Matheson CJ, Backos DS, Reigan P. Evaluation of quantitative assays for the identification of direct signal transducer and activator of transcription 3 (STAT3) inhibitors. *Oncotarget* (2016) 7:77998–8008. doi: 10.18632/oncotarget.12868
52. Arpin CC, Mac S, Jiang Y, Cheng H, Grimard M, Page BD, et al. Applying small molecule Signal Transducer and Activator of Transcription-3 (STAT3) protein inhibitors as pancreatic cancer therapeutics. *Mol Cancer Ther.* (2016) 15:794–805. doi: 10.1158/1535-7163.MCT-15-0003
53. Bill MA, Nicholas C, Mace TA, Etter JP, Li C, Schwartz EB, et al. Structurally modified curcumin analogs inhibit STAT3 phosphorylation and promote apoptosis of human renal cell carcinoma and melanoma cell lines. *PLoS ONE* (2012) 7:e40724. doi: 10.1371/journal.pone.0040724
54. Shin DS, Kim HN, Shin KD, Yoon YJ, Kim SJ, Han DC, et al. Cryptotanshinone inhibits constitutive signal transducer and activator of transcription 3 function through blocking the dimerization in DU145 prostate cancer cells. *Cancer Res.* (2009) 69:193–202. doi: 10.1158/0008-5472.CAN-08-2575
55. Capiralla H, Vingtdeux V, Zhao H, Sankowski R, Al-Abed Y, Davies P, et al. Resveratrol mitigates lipopolysaccharide- and Abeta-mediated microglial inflammation by inhibiting the TLR4/NF-kappaB/STAT signaling cascade. *J Neurochem.* (2012) 120:461–72. doi: 10.1111/j.1471-4159.2011.07594.x
56. Sanseverino I, Purificato C, Gauzzi MC, Gessani S. Revisiting the specificity of small molecule inhibitors: the example of stattic in dendritic cells. *Chem Biol.* (2012) 19:1213–4; author reply 1215–1216. doi: 10.1016/j.chembiol.2012.08.021
57. Debnath B, Xu S, Neamati N. Small molecule inhibitors of signal transducer and activator of transcription 3 (Stat3) protein. *J Med Chem.* (2012) 55:6645–68. doi: 10.1021/jm300207s
58. Bill MA, Fuchs JR, Li C, Yui J, Bakan C, Benson DM Jr, et al. The small molecule curcumin analog FLLL32 induces apoptosis in melanoma cells via STAT3 inhibition and retains the cellular response to cytokines with anti-tumor activity. *Mol Cancer* (2010) 9:165. doi: 10.1186/1476-4598-9-165
59. Dutzmann J, Daniel JM, Bauersachs J, Hilfiker-Kleiner D, Sedding DG. Emerging translational approaches to target STAT3 signalling and its impact on vascular disease. *Cardiovasc Res.* (2015) 106:365–74. doi: 10.1093/cvr/cvv103
60. Voraberger G, Schafer R, Stratowa C. Cloning of the human gene for intercellular adhesion molecule 1 and analysis of its 5'-regulatory region. Induction by cytokines and phorbol ester. *J Immunol.* (1991) 147:2777–86.
61. Lowenstein CJ, Alley EW, Raval P, Snowman AM, Snyder SH, Russell SW, et al. Macrophage nitric oxide synthase gene: two upstream regions mediate induction by interferon gamma and lipopolysaccharide. *Proc Natl Acad Sci USA.* (1993) 90:9730–4.
62. Jahnke A, Johnson JP. Synergistic activation of intercellular adhesion molecule 1 (ICAM-1) by TNF-alpha and IFN-gamma is mediated by p65/p50 and p65/c-Rel and interferon-responsive factor Stat1 alpha (p91) that can be activated by both IFN-gamma and IFN-alpha. *FEBS Lett.* (1994) 354:220–6.
63. Ohmori Y, Hamilton TA. The interferon-stimulated response element and a kappa B site mediate synergistic induction of murine IP-10 gene transcription by IFN-gamma and TNF-alpha. *J Immunol.* (1995) 154:5235–44.
64. Ohmori Y, Schreiber RD, Hamilton TA. Synergy between interferon-gamma and tumor necrosis factor-alpha in transcriptional activation is mediated by cooperation between signal transducer and activator of transcription 1 and nuclear factor kappaB. *J Biol Chem.* (1997) 272:14899–907.
65. Pine R. Convergence of TNFalpha and IFNgamma signalling pathways through synergistic induction of IRF-1/ISGF-2 is mediated by a composite GAS/kappaB promoter element. *Nucleic Acids Res.* (1997) 25:4346–54.
66. Ohmori Y, Hamilton TA. Requirement for STAT1 in LPS-induced gene expression in macrophages. *J Leukoc Biol.* (2001) 69:598–604. doi: 10.1189/jlb.69.4.598
67. Naschberger E, Werner T, Vicente AB, Guenzi E, Topolt K, Leubert R, et al. Nuclear factor-kappaB motif and interferon-alpha-stimulated response element co-operate in the activation of guanylate-binding protein-1 expression by inflammatory cytokines in endothelial cells. *Biochem J.* (2004) 379(Pt 2):409–20. doi: 10.1042/BJ20031873
68. Wienerroither S, Shukla P, Farlik M, Majoros A, Stych B, Vogl C, et al. Cooperative transcriptional activation of antimicrobial genes by STAT and NF-kappaB pathways by concerted recruitment of the mediator complex. *Cell Rep.* (2015) 12:300–12. doi: 10.1016/j.celrep.2015.06.021
69. Sikorski K, Chmielewski S, Olejnik A, Wesoly JZ, Heemann U, Baumann M, et al. STAT1 as a central mediator of IFNgamma and TLR4 signal integration in vascular dysfunction. *JAKSTAT* (2012) 1:241–9. doi: 10.4161/jkst.22469
70. O'Shea JJ, Ma A, Lipsky P. Cytokines and autoimmunity. *Nat Rev Immunol.* (2002) 2:37–45. doi: 10.1038/nri702
71. Sikorski K, Wesoly J, Bluyssen HA. Data mining of atherosclerotic plaque transcriptomes predicts STAT1-dependent inflammatory signal integration in vascular disease. *Int J Mol Sci.* (2014) 15:14313–31. doi: 10.3390/ijms150814313
72. Van Hinsbergh VW, Tasev D. Platelets and thromboxane receptors: pivotal players in arteriogenesis. *Cardiovasc Res.* (2015) 107:400–2. doi: 10.1093/cvr/cvv194
73. Schindler C, Levy DE, Decker T. JAK-STAT signaling: from interferons to cytokines. *J Biol Chem.* (2007) 282:20059–63. doi: 10.1074/jbc.R700016200

74. Wesoly J, Szweykowska-Kulinska Z, Bluyssen HA. STAT activation and differential complex formation dictate selectivity of interferon responses. *Acta Biochim Pol.* (2007) 54:27–38.
75. Lopez-Pelaez M, Lamont DJ, Peggie M, Shpiro N, Gray NS, Cohen P. Protein kinase IKKbeta-catalyzed phosphorylation of IRF5 at Ser462 induces its dimerization and nuclear translocation in myeloid cells. *Proc Natl Acad Sci USA.* (2014) 111:17432–7. doi: 10.1073/pnas.1418399111
76. Caldenhoven E, Coffer P, Yuan J, Van de Stolpe A, Horn F, Kruijer W, et al. Stimulation of the human intercellular adhesion molecule-1 promoter by interleukin-6 and interferon-gamma involves binding of distinct factors to a palindromic response element. *J Biol Chem.* (1994) 269:21146–54.
77. Kuhlencordt PJ, Chen J, Han F, Astern J, Huang PL. Genetic deficiency of inducible nitric oxide synthase reduces atherosclerosis and lowers plasma lipid peroxides in apolipoprotein E-knockout mice. *Circulation* (2001) 103:3099–104. doi: 10.1161/circ.103.25.3099
78. Niu XL, Yang X, Hoshiai K, Tanaka K, Sawamura S, Koga Y, et al. Inducible nitric oxide synthase deficiency does not affect the susceptibility of mice to atherosclerosis but increases collagen content in lesions. *Circulation* (2001) 103:1115–20. doi: 10.1161/circ.103.8.1115
79. Farlik M, Reutterer B, Schindler C, Greten F, Vogl C, Muller M, et al. Nonconventional initiation complex assembly by STAT and NF-kappaB transcription factors regulates nitric oxide synthase expression. *Immunity* (2010) 33:25–34. doi: 10.1016/j.immuni.2010.07.001
80. Darnell JEJr, Kerr IM, Stark GR. Jak-STAT pathways and transcriptional activation in response to IFNs and other extracellular signaling proteins. *Science* (1994) 264:1415–21.
81. Johnson AW, Kinzenbaw DA, Modrick ML, Faraci FM. Small-molecule inhibitors of signal transducer and activator of transcription 3 protect against angiotensin II-induced vascular dysfunction and hypertension. *Hypertension* (2013) 61:437–42. doi: 10.1161/HYPERTENSIONAHA.111.00299
82. Horiuchi M, Cui TX, Li Z, Li JM, Nakagami H, Iwai M. Fluvastatin enhances the inhibitory effects of a selective angiotensin II type 1 receptor blocker, valsartan, on vascular neointimal formation. *Circulation* (2003) 107:106–12. doi: 10.1161/01.CIR.0000043244.13596.20
83. Banes-Berceli AK, Ketsawatsomkron P, Ogbi S, Patel B, Pollock DM, Marrero MB. Angiotensin II and endothelin-1 augment the vascular complications of diabetes via JAK2 activation. *Am J Physiol Heart Circ Physiol.* (2007) 293:H1291–9. doi: 10.1152/ajpheart.00181.2007
84. Wincewicz A, Sulkowska M, Rutkowski R, Sulkowski S, Musiatowicz B, Hirnle T, et al. STAT1 and STAT3 as intracellular regulators of vascular remodeling. *Eur J Int Med.* (2007) 18:267–71. doi: 10.1016/j.ejim.2006.12.007
85. Jiao S, Zheng X, Yang X, Zhang J, Wang L. Losartan inhibits STAT1 activation and protects human glomerular mesangial cells from angiotensin II induced premature senescence. *Can J Physiol Pharmacol.* (2012) 90:89–98. doi: 10.1139/y11-105
86. Agudelo-Garcia PA, De Jesus JK, Williams SP, Nowicki MO, Chiocca EA, Liyanarachchi S, et al. Glioma cell migration on three-dimensional nanofiber scaffolds is regulated by substrate topography and abolished by inhibition of STAT3 signaling. *Neoplasia* (2011) 13:831–40. doi: 10.1593/neo.11612
87. Lin L, Liu A, Peng Z, Lin HJ, Li PK, Li C, et al. STAT3 is necessary for proliferation and survival in colon cancer-initiating cells. *Cancer Res.* (2011) 71:7226–37. doi: 10.1158/0008-5472.CAN-10-4660
88. Katz E, Sims AH, Sproul D, Caldwell H, Dixon MJ, Meehan RR, et al. Targeting of Rac GTPases blocks the spread of intact human breast cancer. *Oncotarget* (2012) 3:608–19. doi: 10.18632/oncotarget.520
89. Adachi M, Cui C, Dodge CT, Bhayani MK, Lai SY. Targeting STAT3 inhibits growth and enhances radiosensitivity in head and neck squamous cell carcinoma. *Oral Oncol.* (2012) 48:1220–6. doi: 10.1016/j.oraloncology.2012.06.00
90. Braun DA, Fribourg M, Sealfon SC. Cytokine response is determined by duration of receptor and signal transducers and activators of transcription 3 (STAT3) activation. *J Biol Chem.* (2013) 288:2986–93. doi: 10.1074/jbc.M112.386573
91. Han X, Boisvert WA. Interleukin-10 protects against atherosclerosis by modulating multiple atherogenic macrophage function. *Thromb Haemost.* (2015) 113:505–12. doi: 10.1160/TH14-06-0509

14

Recent Developments on the Crosstalk Between STAT3 and Inflammation in Heart Function and Disease

Mazen Kurdi[1]*, Carlos Zgheib[2] and George W. Booz[3]

[1] Faculty of Sciences, Department of Chemistry and Biochemistry, and The Laboratory of Experimental and Clinical Pharmacology, Lebanese University, Beirut, Lebanon, [2] Laboratory for Fetal and Regenerative Biology, Department of Surgery, School of Medicine, University of Colorado Denver, Anschutz Medical Campus and Colorado Children's Hospital, Aurora, CO, United States, [3] Department of Pharmacology and Toxicology, University of Mississippi Medical Center, Jackson, MS, United States

***Correspondence:**
Mazen Kurdi
mkurdi@ul.edu.lb

The transcription factor STAT3 has a protective function in the heart. Until recently, the role of STAT3 in hypertension-induced cardiac hypertrophy was unsettled. Earlier studies revealed that global reduction of STAT3 activity reduced cardiac hypertrophy with hypertension, but caused a disruption of myofilaments and increased contractile dysfunction. However, newer studies with cardiomyocyte-specific deletion of STAT3 indicate that STAT3 does not cause cardiac hypertrophy with increased blood pressure. Rather, cardiac STAT3 is important for maintaining metabolic homeostasis, and loss of STAT3 in cardiomyocytes makes the heart more susceptible to chronic pathological insult, for example by disrupting glucose metabolism and protective signaling networks via the upregulation of certain microRNAs. This scenario has implications for understanding peripartum cardiomyopathy as well. In viral myocarditis, STAT3 opposes the initiation of the dilated phenotype by maintaining membrane integrity via the expression of dystrophin. STAT3 signaling was also found to attenuate myocarditis by polarizing macrophages to a less inflammatory phenotype. On the other hand, STAT3 contributes to immune-mediated myocarditis due to IL-6-induced complement component C3 production in the liver, as well as the differentiation of Th17 cells, which play a role in initiation and development of myocarditis. Besides canonical signaling pathways, unphosphorylated STAT3 (U-STAT3) and redox-activated STAT3 have been shown to couple to transcription in the heart. In addition, tissue signaling cytokines such as IL-22 and IL-17 have been proposed to have actions on the heart that involve STAT3, but are not fully defined. Understanding the novel and often protective aspects of STAT3 in the myocardium could lead to new therapeutic approaches to treat heart disease.

Keywords: cardiac remodeling, myocarditis, heart failure, peripartum cardiomyopathy, cytokines, immunity

INTRODUCTION

The transcription factor signal transducer and activator of transcription 3 (STAT3) continues to excite much interest in heart research. A PubMed search on August 7, 2018 using the terms "STAT3 and (cardiac or heart)" shows a steady increase in the number of publications over time (**Figure 1**). The total number was more than 4.4 times that of STAT1 and 6.3 times that of STAT5. Activation of STAT3 in the heart has been linked to cardiac protective mechanisms that constitute the various forms of pre-and post-conditioning to protect against ischemia-reperfusion injury (1). Much of the protective actions of STAT3 are attributable to the induction of anti-inflammatory and survival genes. Besides that, STAT3 has been demonstrated to have direct protective effects in mitochondria, which were first demonstrated in cardiomyocytes (2). The reader is directed to several recent reviews that tackle these aspects of STAT3 signaling in the heart, as well as covering the topic of its posttranslational modifications (1–3). In the present review, we focus on recent developments addressing the importance of STAT3 in cardiac hypertrophy, myocardial infarction (MI), heart failure, and peripartum cardiomyopathy, with particular focus on the contribution of immunity and inflammation. Related to this, we provide an update on novel aspects of nuclear STAT3 signaling, namely its redox activation and unphosphorylated (U-STAT3) signaling, as well as the role of STAT3 in the actions of IL-22 and IL-17 on the heart.

CARDIAC HYPERTROPHY AND HEART FAILURE

In response to increased blood pressure, the heart undergoes cardiac hypertrophy, which is an independent risk factor for morbidity and mortality. While initially beneficial by normalizing wall stress, this hypertrophy may progress to heart failure through unidentified means (4). Although early studies showed that transgenic overexpression of STAT3 in mouse hearts induced pathological cardiac hypertrophy (5), the role of this transcription factor in hypertension-induced cardiac remodeling is still unsettled.

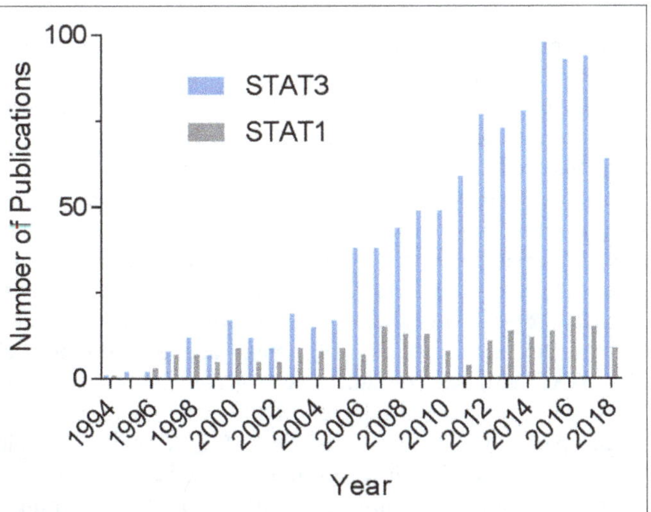

FIGURE 1 | Historical record of STAT3-related publications in the heart. The PubMed databased was searched on August 7, 2018 using the terms "STAT3 and (cardiac or heart)" or, for comparison, "STAT1 and (cardiac or heart)."

The original suspicion that STAT3 was positively linked to cardiac hypertrophy arose from observations that several members of the IL-6 family of cytokines induced growth of isolated neonatal rat ventricular myocytes. Yet, conflicting findings were reported on consequence of IL-6 deletion on left ventricular hypertrophy and dysfunction resulting from transverse aortic constriction (TAC) (6, 7). Moreover, our lab observed that chronic treatment of mice with the IL-6 family cytokine, leukemia inhibitory factor (LIF) did not induce cardiac hypertrophy (8). More recently, deletion of IL-6 was reported to inhibit cardiac inflammation, fibrosis, and dysfunction in an angiotensin II (AngII) and high salt-induced model of hypertension, without affecting cardiac hypertrophy (9). On the other hand, cardiac-specific overexpression of the STAT3 gene was found to induce hypertrophy of the heart, as well as protection against doxorubicin-induced cardiomyopathy (5).

Recent gene deletion studies suggest that STAT3 at endogenous levels does not couple to cardiac hypertrophy. Zhang et al. found that cardiomyocyte-restricted STAT3 knockout (KO) mice exhibited marked cardiomyocyte hypertrophy, as well as cell death and associated cardiac fibrosis, in response to chronic β-adrenergic stimulation with isoproterenol (10). The progression of cardiac hypertrophy to heart failure was attributed to an increase in T-type Ca^{2+} channels with subsequent engagement of the hypertrophic transcription factor NFAT (nuclear factor of activated T-cells), as well as the loss of the pro-survival factor Bcl-xl. Acute stimulation was associated with reduced cardiac contractility due to the downregulation of β1-adrenergic receptors, protein kinase A, and several other downstream effectors (**Figure 2**).

Comparable findings were reported in an AngII-induced model of hypertension (11). In this study, cardiac STAT3 KO mice showed reduced contractile function, but similar hypertrophy as control mice. Moreover, STAT3 deficiency promoted a shift toward increased glucose utilization with cardiac hypertrophy. The results of both of these studies support the idea that STAT3 serves to maintain normal cardiac function in the heart, rather than promoting pathological cardiac growth (**Figure 2**). However, an earlier study that infused AngII into mice with a global S727A mutation that impedes STAT3 activation showed reduced cardiac hypertrophy and increased reparative patches of fibrosis in the heart (12). The most straightforward explanation for these results is a contribution of non-cardiomyocyte STAT3 to the myocardium under stress conditions.

For a number of reasons the findings arguing against a role for STAT3 in cardiac hypertrophy that are based on its targeted KO in cardiomyocytes may not be definitive, and intriguing reports persists suggesting that STAT3 does play a more active role depending upon the circumstances. Granted

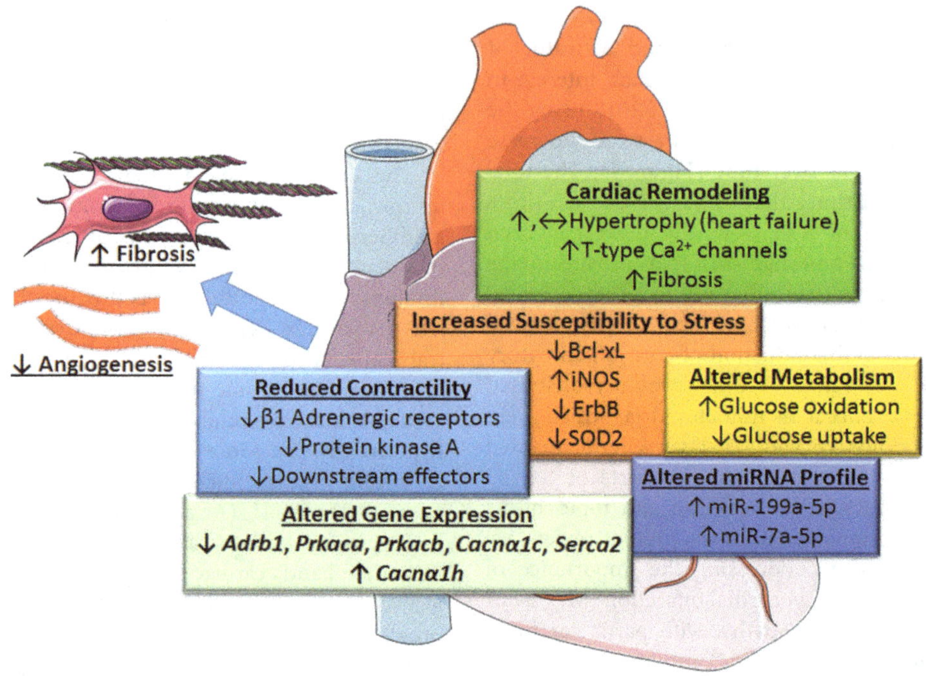

FIGURE 2 | Role of STAT3 in protecting the heart from increased blood pressure revealed by cardiac myocyte-targeted STAT3 deletion. Loss of cardiac STAT3 was found to reduce contractility from β1-adrenergic stimulation and increase susceptibility of the heart to stress by altering gene expression. Under basal conditions, the following genes are downregulated in cardiomyocyte-targeted hearts (↓): β1 adrenergic receptor (*Adrb1*), protein kinase A (PKA) catalytic subunit α and β (*Prkaca* and *Prkacb*), L-type calcium channel subunit (*Cacnα1c*), and Serca2; whereas, α-subunit of voltage-gated T-type Ca^{2+} channel (*Cacnα1h*) is upregulated (↑). Enhanced levels of certain microRNAs (miRNA-199a-5p and miRNA-7a-5p) induced oxidative stress due to altered glucose metabolism under stress conditions and diminished protective neuregulin-ErbB signaling. Overall, loss of cardiac myocyte STAT3 has a neutral or positive effect (possibly through an increase in T-type Ca^{2+} channels and NFAT activation) on cardiac hypertrophy and associated fibrosis. Evidence suggests, however, that STAT3-deficient cardiac myocytes produce unidentified paracrine factors that attenuate capillary formation and promote fibrosis with aging. Images adapted from Servier Medical Art (https://smart.servier.com/).

many of these studies are also less than definitive as they base their conclusions on an association of STAT3 activity levels with cardiac hypertrophy and/or use a pharmacological inhibitor. Nonetheless, the choice of experimental model may be a determining factor in whether STAT3 contributes to hypertrophy. STAT3 was recently implicated in the mouse heart in ischemia-induced cardiac hypertrophy downstream of heat-shock transcription factor 1 (13). In a mouse model of abdominal aortic constriction, which results in a more gradual increase in pressure overload to the heart and perhaps better mimics the effect of hypertension on the human heart, cardiac hypertrophy was dependent upon poly(ADP-ribose) polymerase 1 (PARP1), in part through its physical interaction with STAT3 and the resultant nuclear accumulation of phosphorylated STAT3 (14). Others have recently reported that endogenous activation of the oxoglutarate receptor 1 (OXGR1) during pressure overload from TAC attenuated cardiac hypertrophy in the mouse by suppressing STAT3 activity (15). OXGR1 is a G protein-coupled receptor that is activated by α-ketoglutaric acid and leukotriene E4. In addition, STAT3 in other cell types besides cardiomyocytes may be important for cardiac hypertrophy. STAT3 in cardiac fibroblasts was linked to the production of paracrine hypertrophic factors, such as ACE and IL-6 (16). Finally, cardiomyocyte targeted STAT3 KO was associated with slowly evolving reduced capillary density after birth (17), indicating other factors may contribute to the phenotype of this model. In this regard, a targeted and inducible knockout model may be more desirable to assess the role of STAT3 in hypertension.

It cannot be discounted that while STAT3 may be pro-hypertrophic it normally inhibits another signaling pathway in cardiac myocytes that couples to hypertrophic growth. Thus, loss of STAT3 and its input into cardiac hypertrophy would be compensated for by activation of this pathway. In this context, the role of STAT3 in regulating mitochondrial function and reactive oxygen species (ROS) formation may be a consideration. In fact, mitochondrial dysfunction is linked to cardiac hypertrophy and heart failure through ROS generation (18). In cardiac myocytes, STAT3 protects mitochondria indirectly via transcriptional means, such as upregulation of the anti-apoptotic protein Bcl2 (19). STAT3 also helps modulate electron complex formation and ROS production via its interaction with the structural subunit of complex 1 GRIM19 or NDUFA13 (20). STAT3 also helps preserve mitochondrial integrity and limit ROS generation via its interaction with cyclophilin D and inhibition of the opening of the mitochondrial permeability transition pore, mPTP (21, 22). Further discussion of the pathophysiological aspects of these extra-genomic actions of STAT3 can be found elsewhere (1, 2).

There is reason to think that endogenous STAT3 may attenuate cardiac hypertrophy in certain cases. An early study showed that IL-10 inhibited isoproterenol- and TAC-induced cardiac hypertrophy (23). Evidence suggested that this was due to inhibition of NF-κB (nuclear factor kappa-light-chain-enhancer of activated B cells) activation, and possibly that of p38, through interaction with STAT3. The observation that left ventricular dysfunction, remodeling (fibrosis and hypertrophy), and fetal gene expression were greater in IL-10 KO mice, supports the physiological relevance of this signaling pathway. A recent study provides evidence for natural killer T (NKT) cells as the source of IL-10 in AngII-induced cardiac remodeling in the mouse (24).

Overall, the findings summarized here indicate that cardiac myocyte-specific STAT3 may not be responsible for hypertrophic growth of the heart in response to a rapid increase in blood pressure. Rather, STAT3 is important for maintaining contractile function and metabolic homeostasis with hypertension. Indeed, endogenous cardiac myocyte STAT3 may attenuate hypertrophy under certain conditions and, in cardiac myofibroblasts, STAT3 likely contributes to extracellular matrix remodeling.

CARDIAC FIBROSIS

Besides an increase in the size of individual cardiomyocytes, pathological cardiac remodeling involves increased fibrosis, which is characterized either as reactive or as reparative when replacement of dead myocardium occurs. Multiple lines of evidence indicate that STAT3 is an important contributor to collagen synthesis and cardiac fibrosis (25, 26). New aspects of which are still being discovered and are cited here. With cardiomyocyte-targeted STAT3 deletion, hyper-activated STAT3 was noted in vascular and interstitial myofibroblasts of mouse hearts with chronic β-adrenergic stimulation (10). Relaxin was found to inhibit TGF-β1-induced cardiac fibrosis by blocking STAT3-dependent autophagy in cardiac fibroblasts (27). AngII stimulated STAT3 activation in atrial fibroblasts through an indirect paracrine effect, which was linked to atrial collagen synthesis and fibrosis in the rat (28). In addition, evidence was recently reported that the cell surface transmembrane ligand EphrinB2 in cardiac fibroblasts has pro-fibrotic actions via its synergistic activation of STAT3 and Smad3, and their subsequent association (29).

A complicated interaction involving STAT3 occurs between cardiac myocytes and fibroblasts in regulating fibrosis of the heart under pathological conditions. In cardiomyocytes of mouse hearts subjected to TAC, displacement of STAT3 from the cytoskeletal protein β_{IV}-spectrin at intercalated discs, downstream of Ca^{2+}/calmodulin-dependent kinase II (CaMKII) activation, was implicated in cardiac fibrosis and loss of cardiac function, but not hypertrophy (30). CaMKII-mediated phosphorylation of β_{IV}-spectrin caused displacement of STAT3, resulting in its translocation to the nucleus and induction of profibrotic genes. In another study, cardiac fibrosis in the rat resulting from ligation of the renal artery was attributed to Hsp90-mediated orchestration of IL-6 synthesis by cardiac myocytes, along with its release in exosomal vesicles (31). The resultant biphasic activation of STAT3 in cardiac fibroblasts was implicated in enhanced collagen expression.

MYOCARDIAL INFARCTION

Cardiomyocyte STAT3 plays an essential role in regulating cardiac remodeling during the subacute phase following an MI (32), although unbridled STAT3 activation is detrimental (33). In part, this involves monocytes/macrophages, which play an essential role in healing the injured heart after MI. Notably, their recruitment to the heart post-MI was found to be facilitated by the secretion of Reg3β by cardiac myocytes in response to the gp130-family cytokine oncostatin M (OSM), and STAT3 was shown to be required for its expression (34). A positive feedback loop sustained by OSM release by infiltrating neutrophils and macrophages was found necessary for proper healing of the infarcted heart.

The initial inflammatory response following an MI is followed sequentially by its suppression and resolution. Proper wound healing is dependent upon reparative macrophages of the M2 phenotype for the repression of inflammation, removal of dead cells and debris, and orchestration of collagen deposition by cardiac fibroblasts (35). Accumulating evidence indicates that STAT3 is a key factor in determining the polarization of macrophages to the M2 phenotype (36). For example, expression of the galectin-3—osteopontin axis by a subset of IL-10-responsive M2 macrophages in the infarcted mouse heart was recently shown to be dependent upon STAT3 (37). Secreted galectin-3 and osteopontin promote the proliferation of fibroblasts and their transformation to myofibroblasts, with collagen synthesis and accumulation, while intracellular galectin-3 promotes osteopontin expression in macrophages. Both proteins also stimulate phagocytosis by macrophages. Others recently reported that in the infarcted rat heart a SGLT2 inhibitor, likely acting as an anti-oxidant, induced the polarization of macrophages to a reparative M2c phenotype that produces IL-10 downstream of enhanced STAT3 activation (38). Fibroblast activation and fibrosis was attenuated by this phenotype by the suppressor cytokine IL-10, as well as by the absence of arginase-1 (an M2a marker) induction, which contributes to collagen deposition and fibrosis.

Unlike the adult heart, the fetal mammalian heart exhibits a regenerative response to MI (39). This response depends upon early resolution of inflammation and expression of the STAT3 target gene VEGFA. The neonatal mouse heart also demonstrates regenerative capacity following the resection of the left ventricular apex. Evidence indicates that cardiac regeneration in this case is a direct transcriptional reversion of the differentiation process that is driven by the Th2 cytokine IL-13, which induces cardiomyocyte cell cycle entry in part via a STAT3-induced periostin pathway (40). This findings is reminiscent of the regenerative program that is initiated by injury in the adult heart of the zebrafish (41). In this model, STAT3 is required for cardiac myocyte proliferation due to the upregulation of the *rln3a* gene, which encodes the hormone Relaxin 3a.

PERIPARTUM REMODELING

Peripartum cardiomyopathy (PPCM) is a life-threatening condition, which may affect women in the last month of pregnancy or the first months after giving birth. Female mice with cardiac myocyte-specific STAT3 deletion develop a form of PPCM (42). This is associated with blunted superoxide dismutase 2 (SOD2) expression, a gene target of STAT3 (43). The associated increase in oxidative stress leads to increased cathepsin D expression and activity. This in turn forms a pro-apoptotic, anti-angiogenic cleaved form of the nursing hormone prolactin. The 16 kDa shortened form of prolactin leads to increased miR-146a expression in endothelial cells, which exerts angiotoxic effects and upon release in exosomes impairs metabolic activity of cardiomyocytes and reduces their expression of Erbb4, Notch1, and Irak1 (43, 44). Paradoxically, enhanced Akt activity in PPCM, downstream of prolactin or interferon-gamma (IFN-γ), further exacerbates the redox imbalance and loss of SOD2, due to activation of p66SHC and down-regulation of anti-oxidative transcription factor FoxO3A (43). In addition, activation of Akt sustains cardiac inflammation by leading to the induction of the pro-inflammatory chemokine CCL2, which among several actions serves to recruit macrophages. Serum levels of activated cathepsin D and the cleaved prolactin are elevated in PPCM patients (43) and left ventricular STAT3 protein levels are decreased in patients with end-stage heart failure due to PPCM (42).

Low STAT3 ventricular levels were also found to compromise glucose uptake and thereby sensitize the normal and peripartum heart to the toxic effects of chronic β-adrenergic signaling by contributing to a state of energy depletion and associated increased generation of ROS (45). This was accomplished in STAT3 KO hearts by the upregulation of two microRNAs: miRNA-199a-5p, which suppressed glucose transporter-4 (GLUT4) levels, and miRNA-7a-5p, which suppressed expression of the cardioprotective receptor for neuregulin, ErbB. Overall, glucose uptake and oxidation by the heart are reduced upon chronic stimulation with the β-adrenergic agonist isoproterenol. Cardiac myocytes are more reliant on glucose oxidation under these conditions, as isoproterenol depletes serum free fatty acids, and cardiac free fatty acids uptake and triglycerides. Evidence was reported that inadequate glucose uptake by cardiac myocytes from loss of STAT3 was associated with increased mitochondrial ROS formation due to insufficient NADPH generation needed to maintain adequate GSH recycling in mitochondria.

MYOCARDITIS

Myocarditis or inflammatory cardiomyopathy is most often caused by a viral infection, commonly involving coxsackievirus. Although all ages are at risk, myocarditis commonly affects the young. In most cases, myocarditis resolves spontaneously, but more than 40% of affected individuals progress from increased cardiac hypertrophy, apoptosis, and fibrosis to a dilated cardiomyopathy with reduced contractility (46). Nearly 20% of sudden death among young adults are attributable to myocarditis. Evidence indicates STAT3 couples to potent protective innate immune response in the context of myocarditis. Decreasing IL-6 family cytokine signaling in mice by either cardiac-specific suppressor of cytokine signaling 3 (SOCS3) overexpression or gp-130 knockout was found to increase susceptibility of the heart to coxsackievirus B3 (CVB3) infection, even though an intact IFN-mediated antiviral response was still present. The protective effects of gp-130 signaling was attributed to STAT3-mediated maintenance of dystrophin expression after virus expression, which is important for membrane integrity, as well as STAT3 contributing toward endogenous α-sarcoglycan levels (47). Disruption of the sarcolemmal membrane due to dystrophin cleavage was linked to CVB3-induced death of cardiac myocytes. Mice with cardiac-specific STAT3 depletion exhibited a long-term decrease in cardiac function after virus infection that was associated with cardiac fibrosis due to increased expression of collagen I and reduced matrix degradation (48).

In contrast, genetically prolonged and enhanced STAT3 activity in cardiac myocyte was associated with greater inflammation, left ventricular rupture, and worse outcome following subacute MI (33). Thus, the degree of STAT3 activation in the heart likely has an impact on outcome. In addition, this finding likely illustrates the contribution of spatiotemporal context and concurrent signaling in the outcome elicited by STAT3 activation (49).

Other cell types are involved in the pathogenesis of myocarditis as well, further complicating the role of STAT3. Evidence was reported that STAT3 contributes to immune-mediated myocarditis in mice due to enhanced hepatic and cardiac IL-6 production, as well as IL-6-induced complement component C3 production in the liver (50). STAT3 is also important for the differentiation of Th17 cells, which play a major role in the initiation and development of myocarditis (51). Recently, evidence was reported that strategies to enhance the cholinergic anti-inflammatory pathway in the heart by left stellectomy or treatment with an α7nAchR agonist alleviated viral myocarditis (52, 53). These protective actions have been attributed to activation of Jak2-STAT3 signaling in macrophages and attenuation of inflammatory effects via SOCS3 induction, blockade of NF-κB nuclear translocation via formation of an unphosphorylated STAT3-NF-κB complex, or production of tristetraprolin, an AU-rich element (ARE)-binding protein that destabilizes pro-inflammatory transcripts with AREs in the 3'-untranslated region (54). The disparate roles of STAT3 in myocarditis are summarized in **Figure 3**.

ADDITIONAL NOVEL MECHANISMS

Nuclear U-STAT3

In the heart, STAT3 uses two mechanisms, canonical and U-STAT3, to regulate the expression of two different pools of genes (1). Canonical signaling entails STAT3 parallel dimers, which form upon Y705 phosphorylation, and tightly bind GAS elements in promoters. Canonical signaling is associated with inflammation (1) and protection from acute ischemic stress by upregulation of cardioprotective and anti-apoptotic proteins, including HO-1, COX-2, Bcl-xL, Mcl-1, c-FLIPS, and c-FLIPL (55–57). Phosphorylation of S727 enhances canonical

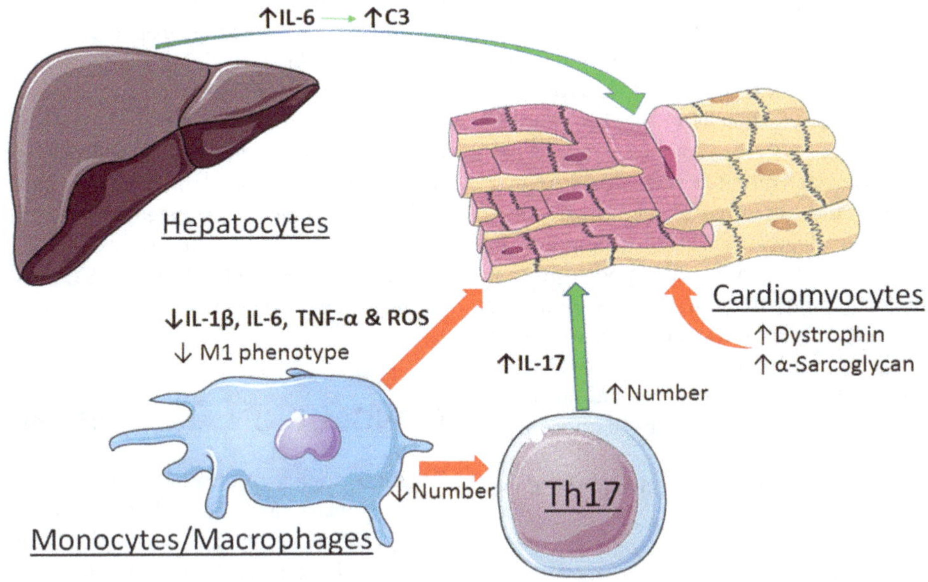

FIGURE 3 | Contrasting roles of STAT3 in viral myocarditis. Cardiac myocyte-specific STAT3 protects against the initiation and development if the dilated phenotype by maintaining expression levels of dystrophin and α-sarcoglycan. Activation of STAT3 by stimulation of the α7nAchR in macrophages alleviates myocarditis by favoring a less inflammatory phenotype. In contrast, STAT3 contributes to myocarditis due to enhanced hepatic and cardiac IL-6 production, as well as IL-6-induced complement component C3 production in the liver. STAT3 also contributes to the differentiation and expansion of Th17 cells that have a role in the development of myocarditis. See text for additional details. Images adapted from Servier Medical Art (https://smart.servier.com/).

transcription by increasing recruitment of transcriptional coactivators (2, 58), or attenuates signaling by recruitment of a tyrosine phosphatase (59, 60).

U-STAT3 signaling occurs as a consequence of canonical STAT3 signaling-induced STAT3 expression and is proposed to prolong the inflammatory response initiated by canonical signaling (61). Elevated U-STAT3 levels were found in the nuclei of AngII receptor type 1 (AT1) overexpressing mouse hearts and AngII-treated neonatal rat ventricular myocytes (62). U-STAT3 levels correlated with the degree of hypertrophy, and U-STAT3 was postulated to induce a subset of inflammatory and pro-hypertrophic genes in the heart, including osteopontin and regulator of G protein signaling 2 (62).

Some genes are activated by U-STAT3 via a complex with the unphosphorylated p65 subunit of NF-κB. Binding does not involve GAS elements, but rather a specific DNA element that supports binding of p65 homodimers and cooperativity with U-STAT3 (63). STAT3 S727 phosphorylation is not involved, at least for the interaction of U-STAT3 and p65 subunit (63). The importance of S727 phosphorylation in U-STAT3-induced gene expression is not thoroughly studied, but evidence indicates that it is not important (62, 63).

The mechanism by which U-STAT3 activates target genes not requiring NF-κB is unknown (61), but may involve binding of U-STAT3 to a GAS or GAS-like element. Recently, STAT3 K685 acetylation was found to be required for expression of most U-STAT3-dependent genes, while playing a minor role in the expression of genes by canonical STAT3 signaling (64). It was suggested that K685 acetylation is important for recruitment of p300 or may facilitate STAT3 parallel dimer formation in the absence of Y705 phosphorylation. The possibility that U-STAT3, which tends to form anti-parallel dimers, also acts as a dominant negative mutant protein is a consideration (62).

U-STAT3 also binds to AT-rich DNA sequence sites and sequences implicated in chromatin organization, as well as DNA structures involved in nucleosomal structure and assembly (65). These observations suggest that U-STAT3 may influence chromatin organization. Deletion of Drosophila STAT homolog Stat92E was reported to disrupt heterochromatin integrity and result in transcriptional activation of genes that are not its direct target (66). Stat92E also regulates histone 1 (HI) and histone 3 (H3) function by interacting with heterochromatin protein 1 (HP1) (67, 68). This epigenetic role is disrupted by Stat92E tyrosine phosphorylation and its subsequent translocation to target genes (67). Notably, STAT3 also has a conserved pentapeptide motif (PxVxI) for potential binding of HP1.

Redox Signaling

Nine of STAT3's 14 highly conserved cysteine residues are redox-sensitive and control its transcriptional activity (1). In many cases, at least *in vitro*, oxidative stress was reported to inhibit canonical STAT3 transcriptional activity. We previously reported that levels of monomeric STAT3 measured under non-reducing conditions were decreased in a redox-sensitive manner in the $G_{\alpha q}$ model of heart failure (69), although the pathophysiological relevance of this observation was not established. Recent evidence suggests that the redox-sensitivity of STAT3 may be a regulated process controlling its transcriptional actions. In response to stimulation with IL-6 or oncostatin M, STAT3 associated with the anti-oxidant and protective protein peroxiredoxin-2 in HEK293T cells (70). This resulted in the oxidation of multiple cysteine residues in STAT3's DNA binding, linker, and transactivation domains, with higher order complex formation and attenuated gene expression. In a model of enhanced endogenous H_2O_2 generation in cardiac myocytes due to a deficiency in a support protein of mitochondrial complex I, peroxiredoxin-2 expression was elevated, as was dimerized STAT3 (19). These hearts were more resistant to ischemia-reperfusion injury because of STAT3-mediated induction of protective proteins, including Bcl2. Given the importance of oxidative stress in the pathogenesis of cardiac hypertrophy and heart failure, it seems likely that STAT3 redox signaling has functional ramifications under these conditions.

Tissue-Signaling Cytokines

Recent interest has been focused on cytokines of the innate and adaptive immune systems that mostly target tissue cells, with little if any action on immune cells. Two such cytokines are of particular interest in pathological cardiac remodeling, IL-22 and IL-17. Both are produced by different types of innate/adaptive leukocytes, but exert different actions that are influenced by the tissue inflammatory milieu (71, 72). IL-22 is generally considered protective and regenerative, but can synergize with TNF-α, IFN-γ, and IL-17 under pro-inflammatory conditions. It binds to a heterodimer of the IL-10Rβ-chain and IL-22R, thereby inducing the phosphorylation of the associated tyrosine JAK kinases and activating STAT3, as well as STAT1 or STAT5 depending upon the cell type. IL-22 induces the principal MAPKs as well. Serum IL-22 levels were recently shown to be positively correlated with blood pressure, and in AngII-induced hypertensive mice, evidence was found that IL-22 contributes to systemic and local inflammation, endothelial dysfunction, and increased blood pressure (73). The STAT3 pathway was shown to mediate the effect of IL-22 on endothelial function and blood pressure. Another study showed increased IL-22 and IL-22R1 levels in the hearts of AngII-infused mice (74). Treatment with an IL-22 neutralizing antibody attenuated cardiac hypertrophy, fibrosis, and contractile dysfunction, although a reduction in blood pressure may have contributed to these actions.

IL-17 (in particular IL-17A and IL-17F) is pro-inflammatory and implicated in adverse remodeling of the heart associated with hypertension and viral myocarditis (75, 76). It was recently shown to contribute to inflammatory dilated cardiomyopathy, a major cause of heart failure in persons under 40 years of age (77). This was attributed to the stimulation of cardiac fibroblasts to produce chemokines and cytokines that recruit monocytes/macrophages and polarize them toward a pro-inflammatory phenotype. IL-17 signals through a receptor complex linked via TNF receptor associated factor 6 (TRAF6) and receptor-interacting protein kinase (RIP) to the activation of MAPKs, AP-1, and NF-κB. IL-17A was recently reported to cause apoptosis of cardiomyocytes *in vitro* by inducing expression of inducible nitric oxide synthase (iNOS); however, its simultaneous activation of STAT3 and STAT3's binding to the promoter region damped iNOS gene induction (78). The pathophysiological relevance of this inhibitory mechanism was shown *in vivo* using a mouse myocardial ischemia-reperfusion injury model, where inhibition of STAT3 caused increased iNOS expression and worsened cardiomyocyte apoptosis.

CONCLUSION AND PERSPECTIVES

Recent evidence indicates that endogenous levels of STAT3 in the heart are needed to maintain normal structure, contractile function, and metabolism under stress conditions. This conclusion has importance for hypertension, peripartum cardiac remodeling, and viral myocarditis. A growing theme is that STAT3 may also have benefit in the heart by repressing certain genes, and a better understanding of how that is accomplished is needed. The importance of STAT3 in immune cells and in crosstalk among the various cell types of the heart ought to be resolved, as well as how the various cellular subcompartments of STAT3 are integrated in controlling the genomic and non-genomic actions of STAT3 in response to stress or injury. Network analysis of STAT3 as a sentinel at intercalated discs, mitochondria, sarcoplasmic reticulum, and nuclei under stress conditions ought to be performed. In addition, novel signaling aspects of STAT3, such as U-STAT3, its redox-sensitivity, and the importance of STAT3 in chromatin organization have been described, but their implications for cardiac function and response to stress are not fully understood. Lastly, the role of STAT3 in the heart in response to tissue-specific cytokines is an area that requires further investigation. Understanding the novel and protective aspects of STAT3 in the myocardium could lead to new therapeutic approaches to treat heart disease.

AUTHOR CONTRIBUTIONS

MK, CZ, and GB helped write the manuscript and create the figures. GB edited the text.

ACKNOWLEDGMENTS

GB acknowledges the support of the Department of Pharmacology and Toxicology of the University of Mississippi Medical Center.

REFERENCES

1. Zouein FA, Altara R, Chen Q, Lesnefsky EJ, Kurdi M, Booz GW. Pivotal importance of STAT3 in protecting the heart from acute and chronic stress: new advancement and unresolved issues. *Front Cardiovasc Med.* (2015) 2:36. doi: 10.3389/fcvm.2015.00036
2. Zouein FA, Kurdi M, Booz GW. Dancing rhinos in stilettos: The amazing saga of the genomic and nongenomic actions of STAT3 in the heart. *JAKSTAT* (2013) 2:e24352. doi: 10.4161/jkst.24352
3. Kurdi M, Booz GW. JAK redux: a second look at the regulation and role of JAKs in the heart. *Am J Physiol Heart Circ Physiol.* (2009) 297:H1545–56. doi: 10.1152/ajpheart.00032.2009
4. Booz GW. Putting the brakes on cardiac hypertrophy: exploiting the NO-cGMP counter-regulatory system. *Hypertension* (2005) 45:341–6. doi: 10.1161/01.HYP.0000156878.17006.02
5. Kunisada K, Negoro S, Tone E, Funamoto M, Osugi T, Yamada S, et al. Signal transducer and activator of transcription 3 in the heart transduces not only a hypertrophic signal but a protective signal against doxorubicin-induced cardiomyopathy. *Proc Natl Acad Sci USA.* (2000) 97:315–9. doi: 10.1073/pnas.97.1.315
6. Zhao L, Cheng G, Jin R, Afzal MR, Samanta A, Xuan YT, et al. Deletion of Interleukin-6 attenuates pressure overload-induced left ventricular hypertrophy and dysfunction. *Circ Res.* (2016) 118:1918–29. doi: 10.1161/CIRCRESAHA.116.308688
7. Lai NC, Gao MH, Tang E, Tang R, Guo T, Dalton ND, et al. Pressure overload-induced cardiac remodeling and dysfunction in the absence of interleukin 6 in mice. *Lab Invest.* (2012) 92:1518–26. doi: 10.1038/labinvest.2012.97
8. Zgheib C, Zouein FA, Kurdi M, Booz GW. Chronic treatment of mice with leukemia inhibitory factor does not cause adverse cardiac remodeling but improves heart function. *Eur Cytokine Netw.* (2012) 23:191–7. doi: 10.1684/ecn.2012.0319
9. Gonzalez GE, Rhaleb NE, D'Ambrosio MA, Nakagawa P, Liu Y, Leung P, et al. Deletion of interleukin-6 prevents cardiac inflammation, fibrosis and dysfunction without affecting blood pressure in angiotensin II-high salt-induced hypertension. *J Hypertens.* (2015) 33:144–52. doi: 10.1097/HJH.0000000000000358
10. Zhang W, Qu X, Chen B, Snyder M, Wang M, Li B, et al. Critical Roles of STAT3 in beta-adrenergic functions in the heart. *Circulation* (2016) 133:48–61. doi: 10.1161/CIRCULATIONAHA.115.017472
11. Altara R, Harmancey R, Didion SP, Booz GW, Zouein FA. Cardiac STAT3 deficiency impairs contractility and metabolic homeostasis in hypertension. *Front Pharmacol.* (2016) 7:436. doi: 10.3389/fphar.2016.00436
12. Zouein FA, Zgheib C, Hamza S, Fuseler JW, Hall JE, Soljancic A, et al. Role of STAT3 in angiotensin II-induced hypertension and cardiac remodeling revealed by mice lacking STAT3 serine 727 phosphorylation. *Hypertens Res.* (2013) 36:496–503. doi: 10.1038/hr.2012.223
13. Yuan L, Qiu L, Ye Y, Wu J, Wang S, Wang X, et al. Heat-shock transcription factor 1 is critically involved in the ischaemia-induced cardiac hypertrophy via JAK2/STAT3 pathway. *J Cell Mol Med.* (2018) 22:4292–303. doi: 10.1111/jcmm.13713
14. Wang L, Li Z, Tan Y, Li Q, Yang H, Wang P, et al. PARP1 interacts with STAT3 and retains active phosphorylated-STAT3 in nucleus during pathological myocardial hypertrophy. *Mol Cell Endocrinol.* (2018) 474:137–50. doi: 10.1016/j.mce.2018.02.020
15. Omede A, Zi M, Prehar S, Maqsood A, Stafford N, Mamas M, et al. The oxoglutarate receptor 1 (OXGR1) modulates pressure overload-induced cardiac hypertrophy in mice. *Biochem Biophys Res Commun.* (2016) 479:708–14. doi: 10.1016/j.bbrc.2016.09.147
16. Ohkura SI, Usui S, Takashima SI, Takuwa N, Yoshioka K, Okamoto Y, et al. Augmented sphingosine 1 phosphate receptor-1 signaling in cardiac fibroblasts induces cardiac hypertrophy and fibrosis through angiotensin II and interleukin-6. *PLoS ONE* (2017) 12:e0182329. doi: 10.1371/journal.pone.0182329
17. Hilfiker-Kleiner D, Hilfiker A, Fuchs M, Kaminski K, Schaefer A, Schieffer B, et al. Signal transducer and activator of transcription 3 is required for myocardial capillary growth, control of interstitial matrix deposition, and heart protection from ischemic injury. *Circ Res.* (2004) 95:187–95. doi: 10.1161/01.RES.0000134921.50377.61
18. Siasos G, Tsigkou V, Kosmopoulos M, Theodosiadis D, Simantiris S, Tagkou NM, et al. Mitochondria and cardiovascular diseases-from pathophysiology to treatment. *Ann Transl Med.* (2018) 6:256. doi: 10.21037/atm.2018.06.21
19. Hu H, Nan J, Sun Y, Zhu D, Xiao C, Wang Y, et al. Electron leak from NDUFA13 within mitochondrial complex I attenuates ischemia-reperfusion injury via dimerized STAT3. *Proc Natl Acad Sci USA.* (2017) 114:11908–13. doi: 10.1073/pnas.1704723114
20. Wegrzyn J, Potla R, Chwae YJ, Sepuri NB, Zhang Q, Koeck T, et al. Function of mitochondrial Stat3 in cellular respiration. *Science* (2009) 323:793–7. doi: 10.1126/science.1164551
21. Meier JA, Hyun M, Cantwell M, Raza A, Mertens C, Raje V, et al. Stress-induced dynamic regulation of mitochondrial STAT3 and its association with cyclophilin D reduce mitochondrial ROS production. *Sci Signal.* (2017) 10:2588. doi: 10.1126/scisignal.aag2588
22. Boengler K, Hilfiker-Kleiner D, Heusch G, Schulz R. Inhibition of permeability transition pore opening by mitochondrial STAT3 and its role in myocardial ischemia/reperfusion. *Basic Res Cardiol.* (2010) 105:771–85. doi: 10.1007/s00395-010-0124-1
23. Verma SK, Krishnamurthy P, Barefield D, Singh N, Gupta R, Lambers E, et al. Interleukin-10 treatment attenuates pressure overload-induced hypertrophic remodeling and improves heart function via signal transducers and activators of transcription 3-dependent inhibition of nuclear factor-kappaB. *Circulation* (2012) 126:418–29. doi: 10.1161/CIRCULATIONAHA.112.112185
24. Wang HX, Li WJ, Hou CL, Lai S, Zhang YL, Tian C, et al. CD1d-dependent natural killer T cells attenuate angiotensin II-induced cardiac remodeling via IL-10 signaling in mice. *Cardiovasc Res.* (2018). doi: 10.1093/cvr/cvy164. [Epub ahead of print].
25. Mir SA, Chatterjee A, Mitra A, Pathak K, Mahata SK, Sarkar S. Inhibition of signal transducer and activator of transcription 3 (STAT3) attenuates interleukin-6 (IL-6)-induced collagen synthesis and resultant hypertrophy in rat heart. *J Biol Chem.* (2012) 287:2666–77. doi: 10.1074/jbc.M111.246173
26. Dai B, Cui M, Zhu M, Su WL, Qiu MC, Zhang H. STAT1/3 and ERK1/2 synergistically regulate cardiac fibrosis induced by high glucose. *Cell Physiol Biochem.* (2013) 32:960–71. doi: 10.1159/000354499
27. Yuan Y, Zhang Y, Han X, Li Y, Zhao X, Sheng L, et al. Relaxin alleviates TGFbeta1-induced cardiac fibrosis via inhibition of Stat3-dependent autophagy. *Biochem Biophys Res Commun.* (2017) 493:1601–7. doi: 10.1016/j.bbrc.2017.09.110
28. Tsai CT, Lai LP, Kuo KT, Hwang JJ, Hsieh CS, Hsu KL, et al. Angiotensin II activates signal transducer and activators of transcription 3 via Rac1 in atrial myocytes and fibroblasts: implication for the therapeutic effect of statin in atrial structural remodeling. *Circulation* (2008) 117:344–55. doi: 10.1161/CIRCULATIONAHA.107.695346
29. Su SA, Yang D, Wu Y, Xie Y, Zhu W, Cai Z, et al. EphrinB2 Regulates Cardiac Fibrosis Through Modulating the Interaction of Stat3 and TGF-beta/Smad3 Signaling. *Circ Res.* (2017) 121:617–27. doi: 10.1161/CIRCRESAHA.117.311045
30. Unudurthi SD, Nassal D, Greer-Short A, Patel N, Howard T, Xu X, et al. βIV-Spectrin regulates STAT3 targeting to tune cardiac response to pressure overload. *J Clin Invest.* (2018) 128:5561–72. doi: 10.1172/JCI99245
31. Datta R, Bansal T, Rana S, Datta K, Datta Chaudhuri R, Chawla-Sarkar M, et al. Myocyte-derived Hsp90 modulates collagen upregulation via biphasic activation of STAT-3 in fibroblasts during cardiac hypertrophy. *Mol Cell Biol.* (2017) 37:e00611-16. doi: 10.1128/MCB.00611-16
32. Enomoto D, Obana M, Miyawaki A, Maeda M, Nakayama H, Fujio Y. Cardiac-specific ablation of the STAT3 gene in the subacute phase of myocardial infarction exacerbated cardiac remodeling. *Am J Physiol Heart Circ Physiol.* (2015) 309:H471–80. doi: 10.1152/ajpheart.00730.2014
33. Hilfiker-Kleiner D, Shukla P, Klein G, Schaefer A, Stapel B, Hoch M, et al. Continuous glycoprotein-130-mediated signal transducer and activator of transcription-3 activation promotes inflammation, left ventricular rupture, and adverse outcome in subacute myocardial infarction. *Circulation* (2010) 122:145–55. doi: 10.1161/CIRCULATIONAHA.109.933127
34. Lorchner H, Poling J, Gajawada P, Hou Y, Polyakova V, Kostin S, et al. Myocardial healing requires Reg3beta-dependent accumulation of macrophages in the ischemic heart. *Nat Med.* (2015) 21:353–62. doi: 10.1038/nm.3816

35. Altara R, Manca M, Sabra R, Eid AA, Booz GW, Zouein FA. Temporal cardiac remodeling post-myocardial infarction: dynamics and prognostic implications in personalized medicine. *Heart Fail Rev.* (2016) 21:25–47. doi: 10.1007/s10741-015-9513-8
36. Ma Y, Mouton AJ, Lindsey ML. Cardiac macrophage biology in the steady-state heart, the aging heart, and following myocardial infarction. *Transl Res.* (2018) 191:15–28. doi: 10.1016/j.trsl.2017.10.001
37. Shirakawa K, Endo J, Kataoka M, Katsumata Y, Yoshida N, Yamamoto T, et al. IL (Interleukin)-10-STAT3-Galectin-3 axis is essential for osteopontin-producing reparative macrophage polarization after myocardial infarction. *Circulation* (2018) 138:2021–35. doi: 10.1161/CIRCULATIONAHA.118.035047
38. Lee TM, Chang NC, Lin SZ. Dapagliflozin, a selective SGLT2 Inhibitor, attenuated cardiac fibrosis by regulating the macrophage polarization via STAT3 signaling in infarcted rat hearts. *Free Radic Biol Med.* (2017) 104:298–310. doi: 10.1016/j.freeradbiomed.2017.01.035
39. Zgheib C, Hodges MM, Allukian MW, Xu J, Spiller KL, Gorman JH, et al. Cardiac progenitor cell recruitment drives fetal cardiac regeneration by enhanced angiogenesis. *Ann Thorac Surg.* (2017) 104:1968–75. doi: 10.1016/j.athoracsur.2017.05.040
40. O'Meara CC, Wamstad JA, Gladstone RA, Fomovsky GM, Butty VL, Shrikumar A, et al. Transcriptional reversion of cardiac myocyte fate during mammalian cardiac regeneration. *Circ Res.* (2015) 116:804–15. doi: 10.1161/CIRCRESAHA.116.304269
41. Fang Y, Gupta V, Karra R, Holdway JE, Kikuchi K, Poss KD. Translational profiling of cardiomyocytes identifies an early Jak1/Stat3 injury response required for zebrafish heart regeneration. *Proc Natl Acad Sci USA.* (2013) 110:13416–21. doi: 10.1073/pnas.1309810110
42. Hilfiker-Kleiner D, Kaminski K, Podewski E, Bonda T, Schaefer A, Sliwa K, et al. A cathepsin D-cleaved 16 kDa form of prolactin mediates postpartum cardiomyopathy. *Cell* (2007) 128:589–600. doi: 10.1016/j.cell.2006.12.036
43. Ricke-Hoch M, Bultmann I, Stapel B, Condorelli G, Rinas U, Sliwa K, et al. Opposing roles of Akt and STAT3 in the protection of the maternal heart from peripartum stress. *Cardiovasc Res.* (2014) 101:587–96. doi: 10.1093/cvr/cvu010
44. Halkein J, Tabruyn SP, Ricke-Hoch M, Haghikia A, Nguyen NQ, Scherr M, et al. MicroRNA-146a is a therapeutic target and biomarker for peripartum cardiomyopathy. *J Clin Invest.* (2013) 123:2143–54. doi: 10.1172/JCI64365
45. Stapel B, Kohlhaas M, Ricke-Hoch M, Haghikia A, Erschow S, Knuuti J, et al. Low STAT3 expression sensitizes to toxic effects of beta-adrenergic receptor stimulation in peripartum cardiomyopathy. *Eur Heart J.* (2017) 38:349–61. doi: 10.1093/eurheartj/ehw086
46. Vdovenko D, Eriksson U. Regulatory Role of CD4(+) T cells in myocarditis. *J Immunol Res.* (2018) 2018:4396351. doi: 10.1155/2018/4396351
47. Yajima T, Yasukawa H, Jeon ES, Xiong D, Dorner A, Iwatate M, et al. Innate defense mechanism against virus infection within the cardiac myocyte requiring gp130-STAT3 signaling. *Circulation* (2006) 114:2364–73. doi: 10.1161/CIRCULATIONAHA.106.642454
48. Lindner D, Hilbrandt M, Marggraf K, Becher PM, Hilfiker-Kleiner D, Klingel K, et al. Protective function of STAT3 in CVB3-induced myocarditis. *Cardiol Res Pract.* (2012) 2012:437623. doi: 10.1155/2012/437623
49. Zgheib C, Zouein FA, Kurdi M, Booz GW. Differential STAT3 signaling in the heart: Impact of concurrent signals and oxidative stress. *JAKSTAT* (2012) 1:101–10. doi: 10.4161/jkst.19776
50. Camporeale A, Marino F, Papageorgiou A, Carai P, Fornero S, Fletcher S, et al. STAT3 activity is necessary and sufficient for the development of immune-mediated myocarditis in mice and promotes progression to dilated cardiomyopathy. *EMBO Mol Med.* (2013) 5:572–90. doi: 10.1002/emmm.201201876
51. Yuan J, Yu M, Lin QW, Cao AL, Yu X, Dong JH, et al. Th17 cells contribute to viral replication in coxsackievirus B3-induced acute viral myocarditis. *J Immunol.* (2010) 185:4004–10. doi: 10.4049/jimmunol.1001718
52. Park H, Park H, Mun D, Kim M, Pak HN, Lee MH, et al. Sympathetic nerve blocks promote anti-inflammatory response by activating the JAK2-STAT3-mediated signaling cascade in rat myocarditis models: A novel mechanism with clinical implications. *Heart Rhythm* (2018) 15:770–9. doi: 10.1016/j.hrthm.2017.09.039
53. Cheng Z, Li-Sha G, Jing-Lin Z, Wen-Wu Z, Xue-Si C, Xing-Xing C, et al. Protective role of the cholinergic anti-inflammatory pathway in a mouse model of viral myocarditis. *PLoS ONE* (2014) 9:e112719. doi: 10.1371/journal.pone.0112719
54. Baez-Pagan CA, Delgado-Velez M, Lasalde-Dominicci JA. Activation of the Macrophage alpha7 Nicotinic Acetylcholine Receptor and Control of Inflammation. *J Neuroimmune Pharmacol.* (2015) 10:468–76. doi: 10.1007/s11481-015-9601-5
55. Bolli R, Stein AB, Guo Y, Wang OL, Rokosh G, Dawn B, et al. A murine model of inducible, cardiac-specific deletion of STAT3: its use to determine the role of STAT3 in the upregulation of cardioprotective proteins by ischemic preconditioning. *J Mol Cell Cardiol.* (2011) 50:589–97. doi: 10.1016/j.yjmcc.2011.01.002
56. Oba T, Yasukawa H, Hoshijima M, Sasaki K, Futamata N, Fukui D, et al. Cardiac-specific deletion of SOCS-3 prevents development of left ventricular remodeling after acute myocardial infarction. *J Am Coll Cardiol.* (2012) 59:838–52. doi: 10.1016/j.jacc.2011.10.887
57. Nagata T, Yasukawa H, Kyogoku S, Oba T, Takahashi J, Nohara S, et al. Cardiac-Specific SOCS3 deletion prevents *In Vivo Myocardial Ischemia* reperfusion injury through sustained activation of cardioprotective signaling molecules. *PLoS ONE* (2015) 10:e0127942. doi: 10.1371/journal.pone.0127942
58. Schuringa JJ, Schepers H, Vellenga E, Kruijer W. Ser727-dependent transcriptional activation by association of p300 with STAT3 upon IL-6 stimulation. *FEBS Lett.* (2001) 495:71–6. doi: 10.1016/S0014-5793(01)02354-7
59. Booz GW, Day JN, Baker KM. Angiotensin II effects on STAT3 phosphorylation in cardiomyocytes: evidence for Erk-dependent Tyr705 dephosphorylation. *Basic Res Cardiol.* (2003) 98:33–8. doi: 10.1007/s00395-003-0387-x
60. Ng IH, Bogoyevitch MA, Jans DA. Cytokine-induced slowing of STAT3 nuclear import; faster basal trafficking of the STAT3β isoform. *Traffic* (2014) 15:946–60. doi: 10.1111/tra.12181
61. Cheon H, Yang J, Stark GR. The functions of signal transducers and activators of transcriptions 1 and 3 as cytokine-inducible proteins. *J Interferon Cytokine Res.* (2011) 31:33–40. doi: 10.1089/jir.2010.0100
62. Yue H, Li W, Desnoyer R, Karnik SS. Role of nuclear unphosphorylated STAT3 in angiotensin II type 1 receptor-induced cardiac hypertrophy. *Cardiovasc Res.* (2010) 85:90–9. doi: 10.1093/cvr/cvp285
63. Yang J, Liao X, Agarwal MK, Barnes L, Auron PE, Stark GR. Unphosphorylated STAT3 accumulates in response to IL-6 and activates transcription by binding to NFκB. *Genes Dev.* (2007) 21:1396–408. doi: 10.1101/gad.1553707
64. Dasgupta M, Unal H, Willard B, Yang J, Karnik SS, Stark GR. Critical role for lysine 685 in gene expression mediated by transcription factor unphosphorylated STAT3. *J Biol Chem.* (2014) 289:30763–71. doi: 10.1074/jbc.M114.603894
65. Timofeeva OA, Chasovskikh S, Lonskaya I, Tarasova NI, Khavrutskii L, Tarasov SG, et al. Mechanisms of unphosphorylated STAT3 transcription factor binding to DNA. *J Biol Chem.* (2012) 287:14192–200. doi: 10.1074/jbc.M111.323899
66. Yan SJ, Lim SJ, Shi S, Dutta P, Li WX. Unphosphorylated STAT and heterochromatin protect genome stability. *FASEB J.* (2011) 25:232–41. doi: 10.1096/fj.10-169367
67. Shi S, Larson K, Guo D, Lim SJ, Dutta P, Yan SJ, et al. Drosophila STAT is required for directly maintaining HP1 localization and heterochromatin stability. *Nat Cell Biol.* (2008) 10:489–96. doi: 10.1038/ncb1713
68. Xu N, Emelyanov AV, Fyodorov DV, Skoultchi AI. Drosophila linker histone H1 coordinates STAT-dependent organization of heterochromatin and suppresses tumorigenesis caused by hyperactive JAK-STAT signaling. *Epigenetics Chromatin.* (2014) 7:16. doi: 10.1186/1756-8935-7-16
69. Zgheib C, Kurdi M, Zouein FA, Gunter BW, Stanley BA, Zgheib J, et al. Acyloxy nitroso compounds inhibit LIF signaling in endothelial cells and cardiac myocytes: evidence that STAT3 signaling is redox-sensitive. *PLoS ONE* (2012) 7:e43313. doi: 10.1371/journal.pone.0043313
70. Sobotta MC, Liou W, Stocker S, Talwar D, Oehler M, Ruppert T, et al. Peroxiredoxin-2 and STAT3 form a redox relay for H_2O_2 signaling. *Nat Chem Biol.* (2015) 11:64–70. doi: 10.1038/nchembio.1695
71. Eyerich S, Eyerich K, Cavani A, Schmidt-Weber C. IL-17 and IL-22: siblings, not twins. *Trends Immunol.* (2010) 31:354–61. doi: 10.1016/j.it.2010.06.004

72. Alabbas SY, Begun J, Florin TH, Oancea I. The role of IL-22 in the resolution of sterile and nonsterile inflammation. *Clin Transl Immunol.* (2018) 7:e1017. doi: 10.1002/cti2.1017
73. Ye J, Ji Q, Liu J, Liu L, Huang Y, Shi Y, et al. Interleukin 22 Promotes Blood pressure elevation and endothelial dysfunction in angiotensin II-treated mice. *J Am Heart Assoc.* (2017) 6:5875. doi: 10.1161/JAHA.117.005875
74. Ye J, Liu L, Ji Q, Huang Y, Shi Y, Shi L, et al. Anti-Interleukin-22-Neutralizing antibody attenuates angiotensin II-induced cardiac hypertrophy in mice. *Media Inflamm.* (2017) 2017:5635929. doi: 10.1155/2017/5635929
75. Liu W, Wang X, Feng W, Li S, Tian W, Xu T, et al. Lentivirus mediated IL-17R blockade improves diastolic cardiac function in spontaneously hypertensive rats. *Exp Mol Pathol.* (2011) 91:362–7. doi: 10.1016/j.yexmp.2011.04.003
76. Xie Y, Li M, Wang X, Zhang X, Peng T, Yang Y, et al. *In vivo* delivery of adenoviral vector containing interleukin-17 receptor a reduces cardiac remodeling and improves myocardial function in viral myocarditis leading to dilated cardiomyopathy. *PLoS ONE* (2013) 8:e72158. doi: 10.1371/journal.pone.0072158
77. Wu L, Ong S, Talor MV, Barin JG, Baldeviano GC, Kass DA, et al. Cardiac fibroblasts mediate IL-17A-driven inflammatory dilated cardiomyopathy. *J Exp Med.* (2014) 211:1449–64. doi: 10.1084/jem.20132126
78. Su SA, Yang D, Zhu W, Cai Z, Zhang N, Zhao L, et al. Interleukin-17A mediates cardiomyocyte apoptosis through Stat3-iNOS pathway. *Biochim Biophys Acta* (2016) 1863:2784–94. doi: 10.1016/j.bbamcr.2016.08.013

15

Regulatory Networks Involving STATs, IRFs and NFκB in Inflammation

Ekaterini Platanitis and Thomas Decker*

Max F. Perutz Laboratories, Department of Microbiology, Immunobiology and Genetics, University of Vienna, Vienna, Austria

***Correspondence:**
Thomas Decker
thomas.decker@univie.ac.at

Cells engaging in inflammation undergo drastic changes of their transcriptomes. In order to tailor these alterations in gene expression to the requirements of the inflammatory process, tight and coordinate regulation of gene expression by environmental cues, microbial or danger-associated molecules or cytokines, are mandatory. The transcriptional response is set off by signal-regulated transcription factors (SRTFs) at the receiving end of pathways originating at pattern recognition- and cytokine receptors. These interact with a genome that has been set for an appropriate response by prior activity of pioneer or lineage determining transcription factors (LDTFs). The same types of transcription factors are also critical determinants of the changes in chromatin landscapes and transcriptomes that specify potential consequences of inflammation: tissue repair, training, and tolerance. Here we focus on the role of three families of SRTFs in inflammation and its sequels: signal transducers and activators of transcription (STATs), interferon regulatory factors (IRFs), and nuclear factor κB (NFκB). We describe recent findings about their interactions and about their networking with LDTFs. Our aim is to provide a snapshot of a highly dynamic research area.

Keywords: inflammation, macrophage, transcription, STAT, IRF, NFκB, epigenetic, chromatin

INTRODUCTION

Inflammation is a rapid response of the innate immune system to infection or sterile causes of trauma and tissue damage. Its main purpose is to alert, recruit, and activate cells of the immune system, mobilize the adaptive immune system, remove the infectious agent or other proinflammatory stimuli and, ultimately, repair the tissue damage inflicted by both the trigger of inflammation and the inflammatory process (1). These events require the coordinate action of a multitude of different cell types of the immune system and the inflamed tissue. Inflammation ensues when cells sense microorganisms by means of microbe-associated molecular patterns (MAMPs) or damaged tissue by the release of damage (or danger)- associated molecular patterns (DAMPs). Both MAMPs and DAMPs are recognized by binding to one or more pattern recognition receptors (PRR). Signal transduction by these receptors enables cells to mobilize a proinflammatory gene expression program (2, 3). As a corollary, antimicrobial effector mechanisms are activated and immune mediators are released that prepare the surrounding tissue for inflammation, cause influx of leukocytes from the blood and allow for the recruited cells to adopt an immunologically activated state.

The progression to a proinflammatory state necessitates dramatic transcriptome changes of the participating cells. Cells such as macrophages with a pivotal role in orchestrating inflammation acquire an appropriately structured genome during differentiation (4). In molecular terms this means that their chromatin ensures accessibility of critical regulatory DNA, thus allowing for an immediate transcriptional response of proinflammatory genes. Cell lineage specificity of genome accessibility requires a compatible (lack of) genome compaction and 3D structure, but also the activity of lineage-determining transcription factors (LDTFs). LTDFs belong to the larger group of pioneer transcription factors with the ability to bind enhancer elements within nucleosomal DNA. Their association with DNA causes nucleosome rearrangement and, at neighboring histones, the deposition of posttranslational modifications (marks) characteristic of accessible or poised enhancers. To initiate a proinflammatory response, MAMPs, DAMPs, or activating cytokines such as interferon γ (IFNγ) cause the synthesis and activation of signal-regulated transcription factors (SRTFs) that interact with the prearranged genome to cause a stimulus and cell-type specific transcriptome change (5). Likewise, suppression and resolution of inflammation and tissue repair result from signals targeting a different set of SRTFs to produce an anti-inflammatory response tailored to a particular cell-lineage by a permissive genome structure.

Signal transducers and activators of transcription (STATs), interferon regulatory factors (IRFs) and nuclear factor κB (NFκB) are major players among SRTFs. Different family members function in the establishment as well as the resolution or prevention of inflammation. This dual mode of macrophage activity during inflammation is represented by the polarization of macrophages into the proinflammatory M1 type and the inflammation-resolving M2 type. While these types, generated *in vitro* by using IFNγ/LPS (M1) or IL4 (M2), represent extremes with most likely no direct *in-vivo* equivalent (6–9), they establish a useful heuristic concept that has produced much insight how macrophages realize their pro- and anti-inflammatory potential.

STATs, IRFs, AND NFκB, A BRIEF OVERVIEW

For in-depth information and additional references concerning these transcription factor families the reader is referred to comprehensive reviews (10–15).

STATs

STATs form a family of 7 members (STATs 1-4, STATs 5a and 5b, STAT6). All family members function predominantly in the context of cytokine-responsive, two-component JAK-STAT pathways. When cytokine receptors bind their cognate ligands, one or more receptor-associated Janus protein tyrosine kinases (JAKs) are activated and phosphorylate latent STATs on a single tyrosine residue. In some STATs this leads to a reorientation of preformed dimers into a parallel arrangement (16) whereas others may dimerize *de-novo*. Dimerization is stabilized by reciprocal phosphotyrosine (pY) interactions with SH2 domains which are, among transcription factors, a distinguishing feature of STATs (**Figure 1**). pY-mediated dimerization exposes an unconventional nuclear localization signal that shifts the subcellular localization of STATs to the nucleus (26). Homo-or heterodimeric STATs recognize a DNA sequence called gamma-interferon-activated sequence [GAS, TTCN_{3-4}GAA; (17)]. In contrast, STATs able to form a complex with a non-STAT subunit, IRF9, bind to a distinct sequence, the interferon-stimulated response element [ISRE; (27)]. The ISRE is a hallmark of all type I and type III IFN-responsive genes (ISG) and a large fraction of IFNγ-inducible genes. Both type I IFN (IFN-I: IFNα, IFNβ, others) and type III IFN (IFN-III: IFNλ) cause tyrosine phosphorylation of STAT1 and STAT2, the resulting heterodimer forms an ISRE-dependent complex with IRF9 called ISGF3. As an addendum to this original paradigm of IFN-I signaling, research in recent years has produced a variety of activities of IRF9-containing complexes other than ISGF3 and of unphosphorylated STATs (U-STATs), both as transcriptional regulators and in non-nuclear contexts (28–30). We and others have recently reviewed these non-canonical STAT activities (31–33). Unlike IFN-I and IFN-III, the IFNγ-stimulated JAK-STAT pathway produces a STAT1 dimer, the gamma-interferon-activated factor (GAF), in addition to a very low level of ISGF3. This difference in STAT activation is one of the factors responsible for overlapping, yet discrete IFN-I and IFNγ-induced transcriptomes (29).

IRFs

The original description and eponymous function of IRFs derives from their activity as regulators of the genes encoding type I IFN (34). The minimal IRF binding site of the IFNβ promoter, characterized by 5′-GAAA-3′ motifs (35) is part of many ISRE sequences (5′-PuPuAAANNGAAAPyPy-3′). Not surprisingly therefore, a second identification of IRFs resulted from the purification of ISRE-associated proteins (36). Subsequent work revealed a total of 9 family members in mice and men (IRF1-9). Common structural features of IRFs include an N-terminal DNA-binding domain with 5 characteristically spaced tryptophanes and one of two structurally distinct C-terminal IRF association domains (IAD; **Figure 1**). In IRF9, but not other IRFs, the IAD contains a binding site for STAT2 (37). The regulation of IRF transcriptional activity requires for some IRFs (IRF3, IRF5, IRF7) the phosphorylation of serine residues within the IAD and C-terminus for dimerization and activation. For others (IRF1, IRF2, IRF4, IRF8), sporadic reports of phosphorylation events exist (38, 39), but this modification is most likely not generally necessary to regulate transcriptional activity. IRF9 is unique as it has no known transcriptional activity on its own and is so far characterized exclusively as a subunit of ISGF3 or other complexes containing either STAT1 or STAT2.

Phosphorylation-dependent IRFs function downstream of toll-like receptors (TLR) and cytosolic nucleic acid receptors (2, 3). The established serine kinases are IKKβ [IRF5; (40)] and the non-canonical IKKs TBK1 and IKKε (41). IRF3 and IRF7 are the main regulators of IFN-I gene expression, whereas IRF5's main activity appears to be in the regulation of typical proinflammatory genes [although IRF5 may in some situations also contribute to IFN-I regulation; (42)]. With the notable exception of IRF3 all IRF family members are cytokine-inducible and have important functions in cytokine responses. Particularly

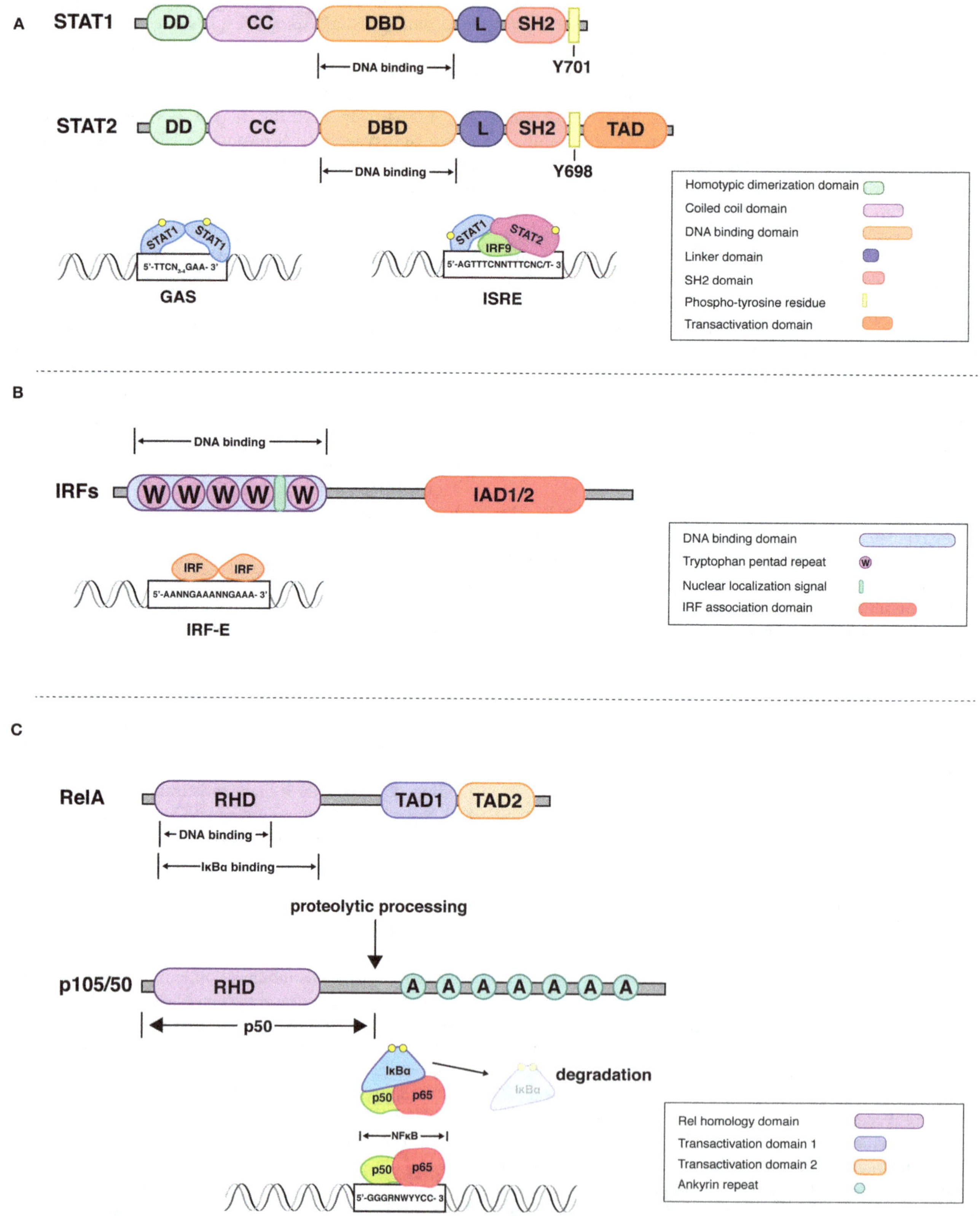

FIGURE 1 | Structural attributes of STAT-, IRF-, and Rel family transcription factors. **STATs**. All mammalian STAT members share a common structural motif consisting of an N-terminal domain, which plays a role in dimerization (DD), followed by a coiled-coil domain (CC), that can be involved in interactions with other proteins, a DNA-binding domain (DBD), a linker domain (L), an SH2 domain for reciprocal phospho-tyrosine interaction and a transactivation domain (10, 11). Upon receptor

(Continued)

FIGURE 1 | engagement Janus kinases lead to the activation of the latent cytoplasmic STATs, via phosphorylation on single tyrosine residues (Y701 on STAT1 and Y690 on STAT2). The STAT1-STAT2 dimer associates with interferon regulatory factor 9 (IRF9) to form a transcriptionally active IFN-stimulated gene factor 3 (ISGF3). This complex controls gene expression by binding to interferon-stimulated response elements (ISRE) present in promoters of IFN stimulated gene (ISG). Additionally, STAT1 homodimers, translocate to the nucleus and stimulate ISG expression by binding to gamma interferon-activated sites (GAS) (17). **IRFs.** All IRFs harbor a conserved N-terminal DNA-binding domain (DBD), which forms a helix-turn-helix domain with a conserved tryptophan cluster that recognizes DNA sequences in interferon induced genes (18). An analysis of the crystal structure of the DBD of IRF1 bound to the Ifnb promoter revealed that 5′-GAAA-3′ is the consensus sequence recognized by the helix-turn-helix motif of IRF1 (19). This DNA motif is known as the IRF-element (IRF-E) (20). All IRFs harbor a C-terminal IRF association domain (IAD), which is responsible for homo- and heteromeric interactions with other family members or transcription factors (21, 22). IAD1 and IAD2 domains can be distinguished by structural criteria and are found, respectively, in IRF1 and IRF2 or all other IRFs. **Rel (NFκB).** One of the best studied NFκB dimers is the p50/p65 heterodimer, whose crystal structure has been solved (23). NFκB recognizes 9–11 bp (base pair) DNA-elements, which are often located within promoters and enhancers of NFκB target genes. The consensus sequence 5′-GGGRNWYYCC-3′, where R denotes a purine base, N means any base, W stands for adenine or thymine and Y represents a pyrimidine base, is recognized by the Rel-homology domain [RHD; (12)]. The C-terminal domain of RelA (p65) contains two strong and independent transactivation domains (TAD) providing full transcriptional activity (24). The p100 precursor protein is proteolytically processed to the NFκB subunit p50. The mature p50 protein contains the RHD followed by glycine-rich region, a region that is essential for directing the cleavage and proteolytic processing of a long IκB-like C-terminal part of the precursors (25). IκBα regulates rapid and transient induction of NFκB activity. The crystal structure of IκBα bound to the p65/p50 heterodimer revealed that one IκBα molecule binds to an NFκB dimer and masks the NLS of p65. IKKβ is necessary and sufficient for phosphorylation of IκBα, leading to IκBα ubiquitination, and further degradation by the proteasome.

IRF4 and IRF8 are important for the specification of immune cell lineages and/or as determinants of their functional attributes. IRF6 is the only family member with a function in embryonic development.

NFκB

Various canonical and non-canonical NFκB complexes are formed by members of the Rel family of transcription factors which contain a Rel homology domain (RHD) for DNA binding and, in case of the RelA, RelB, and c-Rel family members, a C-terminal transactivation domain (12). The p52 and p50 proteins are formed from larger precursor protein (p100 and p105, respectively) by proteolytic processing. The major player among proinflammatory NFκBs, and the only one discussed here, is the heterodimer of RelA/p65 and p50. Its nuclear activity is restricted by inhibitors of NFκB (IκB, mainly IκBα) through a direct interaction that masks the nuclear localization signal. Activation of the IκB kinase complex (IKK complex, consisting of IKKα, IKKβ, and IKKγ/NEMO) causes the phosphorylation of IkBα on two critical serines which leads to its ubiquitination and subsequent degradation. In the innate immune system activation of the IKK complex is caused by all PRR, and by TNF receptor- as well as CD40-related receptor families. In the adaptive immune system NFκB is activated by these same receptor families and also by lymphocyte antigen receptors.

TABLE 1 | Different molecular principles guiding the interaction between transcription factors (TFs) of the STAT, IRF and Rel/NFκB families.

Mode of interaction	Example	References
TF1 regulates TF2 synthesis	• STAT1 regulates IRF1 and IRF8 synthesis • NFκB regulates IRF1 synthesis	(43) (44) (45)
Promoter occupancy of TF1 required for binding of TF2	• IRF8 required for NFκB/IRF3/7-dependent Ifnb enhanceosome assembly by LPS • IRF8 enhances IFNγ-induced gene transcription by STAT1 and IRF1 in myeloid cells	(46) (47) (48)
Promoter co-occupancy by TFs required for transcriptional activation	• ISGF3 and NFκB cooperate at iNOS and IL6 promoters • STAT1 and IRF1 cooperate in IFNγ-induced transcription	(49) (50) (51) (52)
Physical interaction of TFs	• IRF9 binds to STAT2 • IRF3 associates with RelA/p65 to function as coactivator at NFκB sites. Conversely, RelA/p65 functions as IRF3 coactivator at ISREs • U-STAT2 associates with RelA/p65 to induce IL6 transcription	(10) (37) (53) (54) (55)
TF competition for promoter binding (direct or indirect)	• STAT6 prevents NFκB binding at overlapping sites • STAT5 prevents STAT1 association at IRF8 promoter	(56) (57) (58)

TRANSCRIPTION FACTOR NETWORKS INVOLVING STATs, IRFs, AND NFκB IN MACROPHAGES

There are several conceptual possibilities how transcription factors form networks (**Table 1**). Networking may result from a common functional context such as inflammation, but result from independent action. On the other hand, there are several ways to directly link the activity of one transcription factor to the activity of the other. For example, networking transcription factors may regulate each other's synthesis or activation or, alternatively, converge at promoter level to cooperate or antagonize each other in the regulation of a common set of genes. Such agonistic or antagonistic action can result from direct physical contacts or from complementing each other in different steps of promoter activation such as chromatin remodeling and modification or the formation of a transcriptional initiation complex. In one way or another all these possibilities contribute to networks containing STATs, IRFs, and NFκB.

Establishment of Enhancers Controlling Inflammatory Gene Expression

The changes in genome structure occurring during macrophage differentiation set the stage for appropriate responses of the mature cells to challenges such as infection or inducers of sterile inflammation (**Figure 2**). As outlined above, this relies on the activity of LDTFs that generate poised enhancers with typical histone marks such as H3K4me1. Activation of these enhancers in differentiated cells is accompanied by the binding of a variable number of SRTFs and the deposition of additional histone modifications including the characteristic H3K27ac mark. While several LDTFs such as C/EBPα and AP1 family TFs are associated with poised enhancers in differentiating macrophages, the most prominent role in the script belongs to the Ets protein Pu.1 (59–61). Many of the Pu.1 binding sites occupied during differentiation represent EICE elements that allow for concomitant association of both Pu.1 and IRF8 [5′-GGAANNGGAAA-3′; (62)]. Thus, Pu.1 and IRF8, by specifying which of the thousands of potential enhancer sequences are accessible for transcription control, are critical in shaping a macrophage-specific chromatin landscape and the response to inflammatory stimuli. By interacting with LDTFs, IRFs, STATs, and NFκB play prominent roles in converting these enhancers into an active state that allows for contacts with the transcriptional machinery at the transcription start site (TSS). Studies such as that by Kaikkonen suggest that enhancer transcription precedes their engagement in the formation of transcription initiation complexes (61).

Not all enhancers of inflammatory gene expression are established during differentiation. Activation of terminally differentiated macrophages also causes the binding of both LDTFs and SRTFs to "latent" enhancers, i.e., sequences embedded into nucleosomes that have not been previously remodeled and marked by deposition of H3K4me1. Both IFNγ and the alternative M2 polarization factor IL4 (see below) convert latent into active enhancers by providing STAT1 and STAT6, respectively (63). Unexpectedly, the binding site in the IFNγ-activated latent enhancers is an ISRE, not a GAS sequence suggesting the participation of ISGF3 or STAT2-IRF9 complexes (29). Once activated, latent enhancers persist for some time to generate a transcriptional memory effect for subsequent stimulation. In LPS-stimulated cells composite binding sites for AP1 family and IRF8 play a prominent role in the mobilization of latent enhancers (47).

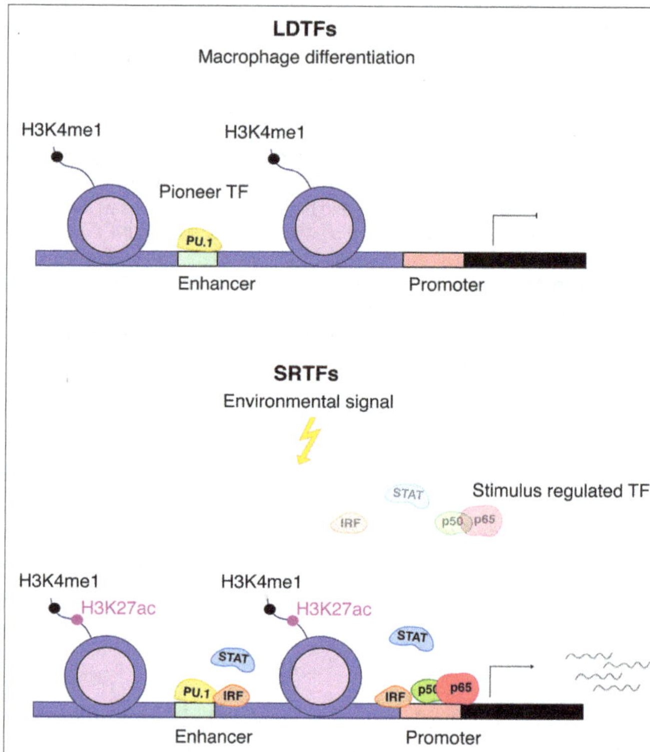

FIGURE 2 | Interplay between LDTFs and SRTFs. Pu.1 is an important macrophage lineage-determining factor (LDTF) and a major driving force behind setting up macrophage enhancers for further action by SRTFs. Enhancers are distinguished by high levels of H3K4me1 and are primed by LDTFs, which further displace nucleosomes. Stimulus responsive enhancers and promoters are bound by stimulus-regulated transcription factors (SRTFs), such as STAT, NFκB, and IRF transcription factors, to direct transcriptional responses in the course of inflammation. The binding of SRTFs to primed promoters and enhancers leads to further recruitment of co-activators that deposit the activation mark H3K27ac (5).

Macrophage Activation and M1 Polarization

In a simplified view macrophage activation results from signals generated by PRR such as the LPS receptor TLR4, which are amplified via JAK-STAT signal transduction by the IFNγ receptor. Polarization expresses the fact that one of several possible physiological states of a macrophage is more or less transiently established with a concomitant suppression of others (**Figure 3**). In case of the M1 macrophage this state is proinflammatory as well as antimicrobial and TNF/NFκB play a role in suppressing the competing M2 fate. Recent studies show that ablation of TNF responsiveness in tumor-associated macrophages (TAMs) suppresses the M1 component of their transcriptome. Further evidence for this concept comes from a report showing that the lack of TNF corresponds with an increased expression of M2 marker genes during infection with *Leishmania major* (7, 66). According to work by van den Bossche M1 polarized macrophages cannot be repolarized to M2 by IL4 treatment because the M1-typic shut-down of mitochondrial oxidative phosphorylation prevents this. The iNOS product NO plays an important role in inhibiting OxPhos, as iNOS inhibition allowed for a partial rescue of IL4-induced alternative activation in M1-polarized cells (67).

IFNγ-Independent Pathways of Macrophage Activation and M1 Polarization

The signaling network operating in IFNγ/LPS-stimulated macrophages produces several types of active SRTFs that include NFκB, IRFs, and STATs. However, many MAMPs alone produce these transcription factor activities without requiring exogenous supplies of IFNγ as follows. LPS activates NFκB both through the MyD88 and TRIF pathways downstream of its receptor TLR4. NFκB is subsequently involved in both immediate, primary, and delayed, secondary expression of proinflammatory LPS

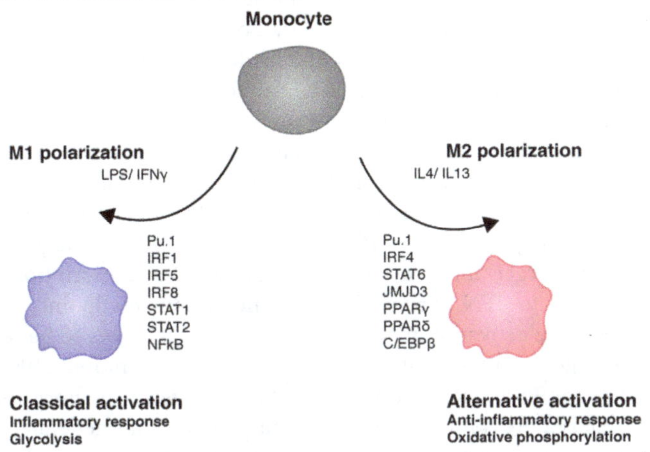

FIGURE 3 | Transcription factors shaping macrophage polarity. M1 stimuli lipopolysaccharide (LPS) and interferon γ (IFNγ) trigger the activation of several transcription factors such as IRF1, IRF5, IRF8 STAT1, STAT2, and NFκB (64). M1 macrophages play key roles in inflammation as well as antibacterial responses. IL4 and IL13 induce M2 polarity in macrophages. M2 transcriptomes are determined by different transcription factors such as IRF4, STAT6, JMJD3, PPARγ, PPARδ, and C/EBPβ. M2 macrophages exert anti-inflammatory activities such as tissue repair. M1 macrophages are glycolytic whereas mitochondrial oxidative phosphorylation is required for M2 macrophage development (65).

target genes (68). Primary and secondary response genes can be distinguished by a differential need for SRTF-dependent chromatin remodeling at the transcription starts (TSS) and proximal promoters (69, 70). These regions contain a high CpG content at primary response genes which impedes nucleosome formation, leaving the TSS, and promoter-proximal transcription factor binding sites accessible for initiation complex formation. In fact, many of these promoters contain paused RNA polymerases. By supporting the binding of elongation factor pTEFb to its recruitment factor, the BET protein BRD4, NFκB helps to remove the DSIF/NELF elongation block for mRNA transcription (70–73). Secondary response genes show a more delayed response, consistent with the need to restructure/modify promoter chromatin in a signal-dependent manner (68–70). Initiation complexes at these genes are established de novo. Secondary responses can be generated via regulatory feed-forward loops, i.e., the synthesis of a secondary mRNA with a transcription factor either encoded by a primary response gene, or activated by a primary response product such as TNF. An example of the former situation is the synthesis of IRF1 in the primary, STAT1-dependent response to IFNγ (52). Interactivity between NFκB and STAT/IRF pathways occurs both at primary and secondary response genes.

While TLR4 is not directly connected to a JAK-STAT pathway, the downstream TRIF pathway targets the IRF3 kinases TBK1 and IKKε, and hence the IFN-I genes (74). LPS-stimulated cells thus accumulate active STATs as a secondary response resulting from signaling by the IFN-I receptor. The same holds true for endosomal TLRs that either use the TRIF adapter for signaling (TLR3) or that form a complex containing IRF7 around the MyD88 adapter (2). In this signalosome IRF7 is phosphorylated by IKKα (75). IFN-I synthesis is also an essential outcome of signaling by all cytosolic nucleic acid receptors that signal via platforms containing the adapters MAVS or STING (3). Therefore, active NFkB, IRFs and STATs are hallmarks of pathogen-exposed macrophages even in the absence of cytokines derived from external sources such as IFNγ. The relevance of this attribute of infected or infection-exposed cells is the ability of IFN-I to provide a priming signal for resting macrophages and other cell types either resident in the surrounding tissue, or entering infected tissue in the process of inflammation (49, 76). Owing to the cooperativity between STATs and IRFs or NFκB, the deposition of ISGF3 during IFN-I priming allows for more vigorous responses to an inflammatory stimulus.

Transcription control of IFN-I genes, particularly Ifnb, is one prominent example of the interaction between different IRFs as well as between IRFs and NFκB. In macrophages the gene is constitutively bound by Pu.1/IRF8 and induction by LPS is strongly reduced in cells lacking functional IRF8 (47). LPS or viral infection stimulate the promoter binding of IRF3 and/or IRF7 as well as NFκB and the subsequent recruitment of chromatin remodeling and modifying enzymes (77). The analysis of the active Ifnb promoter culminated in an atomic model of its enhanceosome (78). It contains not only IRFs3/7 and NFκB, but also the AP1 family members ATF2 and c-Jun.

The cooperation between NFκB and IRF3 shows additional levels of complexity in TLR responses of macrophages. Two studies are consistent with the idea that the two transcription factors can act as coactivators for each other. On the one hand, NFκB function at a subset of its binding sites requires direct interaction with IRF3 (53). On the other hand, p65 is tethered to ISRE subsets during macrophage TLR4 or TLR9 signaling. In LPS-treated macrophages around 100 ISREs bound these complexes and the corresponding genes were selectively inhibited by agonists of the glucocorticoid receptor [GR; (54)]. The data further demonstrate sensitivity of the interaction between IRF3 and the RelA RHD to disruption by the GR *in vitro*. The two studies reveal that some inflammatory genes are controlled by NFκB/IRF interaction without having promoter binding sites for both. Genome-wide DNA binding data in virus-infected cells further confirmed the impact of gene co-regulation by IRF3 and NFκB (79). An alternative experimental approach supports the importance of this finding by using a virus mutant with reduced ability to suppress NFκB activation. In IRF7-deficient cells the increased NFκB activation compared to wt virus partially rescued inflammatory gene expression and antiviral immunity (80), suggesting that a higher dose of NFκB activity compensates for the loss of IRF7 at coregulated genes.

Similar to IRF3, IRF5 is recruited to inflammatory genes and is essential for their efficient transcription. In LPS-treated macrophages NFκB assists IRF5 in binding to DNA, and the two factors set up a unique "inflammatory" IRF5-RelA cistrome which is best explained by the presence of consensus NF-κB and a composite Pu.1-ISRE element (81). Conditional deletion of IRF5 in macrophages is incompatible with M1 polarization (82).

IFN-I production in response to inflammatory stimuli produces transcriptional activity of transcription factor ISGF3, the STAT1/STAT2/IRF9 heterotrimer. ISGF3 exemplifies a direct physical STAT/IRF contact (37). According to the JAK-STAT paradigm described above, ISGF3 is the terminal component of IFN-I and IFN-III signaling. Whereas, a large fraction of IFNγ-inducible genes essentially depends on multimerized STAT1 dimers (83), there is currently no evidence that STAT1 dimers make important contributions to IFN-I or IFN-III signaling. As will be discussed in more detail below, genes regulated by STAT1 dimers are characterized by frequent cooperativity with IRF1, IRF8 and, at least for some genes, IRF7 (48, 52, 84–86). Conventional ISGs, i.e. ISGF3-dependent genes responding with a strong transcriptional increase to IFN-I do not require IRF1 (87), but a large fraction shows ISGF3 binding at or near Pu.1 and IRF8 (47, 62). Correspondingly, about 20% of total ISGs show diminished responses to IFNβ in cells expressing the IRF8 R294C mutant which is unable to interact with Ets family proteins and thus strongly impaired in its ability to bind DNA at composite binding sites (88). The ISREs of such ISGs contain the expected 5′ GGAA motif that allows for simultaneous association of IRF8 and Pu.1. Notwithstanding the neighborhood of ISGF3 and IRF8 at macrophage promoters, activity of the ISGF3 complex shows greater independence from ancillary IRFs than STAT1 dimers. One reason for this is the potent transactivating domain (TAD) of STAT2 compared with that of STAT1 (89). In fact, expression of a fusion protein of IRF9 with the STAT2 TAD largely recapitulates the transcriptional response to IFN-I (90).

In non-hematopoietic cells ISGs require a signal-independent nucleosome rearrangement prior to ISGF3 binding. It is executed by the mammalian SWI/SNF (or BAF) remodeling complex including the ATPase BRG1 (91). In addition, recent work has shown that ISGF3 binding causes additional IFN-dependent remodeling, shown by the appearance of open chromatin regions in ATAC-Seq or MNase I sensitivity experiments (92, 93). Histone exchange also takes place and results in the removal of the repressive variant H2A.Z. It will be interesting to determine how these non-hematopoietic remodeling events compare to chromatin opening during macrophage differentiation.

Despite the largely self-sufficient mode of ISGF3 action at many conventional ISGs, some genes expressed in MAMP-exposed or infected macrophages demonstrate a different behavior. These genes are referred to as unconventional ISGs (76) or synergy genes (50) because they respond poorly to IFN-I alone, instead requiring an additional PRR-derived signal. In many cases NFκB is essential to provide this second signal (50). By conservative estimate around 130 unconventional ISGs show synergistic transcriptional responses owing to ISGF3 and NFκB occupancy in macrophages infected with the intracellular bacterial pathogen *Listeria monocytogenes*. They include the genes encoding iNOS (NOS2) or IL6. Mechanistically the cooperativity at these two genes is explained by NFκB predominance in the recruitment of histone-modifying enzymes, the BET protein Brd4 and the TFIIH and pTEFb complexes needed for the phosphorylation of the RNA polymerase II (Pol II) carboxyterminal domain (CTD; **Figure 4A**). In contrast, ISGF3 plays a dominant role in the promoter recruitment of the general transcription factor TFIID and the formation of a complete initiation complex including Pol II. Both transcription factors cooperate in the recruitment of the mediator complex with core and kinase modules (49–51). Whether these mechanisms apply to all or a majority of genes showing NFκB/ISGF3 cooperativity remains to be determined. We have found that some of the conventional ISGs such as Isg15, Gbp, or Stat1 also have binding sites for NFκB and these sites are occupied during infection with *L. monocytogenes* [**Figure 4B**, data set as in (50)]. This suggests an even larger input of NFκB signaling into transcriptional responses to IFN. From the immunological standpoint the cooperative activation mode is useful because it allows to better dose signal strength at promoter level. Furthermore, NFκB can generate a state of transcriptional short-term memory for ISGF3, i.e., providing an NFκB-inducing signal alone generates a cooperative response even when the IFN signal follows up to 24 h later (49). This effect is similar to the latent enhancer activation described above, or to the priming effect of IFNγ described below. During an inflammatory response the kinetics of exposure to the many environmental signals differ for individual cells, thus these memory mechanisms appear highly advantageous. In support of this notion a study by Park et al. confirms the ability of both TNF and IFNα to reprogram the human macrophage epigenome, thus altering inflammatory responses to TLR4 stimulation. Preexposure with TNF may tolerize genes with NFκB sites or lead to synergism with LPS in genes with ISRE/IRF and AP1 elements. IFN pretreatment can counteract the tolerizing effects of TNF (76).

The Transcriptional Response to IFNγ–Its Contribution to Macrophage Activation and Inflammation

IFNγ is the macrophage-activating cytokine produced in the course of an inflammatory responses by innate lymphocytes such as NK or ILC1 cells, but also via an innate response of T lymphocytes. Immunological effects of IFNγ are to a large extent established *de novo* and require extensive chromatin landscape changes (94). Formation of STAT1 dimers (or GAF) by the IFNγ receptor complex is sufficient for the transcription of a relatively small number of primary response genes with GAS promoter elements. Among these are the Irf1 and Irf8 genes. IRF1 and IRF8 production is necessary for a delayed transcriptional of many secondary IFNγ-induced genes, represented by e.g., the GBP family, the gp91Phox, Nos2 (iNOS), or the Ciita gene encoding the master regulator of MHC II expression (48, 52, 84, 85, 95–97). In addition, our recent data in IFNγ-treated macrophages reveal a surprisingly large contribution of ISGF3 to the IFNγ-induced transcriptome (29).

Increased amounts of IRF8 in LPS or IFNγ-treated cells allow the transcription factor to occupy landing sites in addition to those established during macrophage differentiation. This is important because similar to ISGs, many IFNγ-inducible promoters are prebound with Pu.1 and a subfraction of these are associated with Pu.1/IRF8. In this situation Pu.1/IRF8 binding occurs via EICE sequences, whereas inducible binding of IRF8 occurs via ISRE, but not via GAS sites (47). IRF1 appears to

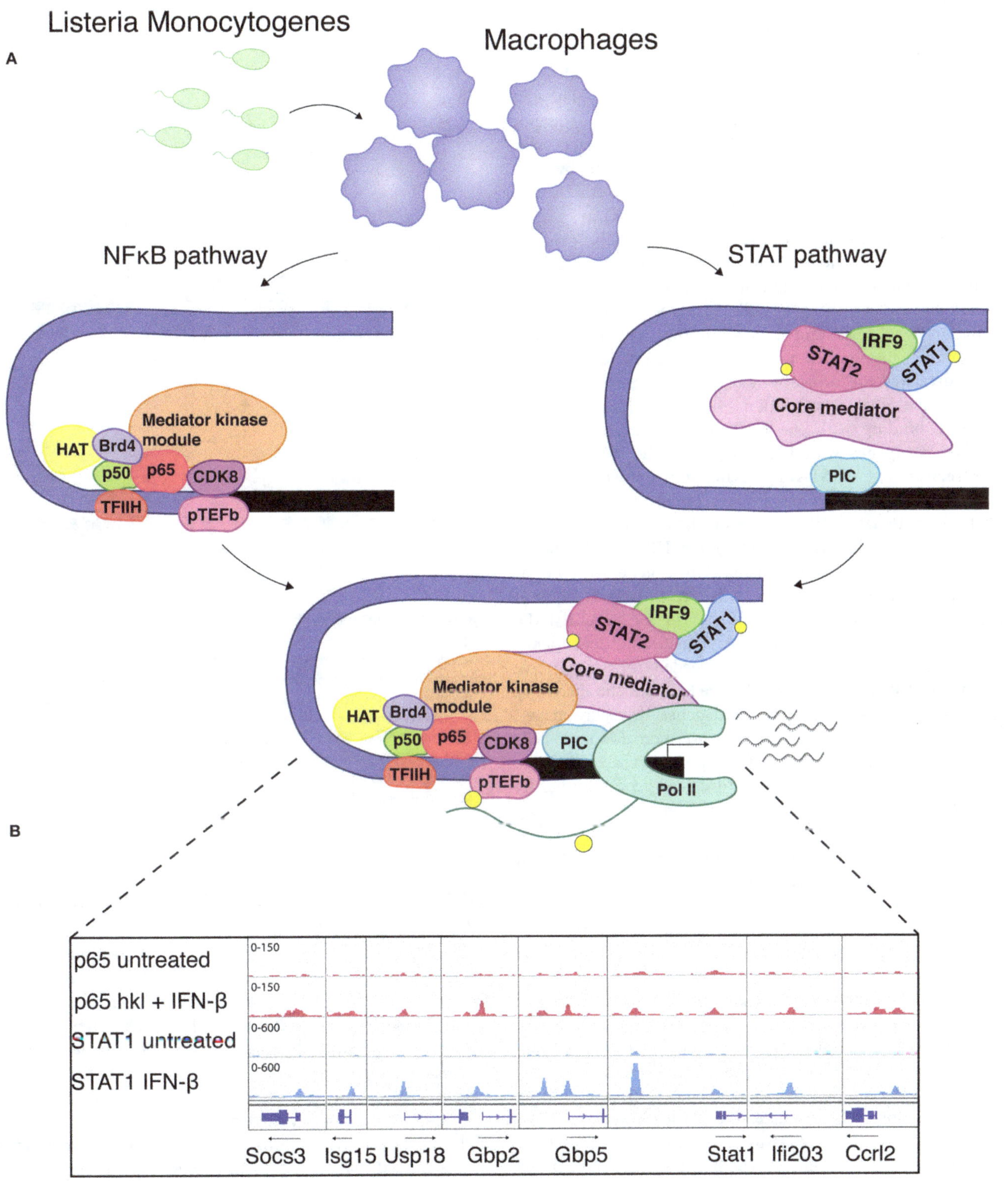

FIGURE 4 | STAT-NFκB cooperativity shapes the transcriptional response to *Listeria monocytogenes*. **(A)** NFκB association with the Nos2 promoter is the initial step and leads to recruitment of TFIIH which is further required for Pol II phosphorylation. Brd4 stabilizes the NFκB-TFIIH complex. In addition, association of HAT and the mediator kinase module (CDK8) strongly depend on NFκB. ISGF3, which recruits the core mediator, is essential for the formation of a pre-initiation complex (PIC) and further provides a critical prerequisite for TFIID and RNA polymerase II (Pol II) binding (49–51). These references also describe the experimental procedures for separate analysis of STAT and NFκB signaling during *L. monocytogenes* infection. **(B)** Binding of NFκB RelA/p65 and STAT1 to promoters of co-regulated ISGs. The igv browser tracks show induced RelA/p65 binding in macrophages treated with IFNβ and heat-killed Listeria (hkl). STAT1 binding sites are shown from IFNβ-stimulated macrophages. A ChIP-seq data set described in reference 50 was used.

have a minor-if any- role in enhancer establishment during differentiation, but its role in signal-dependent gene induction is essential and not redundant with other IRFs. Based on their IRF requirement, a recent report by Langlais and colleagues distinguishes two types of IFNγ-induced gene clusters. The first is characterized by prebound Pu.1/IRF8 and its ISRE sequence will associate with both IRF8 and IRF1 in IFNγ-treated cells. The second type of IFNγ-induced genes is prebound by Pu.1 alone and its ISRE will associate with IRF1 only. Both clusters show a large overlap with STAT1 binding (48). Thus, STAT1 in the IFNγ response acts both as an inducer of the primary response genes IRF1 and IRF8 and then cooperates with these IRFs in the second tier of the transcriptional response. There is a very limited number of studies providing a mechanistic explanation why IRFs and STATs together potently induce transcription where either of them alone fails to do so. Two studies correlated the presence of IRF8 with the establishment of constitutive H3K27 acetylation (47, 48) and one of these links IRF1 binding with the IFNγ-induced increase of this mark (48). At genes with EICE sequences IRF8 participates in the recruitment of STAT1, leaving it open which of the two is the histone acetyl transferase (HAT)-recruiting factor (47). In non-hematopoietic cells our data suggest a crucial role of STAT1 in the recruitment of the HAT CBP/P300 to the promoter of the IFNγ-inducible GBP2 gene with no or very little contribution of IRF1. CBP recruitment required phosphorylation of the C-terminal S727 in the STAT1 TAD. The two transcription factors displayed no interdependence of DNA binding, but were equally needed for cooperative recruitment of RNA Pol II [(52), **Figure 5**]. With the discovery of different clusters of IFNγ-induced genes in macrophages, regulatory heterogeneity may apply to non-hematopoietic cells as well and the data with the GBP promoter are likely to represent only a subfraction of IFNγ-induced genes. Studies by El Hassan et al. in epithelial cells show that IRF1 occupies a large number of sites without STAT1, but, conversely, STAT1 is mostly co-associated with IRF1 [(97), this appears to be different in macrophages (48)]. The larger number of IRF1 binding sites may be explained by a role of IRF1-binding enhancers in the formation of a 3D promoter structure as reported by the same group for the gene encoding the MHC II master regulator CIITA (96).

We have briefly mentioned the participation of IFNγ/STAT1 in the mobilization of latent enhancers in murine macrophages. Consistent with this Qiao et al. report studies in human macrophages showing that IFNγ primes LPS-responsive genes with STAT/IRF binding sites without necessarily activating their transcription (98). Examples are the genes encoding IL6 and IL12. IFNγ priming leads to a massive increase in their subsequent LPS responsiveness. Whether this is mechanistically related to the priming of the Il6 and Nos2 (iNOS) genes by type I IFN remains to be determined. However, the data suggest that cooperativity between NFκB and STATs may contribute to the increased inflammatory response after priming with IFNγ from exogenous sources much as it does in case of proinflammatory stimuli and endogenously produced IFN-I.

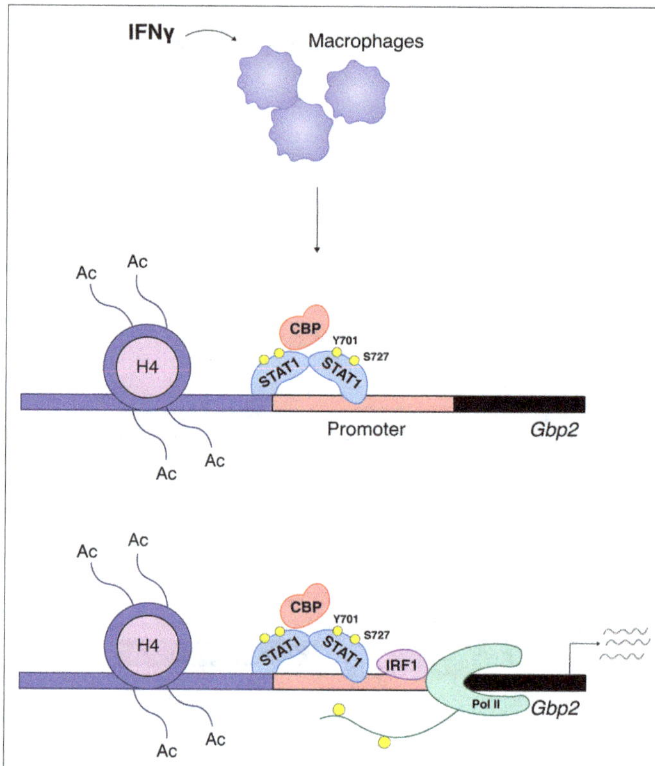

FIGURE 5 | STAT1 and IRF1 synergistically drive expression of Gbp2. A large group of IFNγ-induced genes such as Gbp2 requires both STAT1 and IRF1 for transcriptional activation (52). STAT1 associates with the Gbp2 promoter and is responsible for the ordered recruitment of the coactivator/histone acetyl transferase CREB-binding protein (CBP) and histone hyperacetylation. CBP recruitment requires phosphorylation of the STAT1 TAD at S727. Irf1 is a STAT1 target gene and, following IRF1 synthesis, its association with the Gbp2 promoter follows that of STAT1, but in respective knockout cells the two transcription factors bind without requiring each other's presence. RNA polymerase II (Pol II) association with the Gbp2 promoter requires both STAT1 and IRF1, but only IRF1 is found in a complex with RNA polymerase II.

M2 Polarization-the Cross-Repression of M1 and M2 Genes

Macrophages undergo "alternative" activation and M2 polarization when exposed to the type II immunity cytokines IL4 and IL13. They lack proinflammatory gene expression and have strongly reduced antimicrobial effector functions. Instead, they typically express genes allowing for tissue repair and fibrosis. M2 type genes such as Arginase1 (Arg1) or the mannose receptor Mrc1 are expressed in adipose tissue macrophages, but also in tumor-associated macrophages or in macrophages fighting parasitic infections (8, 64). Unlike M1 polarization, M2-polarized macrophages can be converted to an M1 type *in vitro* by treatment with IFNγ/LPS (67).

The apical transcription factor specifying the M2 state is STAT6, activated by the IL4 and IL13 receptors. Many of the typical M2 genes are direct targets of STAT6. IL4 also induces an IRF family member, IRF4. The human Irf4 gene contains a GAS element, suggesting it is under direct control of STAT6 (99, 100). Transcriptional induction of the Irf4 gene also requires the histone demethylase JMJD3 to remove the repressive H3K27me3 histone mark in the vicinity of the Irf4 transcription start. This demethylation step is of critical importance as Jmjd3$^{-/-}$ macrophages do not undergo M2 polarization during helminth infection (101). More recent knockdown studies in human monocytes suggest an enhancement of JMJD3 expression by STAT6 (100). This suggests that STAT6 is apical to both JMJD3 and IRF4. In specifying M2 transcriptomes STAT6 and IRF4 interact with other transcription factors, particularly PPARγ, C/EBPβ, and KLF4. Gene deficiencies for these transcription factors reduce the M2 potential, as do those for STAT6 and IRF4 (8). Different combinations of these transcription factors may specify distinct M2ish transcriptomes in animals (64). For example, PPARγ is instrumental in arranging the lipid metabolism of adipose tissue macrophages.

STAT6 is unique among STATs by preferentially associating with GAS containing 4 spacer nucleotides between half sites (5′-TTCN$_4$GAA-3′). This explains in part why its target genes are different from those activated by STAT1. On the other hand, genome-wide analysis of STAT1 and STAT6 binding to GAS elements revealed a large number of sites occupied by STAT1 and STAT6, respectively, in IFNγ or IL4-stimulated cells (102). Thus, epigenetic mechanisms and/or the cooperation with other M2 transcription factors are likely to further contribute to the distinction between STAT6 and STAT1-induced transcriptome changes. Although IRF4 is most likely a primary STAT6 target in analogy to the situation with STAT1 and IRF1/IRF8, we are not aware of a similarly important interaction of STAT6 and IRF4 at the level of common target promoters. In a recent study, an important function is assigned to STAT6 in cross-repressing M1 genes. In IL4-treated macrophages STAT6 represses genes at steady state and, in addition, renders proinflammatory genes unresponsive to a subsequent LPS challenge. Suppression requires HDAC3 activity and causes decreased promoter binding of LDTFs (e.g., Pu.1, C/EBP) as well as the p300 histone acetyl transferase. More than 600 LPS-induced genes show an overlap of NFκB and STAT6 binding sites (GAS), 70% of which are inhibited by IL4 and in 11.5% of them IL4 inhibited RelA/p65 binding (57). These genome-wide data are consistent with a model of competitive enhancer association as one of several mechanisms by which STAT6 represses NFκB activity. This model agrees with an earlier study of the E- selectin promoter suggesting direct competition of STAT6 and NFκB at overlapping binding sites (56). IRF4 stimulates gene expression via ISRE elements. It forms ternary complexes with Pu.1 and IRF8 on composite ISREs. However, the data are conflicting with regard to the outcome of complex formation on ISG transcription with some suggesting an inhibitory activity and repression of IRF1 activity (103, 104) and others supporting a stimulatory role (105).

Just as M1 genes are suppressed in M2 macrophages, the inverse situation is established in M1 polarized cells. In human macrophages transcription factor MAF regulates the expression of a subset of M2 genes. Fifteen percent of the genes repressed by IFNγ treatment are MAF targets. MAFb is a bZip transcription factor important for the development of macrophage-dendritic cell progenitors to monocytes (106). The work of Kang et al. demonstrates that IFNγ treatment causes a disassembly of MAF-associating enhancer sequences. Accompanying changes were a loss of enhancer transcription, of LDTF binding (Pu.1, CEBPβ), cohesin association and of the H3K27ac mark as a beacon of transcriptionally active genes. At the same time IFNγ deposits LDTFs at latent enhancers. Disassembled MAF enhancers also lose accessibility, determined by the disappearance of ATACseq signals. Chromatin closing at MAF enhancers contrasts with the majority of IFNγ-repressed genes that appear to be subject to a different inhibitory mechanism. A complex enhancer regulating MAF expression loses activating histone marks upon IFNγ treatment, consistent with decreased MAF levels in such cells. MAF family members are known to interact with Ets family proteins, suggesting that M2 enhancer accessibility may be regulated via Pu.1/MAF interaction. Another report by Ivashkiv's group showed that in human macrophages a small number of genes is stably repressed by IFNγ via H3K27me3 deposition by the PRC2 complex including the histone methylase EZH2 (107). These elegant studies provide important insight how IFNγ tips the polarity balance by repressing M2 genes. The studies do not address how the repressive mechanisms are linked to signals from the IFNγ receptor or the STAT/IRF network it activates. This will be an important task for future work. Likewise, the similarities and differences to mouse macrophages will interesting to decipher.

In a different approach, Piccolo and colleagues addressed the question how mouse macrophages are reprogrammed by a simultaneous encounter with the opposing IFNγ and IL4 (102). The authors report that each cytokine cross-inhibits genes of the opposite pole, but the impact of IFNγ dominates, most likely because it exerts a global effect on the binding of STAT6. In contrast, the repressive effect of IL4 on IFNγ-induced genes is more selective. Promoters containing GAS and ISRE elements only are spared from repression whereas more complex promoters that include sites for AP1 transcription factors with JunB subunits, such as the Nos2 gene, are repressed. In line with the study in human macrophages (108), MAFb-regulated genes are also enriched among IFNγ-repressed genes. The authors speculate that the inability of IL4 to globally suppress all IFNγ activity allows macrophages to maintain essential immunological functions such as the antiviral state. However, an immunological assessment of IL4/IFNγ co-treated macrophages has not been carried out. Interestingly, combining the finding that STAT6 and STAT1 both bind many GAS elements with the observed suppression of STAT6 binding by IFNγ lends further support to the direct competition model as one mechanism explaining the cross inhibition of polarization genes.

Sequels of the Inflammatory Response: LPS Tolerance and Macrophage Training

Chronic stimulation of macrophages with LPS causes a state of tolerance in which many inflammatory genes are refractory to further stimulation with LPS. The mechanisms contributing to this refractory state are manifold and many are not at promoter level, but rather affect TLR signaling and the activation of inflammatory transcription factors (109). A notable exception is the NFκB pathway. NFκB binding sites are enriched in tolerized genes (110), supporting an earlier notion that NFκB1/p50 forms repressive dimers on such sites (111). Macrophages lacking NFκB1 cannot be tolerized by LPS (112). Yan et al further demonstrate that p50 recruits HDAC complexes to tolerized genes. In human monocyte-derived macrophages LPS pretreatment leads to a tolerant state with extensive changes in histone modifications (enhancer marks) in which a fraction of LPS-induced genes shows an absent or reduced response to a second LPS stimulus. IRF (particularly IRF8) and STAT motifs are strongly enriched in genes showing partial unresponsiveness. IRF1, IRF8, STAT2, and STAT5 themselves are among highly tolerized genes. Interestingly, tolerization can to a large extent be reversed by the yeast MAMP β-glucan. This substance is associated with "trained immunity" (113). IFNγ pretreatment reverses effects of the tolerized state by maintaining chromatin remodeling and accessibility at LPS-induced genes (114). A seminal study on the topic showed that chromatin modifications and accessibility acquired during tolerization distinguish between proinflammatory cytokine genes and antimicrobial genes. While the former show a loss of remodeling and activating histone marks, these are retained on the latter. Consistently, the proinflammatory group enters a state of repression while the latter maintains inducibility (115). This suggests that in the tolerant state inflammation is dampened whereas antimicrobial defense remains. However, LPS tolerance is also thought to underlie the immunoparalysis of post-septic patients.

Trained Immunity

Trained immunity denotes a state of innate immunological memory resulting in macrophages and other innate cells from the previous encounter of an inflammatory and activating stimulus (116). LPS tolerance is one form of trained immunity. Training resulting from microbes such as BCG or *Candida albicans* or the yeast-associated molecular pattern β-glucan enhances subsequent responses of the innate immune system to different microbial infections. The trained state is accompanied by persistent metabolic and epigenetic changes. Epigenomic alterations show partial overlap, but are clearly distinct between LPS-tolerized and β-glucan-trained human macrophages (117). At the level of transcription training is explained by persistence of activating chromatin marks and regulatory site accessibility, particularly at previously latent enhancers. The causes for these genome changes are not understood. One study suggests an IFNγ-dependent role for STAT1 in training by *C. albicans*, but not β-glucan (118).

STATs AND IRFs IN DENDRITIC CELL (DC) DEVELOPMENT AND FUNCTION

For a comprehensive review of transcription factors in the development of DC subsets the reader is referred to the following reviews (119, 120).

DC Development

Both STATs and IRFs play important roles in the generation of different DC lineages and both influence each other's activities. STAT3, downstream of the Flt3 receptor, is required for the generation of most likely all DC lineages *in vitro* and has a clear role in plasmacytoid DC (pDC) development *in vivo* (121). Constitutive IRF7 expression is thought to accompany the development of pDC precursors into IFN-I-producing cells (IPC), i.e., cells with the ability to rapidly synthesize large quantities of IFN-I in response to TLR ligands (122). Recent studies suggest that pDC precursors diversify in response to a single TLR ligand and not all the resulting subpopulations are IFN-I-producing cells (123). Single cell RNA sequencing of human pDC suggests that only a small subpopulation is stimulated to produce IFN-I. IFN-I production of this population results from stochastic events rather than from developmental predetermination and IRF7 is indeed not a prognostic marker for future IFN-I production (124). Based on this study the concept how IFN-producing cells arise may have to be revised.

STAT5 is required for the production of myeloid DC by GM-CSF *in vitro*. It also mediates the suppressive function of GM-CSF on pDC development (58). Type I IFN stimulate DC maturation (125) and were shown in a recent study to regulate the glycolytic switch required for DC activation (126). In contrast, IFN-I suppress CD8$^+$ DC generation *in vitro* and during viral infection *in vivo*. Intriguingly, this effect was shown to require STAT2, but not STAT1 (127). The seeding of Payer's patches with pDC also requires IFN-I/STAT activity (128).

As during macrophage polarization, IRF8 and IRF4 determine different DC fates. IRF8 is critical for the development of pDC, tissue-resident CD103$^+$ DC, CD8$^+$ DC and Langerhans cells (129–133). Intriguingly, the R294C mutant allows to distinguish the role of IRF8 in the generation of pDC vs. CD8$^+$ and CD103$^+$ DC with the former being unaffected and development of the latter being inhibited (88, 131, 134). The property of this mutation to disrupt the interaction between IRF8 and Pu.1 (88) supports the assumption that composite Pu.1/IRF8 elements are important for CD103$^+$ and CD8$^+$ DC, but not for pDC. The IRF8 transcriptional network in CD103$^+$ and CD8$^+$ DC includes Id2, BATF3, and Notch2, whereas in pDC IRF8 functionally interacts with E2-2 and Bcl-11a (119). The suppressive effect of GM-CSF on pDC development requires STAT5 binding to a GAS in the IRF8 promoter where it inhibits IFN/STAT1-mediated upregulation of IRF8 expression (58).

IRF4 is expressed in cDC expressing CD4 and CD11b (also called cDC2) in a transcriptional network including RelB and Notch2 (119, 135). IRF4 may support cDC2 function more than their development. cDC2 are linked to both type 2 and type 3 immunity (135).

DC Activation

Similar to the studies defining the hierarchical action of transcription factors and the distinction between LDTFs and SRTFs in macrophages, Garber and colleagues defined analogous networks of preexisting pioneers (LDTFs) for lineage commitment, broad binders for priming, and dynamic factors (SRTFs) for execution (136). The authors used myeloid, IRF4$^+$ DC, generated *in vitro* with GM-CSF, for stimulation with LPS. Prominent LDTFs were Pu.1 and C/EBP as in macrophages. However, whether they occupy different sites in the two cell types has not been determined. In the LPS response the authors distinguished immediate and delayed response gene clusters that differed in priming factors (immediate: IRF4, JUNB, ATF3, EGR2, MAFf; delayed: IRF4, JUNB, ATF3) and dynamic association of the SRTFs IRF1 and NFκB. As might be expected from the kinetics of IFN production during the LPS response, STATs 1 and 2 associated with the delayed, but not the immediate LPS-responsive gene cluster.

The data in DC support the notion that the molecular principles governing enhancer accessibility, priming, and signal-regulated response are very similar between macrophages and DC, although the detailed usage of transcription factors for each stage of the transcriptional response during inflammation may differ.

CONCLUDING REMARKS

This review is focused on the role of macrophages in inflammation, with lesser attention to DC or non-hematopoietic cells. We realize this is only one chapter of a complex story but, based on available data, have focused on the cells allowing for the closest inspection of transcriptional networks in inflammation. Detailed views of the inflammatory response in other cells of the innate immune system are needed. In an organismic context, macrophages are shaped by their local environment (137). The impact of the resulting diversity on inflammatory responses remains to be determined. In future work ongoing large-scale efforts will integrate dynamic changes of the 3D genome structure into current knowledge about regulatory networks (138) and cell atlases based on single cell transcriptomes will further resolve distinct cell populations of the inflammatory response (139). However, while genome-wide perspectives have yielded new insight at an amazing pace in recent years and will continue to do so, future research needs to follow up on these data with biochemical approaches toward mechanisms of transcription factor cooperativity and antagonism. For example, it will be exciting to determine the different modes of action of LDTFs and SRTFs or to provide further insight how combinations of SRTFs feed into a common overall mechanism of promoter activation. Determining dynamic structures of the complexes they form at near atomic resolution will be invaluable support for such efforts (140). Cas9-mediated editing is and will be an extremely useful tool to test the impact of regulatory DNA (141). The recent past has given us a panoply of powerful new tools to advance our understanding of transcriptional mechanisms behind the inflammatory response.

AUTHOR CONTRIBUTIONS

All authors listed have made a substantial, direct and intellectual contribution to the work, and approved it for publication.

ACKNOWLEDGMENTS

Work in TD's laboratory is supported by the Austrian Science Fund (FWF) through grants P25186-B22, P30992-B28, and SFB F6103.

REFERENCES

1. Medzhitov R. Inflammation 2010: new adventures of an old flame. *Cell* (2010) 140:771–6. doi: 10.1016/j.cell.2010.03.006
2. O'Neill LAJ. When signaling pathways collide: positive and negative regulation of toll-like receptor signal transduction. *Immunity* (2008) 29:12–20. doi: 10.1016/j.immuni.2008.06.004
3. Hu M-M, Shu H-B. Cytoplasmic mechanisms of recognition and defense of microbial nucleic acids. *Annu Rev Cell Dev Biol.* (2018) 34: 357–9. doi: 10.1146/annurev-cellbio-100617-062903
4. Natoli G, Ghisletti S, Barozzi I. The genomic landscapes of inflammation. *Genes Dev.* (2011) 25:101–6. doi: 10.1101/gad.2018811
5. Glass CK, Natoli G. Molecular control of activation and priming in macrophages. *Nature Immunol.* (2016) 17:26–33. doi: 10.1038/ni.3306
6. Martinez FO, Gordon S. The M1 and M2 paradigm of macrophage activation: time for reassessment. *F1000Prime Rep.* (2014) 6:13. doi: 10.12703/P6-13
7. Ostuni R, Kratochvill F, Murray PJ, Natoli G. Macrophages and cancer: from mechanisms to therapeutic implications. *Trends Immunol.* (2015) 36:229–39. doi: 10.1016/j.it.2015.02.004
8. Murray PJ. Macrophage polarization. *Annu Rev Physiol.* (2017) 79:541–66. doi: 10.1146/annurev-physiol-022516-034339
9. Chávez-Galán L, Olleros ML, Vesin D, Garcia I. Much more than M1 and M2 macrophages, there are also CD169(+) and TCR(+) macrophages. *Front Immunol.* (2015) 6:263. doi: 10.3389/fimmu.2015.00263
10. Levy DE, Darnell JEJ. Stats: transcriptional control and biological impact. *Nat Rev Mol Cell Biol.* (2002) 3:651–2. doi: 10.1038/nrm909
11. Stark GR, Darnell JE. The JAK-STAT pathway at twenty. *Immunity* (2012) 36:503–14. doi: 10.1016/j.immuni.2012.03.013
12. Hayden MS, Ghosh S. NF-κB, the first quarter-century: remarkable progress and outstanding questions. *Genes Dev.* (2012) 26, 203–14. doi: 10.1101/gad.183434.111
13. Oeckinghaus A, Hayden MS, Ghosh S. Crosstalk in NF-κB signaling pathways. *Nature Immunol.* (2011) 12:695–708. doi: 10.1038/ni.2065
14. Tamura T, Yanai H, Savitsky D, Taniguchi T. The IRF family transcription factors in immunity and oncogenesis. *Ann Rev Immunol.* (2008) 26:535–84. doi: 10.1146/annurev.immunol.26.021607.090400
15. Negishi H, Taniguchi T, Yanai H. The Interferon (IFN) class of cytokines and the IFN regulatory factor (IRF) transcription factor family. *Cold Spring Harb Perspect Biol.* (2017). doi: 10.1101/cshperspect.a028423. [Epub ahead of print].
16. Mertens C, Zhong M, Krishnaraj R, Zou W, Chen X, Darnell JE. Dephosphorylation of phosphotyrosine on STAT1 dimers requires extensive spatial reorientation of the monomers facilitated by the N-terminal domain. *Genes Dev.* (2006) 20:3372–81. doi: 10.1101/gad.1485406
17. Decker T, Kovarik P, Meinke A. Gas elements: a few nucleotides with a major impact on cytokine-induced gene expression. *J Interferon Cytokine Res.* (1997) 17:121–34.
18. Honda K, Taniguchi T. IRFs: master regulators of signalling by Toll-like receptors and cytosolic pattern-recognition receptors. *Nat Rev.* (2006) 6:644–58. doi: 10.1038/nri1900
19. Escalante CR, Yie J, Thanos D, Aggarwal AK. Structure of IRF-1 with bound DNA reveals determinants of interferon regulation. *Nature* (1998) 391:103–06. doi: 10.1038/34224
20. Tanaka N, Kawakami T, Taniguchi T. Recognition DNA sequences of interferon regulatory factor 1 (IRF-1) and IRF-2, regulators of cell growth and the interferon system. *Mol Cell Biol.* (1993) 13:4531–8.
21. Mamane Y, Heylbroeck C, Genin P, Algarte M, Servant MJ, LePage C, et al. Interferon regulatory factors: the next generation. *Gene* (1999) 237:1–14.

22. Taniguchi T, Ogasawara K, Takaoka A, Tanaka N. Irf family of transcription factors as regulators of host defense. *Ann Rev Immunol.* (2001) 19:623–55. doi: 10.1146/annurev.immunol.19.1.623
23. Chen X, Vinkemeier U, Zhao Y, Jeruzalmi D, Darnell JEJ, Kuriyan J. Crystal structure of a tyrosine phosphorylated STAT-1 dimer bound to DNA. *Cell* (1998) 93:827–39.
24. Schmitz ML, Baeuerle PA. The p65 subunit is responsible for the strong transcription activating potential of NF-kappa B. *EMBO J.* (1991) 10:3805–17. doi: 10.1002/j.1460-2075.1991.tb04950.x
25. Ghosh G, Wang VY-F, Huang D-B, Fusco A. NF-κB regulation: lessons from structures. *Immunol Rev.* (2012) 246:36–58. doi: 10.1111/j.1600-065X.2012.01097.x
26. Reich NC, Liu L. Tracking STAT nuclear traffic. *Nat Rev Immunol.* (2006) 6:602–12. doi: 10.1038/nri1885
27. Levy DE, Kessler DS, Pine R, Reich N, Darnell JEJ. Interferon-induced nuclear factors that bind a shared promoter element correlate with positive and negative transcriptional control. *Genes Dev.* (1988) 2:383–93.
28. Mariani M, Dasmeh P, Fortin A, Kalamujic M, Caron E, Harrison AN, et al. RNASeq analysis identifies non-canonical role of STAT2 and IRF9 in the regulation of a STAT1-independent antiviral and immunoregulatory transcriptional program induced by IFNβ and TNFα. *bioRxiv [preprint]* (2018). doi: 10.1101/273623
29. Platanitis E, Demiroz D, Capelle C, Schneller A, Hartl M, Gossenreiter T, et al. Homeostatic and Interferon-induced gene expression represent different states of promoter-associated transcription factor ISGF3. *bioRxiv [preprint]* (2018). doi: 10.1101/377275
30. Cheon H, Stark GR. Unphosphorylated STAT1 prolongs the expression of interferon-induced immune regulatory genes. *Proc Natl Acad Sci USA.* (2009) 106:9373–78. doi: 10.1073/pnas.0903487106
31. Fink K, Grandvaux N. STAT2 and IRF9: Beyond ISGF3. *JAK-STAT* (2013) 2:e27521. doi: 10.4161/jkst.27521
32. Blaszczyk K, Nowicka H, Kostyrko K, Antonczyk A, Wesoly J, Bluyssen HAR. The unique role of STAT2 in constitutive and IFN-induced transcription and antiviral responses. *Cytokine Growth Factor Rev.* (2016) 29:71–81. doi: 10.1016/j.cytogfr.2016.02.010
33. Majoros A, Platanitis E, Kernbauer-Hölzl E, Rosebrock F, Müller M, Decker T. Canonical and non-canonical aspects of JAK–STAT signaling: lessons from interferons for cytokine responses. *Front Immunol.* (2017) 8:29–41. doi: 10.3389/fimmu.2017.00029
34. Miyamoto M, Fujita T, Kimura Y, Maruyama M, Harada H, Sudo Y, et al. Regulated expression of a gene encoding a nuclear factor, IRF-1, that specifically binds to IFN-beta gene regulatory elements. *Cell* (1988) 54:903–13.
35. Goodbourn S, Maniatis T. Overlapping positive and negative regulatory domains of the human beta-interferon gene. *Proc Nat Acad Sci USA.* (1988) 85:1447–51
36. Pine R, Decker T, Kessler DS, Levy DE, Darnell JEJ. Purification and cloning of interferon-stimulated gene factor 2 (ISGF2): ISGF2 (IRF-1) can bind to the promoters of both beta interferon- and interferon-stimulated genes but is not a primary transcriptional activator of either. *Mol Cell Biol.* (1990) 10:2448–57.
37. Rengachari S, Groiss S, Devos JM, Caron E, Grandvaux N, Panne D. Structural basis of STAT2 recognition by IRF9 reveals molecular insights into ISGF3 function. *Proc Nat Acad Sci USA.* (2018) 115:E601–9. doi: 10.1073/pnas.1718426115
38. Sharf R, Meraro D, Azriel A, Thornton AM, Ozato K, Petricoin EF, et al. Phosphorylation events modulate the ability of interferon consensus sequence binding protein to interact with interferon regulatory factors and to bind DNA. *J Biol Chem.* (1997) 272:9785–92.
39. Lin R, Hiscott J. A role for casein kinase II phosphorylation in the regulation of IRF-1 transcriptional activity. *Mol Cell Biochem.* (1999) 191:169–80.
40. Ren J, Chen X, Chen ZJ. IKKβ is an IRF5 kinase that instigates inflammation. *Proc Nat Acad Sci USA.* (2014) 111:17438–43. doi: 10.1073/pnas.1418516111
41. Fitzgerald KA, McWhirter SM, Faia KL, Rowe DC, Latz E, Golenbock DT, et al. IKKepsilon and TBK1 are essential components of the IRF3 signaling pathway. *Nat Immunol.* (2003) 4:491–6.
42. Andrilenas KK, Ramlall V, Kurland J, Leung B, Harbaugh AG, Siggers T. DNA-binding landscape of IRF3, IRF5 and IRF7 dimers: implications for dimer-specific gene regulation. *Nucleic Acids Res.* (2018) 46:2509–20. doi: 10.1093/nar/gky002
43. Pine R, Canova A, Schindler C. Tyrosine phosphorylated p91 binds to a single element in the ISGF2/IRF-1 promoter to mediate induction by IFN alpha and IFN gamma, and is likely to autoregulate the p91 gene. *EMBO J.* (1994) 13:158–67.
44. Pine R. Convergence of TNFa and IFNg signalling pathways through synergistic induction of IRF-1/ISGF-2 is mediated by a composite GAS/kB element. *Nucleic Acids Res.* (1997) 25:4346–54.
45. Kanno Y, Kozak CA, Schindler C, Driggers PH, Ennist DL, Gleason SL, et al. The genomic structure of the murine ICSBP gene reveals the presence of the gamma interferon-responsive element, to which an ISGF3 alpha subunit (or similar) molecule binds. *Mol Cell Biol.* (1993) 13:3951–63.
46. Contursi C, Wang IM, Gabriele L, Gadina M, O'Shea J, Morse HC3, et al. IFN consensus sequence binding protein potentiates STAT1-dependent activation of IFNγ-responsive promoters in macrophages. *Proc Natl Acad Sci USA.* (2000) 97:91–6. doi: 10.1073/pnas.97.1.91
47. Mancino A, Termanini A, Barozzi I, Ghisletti S, Ostuni R, Prosperini E, et al. A dual cis-regulatory code links IRF8 to constitutive and inducible gene expression in macrophages. *Genes Dev.* (2015) 29:394–408. doi: 10.1101/gad.257592.114
48. Langlais D, Barreiro LB, Gros P. The macrophage IRF8/IRF1 regulome is required for protection against infections and is associated with chronic inflammation. *J Exp Med.* (2016) 213:585–603. doi: 10.1084/jem.20151764
49. Farlik M, Reutterer B, Schindler C, Greten F, Vogl C, Müller M, et al. initiation complex assembly by STAT and NF-kappaB transcription factors regulates nitric oxide synthase expression. *Immunity* (2010) 33:25–34. doi: 10.1016/j.immuni.2010.07.001
50. Wienerroither S, Shukla P, Farlik M, Majoros A, Stych B, Vogl C, et al. Cooperative transcriptional activation of antimicrobial genes by STAT and NF-κB pathways by concerted recruitment of the mediator complex. *Cell Rep.* (2015) 12:300–12. doi: 10.1016/j.celrep.2015.06.021
51. Wienerroither S, Rauch I, Rosebrock F, Jamieson AM, Bradner J, Muhar M, et al. Regulation of NO synthesis, local inflammation, and innate immunity to pathogens by BET family proteins. *Mol Cell Biol.* (2014) 34:415–27. doi: 10.1128/MCB.01353-13
52. Ramsauer K, Farlik M, Zupkovitz G, Seiser C, Kröger A, Hauser H, et al. Distinct modes of action applied by transcription factors STAT1 and IRF1 to initiate transcription of the IFN-gamma-inducible gbp2 gene. *Proc Nat Acad Sci USA.* (2007) 104:2849–54. doi: 10.1073/pnas.0610944104
53. Leung TH, Hoffmann A, Baltimore D. One nucleotide in a κB site can determine cofactor specificity for NF-κB dimers. *Cell* (2004) 118:453–64. doi: 10.1016/j.cell.2004.08.007
54. Ogawa S, Lozach J, Benner C, Pascual G, Tangirala RK, Westin S, et al. Molecular determinants of crosstalk between nuclear receptors and toll-like receptors. *Cell* (2005) 122:707–21. doi: 10.1016/j.cell.2005.06.029
55. Nan J, Wang Y, Yang J, Stark GR. IRF9 and unphosphorylated STAT2 cooperate with NF-κB to drive IL6 expression. *Proc Natl Acad Sci USA.* (2018) 115:3906–911. doi: 10.1073/pnas.1714102115
56. Bennett BL, Cruz R, Lacson RG, Manning AM. Interleukin-4 suppression of tumor necrosis factor alpha-stimulated E-selectin gene transcription is mediated by STAT6 antagonism of NF-kappaB. *J Biol Chem.* (1997) 272:10212–19. doi: 10.1074/jbc.272.15.10212
57. Czimmerer Z, Daniel B, Horvath A, Rückerl D, Nagy G, Kiss M, et al. The transcription factor STAT6 mediates direct repression of inflammatory enhancers and limits activation of alternatively polarized macrophages. *Immunity* (2018) 48:75–90.e6. doi: 10.1016/j.immuni.2017.12.010
58. Esashi E, Wang YH, Perng O, Qin XF, Liu YJ, Watowich SS. The signal transducer STAT5 inhibits plasmacytoid dendritic cell development by suppressing transcription factor IRF8. *Immunity* (2008) 28:509–20. doi: 10.1016/j.immuni.2008.02.013
59. Heinz S, Benner C, Spann N, Bertolino E, Yin YC, Laslo P, et al. Simple combinations of lineage-determining transcription factors prime cis-regulatory elements required for macrophage and B cell identities. *Mol Cell.* (2010) 38:576–89. doi: 10.1016/j.molcel.2010.05.004
60. Ghisletti S, Barozzi I, Mietton F, Polletti S, De Santa F, Venturini E, et al. Identification and characterization of enhancers controlling the

inflammatory gene expression program in macrophages. *Immunity* (2010) 32:317–28. doi: 10.1016/j.immuni.2010.02.008

61. Kaikkonen MU, Spann NJ, Heinz S, Romanoski CE, Allison KA, Stender JD, et al. Remodeling of the enhancer landscape during macrophage activation is coupled to enhancer transcription. *Mol Cell* (2013) 51:310–25. doi: 10.1016/j.molcel.2013.07.010
62. Kanno Y, Levi BZ, Tamura T, Ozato K. Immune cell-specific amplification of interferon signaling by the IRF-4/8-PU.1 complex. *J Interferon Cytokine Res.* (2005) 25:770–79. doi: 10.1089/jir.2005.25.770
63. Ostuni R, Piccolo V, Barozzi I, Polletti S, Termanini A, Bonifacio S, et al. Latent enhancers activated by stimulation in differentiated cells. *Cell* (2013) 152:157–71. doi: 10.1016/j.cell.2012.12.018
64. Lawrence T, Natoli G. Transcriptional regulation of macrophage polarization: enabling diversity with identity. *Nat Rev.* (2011) 11:750–61. doi: 10.1038/nri3088
65. O'Neill LAJ, Pearce EJ. Immunometabolism governs dendritic cell and macrophage function. *J Exp Med.* (2016) 213:15–23. doi: 10.1084/jem.20151570
66. Schleicher U, Paduch K, Debus A, Obermeyer S, König T, Kling JC, et al. TNF-mediated restriction of arginase 1 expression in myeloid cells triggers type 2 NO synthase activity at the site of infection. *Cell Rep.* (2016) 15:1062–75. doi: 10.1016/j.celrep.2016.04.001
67. Van den Bossche J, Baardman J, Otto NA, van der Velden S, Neele AE, van den Berg SM, et al. Mitochondrial dysfunction prevents repolarization of inflammatory macrophages. *Cell Rep.* (2016) 17:684–96. doi: 10.1016/j.celrep.2016.09.008
68. Pope SD, Medzhitov R. Emerging principles of gene expression programs and their regulation. *Mol Cell* (2018) 71:389–97. doi: 10.1016/j.molcel.2018.07.017
69. Ramirez-Carrozzi VR, Braas D, Bhatt DM, Cheng CS, Hong C, Doty KR, et al. A unifying model for the selective regulation of inducible transcription by CpG islands and nucleosome remodeling. *Cell* (2009) 138:114–28. doi: 10.1016/j.cell.2009.04.020
70. Hargreaves DC, Horng T, Medzhitov R. Control of inducible gene expression by signal-dependent transcriptional elongation. *Cell* (2009) 138:129–45. doi: 10.1016/j.cell.2009.05.047
71. Nicodeme E, Jeffrey KL, Schaefer U, Beinke S, Dewell S, Chung C-W, et al. Suppression of inflammation by a synthetic histone mimic. *Nature* (2010) 468:1119–23. doi: 10.1038/nature09589
72. Adelman K, Lis JT. Promoter-proximal pausing of RNA polymerase II: emerging roles in metazoans. *Nat Rev Genet.* (2012) 13:720–31. doi: 10.1038/nrg3293
73. Diamant G, Dikstein R. Transcriptional control by NF-κB: elongation in focus. *Biochim et Biophys Acta* (2013) 1829:937–45. doi: 10.1016/j.bbagrm.2013.04.007
74. Hemmi H, Takeuchi O, Sato S, Yamamoto M, Kaisho T, Sanjo H, et al. The roles of two IkappaB kinase-related kinases in lipopolysaccharide and double stranded RNA signaling and viral infection. *J Exp Med.* (2004) 199:1641–50. doi: 10.1084/jem.20040520
75. Hoshino K, Sugiyama T, Matsumoto M, Tanaka T, Saito M, Hemmi H, et al. IκB kinase-α is critical for interferon-α production induced by Toll-like receptors 7 and 9. *Nature* (2006) 440:949–53. doi: 10.1038/nature04641
76. Park S-H, Kang K, Giannopoulou E, Qiao Y, Kang K, Kim G, et al. Type I interferons and the cytokine TNF cooperatively reprogram the macrophage epigenome to promote inflammatory activation. *Nat Immunol.* (2017) 18:1104–16. doi: 10.1038/ni.3818
77. Agalioti T, Lomvardas S, Parekh B, Yie J, Maniatis T, Thanos D. Ordered recruitment of chromatin modifying and general transcription factors to the IFN-beta promoter. *Cell* (2000) 103:667–78. doi: 10.1016/S0092-8674(00)00169-0
78. Panne D, Maniatis T, Harrison SC. An atomic model of the interferon-beta enhanceosome. *Cell* (2007) 129:1111–23. doi: 10.1016/j.cell.2007.05.019
79. Freaney JE, Kim R, Mandhana R, Horvath CM. Extensive cooperation of immune master regulators IRF3 and NFκB in RNA Pol II recruitment and pause release in human innate antiviral transcription. *Cell Rep.* (2013) 4:959–73. doi: 10.1016/j.celrep.2013.07.043
80. Rubio D, Xu R-H, Remakus S, Krouse TE, Truckenmiller ME, Thapa RJ, et al. Crosstalk between the Type 1 interferon and nuclear factor kappa B pathways confers resistance to a lethal virus infection. *Cell Host Microbe* (2013) 13:701–10. doi: 10.1016/j.chom.2013.04.015
81. Saliba DG, Heger A, Eames HL, Oikonomopoulos S, Teixeira A, Blazek K, et al. IRF5:RelA interaction targets inflammatory genes in macrophages. *Cell Rep* (2014) 8:1308–17. doi: 10.1016/j.celrep.2014.07.034
82. Dalmas E, Toubal A, Alzaid F, Blazek K, Eames HL, Lebozec K, et al. Irf5 deficiency in macrophages promotes beneficial adipose tissue expansion and insulin sensitivity during obesity. *Nat Med.* (2015) 21:610–18. doi: 10.1038/nm.3829
83. Begitt A, Droescher M, Meyer T, Schmid CD, Baker M, Antunes F, et al. STAT1-cooperative DNA binding distinguishes type 1 from type 2 interferon signaling. *Nat Immunol.* (2014) 15:168–76. doi: 10.1038/ni.2794
84. Kamijo R, Harada H, Matsuyama T, Bosland M, Gerecitano J, Shapiro D, et al. Requirement for transcription factor IRF-1 in NO synthase induction in macrophages. *Science* (1994) 263:1612–15.
85. Kimura T, Kadokawa Y, Harada H, Matsumoto M, Sato M, Kashiwazaki Y, et al. Essential and non-redundant roles of p48 (ISGF3γ) and IRF-1 in both type I and type II interferon responses, as revealed by gene targeting studies. *Genes Cells* (1996) 1:115–24. doi: 10.1046/j.1365-2443.1996.08008.x
86. Farlik M, Rapp B, Marie I, Levy DE, Jamieson AM, Decker T. Contribution of a TANK-binding kinase 1-interferon (IFN) regulatory factor 7 pathway to IFN-γ-induced gene expression. *Mol Cell Biol.* (2012) 32:1032–43. doi: 10.1128/MCB.06021-11
87. Reis LF, Ruffner H, Stark G, Aguet M, Weissmann C. Mice devoid of interferon regulatory factor 1 (IRF-1) show normal expression of type I interferon genes. *EMBO J.* (1994) 13:4798–806.
88. Tailor P, Tamura T, Morse HC, Ozato K. The BXH2 mutation in IRF8 differentially impairs dendritic cell subset development in the mouse. *Blood* (2008) 111:1942–5. doi: 10.1182/blood-2007-07-100750
89. Shen Y, Darnell JE. Antiviral response in cells containing Stat1 with heterologous transactivation domains. *J Virol.* (2001) 75:2627–33. doi: 10.1128/JVI.75.6.2627-2633.2001
90. Kraus TA, Lau JF, Parisien J-P, Horvath CM. A hybrid IRF9-STAT2 protein recapitulates interferon-stimulated gene expression and antiviral response. *J Biol Chem.* (2003) 278:13033–38. doi: 10.1074/jbc.M212972200
91. Ni Z, Karaskov E, Yu T, Callaghan SM, Der S, Park DS, et al. Apical role for BRG1 in cytokine-induced promoter assembly. *Proc Natl Acad Sci USA.* (2005) 102:14611–16. doi: 10.1073/pnas.0503070102
92. Mostafavi S, Yoshida H, Moodley D, LeBoité H, Rothamel K, Raj T, et al. Parsing the interferon transcriptional network and its disease associations. *Cell* (2016) 164:564–78. doi: 10.1016/j.cell.2015.12.032
93. Au-Yeung N, Horvath CM. Histone H2A.Z suppression of interferon-stimulated transcription and antiviral immunity is modulated by GCN5 and BRD2. *iScience* (2018) 6:68–82. doi: 10.1016/j.isci.2018.07.013
94. Ivashkiv LB. IFNγ: signalling, epigenetics and roles in immunity, metabolism, disease and cancer immunotherapy. *Nat Rev.* (2018) 31:1. doi: 10.1038/s41577-018-0029-z
95. Kumatori A, Yang D, Suzuki S, Nakamura M. Cooperation of STAT-1 and IRF-1 in interferon-gamma-induced transcription of the gp91(phox) gene. *J Biol Chem.* (2002) 277:9103–11. doi: 10.1074/jbc.M109803200
96. Ni Z, Abou El Hassan M, Xu Z, Yu T, Bremner R. The chromatin-remodeling enzyme BRG1 coordinates CIITA induction through many interdependent distal enhancers. *Nat Immunol.* (2008) 9:785–93. doi: 10.1038/ni.1619
97. Hassan El MA, Huang K, Eswara MBK, Xu Z, Yu T, Aubry A, et al. Properties of STAT1 and IRF1 enhancers and the influence of SNPs. *BMC Mol Biol.* (2017) 18:6. doi: 10.1186/s12867-017-0084-1
98. Qiao Y, Giannopoulou EG, Chan CH, Park S-H, Gong S, Chen J, et al. Synergistic activation of inflammatory cytokine genes by interferon-γ-induced chromatin remodeling and toll-like receptor signaling. *Immunity* (2013) 39:454–69. doi: 10.1016/j.immuni.2013.08.009
99. Lehtonen A, Veckman V, Nikula T, Lahesmaa R, Kinnunen L, Matikainen S, et al. Differential expression of IFN regulatory factor 4 gene in human monocyte-derived dendritic cells and macrophages. *J Immunol.* (2005) 175:6570–9. doi: 10.4049/jimmunol.175.10.6570
100. Hsu AT, Lupancu TJ, Lee M-C, Fleetwood AJ, Cook AD, Hamilton JA, et al. Epigenetic and transcriptional regulation of IL4-induced CCL17 production in human monocytes and murine macrophages. *J Biol Chem.* (2018) 293: 11415–23. doi: 10.1074/jbc.RA118.002416

101. Satoh T, Takeuchi O, Vandenbon A, Yasuda K, Tanaka Y, Kumagai Y, et al. The Jmjd3-Irf4 axis regulates M2 macrophage polarization and host responses against helminth infection. *Nat Immunol.* (2010) 11:936–44. doi: 10.1038/ni.1920
102. Piccolo V, Curina A, Genua M, Ghisletti S, Simonatto M, Sabò A, et al. Opposing macrophage polarization programs show extensive epigenomic and transcriptional cross-talk. *Nat Immunol.* (2017) 18:530–40. doi: 10.1038/ni.3710
103. Yamagata M, Merlie JP, Sanes JR. Interspecific comparisons reveal conserved features of the Drosophila Toll protein. *Gene* (1994) 139:223–8.
104. Rosenbauer F, Waring JF, Foerster J, Wietstruk M, Philipp D, Horak I. Interferon consensus sequence binding protein and interferon regulatory factor-4/pip form a complex that represses the expression of the interferon-stimulated gene-15 in macrophages. *Blood* (1999) 94:4274–81.
105. Meraro D, Gleit-Kielmanowicz M, Hauser H, Levi B-Z. IFN-stimulated gene 15 is synergistically activated through interactions between the myelocyte/lymphocyte-specific transcription factors, PU.1, IFN regulatory factor-8/IFN consensus sequence binding protein, and IFN regulatory factor-4: characterization of a new subtype of IFN-stimulated response element. *J Immunol.* (2002) 168:6224–31. doi: 10.4049/jimmunol.168.12.6224
106. Wu X, Briseño CG, Durai V, Albring JC, Haldar M, Bagadia P, et al. Mafb lineage tracing to distinguish macrophages from other immune lineages reveals dual identity of Langerhans cells. *J Exp Med.* (2016) 213:2553–65. doi: 10.1084/jem.20160600
107. Qiao Y, Kang K, Giannopoulou E, Fang C, Ivashkiv LB. IFN-γ induces histone 3 lysine 27 trimethylation in a small subset of promoters to stably silence gene expression in human macrophages. *Cell Rep.* (2016) 16:3121–29. doi: 10.1016/j.celrep.2016.08.051
108. Kang K, Park S-H, Chen J, Qiao Y, Giannopoulou E, Berg K, et al. Interferon-γ represses M2 gene expression in human macrophages by disassembling enhancers bound by the transcription factor MAF. *Immunity* (2017) 47:235–250.e4. doi: 10.1016/j.immuni.2017.07.017
109. Biswas SK, Lopez-Collazo E. Endotoxin tolerance: new mechanisms, molecules and clinical significance. *Trends Immunol.* (2009) 30:475–87. doi: 10.1016/j.it.2009.07.009
110. Yan Q, Carmody RJ, Qu Z, Ruan Q, Jager J, Mullican SE, et al. Nuclear factor-κB binding motifs specify Toll-like receptor-induced gene repression through an inducible repressosome. *Proc Natl Acad Sci USA.* (2012) 109:14140–45. doi: 10.1073/pnas.1119842109
111. Kastenbauer S, Ziegler-Heitbrock HW. NF-kappaB1 (p50) is upregulated in lipopolysaccharide tolerance and can block tumor necrosis factor gene expression. *Infect Immun.* (1999) 67:1553–59.
112. Bohuslav J, Kravchenko VV, Parry GC, Erlich JH, Gerondakis S, Mackman N, et al. Regulation of an essential innate immune response by the p50 subunit of NF-kappaB. *J Clin Invest.* (1998) 102:1645–52. doi: 10.1172/JCI3877
113. Novakovic B, Habibi E, Wang S-Y, Arts RJW, Davar R, Megchelenbrink W, et al. β-Glucan reverses the epigenetic state of lps-induced immunological tolerance. *Cell* (2016) 167:1354–1368.e14. doi: 10.1016/j.cell.2016.09.034
114. Chen J, Ivashkiv LB. IFN-γ abrogates endotoxin tolerance by facilitating Toll-like receptor-induced chromatin remodeling. *Proc Natl Acad Sci USA.* (2010) 107:19438–43. doi: 10.1073/pnas.1007816107
115. Foster SL, Hargreaves DC, Medzhitov R. Gene-specific control of inflammation by TLR-induced chromatin modifications. *Nature* (2007) 447:972–8. doi: 10.1038/nature05836
116. Netea MG, Joosten LAB, Latz E, Mills KHG, Natoli G, Stunnenberg HG, et al. Trained immunity: a program of innate immune memory in health and disease. *Science* (2016) 352:aaf1098. doi: 10.1126/science.aaf1098
117. Saeed S, Quintin J, Kerstens HHD, Rao NA, Aghajanirefah A, Matarese F, et al. Epigenetic programming of monocyte-to-macrophage differentiation and trained innate immunity. *Science* (2014) 345:1251086. doi: 10.1126/science.1251086
118. Ifrim DC, Quintin J, Kessel LM, Plantinga TS, Joosten LAB, van der Meer JWM, et al. Defective trained immunity in patients with STAT-1-dependent chronic mucocutaneaous candidiasis. *Clin Exp Immunol.* (2015) 181:434–40. doi: 10.1111/cei.12642
119. Satpathy AT, Wu X, Albring JC, Murphy KM. Re(de)fining the dendritic cell lineage. *Nat Immunol.* (2012) 13:1145–54. doi: 10.1038/ni.2467
120. Li HS, Watowich SS. A STATus report on DC development. *J Leukocyte Biol.* (2012) 92:445–59. doi: 10.1189/jlb.0212052
121. Laouar Y, Welte T, Fu XY, Flavell RA. STAT3 is required for Flt3L-dependent dendritic cell differentiation. *Immunity* (2003) 19:903–912. doi: 10.1016/S1074-7613(03)00332-7
122. Liu Y-J. IPC: professional type 1 interferon-producing cells and plasmacytoid dendritic cell precursors. *Ann Rev Immunol.* (2005) 23:275–306. doi: 10.1146/annurev.immunol.23.021704.115633
123. Alculumbre SG, Saint-André V, Di Domizio J, Vargas P, Sirven P, Bost P, et al. Diversification of human plasmacytoid predendritic cells in response to a single stimulus. *Nat Immunol.* (2018) 19:63–75. doi: 10.1038/s41590-017-0012-z
124. Wimmers F, Subedi N, van Buuringen N, Heister D, Vivié J, Beeren-Reinieren I, et al. Single-cell analysis reveals that stochasticity and paracrine signaling control interferon-alpha production by plasmacytoid dendritic cells. *Nat Commun.* (2018) 9:3317. doi: 10.1038/s41467-018-05784-3
125. Luft T, Pang KC, Thomas E, Hertzog P, Hart DNJ, Trapani J, et al. Type I IFNs enhance the terminal differentiation of dendritic cells. *J Immunol.* (1998) 161:1947–53.
126. Pantel A, Teixeira A, Haddad E, Wood EG, Steinman RM, Longhi MP. Direct Type I IFN but Not MDA5/TLR3 activation of dendritic cells is required for maturation and metabolic shift to glycolysis after poly ic stimulation. *PLoS Biol.* (2014) 12:e1001759. doi: 10.1371/journal.pbio.1001759
127. Hahm B, Trifilo MJ, Zuniga EI, Oldstone MB. Viruses evade the immune system through type I interferon-mediated STAT2-dependent, but STAT1-independent, signaling. *Immunity* (2005) 22:247–257. doi: 10.1016/j.immuni.2005.01.005
128. Li HS, Gelbard A, Martinez GJ, Esashi E, Zhang H, Nguyen-Jackson H, et al. Cell-intrinsic role for IFN-α-STAT1 signals in regulating murine Peyer patch plasmacytoid dendritic cells and conditioning an inflammatory response. *Blood* (2011) 118:3879–89. doi: 10.1182/blood-2011-04-349761
129. Geissmann F, Gordon S, Hume DA, Mowat AM, Randolph GJ. Unravelling mononuclear phagocyte heterogeneity. *Nat Rev.* (2010) 10:453–60. doi: 10.1038/nri2784
130. Bedoui S, Whitney PG, Waithman J, Eidsmo L, Wakim L, Caminschi I, et al. Cross-presentation of viral and self antigens by skin-derived CD103+ dendritic cells. *Nat Immunol.* (2009) 10:488–95. doi: 10.1038/ni.1724
131. Edelson BT, KC W, Juang R, Kohyama M, Benoit LA, Klekotka PA, et al. Peripheral CD103+ dendritic cells form a unified subset developmentally related to CD8alpha+ conventional dendritic cells. *J Exp Med.* (2010) 207:823–36. doi: 10.1084/jem.20091627
132. Lindstedt M, Lundberg K, Borrebaeck CAK. Gene family clustering identifies functionally associated subsets of human *in vivo* blood and tonsillar dendritic cells. *J Immunol.* (2005) 175: 4839–6. doi: 10.4049/jimmunol.175.8.4839
133. Robbins SH, Walzer T, Dembélé D, Thibault C, Defays A, Bessou G, et al. Novel insights into the relationships between dendritic cell subsets in human and mouse revealed by genome-wide expression profiling. *Genome Biol.* (2008) 9:R17. doi: 10.1186/gb-2008-9-1-r17
134. Ginhoux F, Liu K, Helft J, Bogunovic M, Greter M, Hashimoto D, et al. The origin and development of nonlymphoid tissue CD103+ DCs. *J Exp Med.* (2009) 206:3115–30. doi: 10.1084/jem.20091756
135. Durai V, Murphy KM. Functions of murine dendritic cells. *Immunity* (2016) 45:719–36. doi: 10.1016/j.immuni.2016.10.010
136. Garber M, Nir Y, Goren A, Raychowdhury R, Thielke A, Guttmann M, et al. A high-throughput chromatin immunoprecipitation approach reveals principles of dynamic gene regulation in mammals. a high-throughput chromatin immunoprecipitation approach reveals principles of dynamic gene regulation in mammals. *Mol Cell* (2012) 47:810–22. doi: 10.1016/j.molcel.2012.07.030
137. Amit I, Winter DR, Jung S. The role of the local environment and epigenetics in shaping macrophage identity and their effect on tissue homeostasis. *Nat Immunol.* (2016) 17:18–25. doi: 10.1038/ni.3325

138. Dekker J, Mirny L. The 3D genome as moderator of chromosomal communication. *Cell* (2016) 164:1110–21. doi: 10.1016/j.cell.2016.02.007
139. Rozenblatt-Rosen O, Stubbington MJT, Regev A, Teichmann SA. The human cell atlas: from vision to reality. *Nat News* (2017) 550:451. doi: 10.1038/550451a
140. Murata K, Wolf M. Cryo-electron microscopy for structural analysis of dynamic biological macromolecules. *Biochim Biophys Acta* (2018) 1862:324–34. doi: 10.1016/j.bbagen.2017.07.020
141. Wang H, La Russa M, Qi LS. CRISPR/Cas9 in Genome Editing and Beyond. *Annu Rev Biochem.* (2016) 85:227–64. doi: 10.1146/annurev-biochem-060815-014607

16

The Many Faces of JAKs and STATs within the COVID-19 Storm

*Alice H. Grant, Armando Estrada III, Yoshira M. Ayala-Marin, America Y. Alvidrez-Camacho, Georgialina Rodriguez, Elisa Robles-Escajeda, Denisse A. Cadena-Medina, Alejandro C. Rodriguez and Robert A. Kirken**

Department of Biological Sciences, The University of Texas at El Paso, El Paso, TX, United States

***Correspondence:**
Robert A. Kirken
rkirken@utep.edu

The positive-sense single stranded RNA virus, Severe Acute Respiratory Syndrome Coronavirus 2 (SARS-CoV-2), resulted in a global pandemic with horrendous health and economic consequences not seen in a century. At a finer scale, immunologically, many of these devastating effects by SARS-CoV-2 can be traced to a "cytokine storm" resulting in the simultaneous activation of Janus Kinases (JAKs) and Signal Transducers and Activators of Transcription (STAT) proteins downstream of the many cytokine receptor families triggered by elevated cytokines found in Coronavirus Disease 2019 (COVID-19). In this report, cytokines found in the storm are discussed in relation to the JAK-STAT pathway in response to SARS-CoV-2 and the lessons learned from RNA viruses and previous Coronaviruses (CoVs). Therapeutic strategies to counteract the SARS-CoV-2 mediated storm are discussed with an emphasis on cell signaling and JAK inhibition.

Keywords: JAK, STAT, cytokine, cytokine storm, cytokine release syndrome, JAK inhibitor, COVID-19, SARS-CoV-2

INTRODUCTION

Covid-19 Pathogenesis and the Cytokine Storm

Late 2019 a positive single strand RNA virus crossed over to humans, causing a Coronavirus (CoV) related pneumonia in Wuhan China. The pathogen responsible for the following CoV Disease 2019 (COVID-19) global pandemic was identified as Severe Acute Respiratory Syndrome Coronavirus-2 (SARS-CoV-2) on January 7th, 2020 (1). Unlike past CoVs which can be mildly pathogenic others like SARS-CoV and Middle East Respiratory Syndrome CoV (MERS-CoV) can result in severe disease and fatality (2). SARS-CoV-2 falls into the latter, with an estimated 178,837,204 infected and greater than 3,880,450 deaths worldwide as of June 23rd, 2021 (World Health Organization). For many the cause of death is due to Acute Respiratory Distress Syndrome (ARDS)/respiratory failure, septic shock, or multiorgan system dysfunction (Centers for Disease Control and Prevention). Additionally, COVID-19 related strokes are on the rise likely due to thromboembolism complications (3, 4).

Many of these overt symptoms result from a cytokine release syndrome or "cytokine storm", with uncontrolled anti- and pro-inflammatory components reaching beyond the local site of infection and resulting in systemic collateral damage (5). Disproportional outcomes of COVID-19 pathology are largely attributed to this dysfunctional immune response (6, 7). This notion is supported by findings that asymptomatic individuals display less inflammatory cytokine profiles and a subtle immune response (8).

SARS-CoV-2 infected, hospitalized patients display elevated levels of Interleukins (ILs) IL-2, IL-4, IL-7, IL-9, IL-6, Granulocyte-Colony Stimulating Factor (G-CSF), Granulocyte Macrophage-CSF (GM-CSF), Interferon α2 (IFNα2), Interferon γ (IFNγ), IL-10, IL-1α, IL-1Ra, IL-1β, Macrophage-CSF (M-CSF), IL-12, Tumor Necrosis Factor α (TNFα), IL-17, IL-8, Macrophage Inflammatory Proteins 1A (MIP1A), Macrophage Inflammatory Proteins 1B (MIP1B), Monocyte Chemoattractant Protein-1 (MCP-1), IFNγ-Inducible Protein 10 (IP-10), Fibroblast Growth Factor (FGF), Hepatocyte Growth Factor (HGF), Vascular Endothelial Growth Factor (VEGF), and Platelet-Derived Growth Factor (PDGF) (6, 9). These elevated cytokines subsequently activate multiple cytokine receptor families belonging to the Type I, Type II, Immunoglobulin Superfamily, G-Protein Coupled, TNFα and Growth Factor Receptors. Many of these cytokine receptors rely on the Janus Kinases (JAKs) and Signal Transducers and Activators of Transcription (STAT) proteins to immunologically eradicate the SARS-CoV-2 pathogen and restore immune homeostasis. Cytokines utilizing Type I, Type II and G-Protein Coupled Receptors propagate direct signals through JAKs and STATs and many have been linked to disease severity (**Figure 1**). Others are regulated by or cross-talk with JAK-STAT pathways.

JAK AND STATS

JAKs consist of seven Janus Homology (JH) domains, JH1-JH7, shared across JAK1, JAK2, JAK3 and Tyrosine Kinase 2 (TYK2) (10, 11). JH1 harbors the kinase domain involved in Tyr phosphorylation while the JH2 consists of an "inactive" pseudo-kinase domain regulating overall activity. JH3-JH7 consists of the 4.1R, Ezrin, Radixin, Moesin (FERM) and Src Homology 2 (SH2) domains involved in receptor binding. Canonically, JAKs act by transferring the γ-phosphate of ATP to the hydroxyl side chain of Tyr residues residing on paired receptors, recruiting in SH2 containing proteins, most notably the STATs. Once captured by the receptor, STATs are phosphorylated by the JAKs among other SRC family kinases (12). Subsequent disengagement from the receptor results in STAT dimerization formed by SH2 interactions with phosphorylated Tyr enhancing nuclear translocation and transcriptional activities. The seven STAT family members contain six domains that include the N-terminal, coiled-coil, DNA binding, linker, SH2, and a transactivation domains (10, 13). And although structurally similar, their target genes are overlapping but also unique (14).

JAKS AND THE IMMUNOLOGICAL RESPONSE

The JAK-STAT pathway is essential for various stages of immunity that ranges from initiating signaling events required for innate and adaptive responses to the pathological stage of driving the storm (15, 16). For example, the innate immune system, launches an anti-viral response through JAK dependent IFNs, pro-inflammatory cytokines and chemokines including those found in the cytokine storm (IFNα2, IL-6, IL-8, G-CSF, MCP-1) (17, 18). This initial response seeks to inhibit viral progression and to activate the adaptive immune system. In this second phase, cytokines elicit an appropriate adaptive response to viral infection by facilitating $CD4^+$ T helper (Th) differentiation and or $CD8^+$ T cytotoxic (Tc) and B cell function. Many cytokines cross-talk and are dependent upon the JAK-STAT pathway to affect the spectrum of Th phenotypes that normally respond to a range of pathogenic variation

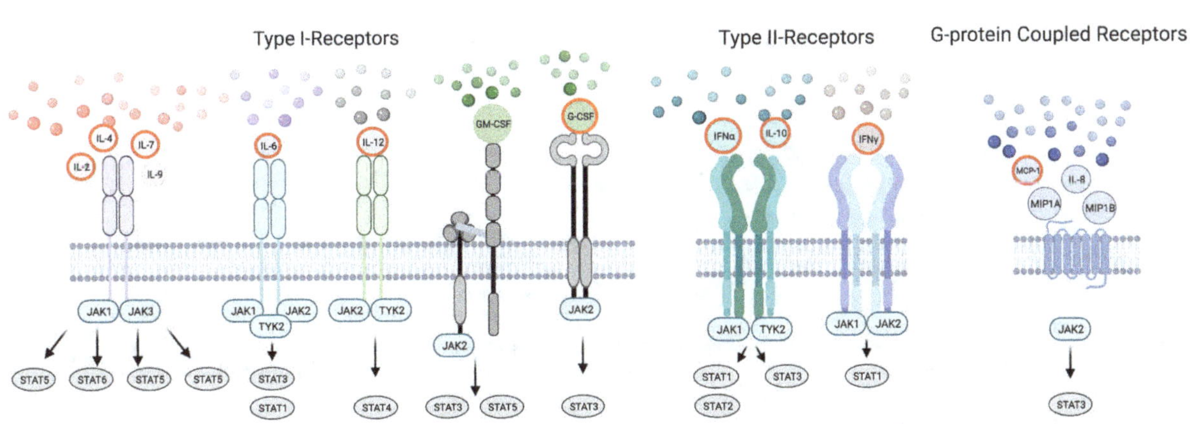

FIGURE 1 | The Cytokine Storm in COVID-19 Utilizes JAKs and STATs. A simple schematic showing elevated cytokines in COVID-19 signaling by Type I, Type II, Immunoglobulin, and G-protein coupled receptors with those correlated to disease severity outlined in red. Paired JAKs are seen signaling immediately downstream of receptors directly activating STATs (solid line).Only the predominantly activated STAT is depicted for shown cytokines.

including among others Th1, Th2, T follicular helper (Tfh), T regulatory (Treg) and Th17 cells (19, 20). Some of these canonical cytokines sway Th differentiation including IFNγ, IL-2, IL-12 towards Th1; IL-2, IL-4 to Th2; IL-12 to Tfh; IL-2 to Treg; and IL-6, IL-1 to Th17 subsets (19). IL-4 and IFNγ inhibit Th1 and Th2 responses respectively (21, 22). Others are produced by Th subtypes including IFNγ, IL-2, TNFα in Th1; IL-4, IL-6, IL-10 in Th2; IL-17 in Th17; and IL-10 in both Tfh and Treg cells. Additionally IL-7, IL-9, MIP1A, MIP1B, MCP-1, and GM-CSF can influence differentiation and adaptive immunity. Failure of the adaptive arm to clear the infection results in a cytokine storm consisting of these latter JAK signaling cytokines (**Figure 2**).

Typically, Th1 cells drive cellular immunity largely accomplished by Tc and NK cells while Th2 and Tfh gear towards humoral immunity utilizing plasma B cells. Treg cells restore and maintain immunological homeostasis (23) while Th17 are crucial in eliciting a response against extracellular pathogens. The signature Th phenotype that succeeds at clearing SARS-CoV-2 infection between asymptomatic, mild/moderate, and severe/critical cases remains elusive. It is implied that asymptomatic and mild to moderate disease achieve viral clearance by intact innate and adaptive responses while hyperinflammation leads to severe/critical disease (24).

It is likely that SARS-CoV-2 immunity in mild to moderate disease is largely accomplished by Th1 responses. Supporting this claim, roughly 70% of non-hospitalized patients that recovered from SARS-CoV-2 infection exhibit virus specific $CD8^+$ Tc cells (25). Furthermore, patients that recovered from past SARS-CoV infection achieve lasting immunity through virus specific memory $CD4^+$ and $CD8^+$ T cells (2). Others have proposed Th2 responses in children translate to the mild outcomes of SARS-CoV-2 infection (26). Although, Tfh and Th2 responses are seen in hospitalized patients (27) with the latter response associated with severe symptoms to SARS-CoV-2 (28). Thus, it is unknown if humoral responses are sufficient to clear SARS-CoV-2 infection (29). Interestingly, unexposed SARS-CoV-2 individuals can present Th cells that recognize the spike viral protein, indicative of past exposure to other CoV (25, 30). Indeed, sera from SARS-CoV-2-uninfected donors contain antibodies against the S2 subunit of the spike protein that can neutralize SARS-CoV-2 (25). SARS-CoV-2–uninfected children and adolescents are more likely than adults to contain these cross reactive and 'protective' antibodies (31). These findings support that immunogenic sites of the spike protein are conserved between other CoV and SARS-CoV-2 (32).

Past CoV have revealed antagonism against the adaptive immune response by impairing $CD4^+$ and $CD8^+$ T cell activation (2). And comparably, severe COVID-19 patients display ineffective Th1 phenotypes indicated by decreased levels of $CD8^+$ Tc cells coupled with markers of exhaustion (33). Lymphopenia in severe COVID-19 patients is met with decreases in both $CD4^+$ and $CD8^+$ T cells (33, 34). Th cells tend to shift towards Th17 cells in severe patients (35, 36) while Tregs are decreased in critically ill patients (35, 37). Details on how Tc and Th cells aid or worsen the progression of COVID-19 are discussed elsewhere (38). Taken together, many severe cases of COVID-19 are accompanied by an uncontrolled immunological response. The latter triggered in part by mechanisms of SARS-CoV-2 immune evasion leading to non-productive cytokine

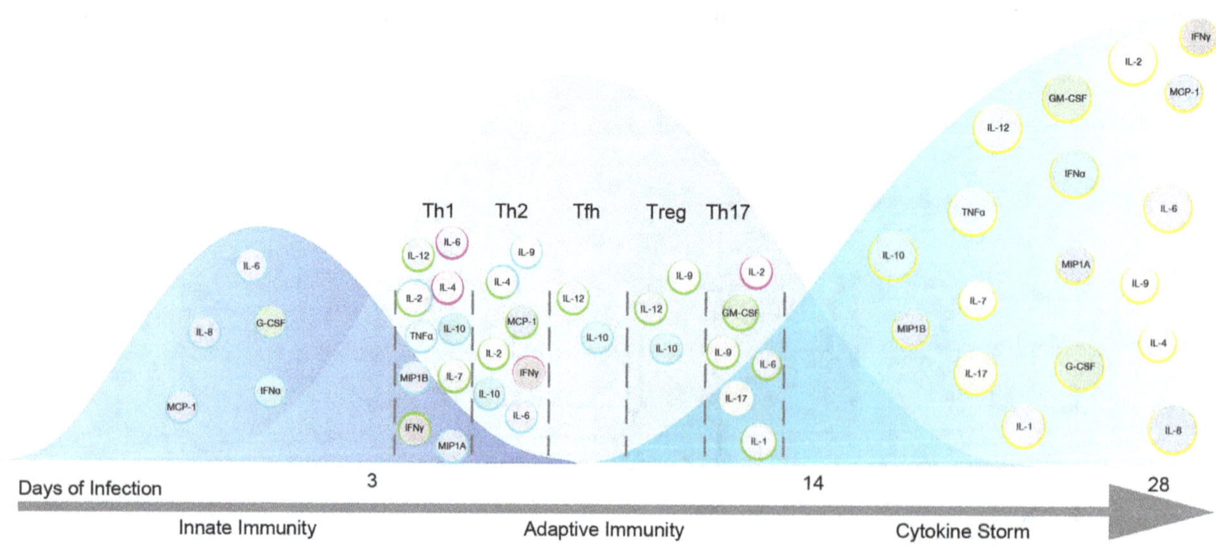

FIGURE 2 | Cytokines within the Storm are Depicted in the Immunological Response to SARS-CoV-2 Infection. A model of the immunological response to SARS-CoV-2 infection displaying cytokines within the storm including those that signal by JAKs and STATs. Cytokines are placed in the immunological timeline based on their expected role in innate and adaptive responses to SARS-CoV-2 infection. Cytokines enhancing immune function are outlined in blue. Cytokines promoting Th differentiation are outlined in green while those inhibiting Th differentiation are outlined in fuchsia. Cytokines are later shown during the COVID-19 cytokine storm outlined in yellow.

profiles (39). Each of these cytokines are discussed below with an emphasis on those that signal through the JAK-STAT pathway.

TYPE I CYTOKINES

γ Chain Family

The common γ chain (γc) cytokines are critical for the survival of T and B cell lineages that generate adaptive immunity to viral infections such as SARS-CoV-2. Emerging data from SARS-CoV-2 patients show increases in nearly all γc cytokines including, IL-2, IL-4, IL-7, and IL-9, were all except IL-9 are associated with disease severity (9, 40). Their respective receptors lacking intrinsic catalytic activity pair with γc and recruit JAK1 and JAK3 to phosphorylate Tyr residues drawing in STAT proteins. Their redundancy ends in part by each STAT protein that is dominantly recruited and phosphorylated in response to a given γc cytokine. Although STATs can be activated at varying degrees, IL-2, IL-7, and IL-9 preferentially activate STAT5A and STAT5B, while IL-4 activates STAT6 (20).

Many γc cytokines are released by naïve or differentiated $CD4^+$ T and $CD8^+$ Tc cells to strengthen the adaptive immune response (41). For example, Th1 cells release IL-2 enhancing Tc differentiation and expansion (42). IL-2 and IL-4 induce Th2 differentiation, where downstream activation of STAT6 by IL-4 regulates Ig gene transcription and switch recombination in plasma B cells (20, 43). IL-7 can induce Th1 differentiation and, like IL-2, is important for the maintenance of memory T cells (44, 45). IL-9, produced by Th2 and Th17 cells has been shown to enhance the suppressive functions of natural Treg cells and promote Th17 differentiation (46, 47).

The simultaneous release of γc cytokines suggests that SARS-CoV-2 fails to generate a single Th phenotype and succeeds at eliciting immunological chaos; perhaps an attempt of redirecting away from cell mediated and humoral responses that aid in viral clearance. Alternatively, elevated levels of γc cytokines in COVID-19, may reflect an attempt to strengthen the adaptive arm of the immune system. Despite the probable increases in γc cytokines acting as growth factors for lymphocytes, lymphopenia is frequently observed in severe COVID-19 patients (33, 34). This paradox has been tackled in depth by others with various explanations (48) including T cell exhaustion. While IL-2 signals are essential for T cell expansion, prolonged IL-2 can mediate exhaustion of $CD8^+$ Tc as well (49, 50).

IL-6

IL-6 is a signature cytokine of inflammation correlating with COVID-19 mortality (51). Binding of IL-6 to its receptor promotes dimerization with gp130 leading to the activation of JAK1, JAK2 and TYK2 (52). JAKs then phosphorylate gp130 to recruit SH2 containing STAT1 and STAT3 that subsequently become phosphorylated. Within various cells, STAT1 and STAT3 form either homo or hetero-dimers acting as transcription factors to regulate expression of multiple genes (53, 54). This in part allows for the pleiotropic activities of IL-6 ranging from polarizing naïve Th cells to supporting differentiation of non-immune cells (55). For example, IL-6 promotes Th2, and Th17 differentiation while inhibiting Th1 responses (56, 57). Among many cytokines discussed hereafter IL-6 also regulates coagulation (58) likely contributing to COVID-19 thrombosis related mortality (59, 60). To ameliorate the effects of IL-6, antibodies generated against IL-6 or its receptor are under clinical trial investigation. However, preliminary data are showing limited efficacy against COVID-19 (61, 62).

IL-12

IL-12 utilizes IL-12p40, IL-12 Receptor β1 (IL-12Rβ1) and IL-12Rβ2 bound to Tyk2 and JAK2, respectively (63). The latter chain creates docking sites for STAT4 that undergoes phosphorylation to regulate transcription and signaling. STAT4 Ser phosphorylation in response to IL-12 has been shown crucial for T cell IFNγ secretion a typical Th1 response (64). IL-12 is also important for Tfh differentiation (65). IL-12p40 mRNA increases rapidly after CNS CoV infection and contributes toward morbidity associated with viral encephalitis (66). Additionally, increased IL-12 expression is correlated with COVID-19 severity (40). Yet, IL-12 is needed by host viral defenses given its influence on Th differentiation. And vaccine development against the SARS-CoV-2 S-protein includes a component of IL-12 based therapy currently in Phase I clinical trials (clinicaltrials.gov).

G-CSF

Severe COVID-19 patients display elevated levels of G-CSF a primary growth factor for neutrophil differentiation (40). G-CSF signaling is mediated through the Tyr receptor kinase G-CSF Receptor (G CSFR) and βc, activating JAK2 and subsequently STAT3 (67, 68). In one study, neutrophilia occurred in more than half of severe COVID-19 patients (69) and is likely attributed in part by the actions of G-CSF.

GM-CSF

GM-CSF also activates JAK2 and STAT3/5 through its GM-CSF Receptor α and βc subunit and is involved in Th17 differentiation (70). Known to link the CNS with inflammation it is perhaps not surprising that elevated levels of GM-CSF are seen in CNS SARS-CoV positive children exhibiting Encephalitis-like syndrome (71). Neurological symptoms seen in SARS-CoV-2 cases have yet to be distinguished as a result from encephalitis, meningitis, or secondary effects of severe infection (72). SARS-CoV-2 viral particles and RNA are observed in neuroanatomical areas that receive olfactory tract projections (73). And other routes of entry for SARS-CoV-2 neuro-invasion have been purposed (74). CNS damage continues to be observed in COVID-19 patients discussed by De Felice et al. (75) and CNS pathologies warrant further investigation.

TYPE II CYTOKINES

Type I and II IFN

Type I IFN (IFN-I) and Type II IFNγ are key in alerting and protecting the body against viral infections (76). Interestingly,

IFNα2 and IFNγ are highly expressed in severe COVID-19 patients. IFN-I acting on their ubiquitously expressed receptors utilize JAK1 and TYK2 for signaling. Once activated the JAKs phosphorylate STAT1 and STAT2, enabling them to complex with IFN Regulatory Factor 9 (IRF9) and initiate transcription of classical IFN stimulated genes involved in antiviral response, immune regulation, and anti-proliferation (76–78). IFNγ utilizes JAK1 and JAK2 signaling to promote STAT1 antiviral activity and drive Th1 differentiation and thus cellular immunity (79, 80). Priming infected cells for destruction, many viruses antagonize IFN responses by targeting the JAK-STAT pathway (81). For example, SARS-CoV Non-Structural Protein 1 (NSP1) acts as a virulence factor for evading the IFN response in part by decreasing phosphorylation of STAT1 (82). STAT3, also downstream of IFN but mainly induced by IL-6, is found dephosphorylated at Tyr 705 in the presence of SARS-CoV (83). Similarly, SARS-CoV-2 ORF3b truncated viral protein in addition to ORF6, and ORF8 can suppress IFN-I signaling (84, 85). Cell lines infected with SARS-CoV-2 show a reduction in JAK1, JAK2, TYK2 and STAT2 protein expression. Moreover, virus-infected cells are not able to induce STAT1, STAT2 and STAT3 phosphorylation to the same extent than non-infected cells in response to IFNα2 (86).

A strategy to harness the initial actions of IFN-I and maintain balance of the immune response, active forms of IFN-I are being investigated in clinical trials against COVID-19 (87, 88). Akin to SARS-CoV, SARS-CoV-2 infection responds similarly to IFN-I therapy, where the timing of its use is critical for efficacy. Specifically, early IFN-I therapy is associated with reduced mortality, while late therapy increases mortality in a retrospective study (89). The timing of effective IFN-I administration is intuitive given its presence in the milieu of cytokines needed to trigger first phase innate immunity, while its delayed presence triggers hyperinflammation (90). However, appealing, IFN-I strategies should be taken with caution given that SARS-CoV-2 can utilize IFNα to induce ACE2 expression, its common route of entry (91).

IL-10

The type II cytokine receptor for IL-10, signals through JAK1 and TYK2 activating STAT3, yet in contrast to IFN yields an anti-inflammatory response inhibiting Th1 differentiation (92). Treg cells achieve their anti-inflammatory effects in part by secreting IL-10 (19). Unlike MERS-CoV, elevated concentrations of IL-10, are seen in SARS-CoV-2 and may be linked to the decreased numbers in CD8$^+$ Tc cells (93, 94). Certain viruses encode IL-10 homologs to suppress the immune system, thus the high levels of IL-10 seen in severe COVID-19 patients likely benefit SARS-CoV-2 (9, 40, 95). However, with the right timing IL-10 can aid in viral clearance when coupled to IFNγ (96). Lastly the anti-inflammatory effects by IL-10 can inhibit coagulation activation and stimulate fibrinolysis (97).

G PROTEIN-COUPLED RECEPTORS

Signaling *via* G-Protein coupled receptors, IL-8, MIP1A, MIP1B, MCP1, IP-10 are elevated in COVID-19 patients (9, 40), conceivably stimulating migration of immune cells to the site of infection. Binding of these chemokines to their respective receptors, IL-8 to CXCR1/CXCR2, MIP1A to CCR1/CCR5, MIP1B to CCR5/CCR8, MCP1 to CCR1/CCR2, and IP-10 to CXCR3 activate the JAK/STAT pathway (98–101) all recruiting JAK2 and STAT3 (98–103), except IP-10. Although IP-10 can indirectly activate downstream STAT1, STAT4 and STAT5 (104). IL-8 acts as a chemoattractant for many immune cells, dominantly recruiting neutrophils for host defense. Although recruited neutrophils are critical for clearing infections, excessive neutrophil invasion could be the culprit of lung injury observed in COVID-19 pneumonia (69). MIP1A and MIP1B, the former linked to COVID-19 severity, are associated with the trafficking of CD8$^+$ and CD4$^+$ T cells, respectively (105, 106). Despite primarily attracting macrophages and lymphocytes (107), MIP1A can also attract neutrophils (108). MCP-1 has been associated with recruiting both pathological macrophages/neutrophils (109) and virus clearing CD8$^+$ Tc cells (110). In addition to acting as a chemoattract, MCP-1 can polarize Th2 responses (98, 111, 112). In contrast, IP-10 stimulates a Th1 response (113) recruiting primarily T cells (114) and its presence correlates with viral load (115–117). Both MCP-1 and IP-10 are linked to COVID-19 severity (9, 40).

REGULATION AND CROSS-TALK WITH JAK-STAT PATHWAYS

Immunoglobulin Superfamily Receptors

IL-1α, IL-1β and IL-1Ra act as damage-associated molecular pattern (DAMP) detectors (118), likely activated by the direct and collateral damage of SARS-CoV-2. Binding IL-1 (IL-1α, IL-1β) to IL-1 receptor type I (IL-1R1) results in a robust pro-inflammatory response (119). In contrast, IL-1Ra produces an anti-inflammatory response (119). Although these factors do not utilize the JAK-STAT pathway, it has been reported that IL-1 inhibits IL-6 driven STAT1 activation (120). M-CSF belongs to the immunoglobulin superfamily and does not cross-talk with the JAK-STAT pathway. Likely propagated by the heightened Th17 response, IL-17 is found at elevated levels in severe COVID-19 patients (40). IL-17A–IL-17F form either homo- or heterodimers and signal through IL-17 Receptor A (IL-17RA) and IL-17RC subunits (121) to promote inflammation. The IL-17RA is relatively expressed in the lungs (http://www.proteinatlas.org) and its activation can promote chemoattractants for neutrophil invasion (122). There is evidence that Th17 responses are implicated in severe lung pathology and mortality induced by CoVs (123). Furthermore, it has been shown to signal in astrocytes *via* an indirect JAK2, STAT1 and STAT3 axis (124, 125).

Tumor Necrosis Factor Receptors

While TNFα does not signal through JAK-STAT proteins, it is discussed here because it is found elevated in COVID-19 patients requiring intensive care (9). TNFα signals through two receptors, TNFR1 and TNFR2 triggering inflammatory pathways, and immune modulation respectively (126). TNFα is also released by differentiated Th1 cells. Cross-talk between TNFα and the JAK-STAT pathway has been suggested by few reports demonstrating changes in STAT3 and STAT5 following activation of TNFR1 and TNFR2 (126, 127). Prothrombotic effects of TNFα are thought to be mediated by TNFR2 rather than TNFR1 (128). Circulating TNFα, IFNγ, IL-1, IL-6, IL-8, and MCP-1 all effect tissue factor expression that initiate coagulation (129, 130). Additionally, TNFα, IL-1, IL-6, IL-12 and IL-2 can induce thrombin (130) which converts fibrinogen to fibrin (131) involved in the cross-linking that stabilizes blood clots. TNFα and IL-1 can also inactivate fibrinolysis (130). Taken together, TNFα along circulating cytokines may contribute to COVID-19 thrombotic complications.

Growth Factor Receptors

Growth factors signal mainly through receptors containing their own intrinsic catalytic activity, bypassing the need for JAKs. Increased levels of growth factor in SARS-CoV-2 patients include VEGF, FGF, HGF and PDGF that are involved in processes such as angiogenesis, morphogenesis and fibrotic remodeling. FGF, VEGF, HGF and PDGF have all been shown to be regulated by or cross-talk with JAK-STAT pathways. For example, VEGF expression along with IL-6 can be induced by IL-17 through STAT1 to promote angiogenesis (125). JAK2 and STAT5 are utilized by FGF receptor 2 (FGFR2) to facilitate morphogenesis (132). HGF stimulates the recruitment and phosphorylation of STAT3 that is also relevant to morphogenesis (133). And PDGF can facilitate airway remodeling by cross-talk *via* a JAK2, STAT1 and STAT3 pathway (134).

TARGETING THE JAK FAMILY

JAKs represent a major therapeutic target for the treatment of COVID-19. However, inhibition of all JAKs might not have beneficial outcomes. Correlating COVID-19 disease severity with elevated cytokines shouldn't imply each cytokine is pathogenic. Cytokines act upon multiple cell types and across distal and proximal sites. In this review the impact of cytokines signaling directly through JAKs were sought to predict their beneficial immunological, ambiguous or pathological responses to SARS-CoV-2 (**Table 1**), color-coded light to dark (respectively), and organized corresponding to JAKs and STATs in **Figure 3A**. IL-2, IL-7, IFNα2, IFNγ, IL-12, IL-10 and MIP1B are predicted to elicit a beneficial immune response against SARS-CoV-2. While IL-6, G-CSF, GM-CSF, and IL-8 might provoke unwanted pathological outcomes. These cytokines utilize different combinations of JAKs and STATs where more often "beneficial" cytokines recruit JAK1 and JAK3 in contrast to "pathogenic" cytokines that predominantly recruit JAK2. The latter being associated with downstream activation of STAT3, also suggested as a plausible target for the treatment of COVID-19 (135). Of note, while few STAT3 direct inhibitors are FDA approved, there are added concerns of inhibitory cross-reactivity with STAT1, critical for antiviral responses (136).

The use of selective JAK inhibitors for the treatment of COVID-19 have conflicting views. Prioritizing IFN antiviral/antibacterial immunity, suggest sparing JAK combinations downstream of IFN-I (JAK1/TYK2) and IFNγ (JAK1/JAK2) (15). In contrast, Schett et al. suggest targeting JAK2, downstream of IL-6 and GM-CSF to ameliorate hyperinflammation, and spare JAK1/JAK3 downstream of IFN-I, IL-2, IL-15, IL-21 and IFNγ involved in viral clearance (137). Others have proposed TYK2 as a target, given that variants effecting expression are related to COVID-19 critical illness (138).

These conflicting views on selective JAK inhibition may be resolved by considering the role of JAK dependent cytokines within the immunological timeline discussed previously (see **Figure 2**). Mild to moderate responses to SARS-CoV-2 are likely associated with intact innate and adaptive responses while severe disease progresses with hyperinflammation brought on by the cytokine storm (24). Thus, strategies to combat SARS-CoV-2 in early mild to moderate disease would benefit from sparing initial (JAK1/TYK2) and (JAK1/JAK2) combinations given IFNs role in innate immunity and transition to Th1 adaptive immunity. However, during the cytokine storm in COVID-19, targeting JAK2 and sparing JAK1/JAK3 combinations may preserve cell mediated and or humoral defenses against SARS-CoV-2. Three FDA approved JAK inhibitors, Tofacitinib, Ruxolitinib and Baricitinib can act on each JAK kinase at varying degrees (**Figure 3B**). Each has undergone clinical trials for treating COVID-19 patients (15) where drug combinations using Baricitinib have been approved by emergency use authorization (139). In agreement with the former analysis, Baricitinib preferentially targets JAK1/JAK2 while somewhat sparing JAK3 inhibition. In general, JAK blockade has shown to reduce recovery time and mortality compared to standard treatments (140).

DISCUSSION

Classic JAK inhibitors exploit the JH1 active site acting as ATP mimetics and because they act on more than one JAK they are casually considered to be pan-inhibitors rather than JAK specific inhibitors (141). The majority of the pipeline of JAK inhibitors are classified as Type I and Type II, depending on whether they target an active or inactive kinase, respectively. The ATP-binding site is highly conserved across kinases allowing them to act broadly. For example, JAK inhibitors are said to cross-react with AP2-associated protein kinase 1 (AAK1) that regulates endocytosis and could thus prevent SARS-CoV-2 entry (142). In contrast, Type III and Type IV inhibitors function to allosterically disrupt either proximal or distal changes to the ATP-binding site respectively (143). These distal and non-entirely conserved regions might be ideal for specific JAK inhibition.

TABLE 1 | Predicted actions of JAK signaling cytokines in SARS-CoV-2 infection.

Consequence	Function	Impact	Collective Consequence
IL-2	Th1 differentiation	1	Beneficial
	Th2 differentiation	0	
	Maintains memory T-cells	1	
	Treg differentiation	1	
	Inhibits Th-17	1	
	Coagulation	-1	
IL-4	Inhibits Th1 differentiation	-1	Ambiguous
	Th2 differentiation	0	
	Immunoglobulin switch	1	
IL-7	Th1 differentiation	1	Beneficial
	Maintains memory T-cells	1	
IL-9	Treg activation	1	Ambiguous
	Released by Th2 cells	0	
	Th17 differentiation	-1	
IL-6	Th2 response	0	Pathological
	Th17 differentiation	-1	
	Coagulation	-1	
IL-12	Th1 differentiation	1	Beneficial
	Tfh differentiation	0	
	T-cell IFN secretion	1	
	Involved in encephalitis	-1	
G-CSF	Neutrophilia	-1	Pathological
GM-CSF	Th17 response	-1	Pathological
	CNS inflammation	-1	
IL-8	Neutrophil recruitment	-1	Ambiguous
MIP1A	Recruits CD8 cells	1	Ambiguous
	Neutrophil recruitment	-1	
MIP1B	Recruits CD4 cells	1	Beneficial
MCP-1	Th2 responses	0	Ambiguous
	Recruits CD8 cells	1	
	Neutrophil recruitment	-1	
	Macrophage recruitment	0	
IFNα2	Antiviral response	1	Beneficial
	Immune regulation	1	
	Anti-proliferation	1	
	ACE2 expression	-1	
IFNγ	Antiviral response	1	Beneficial
	Th1 differentiation	1	
IL-10	Produced by Tregs	1	Beneficial
	Counters coagulation	1	
	Inhibits Th1 differentiation	-1	

1, Predicted to positively affect COVID-19.
0, Predicted to have no or neutral impact on COVID-19.
-1, Predicted to negatively affect COVID-19.

At present, there are limited allosteric JAK inhibitors available and none of which have been approved by the FDA (144). New allosteric strategies might include, exploiting endogenous mechanisms of JAK regulation. For example, small peptide inhibitors mimicking as substrates could accomplish steric hindrance in a JAK specific manner by targeting unique substrate specific residues within the JH1. Additionally, identifying negative regulatory phosphorylation sites within JAKs could be key in determining which kinase specific phosphatases could be effectively inhibited to disrupt subsequent downstream signals. Lastly, the pseudokinase JH2 domain acts as an intrinsic regulator of JAK activity and identifying key residues, or non-conserved motifs, required for negative regulation could be exploited for JAK inhibition.

The use of JAK inhibitors for treating COVID-19 have been met with caution given their potential risk of thrombosis (145–147). Whether these concerns apply to pan-JAK inhibitors and/or specific JAK inhibitors should be addressed. Regardless, the hypercoagulability state that contributes to thrombotic effects in COVID-19 patients may be compounded by pan-JAK inhibition (145, 148). Thus, such patients experiencing complications of thrombosis may not benefit from "pan" JAK inhibitors (15). Perhaps the ability to effectively counter these complications reflects differences in the hemostatic system that differs across age and sex similar to the risk of COVID-19 pathogenesis (6, 149–151). Nevertheless, hospitalized COVID-19 patients can benefit from a recently approved treatment regimen consisting of baricitinib, in combination with remdesivir.

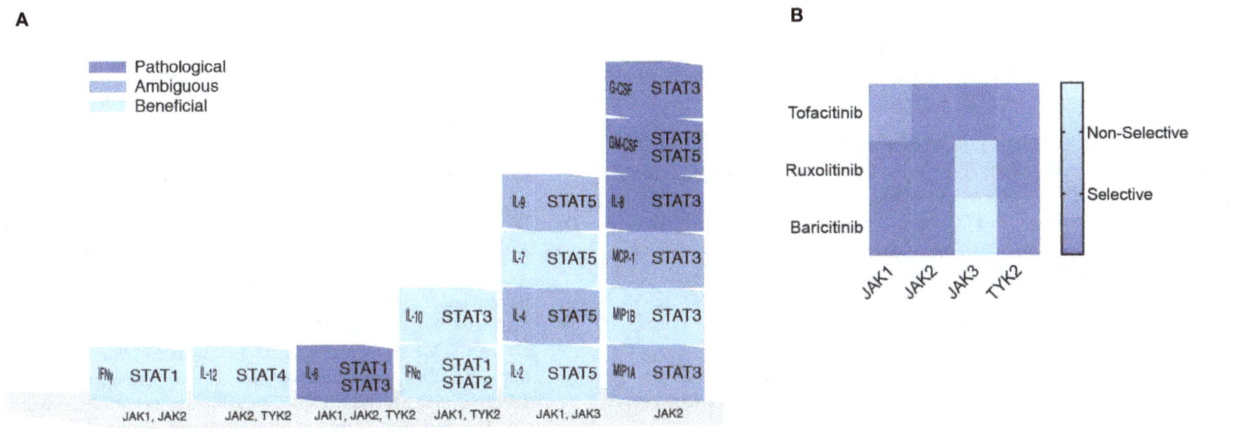

FIGURE 3 | Pathogenicity of the Cytokine Storm Driven by JAKs. **(A)** COVID-19 elevated cytokines directly signaling by the JAK-STAT pathway are shown in a heat map corresponding to their predicted pathogenicity in COVID-19 based on **Table 1**. **(B)** JAK inhibitors are shown with their selectivity of each JAK based on their IC50 values.

The FDA recommends continued efforts in drug strategies to accelerate recovery, slow disease progression and lower mortality in COVID-19. These efforts might benefit from specific JAK2 inhibitors with the rationale as provided in this review. Lastly, it should be noted that JAK inhibition is one of many treatment strategies for COVID-19 patients that are not managed by currently approved treatment strategies. Such efforts must continue during vaccine distribution programs and continued for unvaccinated individuals or when vaccination is ineffective. For now, JAK inhibitors are accessible in this time sensitive fight against SARS-CoV-2 and a path to dodge the storm.

AUTHOR CONTRIBUTIONS

AHG conceived, wrote, and finalized figures of the manuscript. AE contributed writing and generated figures. YA-M, AA-C, GR, and ER-E contributed to writing and editing. DC-M and ACR contributed writing. RAK conceived and critically revised the manuscript. All authors contributed to the article and approved the submitted version.

FUNDING

This work was supported by Grant 5U54MD007592 from the National Institutes on Minority Health and Health Disparities (NIMHD), a component of the National Institutes of Health (NIH) and by the RISE Scholars Program at UTEP from the National Institute of General Medical Sciences (NIGMS) Grant R25GM069621-18.

ACKNOWLEDGMENTS

We would like to thank Dr. Henry Wilson for his helpful discussions on COVID-19 pathology and thrombosis. Figures were created with BioRender.com and Adobe Illustrator 2019.

REFERENCES

1. Wang C, Horby PW, Hayden FG, Gao GF. A Novel Coronavirus Outbreak of Global Health Concern. *Lancet* (2020) 395(10223):470–3. doi: 10.1016/s0140-6736(20)30185-9
2. Channappanavar R, Zhao J, Perlman S. T Cell-Mediated Immune Response to Respiratory Coronaviruses. *Immunol Res* (2014) 59(1-3):118–28. doi: 10.1007/s12026-014-8534-z
3. Spence JD, de Freitas GR, Pettigrew LC, Ay H, Liebeskind DS, Kase CS, et al. Mechanisms of Stroke in COVID-19. *Cerebrovasc Dis* (2020) 49(4):451–8. doi: 10.1159/000509581
4. Helms J, Tacquard C, Severac F, Leonard-Lorant I, Ohana M, Delabranche X, et al. High Risk of Thrombosis in Patients With Severe SARS-CoV-2 Infection: A Multicenter Prospective Cohort Study. *Intensive Care Med* (2020) 46(6):1089–98. doi: 10.1007/s00134-020-06062-x
5. Tay MZ, Poh CM, Renia L, MacAry PA, Ng LFP. The Trinity of COVID-19: Immunity, Inflammation and Intervention. *Nat Rev Immunol* (2020) 20 (6):363–74. doi: 10.1038/s41577-020-0311-8
6. Liu Y, Mao B, Liang S, Yang JW, Lu HW, Chai YH, et al. Association Between Age and Clinical Characteristics and Outcomes of COVID-19. *Eur Respir J* (2020) 55(5):2001112. doi: 10.1183/13993003.01112-2020
7. Jones VG, Mills M, Suarez D, Hogan CA, Yeh D, Bradley Segal J, et al. Covid-19 and Kawasaki Disease: Novel Virus and Novel Case. *Hosp Pediatr* (2020) 10(6):537–40. doi: 10.1542/hpeds.2020-0123
8. Long QX, Tang XJ, Shi QL, Li Q, Deng HJ, Yuan J, et al. Clinical and Immunological Assessment of Asymptomatic SARS-CoV-2 Infections. *Nat Med* (2020) 26(8):1200–4. doi: 10.1038/s41591-020-0965-6
9. Huang C, Wang Y, Li X, Ren L, Zhao J, Hu Y, et al. Clinical Features of Patients Infected With 2019 Novel Coronavirus in Wuhan, China. *Lancet* (2020) 395(10223):497–506. doi: 10.1016/S0140-6736(20) 30183-5
10. Ross JA, Nagy ZS, Cheng H, Stepkowski SM, Kirken RA. Regulation of T Cell Homeostasis by JAKs and Stats. *Arch Immunol Ther Exp (Warsz)* (2007) 55(4):231–45. doi: 10.1007/s00005-007-0030-x
11. McNally R, Eck MJ. JAK-Cytokine Receptor Recognition, Unboxed. *Nat Struct Mol Biol* (2014) 21(5):431–3. doi: 10.1038/nsmb.2824

12. Silva CM. Role of STATs as Downstream Signal Transducers in Src Family Kinase-Mediated Tumorigenesis. *Oncogene* (2004) 23(48):8017–23. doi: 10.1038/sj.onc.1208159
13. Seif F, Khoshmirsafa M, Aazami H, Mohsenzadegan M, Sedighi G, Bahar M. The Role of JAK-STAT Signaling Pathway and its Regulators in the Fate of T Helper Cells. *Cell Commun Signal* (2017) 15(1):23. doi: 10.1186/s12964-017-0177-y
14. Murray PJ. The JAK-STAT Signaling Pathway: Input and Output Integration. *J Immunol* (2007) 178(5):2623–9. doi: 10.4049/jimmunol.178.5.2623
15. Luo W, Li Y-X, Jiang L-J, Chen Q, Wang T, Ye D-W. Targeting JAK-STAT Signaling to Control Cytokine Release Syndrome in COVID-19. *Trends Pharmacol Sci* (2020) 41(8):531–43. doi: 10.1016/j.tips.2020.06.007
16. Ragab D, Salah Eldin H, Taeimah M, Khattab R, Salem R. The COVID-19 Cytokine Storm; What We Know So Far. *Front Immunol* (2020) 11:1446. doi: 10.3389/fimmu.2020.01446
17. Park A, Iwasaki A. Type I and Type Iii Interferons - Induction, Signaling, Evasion, and Application to Combat Covid-19. *Cell Host Microbe* (2020) 27 (6):870–8. doi: 10.1016/j.chom.2020.05.008
18. Goker Bagca B, Biray Avci C. The Potential of JAK/STAT Pathway Inhibition by Ruxolitinib in the Treatment of COVID-19. *Cytokine Growth factor Rev* (2020) 54:51–62. doi: 10.1016/j.cytogfr.2020.06.013
19. Flies A. The Effects of Cytokines on T Cell Differentiation [Whitepaper]. In: *Life Science Industry Research and News*. Newburyport MA: Cell Sciences, Inc. (2017).
20. Rochman Y, Spolski R, Leonard WJ. New Insights Into the Regulation of T Cells by Gamma(C) Family Cytokines. *Nat Rev Immunol* (2009) 9(7):480–90. doi: 10.1038/nri2580
21. Wurtz O, Bajénoff M, Guerder S. Il-4-mediated Inhibition of IFN-γ Production by CD4+ T Cells Proceeds by Several Developmentally Regulated Mechanisms. *Int Immunol* (2004) 16(3):501–8. doi: 10.1093/intimm/dxh050
22. Oriss TB, McCarthy SA, Morel BF, Campana MA, Morel PA. Crossregulation Between T Helper Cell (Th)1 and Th2: Inhibition of Th2 Proliferation by IFN-Gamma Involves Interference With IL-1. *J Immunol* (1997) 158(8):3666–72.
23. Nurieva RI, Chung Y. Understanding the Development and Function of T Follicular Helper Cells. *Cell Mol Immunol* (2010) 7(3):190–7. doi: 10.1038/cmi.2010.24
24. Kaushic C. Understanding Immune Responses to SARS-Cov-2. In: *Rsc COVID-19 Series*. Ottawa, ON: Royal Society of Canada, Voices of the RSC (2020).
25. Grifoni A, Weiskopf D, Ramirez SI, Mateus J, Dan JM, Moderbacher CR, et al. Targets of T Cell Responses to SARS-CoV-2 Coronavirus in Humans With COVID-19 Disease and Unexposed Individuals. *Cell* (2020) 181 (7):1489–1501 e15. doi: 10.1016/j.cell.2020.05.015
26. Steinman JB, Lum FM, Ho PP, Kaminski N, Steinman L. Reduced Development of COVID-19 in Children Reveals Molecular Checkpoints Gating Pathogenesis Illuminating Potential Therapeutics. *Proc Natl Acad Sci USA* (2020) 117(40):24620–6. doi: 10.1073/pnas.2012358117
27. Meckiff BJ, Ramirez-Suastegui C, Fajardo V, Chee SJ, Kusnadi A, Simon H, et al. Imbalance of Regulatory and Cytotoxic Sars-CoV-2-Reactive Cd4(+) T Cells in COVID-19. *Cell* (2020) 183(5):1340–53.e16. doi: 10.1016/j.cell.2020.10.001
28. Gil-Etayo FJ, Suàrez-Fernández P, Cabrera-Marante O, Arroyo D, Garcinuño S, Naranjo L, et al. T-Helper Cell Subset Response is a Determining Factor in COVID-19 Progression. *Front Cell Infect Microbiol* (2021) 11:624483. doi: 10.3389/fcimb.2021.624483
29. Woodruff MC, Ramonell RP, Nguyen DC, Cashman KS, Saini AS, Haddad NS, et al. Extrafollicular B Cell Responses Correlate With Neutralizing Antibodies and Morbidity in COVID-19. *Nat Immunol* (2020) 21(12):1506–16. doi: 10.1038/s41590-020-00814-z
30. Braun J, Loyal L, Frentsch M, Wendisch D, Georg P, Kurth F, et al. SARS-Cov-2-Reactive T Cells in Healthy Donors and Patients With COVID-19. *Nature* (2020) 587(7833):270–4. doi: 10.1038/s41586-020-2598-9
31. Ng KW, Faulkner N, Cornish GH, Rosa A, Harvey R, Hussain S, et al. Preexisting and *De Novo* Humoral Immunity to SARS-CoV-2 in Humans. *Science* (2020) 370(6522):1339–43. doi: 10.1126/science.abe1107
32. Wang C, van Haperen R, Gutiérrez-Álvarez J, Li W, Okba NMA, Albulescu I, et al. A Conserved Immunogenic and Vulnerable Site on the Coronavirus Spike Protein Delineated by Cross-Reactive Monoclonal Antibodies. *Nat Commun* (2021) 12(1):1715. doi: 10.1038/s41467-021-21968-w
33. Diao B, Wang C, Tan Y, Chen X, Liu Y, Ning L, et al. Reduction and Functional Exhaustion of T Cells in Patients With Coronavirus Disease 2019 (Covid-19). *Front Immunol* (2020) 11:827. doi: 10.3389/fimmu.2020.00827
34. Qin C, Zhou L, Hu Z, Zhang S, Yang S, Tao Y, et al. Dysregulation of Immune Response in Patients With Coronavirus 2019 (Covid-19) in Wuhan, China. *Clin Infect Dis* (2020) 71(15):762–8. doi: 10.1093/cid/ciaa248
35. Sadeghi A, Tahmasebi S, Mahmood A, Kuznetsova M, Valizadeh H, Taghizadieh A, et al. Th17 and Treg Cells Function in SARS-CoV2 Patients Compared With Healthy Controls. *J Cell Physiol* (2020) 236 (4):2829–39. doi: 10.1002/jcp.30047
36. De Biasi S, Meschiari M, Gibellini L, Bellinazzi C, Borella R, Fidanza L, et al. Marked T Cell Activation, Senescence, Exhaustion and Skewing Towards TH17 in Patients With COVID-19 Pneumonia. *Nat Commun* (2020) 11 (1):3434. doi: 10.1038/s41467-020-17292-4
37. Rahimzadeh M, Naderi N. Towards Understanding of Regulatory T Cells in COVID-19: A Systematic Review. *J Med Virol* (2021) 93(7):4167–81. doi: 10.1002/jmv.26891
38. Chen Z, John Wherry E. T Cell Responses in Patients With COVID-19. *Nat Rev Immunol* (2020) 20(9):529–36. doi: 10.1038/s41577-020-0402-6
39. Taefehshokr N, Taefehshokr S, Hemmat N, Heit B. Covid-19: Perspectives on Innate Immune Evasion. *Front Immunol* (2020) 11:580641. doi: 10.3389/fimmu.2020.580641
40. Liu Y, Zhang C, Huang F, Yang Y, Wang F, Yuan J, et al. Elevated Plasma Levels of Selective Cytokines in COVID-19 Patients Reflect Viral Load and Lung Injury. *Natl Sci Rev* (2020) 7(6):1003–11. doi: 10.1093/nsr/nwaa037
41. Lin J-X, Leonard WJ. The Common Cytokine Receptor γ Chain Family of Cytokines. *Cold Spring Harbor Perspect Biol* (2018) 10(9):a028449. doi: 10.1101/cshperspect.a028449
42. Boyman O, Sprent J. The Role of Interleukin-2 During Homeostasis and Activation of the Immune System. *Nat Rev Immunol* (2012) 12(3):180–90. doi: 10.1038/nri3156
43. Linehan LA, Warren WD, Thompson PA, Grusby MJ, Berton MT. STAT6 is Required for IL-4-induced Germline Ig Gene Transcription and Switch Recombination. *J Immunol* (1998) 161(1):302–10.
44. Schluns KS, Lefrancois L. Cytokine Control of Memory T-cell Development and Survival. *Nat Rev Immunol* (2003) 3(4):269–79. doi: 10.1038/nri1052
45. Lee LF, Axtell R, Tu GH, Logronio K, Dilley J, Yu J, et al. IL-7 Promotes T(H) 1 Development and Serum IL-7 Predicts Clinical Response to Interferon-Beta in Multiple Sclerosis. *Sci Transl Med* (2011) 3(93):93ra68. doi: 10.1126/scitranslmed.3002400
46. Knoops L, Renauld J-C. IL-9 and its Receptor: From Signal Transduction to Tumorigenesis. *Growth Factors* (2004) 22(4):207–15. doi: 10.1080/08977190410001720879
47. Elyaman W, Bradshaw EM, Uyttenhove C, Dardalhon V, Awasthi A, Imitola J, et al. IL-9 Induces Differentiation of TH17 Cells and Enhances Function of FoxP3+ Natural Regulatory T Cells. *Proc Natl Acad Sci USA* (2009) 106 (31):12885–90. doi: 10.1073/pnas.0812530106
48. Tavakolpour S, Rakhshandehroo T, Wei EX, Rashidian M. Lymphopenia During the COVID-19 Infection: What it Shows and What can be Learned. *Immunol Lett* (2020) 225:31–2. doi: 10.1016/j.imlet.2020.06.013
49. Kalia V, Xiao H, Yuzefpolskiy Y, Sarkar S. Il-2 Signals Program the Fate of Exhausted Cd8 T Cells. *J Immunol* (2019) 202(1 Supplement):181.24–4.
50. Liu Y, Zhou N, Zhou L, Wang J, Zhou Y, Zhang T, et al. IL-2 Regulates Tumor-Reactive CD8+ T Cell Exhaustion by Activating the Aryl Hydrocarbon Receptor. *Nat Immunol* (2021) 22(3):358–69. doi: 10.1038/s41590-020-00850-9
51. Zhou F, Yu T, Du R, Fan G, Liu Y, Liu Z, et al. Clinical Course and Risk Factors for Mortality of Adult Inpatients With COVID-19 in Wuhan, China: A Retrospective Cohort Study. *Lancet* (2020) 395(10229):1054–62. doi: 10.1016/S0140-6736(20)30566-3
52. Heinrich PC, Behrmann I, Haan S, Hermanns HM, Müller-Newen G, Schaper F. Principles of Interleukin (IL)-6-type Cytokine Signalling and its Regulation. *Biochem J* (2003) 374(1):1–20. doi: 10.1042/bj20030407

53. Taga T, Kishimoto T. Gp130 and the Interleukin-6 Family of Cytokines. *Annu Rev Immunol* (1997) 15(1):797–819. doi: 10.1146/annurev.immunol.15.1.797
54. Wang SW, Sun YM. The IL-6/JAK/STAT3 Pathway: Potential Therapeutic Strategies in Treating Colorectal Cancer (Review). *Int J Oncol* (2014) 44 (4):1032–40. doi: 10.3892/ijo.2014.2259
55. Tanaka T, Narazaki M, Kishimoto T. IL-6 in Inflammation, Immunity, and Disease. *Cold Spring Harb Perspect Biol* (2014) 6(10):a016295. doi: 10.1101/cshperspect.a016295
56. Diehl S, Rincon M. The Two Faces of IL-6 on Th1/Th2 Differentiation. *Mol Immunol* (2002) 39(9):531–6. doi: 10.1016/s0161-5890(02)00210-9
57. Dienz O, Rincon M. The Effects of IL-6 on CD4 T Cell Responses. *Clin Immunol* (2009) 130(1):27–33. doi: 10.1016/j.clim.2008.08.018
58. Kerr R, Stirling D, Ludlam CA. Interleukin 6 and Haemostasis. *Br J haematol* (2001) 115(1):3–12. doi: 10.1046/j.1365-2141.2001.03061.x
59. Gu SX, Tyagi T, Jain K, Gu VW, Lee SH, Hwa JM, et al. Thrombocytopathy and Endotheliopathy: Crucial Contributors to COVID-19 Thromboinflammation. *Nat Rev Cardiol* (2020) 18:1–16. doi: 10.1038/s41569-020-00469-1
60. D'Alessandro A, Thomas T, Dzieciatkowska M, Hill RC, Francis RO, Hudson KE, et al. Serum Proteomics in COVID-19 Patients: Altered Coagulation and Complement Status as a Function of IL-6 Level. *J Proteome Res* (2020) 19(11):4417–27. doi: 10.1021/acs.jproteome.0c00365
61. Rosas IO, Bräu N, Waters M, Go RC, Hunter BD, Bhagani S, et al. Tocilizumab in Hospitalized Patients With Severe Covid-19 Pneumonia. *New Engl J Med* (2021) 384(16):1503–16.
62. Della-Torre E, Campochiaro C, Cavalli G, De Luca G, Napolitano A, La Marca S, et al. Interleukin-6 Blockade With Sarilumab in Severe COVID-19 Pneumonia With Systemic Hyperinflammation: An Open-Label Cohort Study. *Ann rheumatic Dis* (2020) 79(10):1277–85. doi: 10.1136/annrheumdis-2020-218122
63. Floss DM, Klöcker T, Schröder J, Lamertz L, Mrotzek S, Strobl B, et al. Defining the Functional Binding Sites of Interleukin 12 Receptor β1 and Interleukin 23 Receptor to Janus Kinases. *Mol Biol Cell* (2016) 27(14):2301–16. doi: 10.1091/mbc.E14-12-1645
64. Morinobu A, Gadina M, Strober W, Visconti R, Fornace A, Montagna C, et al. STAT4 Serine Phosphorylation is Critical for IL-12-induced IFN-Gamma Production But Not for Cell Proliferation. *Proc Natl Acad Sci USA* (2002) 99(19):12281–6. doi: 10.1073/pnas.182618999
65. Schmitt N, Liu Y, Bentebibel S-E, Ueno H. Molecular Mechanisms Regulating T Helper 1 *Versus* T Follicular Helper Cell Differentiation in Humans. *Cell Rep* (2016) 16(4):1082–95. doi: 10.1016/j.celrep.2016.06.063
66. Kapil P, Atkinson R, Ramakrishna C, Cua DJ, Bergmann CC, Stohlman SA. Interleukin-12 (Il-12), But Not IL-23, Deficiency Ameliorates Viral Encephalitis Without Affecting Viral Control. *J Virol* (2009) 83(12):5978–86. doi: 10.1128/JVI.00315-09
67. Barge RM, de Koning JP, Pouwels K, Dong F, Lowenberg B, Touw IP. Tryptophan 650 of Human Granulocyte Colony-Stimulating Factor (G-CSF) Receptor, Implicated in the Activation of JAK2, is Also Required for G-CSF-mediated Activation of Signaling Complexes of the p21ras Route. *Blood* (1996) 87(6):2148–53. doi: 10.1182/blood.V87.6.2148.bloodjournal8762148
68. Yamaguchi T, Mukasa T, Uchida E, Kanayasu-Toyoda T, Hayakawa T. The Role of STAT3 in Granulocyte Colony-Stimulating Factor-Induced Enhancement of Neutrophilic Differentiation of Me2SO-treated Hl-60 Cells. GM-CSF Inhibits the Nuclear Translocation of Tyrosine-Phosphorylated STAT3. *J Biol Chem* (1999) 274(22):15575–81. doi: 10.1074/jbc.274.22.15575
69. Wang J, Li Q, Yin Y, Zhang Y, Cao Y, Lin X, et al. Excessive Neutrophils and Neutrophil Extracellular Traps in COVID-19. *Front Immunol* (2020) 11:2063. doi: 10.3389/fimmu.2020.02063
70. Hercus TR, Thomas D, Guthridge MA, Ekert PG, King-Scott J, Parker MW, et al. The Granulocyte-Macrophage Colony-Stimulating Factor Receptor: Linking its Structure to Cell Signaling and its Role in Disease. *Blood* (2009) 114(7):1289–98. doi: 10.1182/blood-2008-12-164004
71. Li Y, Li H, Fan R, Wen B, Zhang J, Cao X, et al. Coronavirus Infections in the Central Nervous System and Respiratory Tract Show Distinct Features in Hospitalized Children. *Intervirology* (2016) 59(3):163–9. doi: 10.1159/000453066
72. Pouga L. Encephalitic Syndrome and Anosmia in COVID-19: do These Clinical Presentations Really Reflect SARS-CoV-2 Neurotropism? A Theory Based on the Review of 25 COVID-19 Cases. *J Med Virol* (2021) 93(1):550–8. doi: 10.1002/jmv.26309
73. Meinhardt J, Radke J, Dittmayer C, Franz J, Thomas C, Mothes R, et al. Olfactory Transmucosal SARS-CoV-2 Invasion as a Port of Central Nervous System Entry in Individuals With COVID-19. *Nat Neurosci* (2021) 24 (2):168–75. doi: 10.1101/2020.06.04.135012
74. Liu JM, Tan BH, Wu S, Gui Y, Suo JL, Li YC. Evidence of Central Nervous System Infection and Neuroinvasive Routes, as Well as Neurological Involvement, in the Lethality of SARS-CoV-2 Infection. *J Med Virol* (2021) 93(3):1304–13. doi: 10.1002/jmv.26570
75. De Felice FG, Tovar-Moll F, Moll J, Munoz DP, Ferreira ST. Severe Acute Respiratory Syndrome Coronavirus 2 (Sars-CoV-2) and the Central Nervous System. *Trends Neurosci* (2020) 43(6):355–7. doi: 10.1016/j.tins.2020.04.004
76. Li S, Gong M, Zhao F, Shao J, Xie Y, Zhang Y, et al. Type I Interferons: Distinct Biological Activities and Current Applications for Viral Infection. *Cell Physiol Biochem* (2018) 51(5):2377–96. doi: 10.1159/000495897
77. Ma DY, Suthar MS. Mechanisms of Innate Immune Evasion in Re-Emerging RNA Viruses. *Curr Opin Virol* (2015) 12:26–37. doi: 10.1016/j.coviro.2015.02.005
78. Nelemans T, Kikkert M. Viral Innate Immune Evasion and the Pathogenesis of Emerging Rna Virus Infections. *Viruses* (2019) 11(10):961. doi: 10.3390/v11100961
79. Lasfar A, Cook JR, Cohen Solal KA, Reuhl K, Kotenko SV, Langer JA, et al. Critical Role of the Endogenous Interferon Ligand-Receptors in Type I and Type II Interferons Response. *Immunology* (2014) 142(3):442–52. doi: 10.1111/imm.12273
80. Bhat MY, Solanki HS, Advani J, Khan AA, Keshava Prasad TS, Gowda H, et al. Comprehensive Network Map of Interferon Gamma Signaling. *J Cell commun Signaling* (2018) 12(4):745–51. doi: 10.1007/s12079-018-0486-y
81. Nan Y, Wu C, Zhang YJ. Interplay Between Janus Kinase/Signal Transducer and Activator of Transcription Signaling Activated by Type I Interferons and Viral Antagonism. *Front Immunol* (2017) 8:1758. doi: 10.3389/fimmu.2017.01758
82. Wathelet MG, Orr M, Frieman MB, Baric RS. Severe Acute Respiratory Syndrome Coronavirus Evades Antiviral Signaling: Role of Nsp1 and Rational Design of an Attenuated Strain. *J Virol* (2007) 81(21):11620–33. doi: 10.1128/JVI.00702-07
83. Mizutani T, Fukushi S, Murakami M, Hirano T, Saijo M, Kurane I, et al. Tyrosine Dephosphorylation of STAT3 in SARS Coronavirus-Infected Vero E6 Cells. *FEBS Lett* (2004) 577(1-2):187–92. doi: 10.1016/j.febslet.2004.10.005
84. Konno Y, Kimura I, Uriu K, Fukushi M, Irie T, Koyanagi Y, et al. SARS-Cov 2 ORF3b is a Potent Interferon Antagonist Whose Activity is Further Increased by a Naturally Occurring Elongation Variant. *bioRxiv* (2020) 2020:5.11.088179. doi: 10.1101/2020.05.11.088179
85. Li J-Y, Liao C-H, Wang Q, Tan Y-J, Luo R, Qiu Y, et al. The ORF6, ORF8 and Nucleocapsid Proteins of SARS-CoV-2 Inhibit Type I Interferon Signaling Pathway. *Virus Res* (2020) 286:198074–4. doi: 10.1016/j.virusres.2020.198074
86. Chen D-Y, Khan N, Close BJ, Goel RK, Blum B, Tavares AH, et al. Sars-CoV-2 Desensitizes Host Cells to Interferon Through Inhibition of the JAK-STAT Pathway. *bioRxiv* (2020) 2020:10.27.358259. doi: 10.1101/2020.10.27.358259
87. Lokugamage KG, Hage A, de Vries M, Valero-Jimenez AM, Schindewolf C, Dittmann M, et al. Sars-CoV-2 is Sensitive to Type I Interferon Pretreatment. *bioRxiv* (2020) 94(23):e01410-20. doi: 10.1101/2020.03.07.982264
88. Sallard E, Lescure F-X, Yazdanpanah Y, Mentre F, Peiffer-Smadja N. Type 1 Interferons as a Potential Treatment Against COVID-19. *Antiviral Res* (2020) 178:104791-1. doi: 10.1016/j.antiviral.2020.104791
89. Wang N, Zhan Y, Zhu L, Hou Z, Liu F, Song P, et al. Retrospective Multicenter Cohort Study Shows Early Interferon Therapy is Associated With Favorable Clinical Responses in COVID-19 Patients. *Cell Host Microbe* (2020) 28(3):455–464 e2. doi: 10.1016/j.chom.2020.07.005
90. Andreakos E, Tsiodras S. Covid-19: Lambda Interferon Against Viral Load and Hyperinflammation. *EMBO Mol Med* (2020) 12(6):e12465. doi: 10.15252/emmm.202012465

91. Ziegler CGK, Allon SJ, Nyquist SK, Mbano IM, Miao VN, Tzouanas CN, et al. SARS-Cov-2 Receptor Ace2 Is an Interferon-Stimulated Gene in Human Airway Epithelial Cells and Is Detected in Specific Cell Subsets Across Tissues. *Cell* (2020) 181(5):1016–1035 e19. doi: 10.1016/j.cell.2020.04.035
92. Schülke S. Induction of Interleukin-10 Producing Dendritic Cells As a Tool to Suppress Allergen-Specific T Helper 2 Responses. *Front Immunol* (2018) 9:455. doi: 10.3389/fimmu.2018.00455
93. Xu B, Fan CY, Wang AL, Zou YL, Yu YH, He C, et al. Suppressed T Cell-Mediated Immunity in Patients With COVID-19: A Clinical Retrospective Study in Wuhan, China. *J Infect* (2020) 81(1):e51–60. doi: 10.1016/j.jinf.2020.04.012
94. Zhang W, Zhao Y, Zhang F, Wang Q, Li T, Liu Z, et al. The Use of Anti-Inflammatory Drugs in the Treatment of People With Severe Coronavirus Disease 2019 (COVID-19): The Perspectives of Clinical Immunologists From China. *Clin Immunol* (2020) 214:108393. doi: 10.1016/j.clim.2020.108393
95. Slobedman B, Barry PA, Spencer JV, Avdic S, Abendroth A. Virus-Encoded Homologs of Cellular Interleukin-10 and Their Control of Host Immune Function. *J Virol* (2009) 83(19):9618–29. doi: 10.1128/jvi.01098-09
96. Rojas JM, Avia M, Martín V, Sevilla N. Il-10: A Multifunctional Cytokine in Viral Infections. *J Immunol Res* (2017) 2017:6104054–6104054. doi: 10.1155/2017/6104054
97. Pajkrt D, van der Poll T, Levi M, Cutler DL, Affrime MB, van den Ende A, et al. Interleukin-10 Inhibits Activation of Coagulation and Fibrinolysis During Human Endotoxemia. *Blood* (1997) 89(8):2701–5. doi: 10.1182/blood.V89.8.2701
98. Rose CEJr., Sung SS, Fu SM. Significant Involvement of CCL2 (Mcp-1) in Inflammatory Disorders of the Lung. *Microcirculation* (2003) 10(3-4):273–88. doi: 10.1038/sj.mn.7800193
99. Mellado M, Rodríguez-Frade JM, Aragay A, del Real G, Martín AM, Vila-Coro AJ, et al. The Chemokine Monocyte Chemotactic Protein 1 Triggers Janus Kinase 2 Activation and Tyrosine Phosphorylation of the CCR2B Receptor. *J Immunol* (1998) 161(2):805–13.
100. Mueller A, Strange PG. CCL3, Acting Via the Chemokine Receptor CCR5, Leads to Independent Activation of Janus Kinase 2 (JAK2) and Gi Proteins. *FEBS Lett* (2004) 570(1-3):126–32. doi: 10.1016/j.febslet.2004.04.100
101. Soldevila G, García-Zepeda EA. The Role of the Jak-Stat Pathway in Chemokine-Mediated Signaling in T Lymphocytes. *Signal Transduction* (2007) 7(5-6):427–38. doi: 10.1002/sita.200700144
102. Fu X-T, Dai Z, Song K, Zhang Z-J, Zhou Z-J, Zhou S-L, et al. Macrophage-Secreted IL-8 Induces Epithelial-Mesenchymal Transition in Hepatocellular Carcinoma Cells by Activating the JAK2/STAT3/Snail Pathway. *Int J Oncol* (2015) 46(2):587–96. doi: 10.3892/ijo.2014.2761
103. Lien M-Y, Tsai H-C, Chang A-C, Tsai M-H, Hua C-H, Wang S-W, et al. Chemokine CCL4 Induces Vascular Endothelial Growth Factor C Expression and Lymphangiogenesis by miR-195-3p in Oral Squamous Cell Carcinoma. *Front Immunol* (2018) 9:412. doi: 10.3389/fimmu.2018.00412
104. Zohar Y, Wildbaum G, Novak R, Salzman AL, Thelen M, Alon R, et al. CXCL11-Dependent Induction of FOXP3-negative Regulatory T Cells Suppresses Autoimmune Encephalomyelitis. *J Clin Invest* (2014) 124 (5):2009–22. doi: 10.1172/JCI71951
105. Taub DD, Conlon K, Lloyd AR, Oppenheim JJ, Kelvin DJ. Preferential Migration of Activated CD4+ and CD8+ T Cells in Response to MIP-1 Alpha and MIP-1 Beta. *Science* (1993) 260(5106):355–8. doi: 10.1126/science.7682337
106. Glass WG, Lane TE. Functional Expression of Chemokine Receptor CCR5 on CD4+ T Cells During Virus-Induced Central Nervous System Disease. *J Virol* (2003) 77(1):191–8. doi: 10.1128/JVI.77.1.191-198.2003
107. Bhavsar I, Miller CS, Al-Sabbagh M. Macrophage Inflammatory Protein-1 Alpha (MIP-1 Alpha)/CCL3: As a Biomarker. *Gen Methods Biomarker Res their Appl* (2015) 223:49. doi: 10.1007/978-94-007-7696-8_27
108. Tumpey TM, Fenton R, Molesworth-Kenyon S, Oakes JE, Lausch RN. Role for Macrophage Inflammatory Protein 2 (MIP-2), MIP-1alpha, and interleukin-1alpha in the Delayed-Type Hypersensitivity Response to Viral Antigen. *J Virol* (2002) 76(16):8050–7. doi: 10.1128/jvi.76.16.8050-8057.2002
109. Huffnagle GB, Strieter RM, Standiford TJ, McDonald RA, Burdick MD, Kunkel SL, et al. The Role of Monocyte Chemotactic Protein-1 (MCP-1) in the Recruitment of Monocytes and CD4+ T Cells During a Pulmonary Cryptococcus Neoformans Infection. *J Immunol* (1995) 155(10):4790–7.
110. Wang T, Dai H, Wan N, Moore Y, Dai Z. The Role for Monocyte Chemoattractant Protein-1 in the Generation and Function of Memory CD8+ T Cells. *J Immunol* (2008) 180(5):2886–93. doi: 10.4049/jimmunol.180.5.2886
111. Narasaraju T, Ng HH, Phoon MC, Chow VTK. MCP-1 Antibody Treatment Enhances Damage and Impedes Repair of the Alveolar Epithelium in Influenza Pneumonitis. *Am J Respir Cell Mol Biol* (2010) 42(6):732–43. doi: 10.1165/rcmb.2008-0423OC
112. Karpus WJ, Kennedy KJ. Mip-1alpha and MCP-1 Differentially Regulate Acute and Relapsing Autoimmune Encephalomyelitis as Well as Th1/Th2 Lymphocyte Differentiation. *J Leukoc Biol* (1997) 62(5):681–7. doi: 10.1002/jlb.62.5.681
113. Groom JR, Richmond J, Murooka TT, Sorensen EW, Sung JH, Bankert K, et al. CXCR3 Chemokine Receptor-Ligand Interactions in the Lymph Node Optimize CD4+ T Helper 1 Cell Differentiation. *Immunity* (2012) 37 (6):1091–103. doi: 10.1016/j.immuni.2012.08.016
114. Agostini C, Calabrese F, Rea F, Facco M, Tosoni A, Loy M, et al. Cxcr3 and its Ligand CXCL10 are Expressed by Inflammatory Cells Infiltrating Lung Allografts and Mediate Chemotaxis of T Cells at Sites of Rejection. *Am J Pathol* (2001) 158(5):1703–11. doi: 10.1016/S0002-9440(10)64126-0
115. Yang L, Liu S, Liu J, Zhang Z, Wan X, Huang B, et al. Covid-19: Immunopathogenesis and Immunotherapeutics. *Signal Transduct Target Ther* (2020) 5(1):128. doi: 10.1038/s41392-020-00243-2
116. Han C, Fu J, Liu Z, Huang H, Luo L, Yin Z. Dipyrithione Inhibits IFN-gamma-induced JAK/STAT1 Signaling Pathway Activation and IP-10/CXCL10 Expression in RAW264.7 Cells. *Inflammation Res Off J Eur Histamine Res Soc* (2010) 59(10):809–16. doi: 10.1007/s00011-010-0192-6
117. Harris DP, Bandyopadhyay S, Maxwell TJ, Willard B, DiCorleto PE. Tumor Necrosis Factor (TNF)-α Induction of CXCL10 in Endothelial Cells Requires Protein Arginine Methyltransferase 5 (PRMT5)-Mediated Nuclear Factor (NF)-κb p65 Methylation. *J Biol Chem* (2014) 289(22):15328–39. doi: 10.1074/jbc.M114.547349
118. Jain A, Kaczanowska S, Davila E. Il-1 Receptor-Associated Kinase Signaling and Its Role in Inflammation, Cancer Progression, and Therapy Resistance. *Front Immunol* (2014) 5:553. doi: 10.3389/fimmu.2014.00553
119. Dinarello CA. Overview of the IL-1 Family in Innate Inflammation and Acquired Immunity. *Immunol Rev* (2018) 281(1):8–27. doi: 10.1111/imr.12621
120. Deon D, Ahmed S, Tai K, Scaletta N, Herrero C, Lee IH, et al. Cross-Talk Between IL-1 and IL-6 Signaling Pathways in Rheumatoid Arthritis Synovial Fibroblasts. *J Immunol* (2001) 167(9):5395–403. doi: 10.4049/jimmunol.167.9.5395
121. Gaffen SL. Structure and Signalling in the IL-17 Receptor Family. *Nat Rev Immunol* (2009) 9(8):556–67. doi: 10.1038/nri2586
122. Pacha O, Sallman MA, Evans SE. Covid-19: A Case for Inhibiting IL-17? *Nat Rev Immunol* (2020) 20(6):345–6. doi: 10.1038/s41577-020-0328-z
123. Hotez PJ, Bottazzi ME, Corry DB. The Potential Role of Th17 Immune Responses in Coronavirus Immunopathology and Vaccine-Induced Immune Enhancement. *Microbes Infect* (2020) 22(4-5):165–7. doi: 10.1016/j.micinf.2020.04.005
124. Huppert J, Closhen D, Croxford A, White R, Kulig P, Pietrowski E, et al. Cellular Mechanisms of IL-17-induced Blood-Brain Barrier Disruption. *FASEB J* (2010) 24(4):1023–34. doi: 10.1096/fj.09-141978
125. You T, Bi Y, Li J, Zhang M, Chen X, Zhang K, et al. Il-17 Induces Reactive Astrocytes and Up-Regulation of Vascular Endothelial Growth Factor (VEGF) Through JAK/STAT Signaling. *Sci Rep* (2017) 7:41779. doi: 10.1038/srep41779
126. Yang S, Wang J, Brand DD, Zheng SG. Role of TNF-TNF Receptor 2 Signal in Regulatory T Cells and Its Therapeutic Implications. *Front Immunol* (2018) 9:784. doi: 10.3389/fimmu.2018.00784
127. Malemud CJ, Sun Y, Pearlman E, Ginley NM, Awadallah A, Wisler BA, et al. Monosodium Urate and Tumor Necrosis Factor-alpha Increase Apoptosis in Human Chondrocyte Cultures. *Rheumatol (Sunnyvale)* (2012) 2:113. doi: 10.4172/2161-1149.1000113
128. Pircher J, Merkle M, Wörnle M, Ribeiro A, Czermak T, Stampnik Y, et al. Prothrombotic Effects of Tumor Necrosis Factor Alpha *In Vivo* Are Amplified by the Absence of TNF-Alpha Receptor Subtype 1 and Require

TNF-Alpha Receptor Subtype 2. *Arthritis Res Ther* (2012) 14(5):225. doi: 10.1186/ar4064

129. van der Poll T, Herwald H. The Coagulation System and its Function in Early Immune Defense. *Thromb Haemost* (2014) 112(4):640–8. doi: 10.1160/TH14-01-0053
130. van der Poll T, de Jonge E. Cytokines as Regulators of Coagulation. In: *Madame Curie Biosci Database [Internet]*. Austin (TX): Landes Bioscience (2013) p. 1141. Available at: https://www.ncbi.nlm.nih.gov/books/NBK6207/.
131. Weisel JW, Litvinov RI. Fibrin Formation, Structure and Properties. *Fibrous Proteins: Structures Mech* (2017) 82:405–56. doi: 10.1007/978-3-319-49674-0_13
132. Yang X, Qiao D, Meyer K, Friedl A. Signal Transducers and Activators of Transcription Mediate Fibroblast Growth Factor-Induced Vascular Endothelial Morphogenesis. *Cancer Res* (2009) 69(4):1668–77. doi: 10.1158/0008-5472.CAN-07-6385
133. Boccaccio C, Ando M, Tamagnone L, Bardelli A, Michieli P, Battistini C, et al. Induction of Epithelial Tubules by Growth Factor HGF Depends on the STAT Pathway. *Nature* (1998) 391(6664):285–8. doi: 10.1038/34657
134. Simon AR, Takahashi S, Severgnini M, Fanburg BL, Cochran BH. Role of the JAK-STAT Pathway in PDGF-stimulated Proliferation of Human Airway Smooth Muscle Cells. *Am J Physiol Lung Cell Mol Physiol* (2002) 282(6): L1296–304. doi: 10.1152/ajplung.00315.2001
135. Matsuyama T, Kubli SP, Yoshinaga SK, Pfeffer K, Mak TW. An Aberrant STAT Pathway is Central to COVID-19. *Cell Death Differ* (2020) 27 (12):3209–25. doi: 10.1038/s41418-020-00633-7
136. Fagard R, Metelev V, Souissi I, Baran-Marszak F. STAT3 Inhibitors for Cancer Therapy: Have All Roads Been Explored? *JAKSTAT* (2013) 2(1): e22882. doi: 10.4161/jkst.22882
137. Schett G, Sticherling M, Neurath MF. Covid-19: Risk for Cytokine Targeting in Chronic Inflammatory Diseases? *Nat Rev Immunol* (2020) 20(5):271–2. doi: 10.1038/s41577-020-0312-7
138. Pairo-Castineira E, Clohisey S, Klaric L, Bretherick AD, Rawlik K, Pasko D, et al. Genetic Mechanisms of Critical Illness in Covid-19. *Nature* (2020) 591 (7848):92–8. doi: 10.1038/s41586-020-03065-y
139. Kalil AC, Patterson TF, Mehta AK, Tomashek KM, Wolfe CR, Ghazaryan V, et al. Baricitinib Plus Remdesivir for Hospitalized Adults With COVID-19. *N Engl J Med* (2021) 384(9):795–807. doi: 10.1056/NEJMoa2031994
140. Walz L, Cohen AJ, Rebaza AP, Vanchieri J, Slade MD, Dela Cruz CS, et al. Janus Kinase-Inhibitor and Type I Interferon Ability to Produce Favorable Clinical Outcomes in COVID-19 Patients: A Systematic Review and Meta-Analysis. *medRxiv* (2020) 21(1):47. doi: 10.1101/2020.08.10.20172189
141. Kothiwale S, Borza C, Pozzi A, Meiler J. Quantitative Structure-Activity Relationship Modeling of Kinase Selectivity Profiles. *Molecules* (2017) 22 (9):1576. doi: 10.3390/molecules22091576
142. Richardson P, Griffin I, Tucker C, Smith D, Oechsle O, Phelan A, et al. Baricitinib as Potential Treatment for 2019-nCoV Acute Respiratory Disease. *Lancet* (2020) 395(10223):E30–1. doi: 10.1016/S0140-6736(20) 30304-4
143. Roskoski RJr. Classification of Small Molecule Protein Kinase Inhibitors Based Upon the Structures of Their Drug-Enzyme Complexes. *Pharmacol Res* (2016) 103:26–48. doi: 10.1016/j.phrs.2015.10.021
144. Szilveszter KP, Nemeth T, Mocsai A. Tyrosine Kinases in Autoimmune and Inflammatory Skin Diseases. *Front Immunol* (2019) 10:1862. doi: 10.3389/fimmu.2019.01862
145. Mehta P, Ciurtin C, Scully M, Levi M, Chambers RC. JAK Inhibitors in COVID-19: The Need for Vigilance Regarding Increased Inherent Thrombotic Risk. *Eur Respir J* (2020) 56(3):2001919. doi: 10.1183/13993003.01919-2020
146. Verden A, Dimbil M, Kyle R, Overstreet B, Hoffman KB. Analysis of Spontaneous Postmarket Case Reports Submitted to the FDA Regarding Thromboembolic Adverse Events and JAK Inhibitors. *Drug Saf* (2018) 41 (4):357–61. doi: 10.1007/s40264-017-0622-2
147. Magro G. Covid-19: Review on Latest Available Drugs and Therapies Against SARS-CoV-2. Coagulation and Inflammation Cross-Talking. *Virus Res* (2020) 286:198070. doi: 10.1016/j.virusres.2020.198070
148. Spinelli FR, Conti F, Gadina M. HiJAKing SARS-CoV-2? The Potential Role of JAK Inhibitors in the Management of COVID-19. *Sci Immunol* (2020) 5 (47):eabc5367. doi: 10.1126/sciimmunol.abc5367
149. Bhopal SS, Bhopal R. Sex Differential in COVID-19 Mortality Varies Markedly by Age. *Lancet* (2020) 396(10250):532–3. doi: 10.1016/S0140-6736(20)31748-7
150. Abbate R, Prisco D, Rostagno C, Boddi M, Gensini GF. Age-Related Changes in the Hemostatic System. *Int J Clin Lab Res* (1993) 23(1):1–3. doi: 10.1007/BF02592271
151. Ariens RA, Coppola R, Potenza I, Mannucci PM. The Increase With Age of the Components of the Tissue Factor Coagulation Pathway is Gender-Dependent. *Blood Coagul Fibrinolysis* (1995) 6(5):433–7. doi: 10.1097/00001721-199507000-00010

17

TLR3 Activation of Hepatic Stellate Cell Line Suppresses HBV Replication in HepG2 Cells

Biao Zhang[1], *Yu Liu*[1], *Xu Wang*[2], *Jieliang Li*[2], *Xiqiu Xu*[1], *Le Guo*[1] *and Wen-Zhe Ho*[1,2*]

[1] *School of Basic Medical Sciences, Wuhan University, Wuhan, China,* [2] *Department of Pathology and Laboratory Medicine, Temple University Lewis Katz School of Medicine, Philadelphia, PA, United States*

Correspondence:
Wen-Zhe Ho
wenzheho@temple.edu

There is limited information about the role of hepatic stellate cells (HSCs) in the liver innate immunity against hepatitis B virus (HBV) infection. We thus examined whether hepatic stellate cell line (LX-2) can be immunologically activated and produce antiviral factors that inhibit HBV replication in HepG2 cells. We found that LX-2 cells expressed the functional Toll-like receptor 3 (TLR3), activation of which by PolyI:C resulted in the selective induction of interferon-β (IFN-β) and IFN-λs, the phosphorylation of IFN regulatory factor 3 (IRF3) and IRF7. When HepG2 cells were treated with supernatant (SN) from PolyI:C-activated LX-2 cells, HBV replication was significantly inhibited. IFN-β and IFN-λ appeared to contribute to LX-2 SN-mediated HBV inhibition, as the antibodies to IFN-β and IFN-λ receptors could largely block the LX-2 SN action. Mechanistically, LX-2 SN treatment of the HepG2 cells induced a number of antiviral IFN-stimulated genes (ISGs: ISG20, ISG54, ISG56, OAS-1, Trim22, and Trim25) and facilitated the phosphorylation of STATs. These observations support further studies on the role of HSCs in the liver innate immunity against HBV infection.

Keywords: hepatic stellate cells, hepatitis B virus, interferon-β, interferon-λ, Toll-like receptor 3, interferon-stimulated genes

INTRODUCTION

Hepatitis B virus (HBV) infection is a frequent cause of severe liver diseases including liver cirrhosis and hepatocellular carcinoma (1). In infected hepatocytes, HBV DNA can integrate into host cell genome or present as non-integrated covalently closed circular DNA (cccDNA), which serves as a template for virus replication and persistent infection (2). Interferon alpha (IFN-α) and nucleos(t)ide analog-based inhibitors are the current treatment strategies for people infected with HBV (3). To establish and maintain persistent replication, HBV has evolved multiple strategies to evade the host innate and adaptive immune responses (4). Although there is controversy about whether HBV has a negative impact on host cell innate immunity, studies from different laboratories have shown that HBV compromises the immune system and establishes chronic infection. Lebosse et al. reported that the innate immune responses were impaired in untreated patients with chronic HBV infection (5). It has also been documented that the expression of IFN-β was suppressed by HBV infection in tupaia belangeri model (6). Besides, HBV can suppress TLR-mediated innate immune response in the liver cells (7). However, a recent study reported that HBV infection had little effect on signal pathway of pattern recognition receptors, and failed to induce IFN and IFN-stimulated genes in human hepatocytes (8). In addition, Suslov et al. showed that liver tissues from HBV-infected patients did not induce the innate immune response (9). These controversial studies underline the importance of our study which determines whether bystander cells such as stellate cells are involved in the liver innate immunity against HBV infection/replication.

Toll-like receptors (TLRs), the sensors of host cell innate immunity to invading pathogens, play an important role in recognizing pathogen-associated molecular patterns (PAMPs). Among identified human cell TLRs, TLR3 is a key sensor for viral infections, participating in virus-mediated innate immune responses (10, 11). A number of studies have demonstrated the expression of TLR3 in the liver cells, such as primary hepatocytes (12), Kupffer cells (13), hepatic dendritic cells (14). Importantly, TLR3-mediated antiviral function was confirmed by the observation that HBV replication could be inhibited by intravenous injection of the TLR3 ligand in a HBV transgenic mice model (15). The expression of type I IFNs induced by TLR3 ligand polyI:C reduced the cytoplasmic HBV pregenomic RNA (pgRNA)-containing capsids (16). In addition, TLR3 activation of Kupffer cells and sinusoidal endothelial cells potently inhibits HBV replication through production of IFN-β in mice (17).

Hepatic stellate cells (HSCs) are a key nonparenchymal component in the sinusoid compartment with multiple functions in the liver (18). In normal liver, HSCs represent 5–8% of the total number of liver cells (19) and maintain a non-proliferative, quiescent phenotype (20). The most characterized function of HSCs is the ability to transdifferentiate from a quiescent phenotype into highly proliferative, contractile, and wound-healing myofibroblast (21). The activated HSCs produce fibril-forming collagens and promote net deposition of fibrotic extracellular matrix to repair liver injury (21). In addition, accumulating evidence has shown that HSCs can function as antigen-presenting cells that present lipid antigens to natural killer T cells (22). HSCs also act as a regulatory bystander to facilitate differentiation and accumulation of regulatory T cells (Tregs) (23). We demonstrated that TLR3 signaling of a human stellate cell line (LX-2) could inhibit hepatitis C virus infection of hepatocytes (24). Here, we examined whether LX-2 cells have the ability to mount a TLR3 activation-mediated induction of antiviral factors in LX-2 cells and inhibit HBV replication in HepG2 cells.

MATERIALS AND METHODS

Reagent

All culture reagents were purchased from GIBCO (Grand Island, NY, USA). All culture plasticware was obtained from Corning (Corning, NY, USA). LyoVec transfection reagent and polyinosinic-polycytidylic (PolyI:C) were purchased from InvivoGen (San Diego, CA, USA). IFN-β was purchased from Peprotech (Rocky Hill, NJ, USA). The pCMV ayw HBV proviral construct was kindly provided by Dr. Mingyu Lv (Jilin University, China). IFN-λ1 and neutralization antibodies against IFN-β, IL-28Rα, and IL-10Rβ were purchased from R&D (Minneapolis, MH, USA). TCI was obtained from EMD Millipore (Burlington, MA, USA).

Cell Culture

Human hepatic stellate cell line (LX-2) and HepG2 cells were cultured in Dulbecco's modified Eagle medium (DMEM) supplemented with 10% fetal bovine serum, 100 IU/ml Penicillin and 100 μg/ml Streptomycin. Cells were cultured in an incubator at 37°C with 5% CO_2 and 100% humidity. Cell culture medium was changed every 3 days.

Transfection

LX-2 cells were seeded in a 48-well plate (10^4/well) for 12 h. The cells were then transfected with PolyI:C by LyoVec transfection reagent for 4 h. LyoVec-treated cells were used as a vehicle control. The pCMV ayw HBV proviral construct (300 μg/ml) was transfected into HepG2 cells with LyoVec transfection reagent.

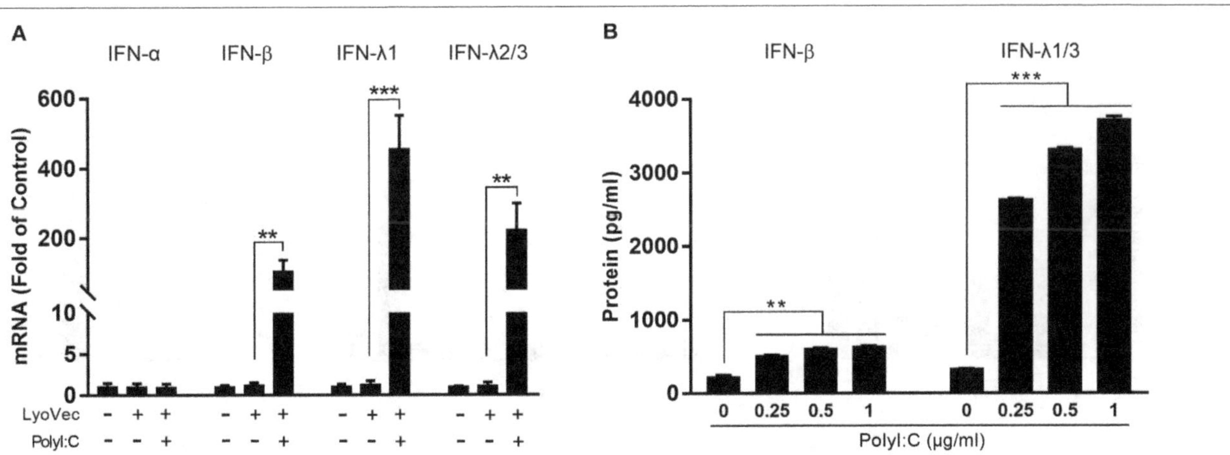

FIGURE 1 | Effect of TLR3 activation on IFN-β and IFN-λ expression in LX-2 cells. **(A)** LX-2 cells were stimulated with PolyI:C (1 μg/ml) for 12 h. Total RNA extracted from cells was subjected to RT-qPCR for the mRNA levels of IFN-α, IFN-β, IFN-λ1, and IFN-λ2/3. **(B)** LX-2 cells were stimulated with different concentrations of PolyI:C (0.25, 0.5, and 1 μg/ml) for 12 h and cultured for 48 h post-stimulation. SN was collected for ELISA to measure the protein levels of IFN-β and IFN-λ1/3. The results are mean ± SD of three different experiments (**$p < 0.01$, ***$p < 0.001$).

The cell cultures was replaced with fresh culture medium 4 h post-transfection.

RNA Extraction and Quantitative Real-Time PCR

Total RNA was extracted from cells with Tri-Reagent (Molecular Research Center, Cincinnati, OH, USA) according to the manufacturer's protocol. Total RNA (1 μg) was subjected to the reverse transcription using reagents purchased from Promega (Fitchburg, WI, USA). The quantitative real-time PCR was performed with iQ SYBR Green Supermix (Bio-Rad Laboratories, Hercules, CA, USA) as previously described (25).

Western Blotting

Total cell lysates from LX-2 cells transfected with PolyI:C or from HepG2 cells treated with supernatant from LX-2 cells cultures were prepared by the cell extraction buffer (Thermo Fisher Scientific, Waltham, MA, USA) according to the manufacturer's instructions. The protein concentrations of cell lysates were measured with BCA Protein Assay Kit (Beyotime, Shanghai, China). Equal amount of protein lysates (30 μg) was separated on 4–12% Bis-Tris gels (Invitrogen, Waltham, MA, USA) and transfected to an Immunobiolon-P membrane (EMD Millipore, Burlington, MA, USA). The membranes (blots) were incubated with primary antibodies (1:1,000 dilution) in 5% non-fat milk in TBS with 0.1% Tween 20 (TBST) overnight at 4°C. Horseradish peroxidase-conjugated rabbit second antibodies were diluted at 1:2,000 to 1:8,000 in 2% non-fat milk TBST. Blots were developed with SuperSignal West Pico Chemiluminescent Substrate (Thermo Fisher Scientific, Waltham, MA, USA). All antibodies were obtained from Cell Signaling Technology (Cell Signaling Technology, Danvers, MA, USA). Densitometric analysis was performed with ImageJ 1.44 software.

ELISA

IFN-β and IFN-λ1/3 protein levels in LX-2 culture SN were measured with ELISA kit (IFN-β: Invitrogen, Waltham, MA, USA; IFN-λ1/3: R&D system Inc., Minneapolis, MN, USA) according to the manufacturer's instructions. HBeAg and HBsAg in HepG2 cell cultures were measured with ELISA kit (Wantai Pharm, Beijing, China) according to the manufacturer's instructions.

Data Analysis

Data were expressed as the mean ± standard deviation, representative of three independent experiments. Statistical significance was measured by Student's *t*-test or one-way analysis of variance followed by the Newman–Keul's test. Statistical significance was defined as $^{*}p < 0.05$, $^{**}p < 0.01$, or $^{***}p < 0.001$.

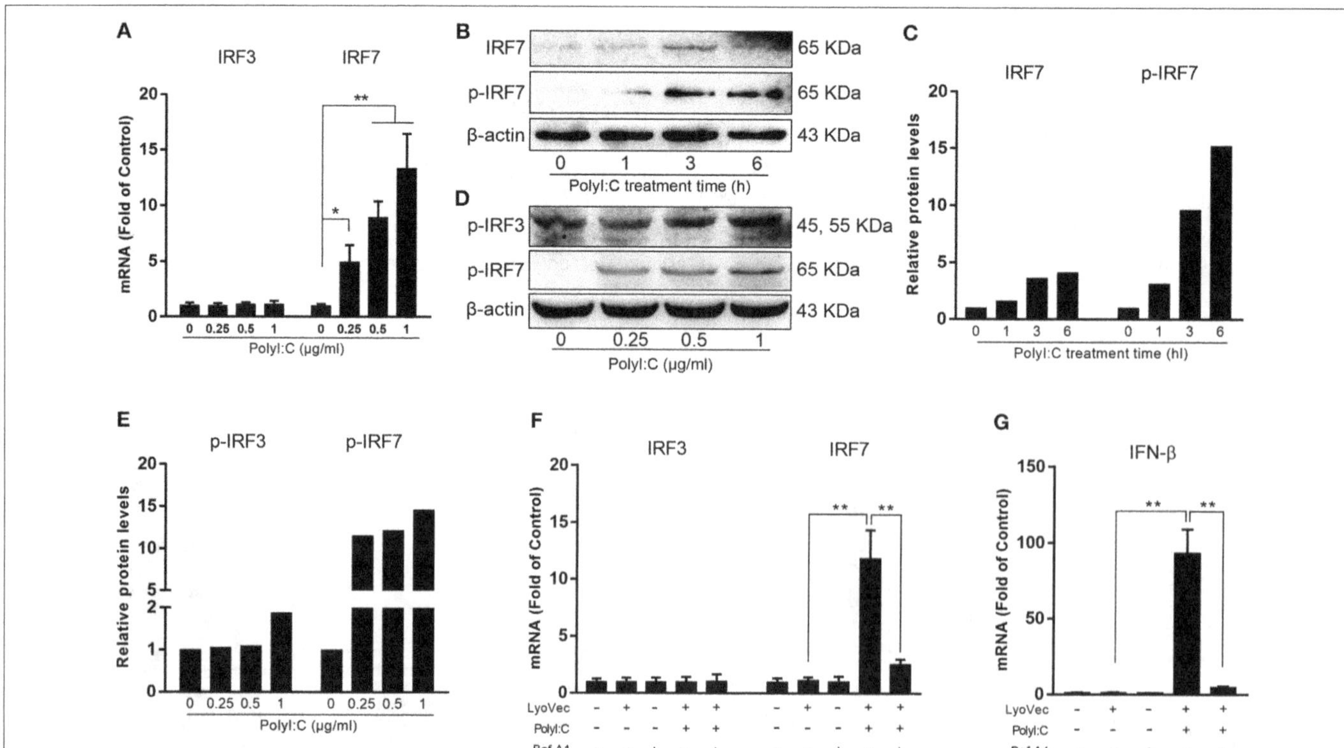

FIGURE 2 | Effect of PolyI:C on the activation of IRF3 and IRF7 expression. **(A)** LX-2 cells were stimulated with PolyI:C (1 μg/ml) for 12 h. Total RNA extracted from cells was subjected to the RT-qPCR for the mRNA levels of IRF3 and IRF7. **(B,C)** LX-2 cells were stimulated with PolyI:C (1 μg/ml) for the indicated time period. Protein extracted from the cells were subjected to Western blotting for IRF7 and p-IRF7. **(D,E)** LX-2 cells were stimulated with PolyI:C (1 μg/ml) for 6 h. Protein extracted from the cells were subjected to Western blotting for p-IRF3 and p-IRF7. Densitometry analysis of the blot was performed with ImageJ 1.44 software. **(F,G)** LX-2 cells were pretreated with or without bafilomycin A1 (100 nM) for 1 h and then transfected with PolyI:C (1 μg/ml), total RNA extracted from cells was subjected to the RT-qPCR for the mRNA levels of IRF3, IRF7, and IFN-β. The results are mean ± SD of three different experiments ($^{*}p < 0.05$, $^{**}p < 0.01$).

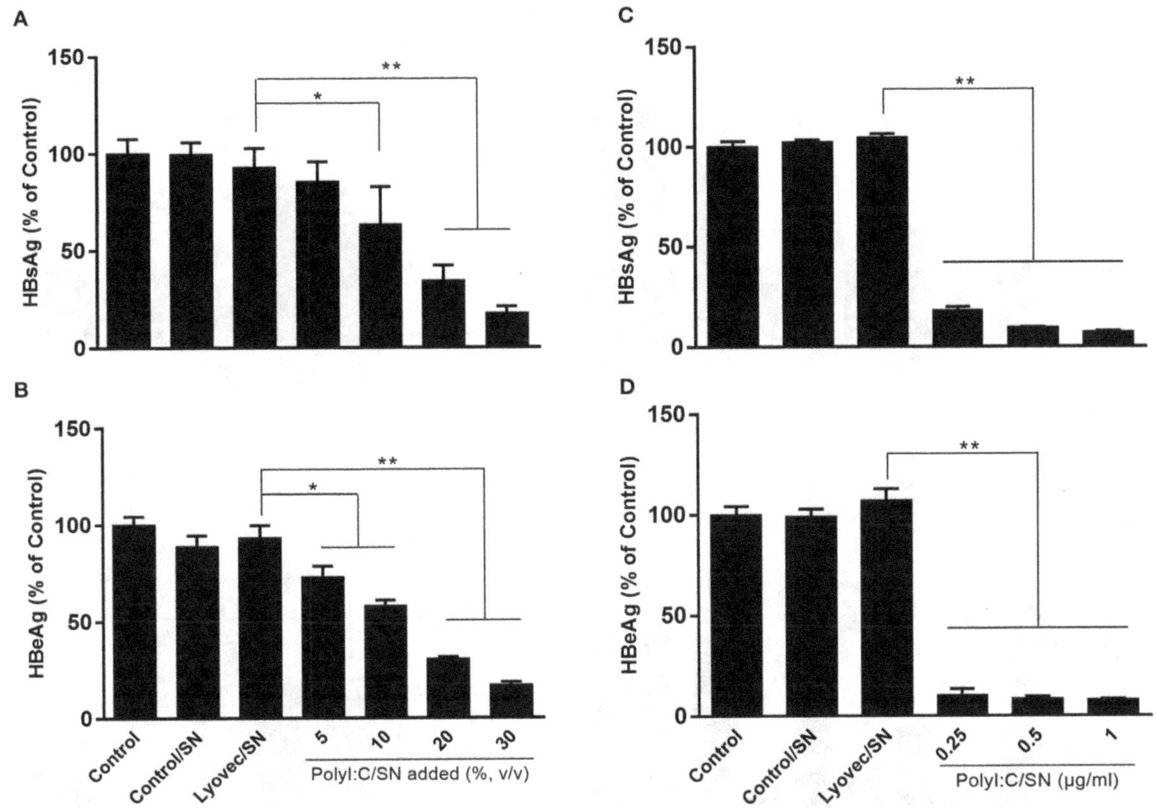

FIGURE 3 | Effect of SN from activated LX-2 cultures on HBV replication in HepG2 cells. HepG2 cells were pretreated with SN from control (Control/SN), LyoVec (LyoVec/SN), or PolyI:C (PolyI:C/SN) -stimulated LX-2 cells cultures for 24 h. HepG2 cells transfected with HBV plasmid (300 ng/ml) were maintained in fresh medium for 48 h. **(A,B)** HepG2 cells were pretreated with indicated volumes of PolyI:C (1 μg/ml)-stimulated LX-2 cultures for 24 h. HBV antigen HBsAg **(A)** and HBeAg **(B)** in SN from HepG2 cultures were detected by ELISA. **(C,D)** HepG2 cells were pretreated with 20% (volume to volume ratio [v/v]) of indicated SNs collected from 0.25, 0.5, or 1 μg/ml PolyI:C-stimulated LX-2 cultures. HBV antigen HBsAg and HBeAg in SN from HepG2 cultures were detected by ELISA. The results are mean ± SD of three different experiments (*$p < 0.05$, **$p < 0.01$).

RESULTS

TLR3 Activation of HSCs Induces IFN-β, IFN-λ, and Phosphorylation of IRF3 and IRF7

We first examined whether PolyI:C could activate TLR3 in human hepatic stellate cells (LX-2). PolyI:C was added into the LX-2 cell cultures and we found it had little effect on TLR3 activation in LX-2 cells (**Supplementary Figure 1**). As shown in **Figure 1**, PolyI:C treatment of LX-2 cells induced IFN-β and IFN-λ expression at both mRNA and protein levels. The effect of PolyI:C on IFN-β and IFN-λ expression was dose-dependent (**Figure 1**). Because IRF3 and IRF7 have a key role in upregulation of type I IFNs, we examined the effect of PolyI:C on the expression of IRF3 and IRF7 in LX-2 cells. While PolyI:C could induce the expression of IRF7, it had little effect on IRF3 (**Figure 2A**). At protein level, PolyI:C significantly upregulated the phosphorylation of IRF7 (**Figures 2B,C**). Phosphorylation level of IRF3 and IRF7 were positively correlated with the concentrations of PolyI:C used to treat LX-2 cells (**Figures 2D,E**). To confirm the role of TLR3 in PolyI:C-stimulated IFN-β expression, LX-2 cells were pretreated with bafilomycin A1, a known inhibitor of TLR3 function, prior to PolyI:C stimulation. As shown in **Figure 2F**, TLR3 activation-mediated IRF expression was compromised by the pretreatment of LX-2 cells with bafilomycin A1. In addition, PolyI:C-mediated IFN-β expression was significantly inhibited by bafilomycin A1 pretreatment (**Figure 2G**). In addition, TCI, a TLR3/dsRNA complex inhibitor (26), also could significantly block the effect of PolyI:C on the induction of IFNs and IRF7 (**Supplementary Figure 2**). HBV containing SN from HepG2 cell cultures had little effect on IFN induction (**Supplementary Figure 3**).

LX-2 SN Inhibits HBV Replication in HepG2 Cells

We then determined whether supernatant (SN) from PolyI:C-stimulated LX-2 cultures inhibits HBV replication in HepG2 cells. As shown in **Figure 3**, pretreatment of HepG2 cells with SN from PolyI:C-stimulated LX-2 cultures significantly inhibited the release of HBeAg and HBsAg from HepG2 cells.

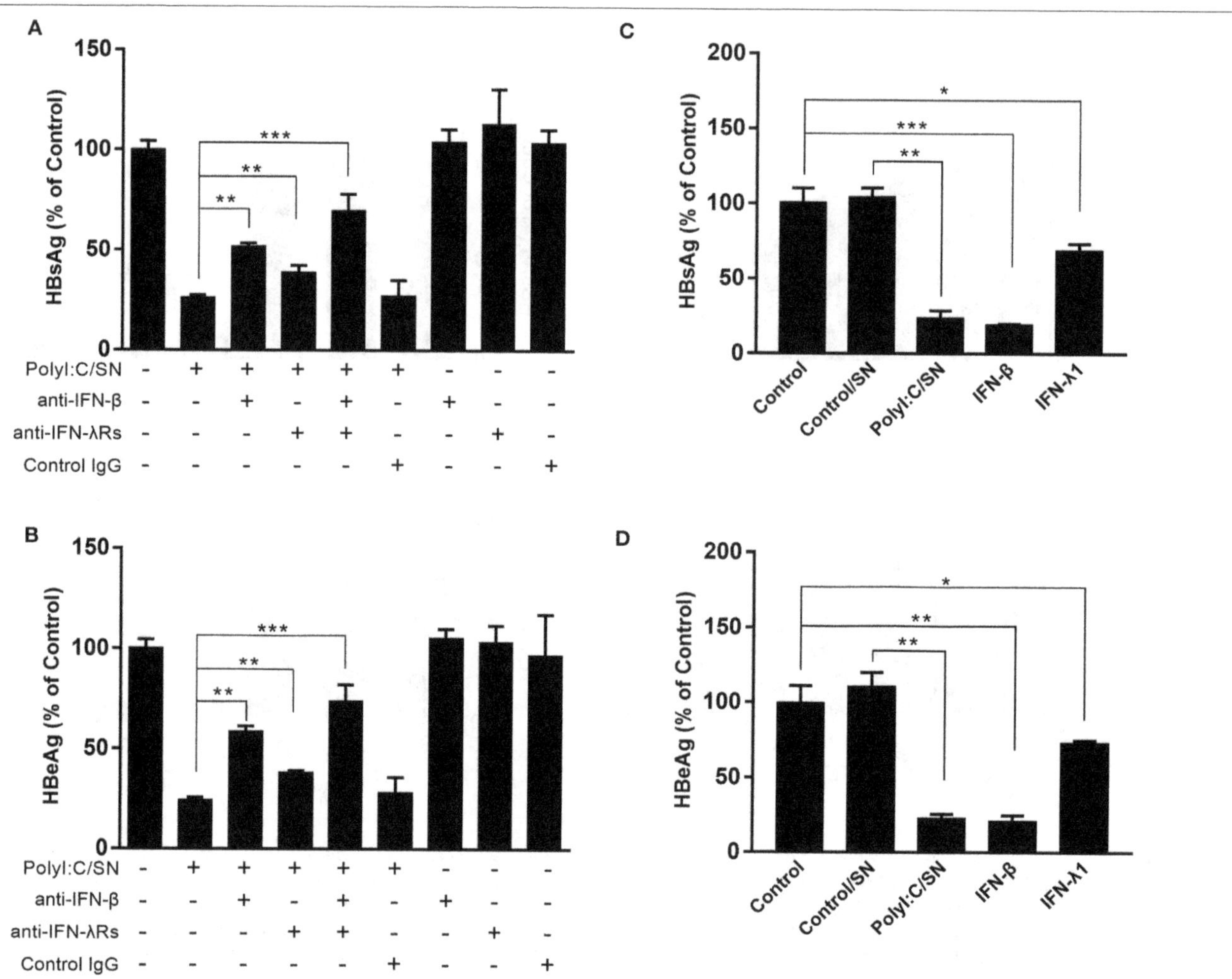

FIGURE 4 | Effect of the antibodies to IFN-β or IFN-λ receptors on LX-2 supernatant (SN)-mediated HBV inhibition. **(A,B)** PolyI:C-stimulated LX-2 culture SN was preincubated with anti-IFN-β neutralization antibody (10 μg/ml) for 1 h and then used to treat HepG2 cells for 24 h prior to HBV plasmid transfection. For IFN-λ receptors pretreatment, the neutralization antibodies against IL-28Rα (25 μg/ml) and IL-10Rβ (10 μg/ml) was added to HepG2 cell cultures for 1 h prior to the addition of LX-2 SN. HBsAg and HBeAg in the culture SN were measured by ELISA 48 h after HBV plasmid transfection. **(C,D)** HepG2 cells were pretreated with exogenous IFN-β (1 ng/ml), IFN-λ (4 ng/ml), and SN from control (Control/SN) or PolyI:C (PolyI:C/SN) -stimulated LX-2 cells cultures for 24 h. HepG2 cells transfected with HBV plasmid (300 ng/ml) were maintained in cultures for 48 h. SN was collected 48 h post-transfection, and HBsAg and HBeAg were measured by ELISA. The results are mean ± SD of three different experiments (*$p < 0.05$, **$p < 0.01$, ***$p < 0.001$).

This inhibitory effect on the HBV antigen expression was dependent on the percentage of SN (from PolyI:C-stimulated LX-2 cultures) added to HepG2 cultures (**Figures 3A,B**) and the concentrations of PolyI:C used to stimulate LX-2 cells (**Figures 3C,D**). The transfection of HBV plasmid into HepG2 cells had little effect on TLR3 activation and IFN induction (**Supplementary Figure 4**).

IFN-β and IFN-λ Are the Key Factors in LX-2 SN-Mediated HBV Inhibition

As shown in **Figure 1**, the TLR3 activation of LX-2 cells induces the expression of both IFN-β and IFN-λ at mRNA and protein levels. To determine the roles of IFNs in LX-2 cells-mediated anti-HBV activity, we used the neutralization antibody to IFN-β to treat the LX-2 SN or antibodies to IFN-λ receptors to treat HepG2 cells. As shown in **Figures 4A,B**, the antibody to IFN-β could largely block the inhibitory effect of SN from PolyI:C-stimulated LX-2 cultures on HBV replication. In addition, the pretreatment of HepG2 cells with the antibodies to IFN-λ receptors (IL-28Rα and IL-10Rβ) also compromised LX-2 SN-mediated HBV suppression, although the extent of the antibodies effect was less than the antibody to IFN-β. As shown in **Figures 4C,D**, IFN-β, IFN-λ1, and SN from PolyI:C-stimulated LX-2 cultures all significantly inhibited the replication of HBV in HepG2 cells. IFN-β was the most potent inhibitor among them.

LX-2 SN Induces ISGs in HepG2 Cells

To determine whether LX-2 SN can induce ISGs in the hepatocytes, we next examined the effect of LX-2 SN on the ISGs expression in HepG2 cells. The mRNAs of ISGs, including ISG20,

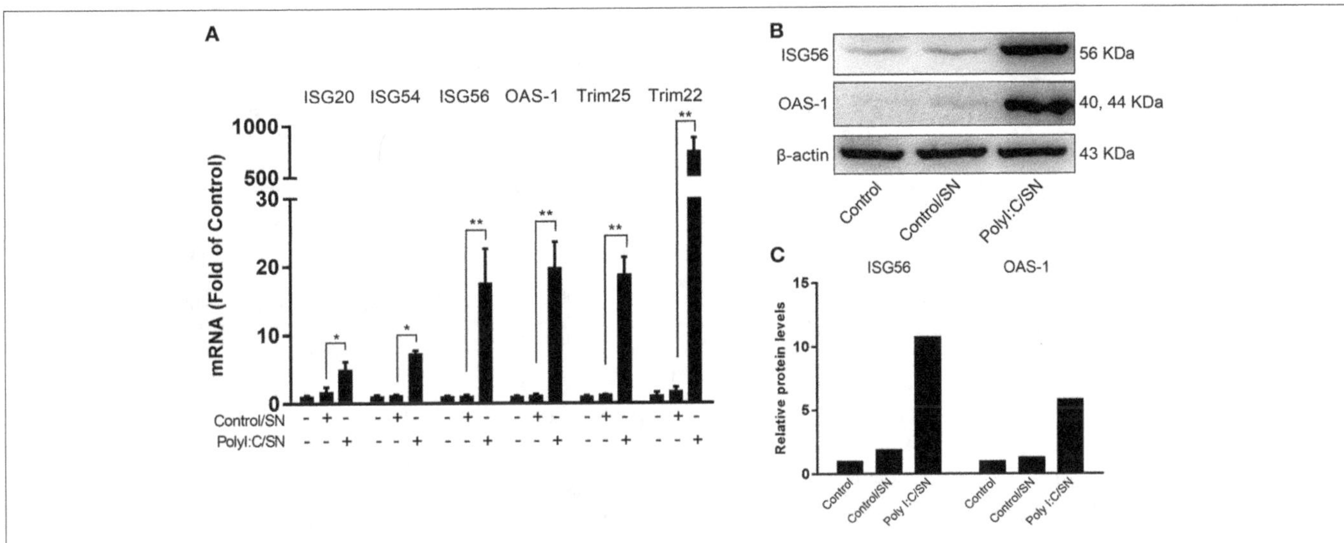

FIGURE 5 | Effect of PolyI:C-stimulated LX-2 culture SN on ISGs expression in HepG2 cells. **(A)** LX-2 cells were stimulated with PolyI:C (1 μg/ml) for 12 h and further incubated to 48 h post-stimulation. Culture SN was collected for treatment of HepG2 cells (20% v/v) for 12 h. RNA was extracted for the expression of the indicated ISGs by RT-qPCR. The results are mean ± SD of three different experiments (*$p < 0.05$, **$p < 0.01$). **(B,C)** HepG2 cells were treated with PolyI:C-stimulated LX-2 culture SN for 24 h and proteins extracted from the cells were subjected to Western blotting for ISG56, OAS-1, and β-actin. Densitometry analysis of the blot was performed with ImageJ 1.44 software.

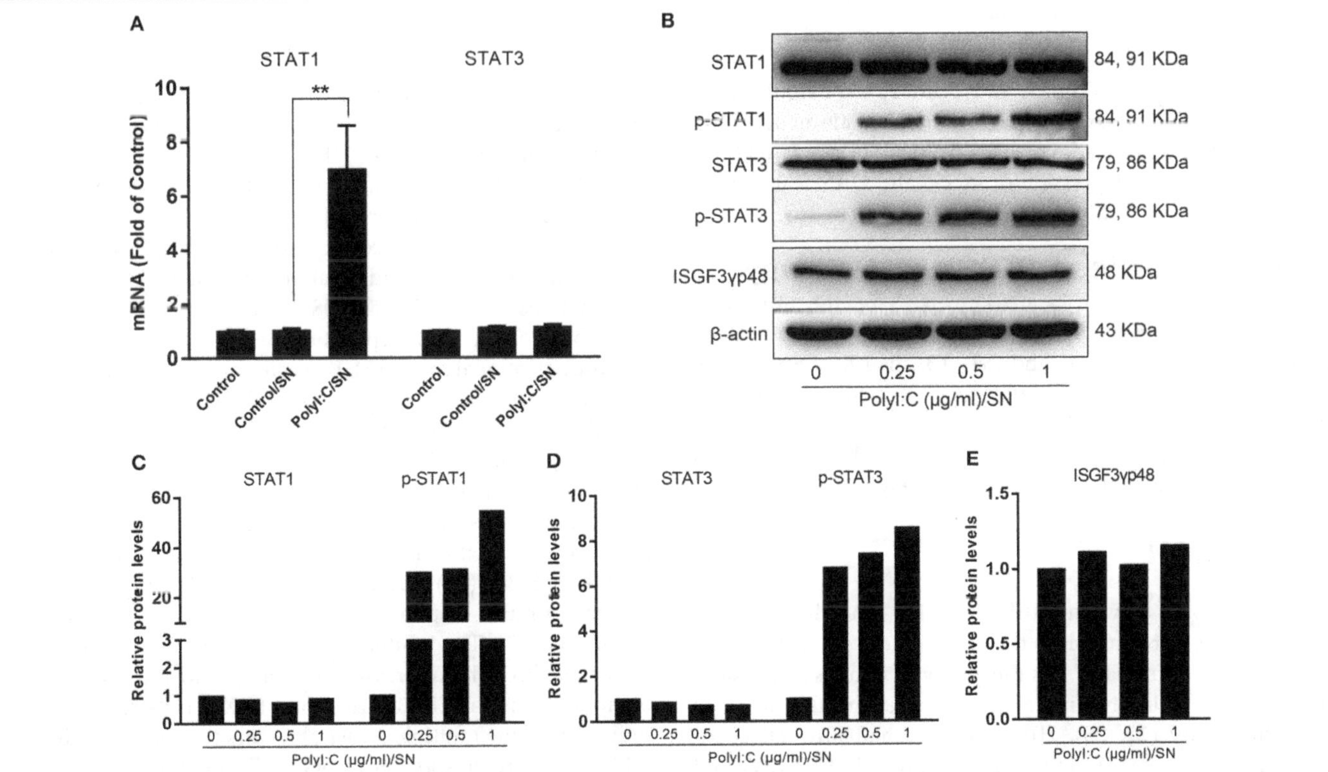

FIGURE 6 | Effect of PolyI:C-stimulated LX-2 culture SN on the activation of STATs in HepG2 cells. LX-2 cells were stimulated with 0.25, 0.5, and 1 μg/ml PolyI:C for 12 h, then washed 3 times, and further incubated in fresh medium to 48 h poststimulation. **(A)** SN from LX-2 cells stimulated with 1 μg/ml PolyI:C was collected to treat HepG2 cells for 12 h (20% v/v). Total RNA extracted from cells was subjected to the RT-qPCR for the mRNA levels of STAT1 and STAT3. The results are mean ± SD of three different experiments (**$p < 0.01$). **(B–E)** SN from LX-2 cells stimulated with indicated concentrations of PolyI:C was collected to treat HepG2 cells for 1 h (20% v/v). Proteins extracted from the cells were subjected to Western blotting for STAT1, p-STAT1, STAT3, p-STAT3, ISGF3γp48, and β-actin. Densitometry analysis of the blot was performed with ImageJ 1.44 software.

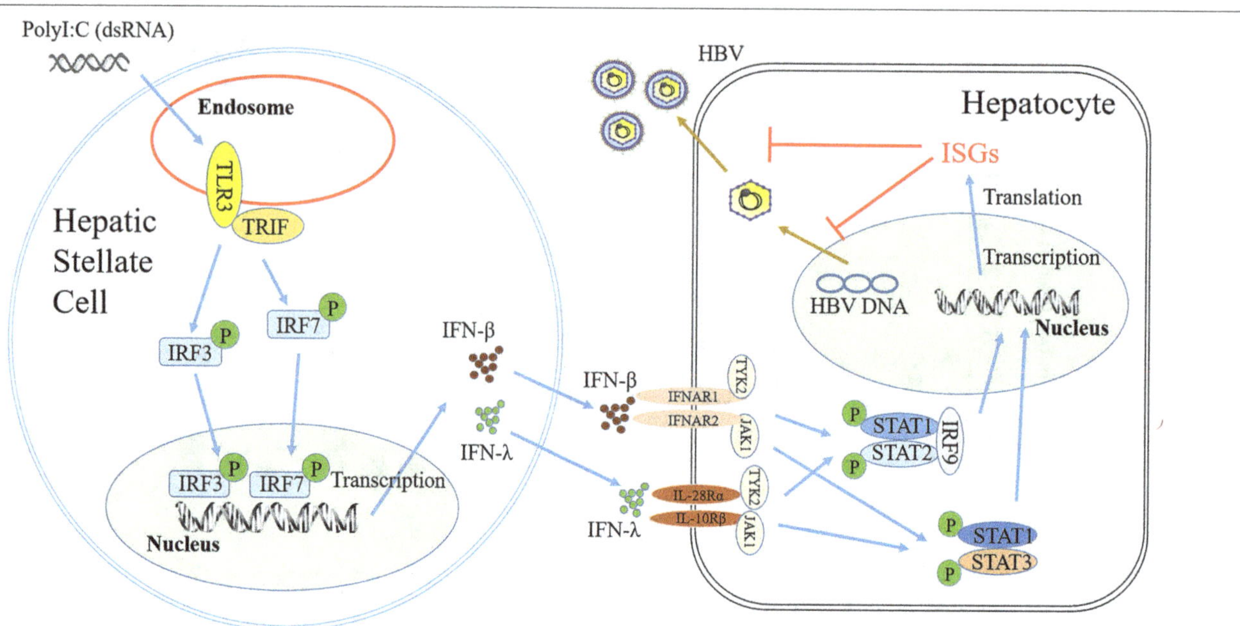

FIGURE 7 | Hypothetical model of anti-HBV mechanism of TLR3 signaling of HSCs. Stimulation of HSCs with PolyI:C (dsRNA) activates TLR3 signal pathway, which facilitates phosphorylation and translocation of IRF3 and IRF7, initiating the production of IFN-β and IFN-λ. IFN-β and IFN-λ released from HSCs could binds to their corresponding receptors in hepatocytes and activate STAT signal pathway, inducing anti-HBV IFN-stimulate genes (ISGs), which can inhibit HBV replication in hepatocytes.

ISG54, ISG56, OAS-1, Trim25, and Trim22, were significantly upregulated in HepG2 cells by SN from PolyI:C-stimulated LX-2 cultures (**Figure 5A**). In addition, SN from TLR3-activated LX-2 cultures induced the expression of ISG56 and OAS-1 at protein level in HepG2 cells (**Figures 5B,C**).

LX-2 SN Activates STAT Signal Pathway

Because STAT1 and STAT3 are known to be the important regulators of ISGs driven by IFN-β and IFN-λ, we also examined the expression of STAT1 and STAT3 in LX-2 SN-treated hepatocytes. As shown in **Figure 6A**, LX-2 SN induced the mRNA expression of STAT1 but not STAT3. However, LX-2 SN could facilitate the phosphorylation of both STAT1 and STAT3 at protein level in a dose-dependent manner (**Figures 6B–E**).

DISCUSSION

The interactions between HBV infection and liver innate immunity have a crucial role in the development of HBV disease. It is well-known that HBV has the ability to establish persistent infection in liver by evading and/or suppressing the host cell innate immunity (27, 28). HBV infection had little effect on host cellular gene expression and induction of IFNs (29) and the ISGs (30). Therefore, to immunologically activate the liver cell-mediated innate immunity suppressed by HBV is of a great interest. In this study, we attempted to determine whether hepatic stellate cells, a non-HBV target in liver, are involved in the innate immunity against HBV infection. We showed that the SN from immunologically activated LX-2 cell cultures potently induced the expression of the antiviral ISGs in HepG2 cells, including ISG20, ISG54, ISG56, OAS-1, Trim25, and Trim22 (**Figure 5**). These antiviral ISGs inhibit HBV replication at different stages of viral life cycle (**Figure 7**). For example, ISG20 has the ability to inhibit HBV replication through degradation of HBV RNA (31), TRIM22 suppresses HBV core promoter activity, thus inhibiting HBV gene expression and viral replication in both vitro and vivo systems (32). ISG54 and ISG56 contribute significantly to the inhibition of HBV replication at both transcriptional and posttranscriptional steps (33). In addition, we found that SN from PolyI:C-stimulated LX-2 cells could facilitate phosphorylation of STAT1 and STAT3 (**Figures 6B–E**), which is likely to be responsible for LX-2 cell SN-mediated the induction of the antiviral ISGs in HepG2 cells.

As the sensors of host cell-mediated innate immunity, TLRs are involved in the immune defense against viral infections, including HBV (34). HBV, however, could counteract to the innate immune response stimulated by TLR3 activation of hepatocytes (7). The inhibitory effect by HBV is at least partially mediated through suppression of IFN-β and the ISGs (7). We demonstrated that TLR3 activation of LX-2 cells resulted in the induction of the multiple antiviral factors that have the ability to inhibit HBV replication in HepG2 cells. Our investigation into the mechanism for the induction n of IFN-β and IFN-λ showed that TLR3 activation of LX-2 cells facilitated the phosphorylation of IRF3 and IRF7 (**Figures 2B–E**), the key positive regulators of IFN signaling pathway. In addition to TLR3, the cytosolic RNA helicases retinoic acid-inducible I (RIG-I) and melanoma differentiation-associated gene 5 (MDA5) also can recognize the dsRNA mimic. To determine which signal pathway plays the major role in PolyI:C-stimulated IFN-β and IFN-λ induction in LX-2 cells, we used the bafilomycin A1, an inhibitor of TLR3 signal pathway, to treat LX-2 cells prior to PolyI:C stimulation. The vacuolar H+ATPases (V-ATPases) are a family of ATP-driven proton pumps responsible for the acidification of a variety of intracellular compartments. V-ATPases provide the acidic environment required for dissociation of internalized ligand-receptor complexes within endosomes (35). TLR3-mediated signaling is initiated from endosomal compartments in cells, requiring endosomal acidification (36). Bafilomycin A1, as a vaculaor H+ATPase inhibitor, can effectively block endosome acidification to inhibit TLR3 signaling. We observed that bafilomycin A1 could suppress the induction of IFN-β and IRF-7 by PolyI:C, indicating that TLR3 is the key sensor responsible for PolyI:C- mediated the induction of IFN-β in LX-2 cells (**Figures 2F,G**). Also, the pretreatment of LX-2 cells with TCI significantly block the induction of IFNs and IRF7 by PolyI:C (**Supplementary Figure 2**).

Because the neutralization antibody to IFN-β could largely block the anti-HBV effect by SN from PolyI:C-activated LX-2 cell cultures, IFN-β is likely to be a major player responsible for the anti-HBV effect. In addition, we observed that the antibodies to IFN-λ receptors could partially block LX-2 SN-mediated HBV inhibition, suggesting that IFN-λ also contributes to the LX-2 SN actions. The role of IFN-β and IFN-λ in LX-2 SN-mediated HBV inhibition was further confirmed by the observation that when added to HBV-infected HepG2 cell cultures, recombinant IFN-β or IFN-λ significantly inhibited the HBV replication (**Figures 4C,D**). These findings are consistent with other studies showing that IFN-β could suppress HBV replication in HepG2 cells and HBV-infected chimeric mice (17, 37, 38). In our previous study, we found that IFN-λ from polyI:C-stimulated LX-2 SN contributed to HCV inhibition in Huh7 cells (24). Several early studies also showed that IFN-λ could inhibit HBV replication in HepG2 cells and HBV-Met cells, a hepatocyte cell line derived from HBV-transgenic mice (39, 40). Recently, Xu et al reported that IFN-λ could inhibit HBV replication in HepG2 cells by inducing the expression of CBFβ (41).

In summary, we provide the experimental evidence to support the notion that the TLR3 signaling of LX-2 cells is beneficial for the immunological control of HBV replication in HepG2 cells. However, future investigations with human liver tissues from people infected with HBV are necessary in order to prove that hepatic stellate cells indeed participate in liver innate immunity against HBV infection. These future studies will determine whether HSCs are a potentially crucial and alternative target for immunological intervention to control HBV infection in liver.

AUTHOR CONTRIBUTIONS

BZ, W-ZH, XW, and JL conceived of and designed the experiments. BZ, YL, XX, and LG performed the experiments. BZ, XW, and W-ZH analyzed the data. BZ made the figures. W-ZH contributed reagents, materials, and analysis tools. BZ and W-ZH wrote the manuscript. All authors reviewed the manuscript.

FUNDING

This work was supported by the National Natural Sciences Foundation of China (81571962), and the National Institutes of Health (DA042373, DA041302, DA045568, DA022177).

REFERENCES

1. Arzumanyan A, Reis HM, Feitelson MA. Pathogenic mechanisms in HBV- and HCV-associated hepatocellular carcinoma. *Nat Rev Cancer* (2013) 13:123–35. doi: 10.1038/nrc3449
2. Nassal M. HBV cccDNA: viral persistence reservoir and key obstacle for a cure of chronic hepatitis B. *Gut* (2015) 64:1972–84. doi: 10.1136/gutjnl-2015-309809
3. Sagnelli E, Sagnelli C, Macera M, Pisaturo M, Coppola N. An update on the treatment options for HBV/HCV coinfection. *Expert Opin Pharmacother.* (2017) 18:1691–702. doi: 10.1080/14656566.2017.1398233
4. Bertoletti A, Ferrari C. Innate and adaptive immune responses in chronic hepatitis B virus infections: towards restoration of immune control of viral infection. *Gut* (2012) 61:1754–64. doi: 10.1136/gutjnl-2011-301073
5. Lebosse F, Testoni B, Fresquet J, Facchetti F, Galmozzi E, Fournier M, et al. Intrahepatic innate immune response pathways are downregulated in untreated chronic hepatitis B. *J Hepatol.* (2017) 66:897–909. doi: 10.1016/j.jhep.2016.12.024
6. Kayesh MEH, Ezzikouri S, Chi H, Sanada T, Yamamoto N, Kitab B, et al. Interferon-beta response is impaired by hepatitis B virus infection in *Tupaia belangeri. Virus Res.* (2017) 237:47–57. doi: 10.1016/j.virusres.2017.05.013
7. Wu J, Meng Z, Jiang M, Pei R, Trippler M, Broering R, et al. Hepatitis B virus suppresses toll-like receptor-mediated innate immune responses in murine parenchymal and nonparenchymal liver cells. *Hepatology* (2009) 49:1132–40. doi: 10.1002/hep.22751
8. Mutz P, Metz P, Lempp FA, Bender S, Qu B, Schoneweis K, et al. HBV bypasses the innate immune response and does not protect hcv from antiviral activity of interferon. *Gastroenterology* (2018) 154:1791–1804.e22. doi: 10.1053/j.gastro.2018.01.044
9. Suslov A, Boldanova T, Wang X, Wieland S, Heim MH. Hepatitis B virus does not interfere with innate immune responses in the human liver. *Gastroenterology* (2018) 154:1778–90. doi: 10.1053/j.gastro.2018.01.034
10. West J, Damania B. Upregulation of the TLR3 pathway by Kaposi's sarcoma-associated herpesvirus during primary infection. *J Virol.* (2008) 82:5440–9. doi: 10.1128/JVI.02590-07
11. Wang N, Liang Y, Devaraj S, Wang J, Lemon SM, Li K. Toll-like receptor 3 mediates establishment of an antiviral state against hepatitis C virus in hepatoma cells. *J Virol.* (2009) 83:9824–34. doi: 10.1128/JVI.01125-09
12. Aly HH, Watashi K, Hijikata M, Kaneko H, Takada Y, Egawa H, et al. Serum-derived hepatitis C virus infectivity in interferon regulatory factor-7-suppressed human primary hepatocytes. *J Hepatol.* (2007) 46:26–36. doi: 10.1016/j.jhep.2006.08.018

13. Tu Z, Bozorgzadeh A, Pierce RH, Kurtis J, Crispe IN, Orloff MS. TLR-dependent cross talk between human Kupffer cells and NK cells. *J Exp Med.* (2008) 205:233–44. doi: 10.1084/jem.20072195
14. Shu SA, Lian ZX, Chuang YH, Yang GX, Moritoki Y, Comstock SS, et al. The role of CD11c(+) hepatic dendritic cells in the induction of innate immune responses. *Clin Exp Immunol.* (2007) 149:335–43. doi: 10.1111/j.1365-2249.2007.03419.x
15. Isogawa M, Robek MD, Furuichi Y, Chisari FV. Toll-like receptor signaling inhibits hepatitis B virus replication *in vivo*. *J Virol.* (2005) 79:7269–72. doi: 10.1128/JVI.79.11.7269-7272.2005
16. Wieland SF, Guidotti LG, Chisari FV. Intrahepatic induction of alpha/beta interferon eliminates viral RNA-containing capsids in hepatitis B virus transgenic mice. *J Virol.* (2000) 74:4165–73. doi: 10.1128/JVI.74.9.4165-4173.2000
17. Wu J, Lu M, Meng Z, Trippler M, Broering R, Szczeponek A, et al. Toll-like receptor-mediated control of HBV replication by nonparenchymal liver cells in mice. *Hepatology* (2007) 46:1769–78. doi: 10.1002/hep.21897
18. Shang L, Hosseini M, Liu X, Kisseleva T, Brenner DA. Human hepatic stellate cell isolation and characterization. *J Gastroenterol.* (2017) 53:1–12. doi: 10.1007/s00535-017-1404-4
19. Geerts A. History, heterogeneity, developmental biology, and functions of quiescent hepatic stellate cells. *Semin Liver Dis.* (2001) 21:311–35. doi: 10.1055/s-2001-17550
20. Tsuchida T, Friedman SL. Mechanisms of hepatic stellate cell activation. *Nat Rev Gastroenterol Hepatol.* (2017) 14:397–411. doi: 10.1038/nrgastro.2017.38
21. Wilson CL, Mann J, Walsh M, Perrugoria MJ, Oakley F, Wright MC, et al. Quiescent hepatic stellate cells functionally contribute to the hepatic innate immune response via TLR3. *PLoS ONE* (2014) 9:e83391. doi: 10.1371/journal.pone.0083391
22. Wang Y, Li J, Wang X, Sang M, Ho W. Hepatic stellate cells, liver innate immunity, and hepatitis C virus. *J Gastroenterol Hepatol.* (2013) 28(Suppl. 1):112–5. doi: 10.1111/jgh.12023
23. Ichikawa S, Mucida D, Tyznik AJ, Kronenberg M, Cheroutre H. Hepatic stellate cells function as regulatory bystanders. *J Immunol.* (2011) 186:5549–55. doi: 10.4049/jimmunol.1003917
24. Wang Y, Li J, Wang X, Ye L, Zhou Y, Ho W. Induction of interferon-lambda contributes to Toll-like receptor-3-activated hepatic stellate cell-mediated hepatitis C virus inhibition in hepatocytes. *J Viral Hepat.* (2013) 20:385–94. doi: 10.1111/jvh.12040
25. Li J, Hu S, Zhou L, Ye L, Wang X, Ho J, et al. Interferon lambda inhibits herpes simplex virus type I infection of human astrocytes and neurons. *Glia* (2011) 59:58–67. doi: 10.1002/glia.21076
26. Cheng K, Wang X, Yin H. Small-molecule inhibitors of the TLR3/dsRNA complex. *J Am Chem Soc.* (2011) 133:3764–7. doi: 10.1021/ja111312h
27. Wieland SF, Chisari FV. Stealth and cunning: hepatitis B and hepatitis C viruses. *J Virol* (2005) 79:9369–80. doi: 10.1128/JVI.79.15.9369-9380.2005
28. Luangsay S, Gruffaz M, Isorce N, Testoni B, Michelet M, Faure-Dupuy S, et al. Early inhibition of hepatocyte innate responses by hepatitis B virus. *J Hepatol.* (2015) 63:1314–22. doi: 10.1016/j.jhep.2015.07.014
29. Dunn C, Peppa D, Khanna P, Nebbia G, Jones M, Brendish N, et al. Temporal analysis of early immune responses in patients with acute hepatitis B virus infection. *Gastroenterology* (2009) 137:1289–300. doi: 10.1053/j.gastro.2009.06.054
30. Wieland S, Thimme R, Purcell RH, Chisari FV. Genomic analysis of the host response to hepatitis B virus infection. *Proc Natl Acad Sci U S A.* (2004) 101:6669–74. doi: 10.1073/pnas.0401771101
31. Liu Y, Nie H, Mao R, Mitra B, Cai D, Yan R, et al. Interferon-inducible ribonuclease ISG20 inhibits hepatitis B virus replication through directly binding to the epsilon stem-loop structure of viral RNA. *PLoS Pathog.* (2017) 13:e1006296. doi: 10.1371/journal.ppat.1006296
32. Gao B, Duan Z, Xu W, Xiong S. Tripartite motif-containing 22 inhibits the activity of hepatitis B virus core promoter, which is dependent on nuclear-located RING domain. *Hepatology* (2009) 50:424–33. doi: 10.1002/hep.23011
33. Pei R, Qin B, Zhang X, Zhu W, Kemper T, Ma Z, et al. Interferon-induced proteins with tetratricopeptide repeats 1 and 2 are cellular factors that limit hepatitis B virus replication. *J Innate Immun.* (2014) 6:182–91. doi: 10.1159/000353220
34. Akira S, Uematsu S, Takeuchi O. Pathogen recognition and innate immunity. *Cell* (2006) 124:783–801. doi: 10.1016/j.cell.2006.02.015
35. Jefferies KC, Cipriano DJ, Forgac M. Function, structure and regulation of the vacuolar (H+)-ATPases. *Arch Biochem Biophys.* (2008) 476:33–42. doi: 10.1016/j.abb.2008.03.025
36. Blasius AL, Beutler B. Intracellular toll-like receptors. *Immunity* (2010) 32:305–15. doi: 10.1016/j.immuni.2010.03.012
37. Yin W, Xu L, Sun R, Wei H, Tian Z. Interleukin-15 suppresses hepatitis B virus replication via IFN-beta production in a C57BL/6 mouse model. *Liver Int.* (2012) 32:1306–14. doi: 10.1111/j.1478-3231.2012.02773.x
38. Tsuge M, Uchida T, Hiraga N, Kan H, Makokha GN, Abe-Chayama H, et al. Development of a novel site-specific pegylated interferon beta for antiviral therapy of chronic hepatitis B virus. *Antimicrob Agents Chemother.* (2017) 61:e00183–17. doi: 10.1128/AAC.00183-17
39. Robek MD, Boyd BS, Chisari FV. Lambda interferon inhibits hepatitis B and C virus replication. *J Virol.* (2005) 79:3851–4. doi: 10.1128/JVI.79.6.3851-3854.2005
40. Doyle SE, Schreckhise H, Khuu-Duong K, Henderson K, Rosler R, Storey H, et al. Interleukin-29 uses a type 1 interferon-like program to promote antiviral responses in human hepatocytes. *Hepatology* (2006) 44:896–906. doi: 10.1002/hep.21312
41. Xu F, Song H, Xiao Q, Li N, Zhang H, Cheng G, et al. Type III interferon-induced CBFbeta inhibits HBV replication by hijacking HBx. *Cell Mol Immunol.* (2018). doi: 10.1038/s41423-018-0006-2. [Epub ahead of print].

Permissions

All chapters in this book were first published Frontiers; hereby published with permission under the Creative Commons Attribution License or equivalent. Every chapter published in this book has been scrutinized by our experts. Their significance has been extensively debated. The topics covered herein carry significant findings which will fuel the growth of the discipline. They may even be implemented as practical applications or may be referred to as a beginning point for another development.

The contributors of this book come from diverse backgrounds, making this book a truly international effort. This book will bring forth new frontiers with its revolutionizing research information and detailed analysis of the nascent developments around the world.

We would like to thank all the contributing authors for lending their expertise to make the book truly unique. They have played a crucial role in the development of this book. Without their invaluable contributions this book wouldn't have been possible. They have made vital efforts to compile up to date information on the varied aspects of this subject to make this book a valuable addition to the collection of many professionals and students.

This book was conceptualized with the vision of imparting up-to-date information and advanced data in this field. To ensure the same, a matchless editorial board was set up. Every individual on the board went through rigorous rounds of assessment to prove their worth. After which they invested a large part of their time researching and compiling the most relevant data for our readers.

The editorial board has been involved in producing this book since its inception. They have spent rigorous hours researching and exploring the diverse topics which have resulted in the successful publishing of this book. They have passed on their knowledge of decades through this book. To expedite this challenging task, the publisher supported the team at every step. A small team of assistant editors was also appointed to further simplify the editing procedure and attain best results for the readers.

Apart from the editorial board, the designing team has also invested a significant amount of their time in understanding the subject and creating the most relevant covers. They scrutinized every image to scout for the most suitable representation of the subject and create an appropriate cover for the book.

The publishing team has been an ardent support to the editorial, designing and production team. Their endless efforts to recruit the best for this project, has resulted in the accomplishment of this book. They are a veteran in the field of academics and their pool of knowledge is as vast as their experience in printing. Their expertise and guidance has proved useful at every step. Their uncompromising quality standards have made this book an exceptional effort. Their encouragement from time to time has been an inspiration for everyone.

The publisher and the editorial board hope that this book will prove to be a valuable piece of knowledge for researchers, students, practitioners and scholars across the globe.

List of Contributors

Alvin Paul, Thean Hock Tang and Siew Kit Ng
Advanced Medical and Dental Institute, Universiti Sains Malaysia, Penang, Malaysia

Ming-Hsun Tsai and Chien-Kuo Lee
Graduate Institute of Immunology, National Taiwan University College of Medicine, Taipei, Taiwan

Li-Mei Pai
Department of Biochemistry and Molecular Biology, Chang Gung University, Taoyuan, Taiwan
Molecular Medicine Research Center, Chang Gung University, Taoyuan, Taiwan
Liver Research Center, Chang Gung Memorial Hospital, Taoyuan, Taiwan

Caroline A. Jefferies
Department of Medicine, Division of Rheumatology and Department of Biomedical Sciences, Cedars Sinai Medical Center, Los Angeles, CA, United States

Patricia López and Ana Suárez
Area of Immunology, Department of Functional Biology, Faculty of Medicine, University of Oviedo, Oviedo, Spain
Instituto de Investigación Sanitaria del Principado de Asturias (ISPA), Oviedo, Spain

Javier Rodríguez-Carrio
Area of Immunology, Department of Functional Biology, Faculty of Medicine, University of Oviedo, Oviedo, Spain
Instituto de Investigación Sanitaria del Principado de Asturias (ISPA), Oviedo, Spain
Bone and Mineral Research Unit, REDinREN del ISCIII, Hospital Universitario Central de Asturias, Oviedo, Spain

Mercedes Alperi-López and Francisco J. Ballina-García
Instituto de Investigación Sanitaria del Principado de Asturias (ISPA), Oviedo, Spain
Department of Rheumatology, Hospital Universitario Central de Asturias, Oviedo, Spain

Luis Caminal-Montero
Area of Immunology, Department of Functional Biology, Faculty of Medicine, University of Oviedo, Oviedo, Spain
Department of Internal Medicine, Hospital Universitario Central de Asturias, Oviedo, Spain

Mazen Kurdi
Faculty of Sciences, Department of Chemistry and Biochemistry, and The Laboratory of Experimental and Clinical Pharmacology, Lebanese University, Beirut, Lebanon

Carlos Zgheib
Laboratory for Fetal and Regenerative Biology, Department of Surgery, School of Medicine, University of Colorado Denver, Anschutz Medical Campus and Colorado Children's Hospital, Aurora, CO, United States

George W. Booz
Department of Pharmacology and Toxicology, University of Mississippi Medical Center, Jackson, MS, United States

Aleksandra Antonczyk, Bart Krist, Malgorzata Sajek, Agata Michalska, Anna Piaszyk-Borychowska, Martyna Plens-Galaska and Hans A. R. Bluyssen
Department of Human Molecular Genetics, Faculty of Biology, Institute of Molecular Biology and Biotechnology, Adam Mickiewicz University, Poznań, Poland

Joanna Wesoly
Laboratory of High Throughput Technologies, Faculty of Biology, Institute of Molecular Biology and Biotechnology, Adam Mickiewicz University, Poznań, Poland

Yu-Ting Kao and Chia-Yi Yu
National Institute of Infectious Diseases and Vaccinology, National Health Research Institutes, Tainan, Taiwan

Michael M. C. Lai
Research Center for Emerging Viruses, China Medical University Hospital, Taichung, Taiwan
Institute of Molecular Biology, Academia Sinica, Taipei, Taiwan

Sarah McKenna, Taylor Burey, Jeryl Sandoval, Leanna Nguyen, Odalis Castro, Suma Gudipati, Jazmin Gonzalez, Karim C. El Kasmi and Clyde J. Wright
Section of Neonatology, Department of Pediatrics, University of Colorado School of Medicine, Aurora, CO, United States

Sebastian Wienerroither, Pavel Kovarik and Thomas Decker
Max F. Perutz Laboratories, University of Vienna, Vienna, Austria

Aida Collado, Patrice Marques and María Jesus Sanz
Department of Pharmacology, Faculty of Medicine, University of Valencia, Valencia, Spain
Institute of Health Research INCLIVA, University Clinic Hospital of Valencia, Valencia, Spain

Susana Vallejo, Mariella Ramos-González and Concepción Peiró
Department of Pharmacology, School of Medicine, Universidad Autónoma de Madrid, Madrid, Spain
Instituto de Investigación Sanitaria Hospital Universitario La Paz (IdiPAZ), Madrid, Spain

Joanna Wesoly
Laboratory of High Throughput Technologies, Institute of Molecular Biology and Biotechnology, Faculty of Biology, Adam Mickiewicz University, Poznan, Poland

Matthias Parrini, Katrin Meissl, Mojoyinola Joanna Ola, Therese Lederer, Ana Puga and Birgit Strobl
Department of Biomedical Sciences, Institute of Animal Breeding and Genetics, University of Veterinary Medicine, Vienna, Austria

Mathias Müller
Department of Biomedical Sciences, Institute of Animal Breeding and Genetics, University of Veterinary Medicine Vienna, Vienna, Austria
University Center Biomodels Austria, University of Veterinary Medicine Vienna, Vienna, Austria

Lajos Széles and Attila Csermely
Department of Biochemistry and Molecular Biology, University of Debrecen, Debrecen, Hungary

Hsin-Chien Chiang and Chien-Kuo Lee
Graduate Institute of Immunology, National Taiwan University College of Medicine, Taipei, Taiwan

Joanna Wesoły
Laboratory of High Throughput Technologies, Adam Mickiewicz University, Poznan, Poland

Laszlo Nagy
Department of Biochemistry and Molecular Biology, University of Debrecen, Debrecen, Hungary
Departments of Medicine and Biological Chemistry, Johns Hopkins All Children's Hospital, Johns Hopkins University School of Medicine, St. Petersburg, FL, United States

Hao-Sen Chiang
Department of Life Science, National Taiwan University, Taipei, Taiwan
Genome and Systems Biology Degree Program, National Taiwan University, Taipei, Taiwan
University School of Medicine, St. Petersburg, FL, United States

Ekaterini Platanitis and Thomas Decker
Max F. Perutz Laboratories, Department of Microbiology, Immunobiology and Genetics, University of Vienna, Vienna, Austria

Anna Piaszyk-Borychowska and Hans A. R. Bluyssen
Department of Human Molecular Genetics, Adam Mickiewicz University, Poznan, Poland

Helene Minyi Liu
Graduate Institute of Biochemistry and Molecular Biology, College of Medicine, National Taiwan University, Taipei, Taiwan

Trine H. Mogensen
Department of Infectious diseases, Aarhus University Hospital, Aarhus, Denmark
Department of Biomedicine, Aarhus University, Aarhus, Denmark
Department of Clinical Medicine, Aarhus University, Aarhus, Denmark

Cherrie D. Thompson, Bharati Matta and Betsy J. Barnes
Center for Autoimmune Musculoskeletal and Hematopoietic Diseases, Feinstein Institute for Medical Research, Manhasset, NY, United States

Alice H. Grant, Armando Estrada III, Yoshira M. Ayala-Marin, America Y. Alvidrez-Camacho, Georgialina Rodriguez, Elisa Robles-Escajeda, Denisse A. Cadena-Medina, Alejandro C. Rodriguez and Robert A. Kirken
Department of Biological Sciences, The University of Texas at El Paso, El Paso, TX, United States

Biao Zhang, Yu Liu, Xiqiu Xu and Le Guo
School of Basic Medical Sciences, Wuhan University, Wuhan, China

Wen-Zhe Ho
School of Basic Medical Sciences, Wuhan University, Wuhan, China
Department of Pathology and Laboratory Medicine, Temple University Lewis Katz School of Medicine, Philadelphia, PA, United States

Xu Wang and Jieliang Li
Department of Pathology and Laboratory Medicine, Temple University Lewis Katz School of Medicine, Philadelphia, PA, United States

Index

www.ingramcontent.com/pod-product-compliance
Lightning Source LLC
LaVergne TN
LVHW060521210926
848485LV00005B/1122